Pediatric Oncology

Gregory H. Reaman • Franklin O. Smith
(Editors)

Childhood Leukemia

A Practical Handbook

Springer

Editors
Gregory H. Reaman
George Washington University School
of Medicine & Health Sciences
The Children's National Medical Center
III Michigan Ave. NW,
Washington, D.C. 20010
greaman@childrensoncologygroup.org

Franklin O. Smith, III
Cincinnati Children's Hospital Medical
Center, University of Cincinnati
Collage of Medicine
3333 Burnett Avenue
Cincinnati, OH, USA
frank.smith@cchmc.org

ISBN 978-3-642-42370-3 ISBN 978-3-642-13781-5 (eBook)
DOI 10.1007/978-3-642-13781-5
Springer Heidelberg Dordrecht London New York

Cover design: eStudioCalamar, Figueres/Berlin

Printed on acid-free paper

Springer is part of Springer Science+Business Media (www.springer.com)

Preface

Among the truly great success stories of modern medicine are the striking improvements in survival and cure rates for children with acute leukemia during the past 4–5 decades. This is particularly, but no longer exclusively, true for acute lymphoblastic leukemia (ALL). Although improvements in supportive care have clearly contributed to this success in both ALL and acute myeloid leukemia (AML), the improvements have largely resulted from specific refinements in anti-leukemia therapy and enhanced biological insights into these diseases. Although definitive mechanisms of causation remain elusive, they are far less so. Genomic interrogation of the leukemias, both the leukemia cell and the affected host, has and will continue to yield much useful insight as to molecular etiology as the technology improves. Such findings have enormous potential for therapeutic exploitation and hopefully, through investigation of gene-environment relationships, provide important information for the generation of risk prevention strategies.

The final common pathway for translating scientific discovery to clinical application is through clinical research and the conduct of controlled clinical trials, ultimately resulting in continually improved standards of care. It has been an honor and immeasurable source of gratification to have played a small role in this success. Despite the success, we remain resolute in advancing science to fight this battle for as long as we are able and until such time that cure is a reality for every child with leukemia.

We are enormously indebted to our legendary teachers and mentors as well as to numerous wonderful colleagues in basic, clinical, statistical, and epidemiologic research, many of whom have contributed to this project. In addition to our scientific colleagues as collaborators, clinical research would be impossible without the effective and essential partnership of patients and families impacted by leukemia who are willing participants in clinical trials. Many have directly benefitted as a result of their participation, and many more have unselfishly contributed to knowledge which has only helped those who have followed them. It is to all of these children and families that we humbly and thankfully dedicate this book.

Gregory H. Reaman
Franklin O. Smith III

Acknowledgments

We would like to express our sincere appreciation for the enormous editorial assistance provided to us by Dr. Judy Racadio, to the untiring efforts of our assistants, Ms. Vaishali Revollo and Ms. Holly Ward, and to the staff at Springer-Verlag. We are also indebted to our wives, Susan and Phyllis, and to our families for their patience and support.

Contents

Part I

Genetics and the Epidemiology of Leukemia in Children

Epidemiology of Acute ChildhoodL eukemia

1

Julie A. Ross, Kimberly J. Johnson,
Logan G. Spector, and John H. Kersey

Contents

J.A.R oss(✉)
Clinical Research, Department of Pediatrics,
University of Minnesota Cancer Center, MMC 422, 420
DelawareSt.S.E. , Minneapolis, MN, 55455 USA
e-mail:ros sx014@umn.edu

K.J.J ohnson
Department of Pediatrics, MMC 715, 420 Delaware St. S.E.,
Minneapolis, MN, 55455 USA
email:john5713@ umn.edu

L.G.Spe ctor
Department of Pediatrics,
University of Minnesota Cancer Center,
MMC 715, 420 Delaware St. S.E., Minneapolis,
MN, 55455 USA
e-mail:s pector@umn.edu

J.H.K ersey
Department of Pediatrics,
University of Minnesota Cancer Center, MMC 86,
420D elawareSt .S .E., Minneapolis, MN, 55455 USA
e-mail:k erse001@umn.edu

1.1 Classification and Natural History

1.1.1 Classification: Immunophenotype, Morphology

All cells that comprise distinct entities in the blood (e.g., platelets, T-cells, etc.) arise from a pluripotent stem cell, which can form lymphoid stem cells or trilineage myeloid stem cells. In the classical model of hematopoiesis, lymphoid stem cells differentiate further into T-cell progenitor and B-cell progenitor cells, which eventually can mature into T- and B-cells, respectively (McKenzie 1996). Myeloid stem cells form myeloid cell progenitors, granulocyte/macrophage progenitors, and eosinophil progenitors, from which mature cells such as erythrocytes, platelets, polymorphonuclear leukocytes, monocytes/macrophages, and eosinophils arise. However, recent data support a more complex model for hematopoiesis, whereby intermediate progenitor cells retain both lymphoid and myeloid potential; thus the developmental potential of cells at various stages is less clear (Ceredig et al. 2009; Kawamoto and Katsura 2009). Nevertheless, acute leukemias that arise in children often occur in the earlier stages of lymphoid or myeloid cell maturation.

Childhood ALL was initially classified using the French-American-British (FAB) Cooperative Group criteria using morphological features (Bennett et al. 1976) and consisted of three subgroups: L1, L2, and

G.H. Reaman and F.O. Smith (eds.), *Childhood Leukemia*,
DOI: 10.1007/978-3-642-13781-5_1, © Springer-Verlag Berlin Heidelberg 2011

L3. The system was lacking, however, in guiding risk stratification for treatment, and it also included the leukemic phase of Burkitt lymphoma (L3). Subsequently, ALL was classified immunologically, given that immunological features were found to be useful in treatment assignment (Kersey et al. 1975). The most recent World Health Organization (WHO) classification for childhood ALL consists of three major subgroups: acute leukemias of ambiguous lineage (rare and not discussed here), B lymphoblastic leukemias/lymphoma, and T lymphoblastic leukemias/lymphoma, where leukemia is distinguished from lymphoma when a mass is present based on the percentage of lymphoblasts in the bone marrow (>25% is generally classified as leukemia). B lymphoblastic leukemias are further subclassified with respect to recurring genetic abnormalities (Vardiman et al. 2009). Molecular and/or genetic classifications of childhood ALL (a few described below) are important in identifying biologically and prognostically distinct subtypes, but, with the exception of infant leukemias, have not been routinely used in epidemiological studies.

Childhood AML has usually been classified into eight different subtypes (M0–M7) using the FAB system, which relies primarily on morphological and cytochemical assessments (Bennett et al. 1976; Bennett et al. 1985; Bennett et al. 1991). However, as with ALL, it is apparent that immunological, molecular, and cytogenetic features can play a role in AML outcome. Thus, the World Health Organization has defined further delineated categories for AML (Vardiman et al. 2009).

1.1.2 Classification: Molecular and Cytogenetics

In addition to morphological and immunological features, most pediatric acute leukemias are characterized by recurring somatic genetic abnormalities in blood cells (most commonly leukocytes) that can often be detected cytogenetically; they can broadly be categorized as those involving: (1) numerical changes in chromosome number (i.e., gain or loss of chromosomes), (2) chromosome structural changes (i.e., translocations, deletions, amplifications, and inversions), or (3) a combination of numerical and structural changes. In addition, gene-specific mutations and epigenetic aberrations contribute to the pathogenesis of acute leukemia (Plass et al. 2008; Garcia-Manero et al. 2009). Leukemia occurs as a consequence of genetic changes that result in altered self-renewal processes, enhanced proliferation, blocked differentiation, and evasion of apoptosis. The genetic abnormalities have prognostic importance and tend to be lineage specific, with distinct genetic abnormalities reported in B-, T-, and myeloid-cell lineage leukemias. In addition, infant leukemia is characterized by a genetic profile that differs from that of older children (Armstrong et al. 2002). Below, an overview of the most commonly occurring genetic abnormalities in each of the major subtypes of acute leukemia, including infant leukemia, is provided. Focusing on these particular subgroups may provide the most relevant information for understanding the etiology of leukemia.

1.1.2.1 AcuteL ymphoidL eukemias

ALL frequently harbors genetic abnormalities involving transcription factors and chromatin modifiers involved in the control of normal B- and T-cell lineage development (Teitell and Pandolfi 2009). The most commonly described genetic abnormalities for B-ALL and T-ALL are shown in Table 1.1 and are discussed below.

B-ALL comprises an estimated 85% of ALL cases. The most common chromosome numerical abnormality in B-ALL is hyperdiploidy, affecting ~30% of B-ALL cases. The *ETV6-RUNX1* (also called *TEL-AML1*) translocation (t(12;21)(p13;q22)) is the most frequent chromosome structural abnormality. Other common genetic abnormalities include the translocations *BCR-ABL* (t(9;22)(q34;q11.2)) and *E2A-PBX* (t(1;19)(q23;p13)) and translocations involving the Mixed Lineage Leukemia (*MLL*) gene located at chromosome 11q23 (Armstrong and Look 2005). Interestingly, translocations involving the *MLL* gene/chromosome band 11q23 (most frequently *MLL-AF4*) are much more common in infant leukemia, being reported in ~75% of cases, while hyperdiploidy and the *ETV6-RUNX1* translocation are very rare in infants (Silverman 2007; Chowdhury and Brady 2008).

T-ALL comprises the remainder of ALL cases and is characterized by genetic abnormalities that are generally distinct from those detected in B-ALL. Common abnormalities found in T-ALL include ectopic

Table1.1 Common genetic abnormalities in childhood acute lymphoblastic leukemia[a]

Genetica bnormality/ genes involved	Cytogenetica berration(s)	Estimated Frequency (%)[b]	Predominant cell type
Hyperdiploidy (>50 chromosomes)	4, 6, 10, 14, 17, 18, 21[c]	25	B-precursor
ETV6-RUNX1	t(12;21)(p13;q22)	22	B-precursor
MLL +pa rtners	t(11q23)	10	B-a ndT -precursor
BCR-ABL	t(9;22)(q34;q11.2)	3	B-precursor
MYC	t(8;14),t (2;8),t (8;22)	2	B-precursor
E2A-PBX1	t(1;19)(q23;p13)	5	B-precursor
TAL1	t(1;14)(p32;q11) t(1;7)(p32;q34)	7	T-precursor
LYL1	t(7;19)(q34;p13)	1.5	T-precursor
HOX11L2	t(5;14)(q35;q32) t(5;14)(q35;q11)	2.5	T-precursor
HOX11	t(7;10)(q35;q24) t(10;14)(q24;q11)	0.7	T-precursor

[a]From Heeremae ta l.(2000), Puie ta l.(2004),A rmstronga ndL ook (2005)
[b]Estimated frequencies are those compiled by Pui et al. (2004)
[c]Mostc ommon

expression of the transcription factor genes *TAL1* (1p32), *HOX11* (10q24), *HOX11L2* (5q35.1), and *LYL1* (19p13) due to illegitimate recombination near enhancers within the TCR β and α/δ chain loci located at 7q34 and 14q11 respectively (Armstrong and Look 2005; Graux et al. 2006). In addition, the *MLL-ENL* (t(11;19)(q23;p13)) translocation that is also observed in B-ALL and AML is found in ~2% of T- ALLs (Armstrong and Look 2005) and mutations in the genes *CDKN2A*, *NOTCH1*, *FBXW7*, and *MYB* have frequently been reported (Van Vlierberghe et al. 2008). Although T-ALL is more common, overall, in males (Raimondi et al. 1988; Pui et al. 1999; Karrman et al. 2009), it is interesting to note that the male:female (M:F) ratio varies by chromosomal abnormality. For example, rearrangements involving the TCR β and α/δ chain loci have been reported in one study to be seven times more common in males than females (Karrman et al. 2009) compared to an overall M:F ratio for T-ALL of 2–3:1 (Raimondi et al. 1988; Pui et al. 1999; Karrman et al. 2009), suggesting that hormonal influences are involved in the etiology of specific translocations.

1.1.2.2 AcuteMyel oidL eukemias

An estimated 200 unique chromosomal abnormalities have been detected in AML cells (Mrozek et al. 2004) and a summary of the most common are shown in Table 1.2. Frequently recurring translocations in AML are *AML1-ETO* t(8;21)(q22;q22) (Martinez-Climent and Garcia-Conde 1999), *PML-RARA* (t(15;17)(q22;q21)), *MYL11-CBFB* (inv(16)(p13q22) and t(16;16)(p13;q22)), and those involving the *MLL* gene (Mrozek et al. 2004; Balgobind et al. 2009), which have been reported in ~13% of AML cases (Mrozek et al. 2004). Similar to ALL, *MLL* translocations are much more common in AMLs affecting infants (Armstrong and Look 2005).

Taken together, the number and complexity of genetic abnormalities found in childhood leukemia make it challenging to design new epidemiological studies and interpret data from existing studies, especially when one considers that specific genetic abnormalities may have distinct etiologies. Nevertheless, these data have been useful in defining the timing of when childhood leukemia likely occurs, and thus can help narrow the focus when searching for potential causes.

Table1.2 Common genetic abnormalities in childhood acute myeloid leukemia

Genetica bnormality/ genes involved	Cytogenetic aberration(s)	Estimated Frequency (%)[a]	AMLF rench American-British type
ETO, AML1	t(8;21)(q22;q22)	10–15	M2
PML, RARA	t(15;17)(q22;q21)	8–15	M3
MYH11, CBFB	inv(16)(p13q22)	6–11	M4Eo
	t(16;16)(p13;q22)		
MLL + partners (AF9, ENL, and AF6)[b]	t(11q23)	13.1	M4/M5,t -AML
	−7/7q−	5–7	AML,t -AML
	+8	5–9.5	AML

[a]Frequenciesr eportedbyM artinez-Climenta ndG arcia-Conde (1999),M rozeke ta l. (2004)
[b]Mostc ommon

1.1.3 Natural History of Leukemia

In the last 15 years, molecular studies have utilized the observations of chromosomal rearrangements in childhood leukemia, which in turn, have elucidated the natural history of the disease. In particular, the timing of the translocation or hyperdiploid event in some childhood leukemia cases has been determined to have a prenatal origin and is considered a first-hit because of the protracted latency that follows in many cases.

One of the most important lines of evidence with regard to in utero initiation of leukemia comes from studies of identical twins. Twins who share a placenta and later develop leukemia often have identical translocation breakpoints, in contrast to the random translocation breakpoints found in dizygotic twins with separate placentas or non-twin siblings. In the seminal study published by Ford et al. (1993), leukemia cells were examined from three pairs of identical twins with pre-B/null ALL. Using restriction enzymes, all three twin pairs demonstrated *MLL* rearrangements. Although the restriction fragments were identical among each twin pair, they differed among the twin pairs and from other leukemic controls. There were no *MLL* rearrangements found in remission or parental blood. Further, two of the three twin pairs demonstrated common allelic immunoglobulin rearrangements, suggesting that the leukemia arose from a single cell clone and subsequently spread to the other twin via shared placental circulation. Additional twin studies, including twins that have developed leukemia several years apart, have confirmed these findings (Greaves et al. 2003; Greaves and Wiemels 2003). Therefore, the presence of identical breakpoints in twins provides strong evidence that the initiating event occurs in utero in one twin and is transferred to the other twin via shared placental circulation (Greaves et al. 2003).

Additional molecular evidence for an in utero origin of leukemic translocations comes from studies of Guthrie cards, or neonatal blood spots (NBS), which are collected at birth to test for metabolic diseases. Using long-range PCR, Gale et al. (1997) identified *MLL* fusion transcripts in Guthrie cards that were obtained retrospectively from three infants who subsequently developed leukemia between 5 months and 2 years. These *MLL-AF4* fusion transcripts were identical to those amplified in the leukemia cells, and provided conclusive evidence that the initiation of leukemia occurred in utero. Subsequent to this landmark study, additional studies have detected several different leukemic translocations in the NBS or reserved cord blood of children with leukemia, in some instances more than 10 years before the onset of disease(M aiae ta l. 2004;G reaves 2005).

These molecular studies provide clear evidence for a prenatal origin, at least in some cases, of childhood leukemia. Interestingly, however, not all individuals with leukemic translocations at birth will subsequently develop leukemia. In a study of cord blood obtained from healthy infants, the *ETV6-RUNX1* translocation was detected in 1% of samples, a frequency 100 times greater than the incidence of childhood leukemia, indicating that secondary hits are involved in *ETV6-RUNX1* leukemogenesis (Mori et al. 2002). The existence of a prenatal origin of genetic abnormalities commonly detected in T-ALLs has not been well studied. However, evidence from four studies suggests that T-ALL can originate in utero, albeit less frequently than B-ALL. In one study of 16 cases that surveyed NBS by PCR for the presence of T-ALL genetic abnormalities, one child had evidence that the leukemia initiated prior to birth (Fischer et al. 2007). In another study of monozygotic twins concordant for T-cell leukemia/lymphoma, their leukemic cells had identical *TCRβ* gene rearrangements (Ford et al. 1997). A third study reported identical *TCRγ* gene rearrangements between the NBS and the leukemic cells at diagnosis in three patients (Fasching et al. 2000). Finally, a fourth study reported detection of a *Notch1* mutation in the NBS of one of three patients, which was also present in the patient's leukemic cells at diagnosis (Eguchi-Ishimae et al. 2008). This is strong evidence that additional environmental and genetic insults must occur before frank leukemia develops in some children.

1.2 Incidence, Survival, and Trends

To begin to understand the potential underlying causes of a disease, epidemiologists often evaluate group level data including rates of incidence and survival to determine if there are differences in person, place, and/or time. These descriptive analyses usually do not allow for evaluation of individual information (e.g., exposures) that can help explain any differences observed (Wakefield 2008); thus they are typically considered hypothesis generating rather than hypothesis confirming.

1.2.1 International Incidence Rates

As shown in Figs. 1.1 and 1.2, respectively, the annual incidence rates for childhood ALL and AML diagnosed from 0–14 years vary considerably by country (International Incidence of Childhood Cancer, 1998; Coebergh et al. 2006; Fajardo-Gutierrez et al. 2007; Michel et al. 2007; Stack et al. 2007; Petridou et al. 2008; Bao et al. 2009). Some of the highest incidence rates for childhood ALL occur in US Hispanics (49.9/million), Costa Rica (46.3/million) and US Whites (45.4/million), as well as in Greece (44.9/million), and Mexico (44.5/million); intermediate rates occur in The Netherlands (30.9/million), Osaka/Japan (28.4/million), and Lima/Peru (25.4/million); low rates occur in US Blacks (18.7/million), Bombay/India (16/million), and Uganda (3.3/million). For AML, highest rates occur in the Maori of New Zealand (14.4/million), US Hawaiians (11.3/million), and Shanghai/China (10.6/million); intermediate rates occur in US blacks (7.1/million), Ireland (6.8/million), and Canada (6.3/million); low rates occur in Greece (5.5/million), India (Bombay) (4.8/million), and Kuwait (2/million Kuwaiti, 1.6/million non-Kuwaiti). While these observations are of interest, it is important to be cautious when considering differences in incidence rates across various countries since cancer registries can vary in scope, completeness, and overall numbers of cases observed. However, the patterns suggest that the highest rates of childhood ALL occur among select ethnic populations in the United States along with people of European origins in developed countries. In contrast, children of African origin, even in developed countries, have low rates. For AML, the highest incidence rates among people of Maori and related ethnic descent are notable, and could suggest environmental and/or genetic contributions to disease risk.

There are also striking differences in incidence rates by age (Parkin et al. 1998). In developed countries, ALL incidence rates peak between the ages of 2 and 5 years (see United States data in Fig. 1.3). Immunophenotyping reveals most cases of this age peak are CD10+ B-cell lineage ALL alone, rather than T-cell or null-cell lineage ALL, and, therefore, are referred to as "common ALL" (cALL) (Greaves et al. 1985). Null cell ALL occurs mainly in infancy, while T-cell ALL is more frequent in adolescents. In contrast, in most developed countries, the incidence of AML is at its maximum in infancy, declines thereafter before rising in adolescence (Parkin et al. 1998).

1.2.2 U.S. Incidence Rates and Trends

The incidence of childhood leukemia has been increasing significantly in the United States; ALL rates increased by an average of 0.8% annually during the period 1973–2006, while those for AML increased by an average of 0.9% annually (Fig. 1.4). Recent analysis of trends since 1992 shows incidence rates continue to rise (Linabery and Ross 2008a). Childhood leukemia has a peak incidence at ~3 years for ALL and 1 year for AML (Fig. 1.3). ALL is more commonly diagnosed in males than females with M:F incidence ratios of 1.2:1

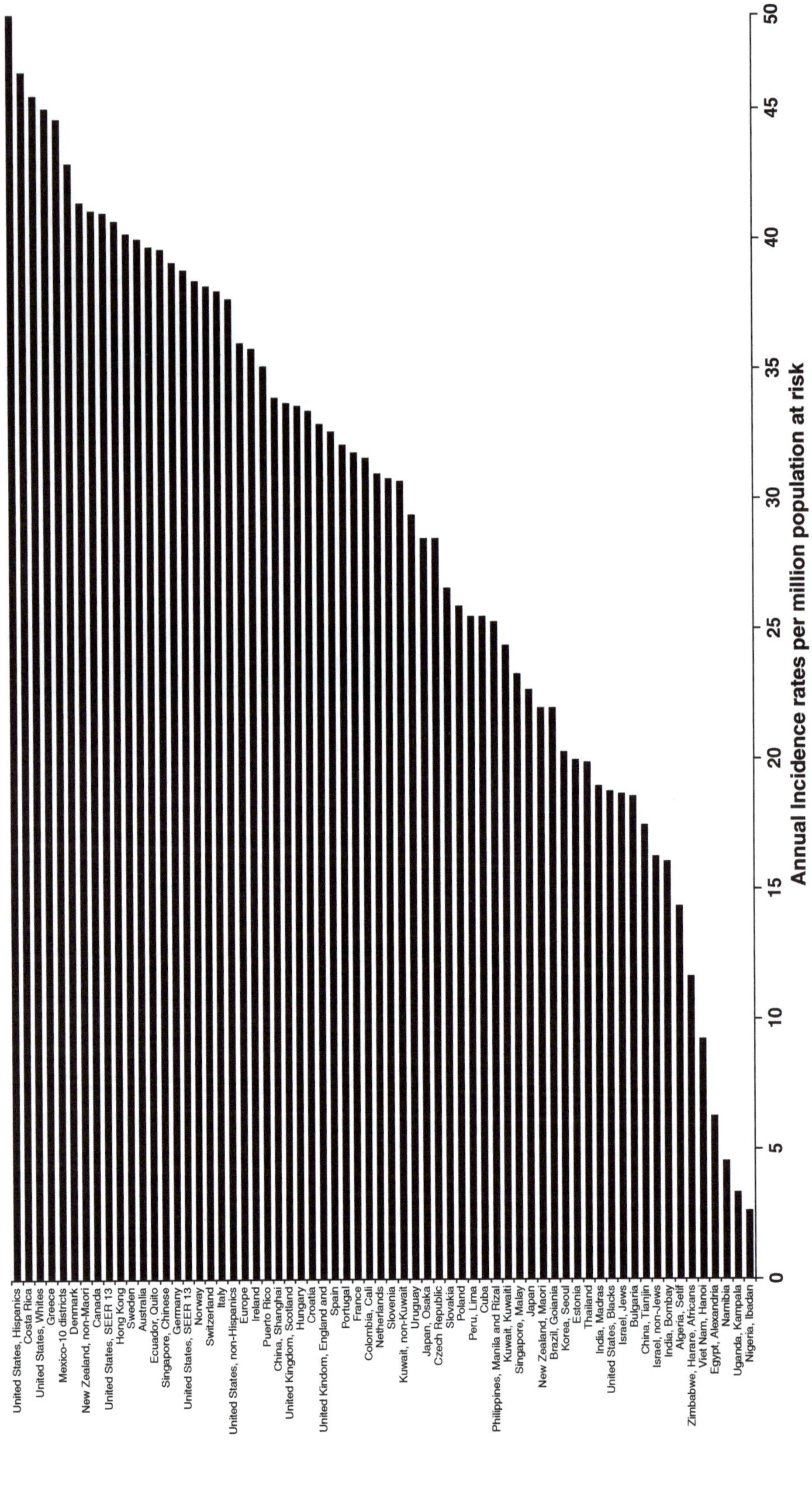

Fig. 1.1 Age adjusted incidence rates for acute lymphoblastic leukemia in children aged 0–14 years. All rates are standardized to the world standard population (International Incidence of Childhood Cancer, 1998; Coebergh et al. 2006; Fajardo-Gutierrez et al. 2007; Michel et al. 2007; Stack et al. 2007; Petridou et al. 2008; Bao et al. 2009)

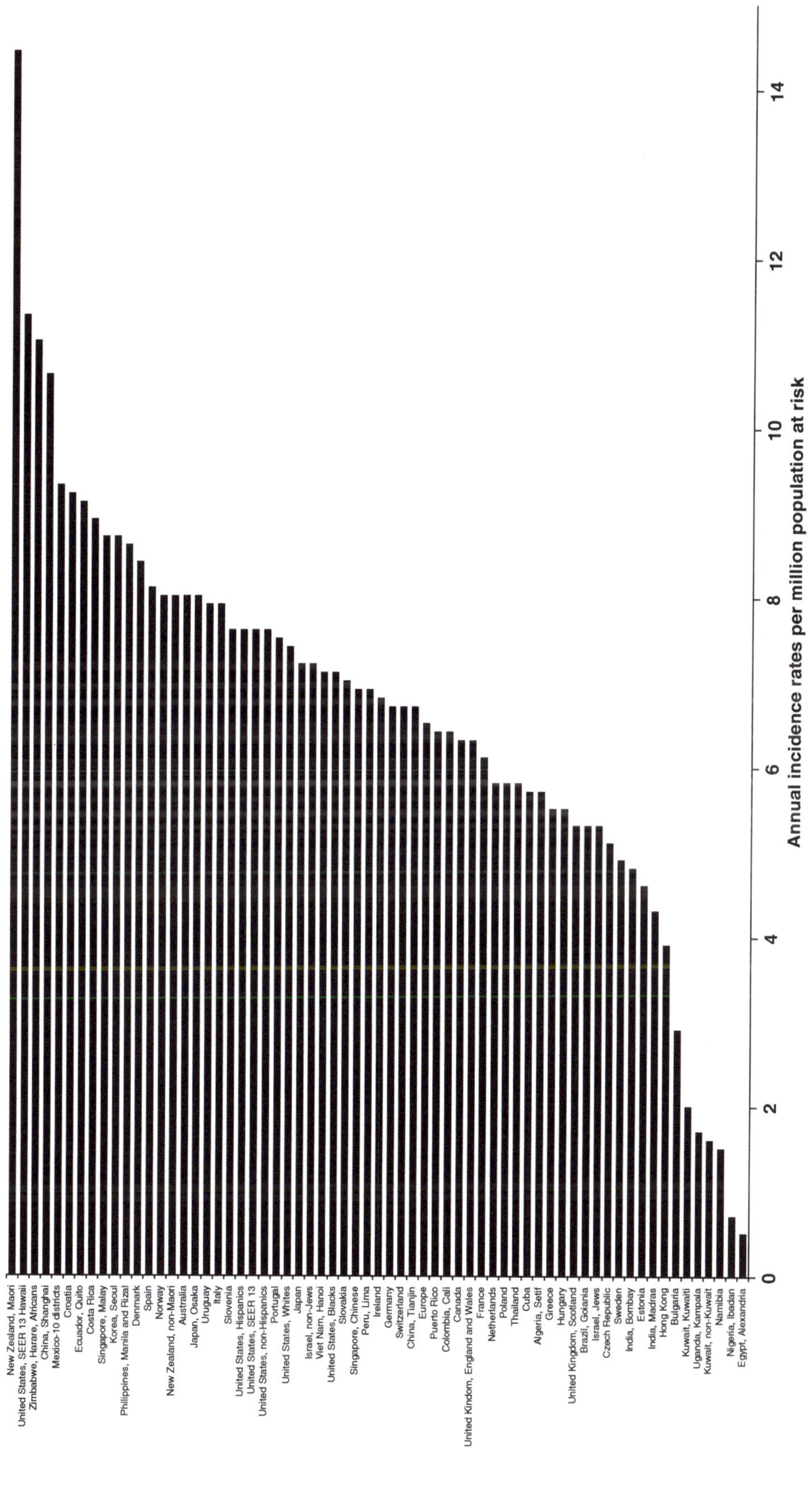

Fig. 1.2 Age adjusted incidence rates for acute myeloid leukemia in children aged 0–14 years. All rates are standardized to the world standard population (International Incidence of Childhood Cancer, 1998; Coebergh et al. 2006; Fajardo-Gutierrez et al. 2007; Michel et al. 2007; Stack et al. 2007; Petridou et al. 2008; Bao et al. 2009)

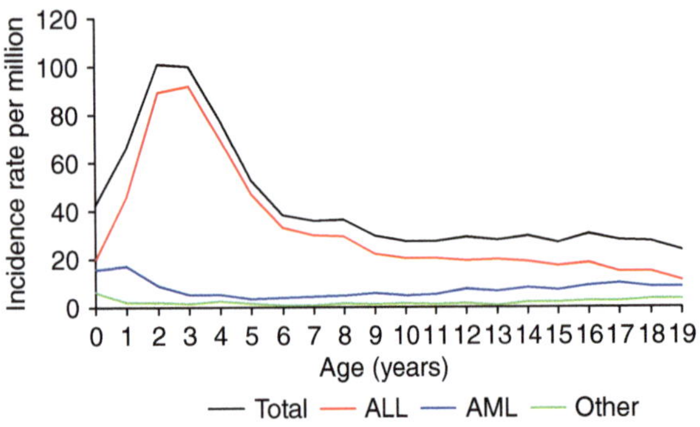

Fig. 1.3 Incidence rates of childhood leukemia by age of diagnosis (from Surveillance, Epidemiology, and End Results 13 registries from 1992–2006). Rates are standardized to the 2000U Ss tandardpopul ation

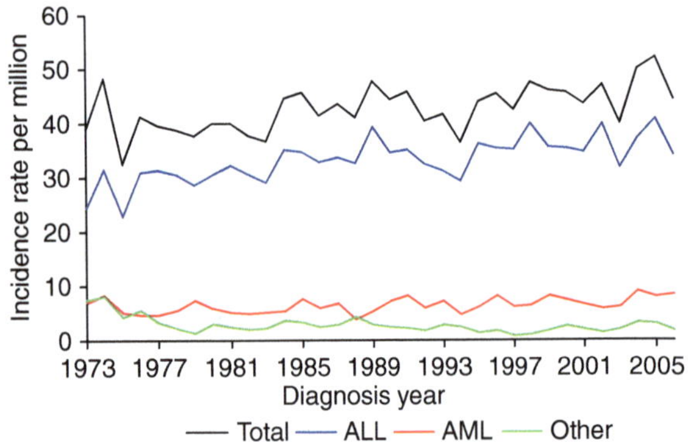

Fig. 1.4 Age-adjusted incidence rates of leukemia in children 0–14 years by year of diagnosis (from SEER 9 registries from 1973–2006). Rates are standardized to the 2000 US standard population

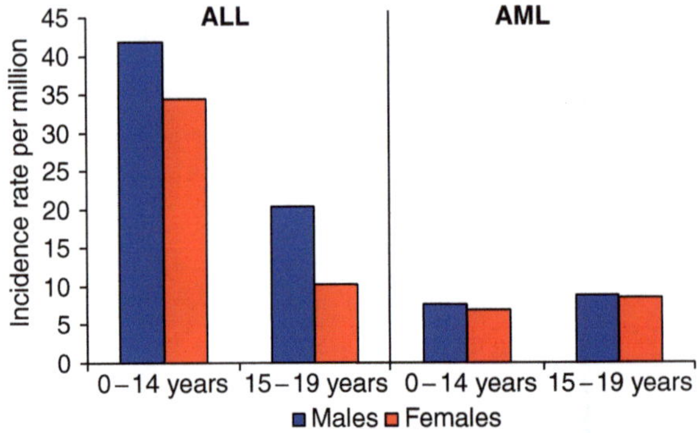

Fig. 1.5 Incidence rates of childhood leukemia by gender (from Surveillance, Epidemiology, and End Results 13 registries from 1992–2006). Rates are standardized to the 2000 US standard population

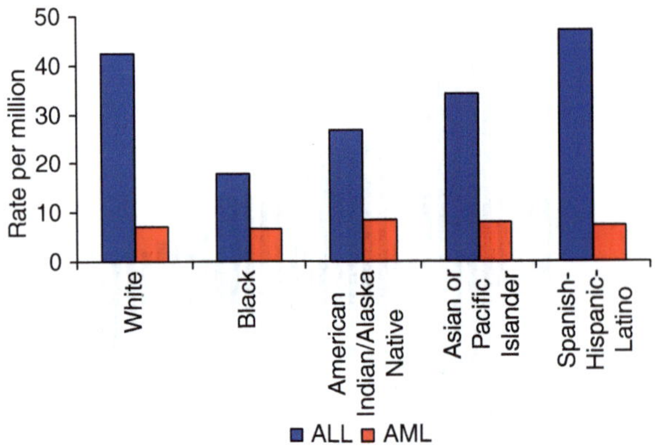

Fig. 1.6 Incidence rates of childhood leukemia diagnosed from 0–14 years by race/ethnicity (from Surveillance, Epidemiology, and End Results 13 registries from 1992–2006). Rates are standardizedt ot he2000U Ss tandardpopul ation

and 2.0:1 for children diagnosed between the ages of 0–14 and 15–19 years, respectively (Fig. 1.5). For AML, incidence rates are also slightly higher in males than females for individuals in the younger, but not the older, age group. The incidence of ALL is highest among whites and lowest among blacks. In contrast, AML incidence rates do not vary markedly by race. By ethnicity, higher ALL rates have been reported for individuals of Spanish-Hispanic-Latino ethnicity than those who do not have this ethnic background (Fig. 1.6).

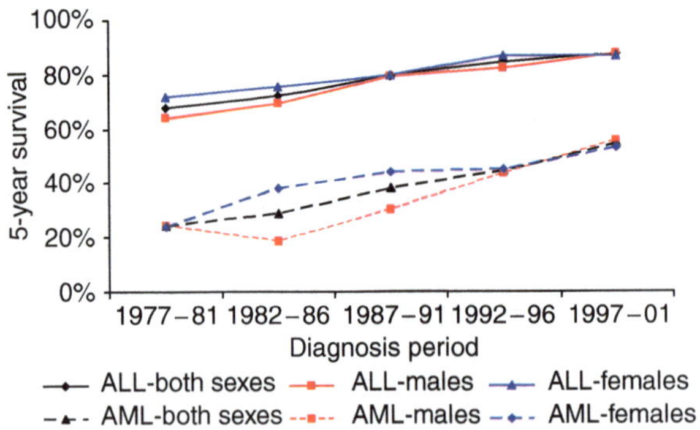

Fig. 1.7 Five-year survival in children diagnosed with acute leukemia from 0–14 years by diagnosis period and sex (from Surveillance, Epidemiology, and End Results 9 registries from 1973–2006). Relative survival rates calculated using the actuarialm ethod

1.2.3 Survival

Survival rates from leukemia have improved significantly over the period from 1977–2001 (Figs. 1.7 and 1.8). For

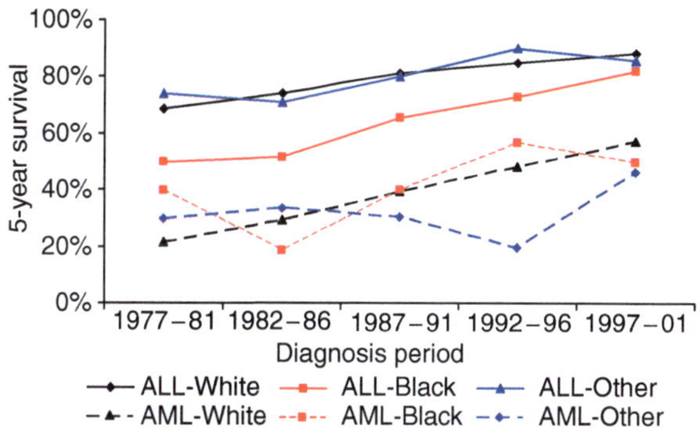

Fig. 1.8 Five-year survival in children diagnosed with acute leukemia from 0–14 years by diagnosis period and race (from Surveillance, Epidemiology, and End Results 9 registries from 1973–2006). Relative survival rates calculated using the actuarial method. "Other" races include American Indian/Alaskan Native, Asian/Pacific Islander, Other unspecified (from 1991), andunkno wn

ALL, 5 year overall survival increased from 68% during 1977–1981 to 86% during 1997–2001. For AML, rates have also improved, with 55% of cases surviving at least 5 years from diagnosis for the latest period compared to only 24% from 1977–1981 (Fig. 1.7). The dramatically improved survival across time is due to therapeutic advances and enrollment in national clinical trials (Reaman 2004; Kumar et al. 2005; Linabery and Ross 2008b). For both ALL and AML, 5 year survival rates are similar between males and females (Fig. 1.7). By race, 5 year survival for ALL was higher for White and children of other races than Black children in the earlier periods with recent rates being similar. For AML, survival rates have been variable with respect to race across time (Fig. 1.8).

1.3 Risk Factors for Childhood Leukemia

1.3.1 Genetic Syndromes

A small proportion of childhood leukemias are associated with predisposing genetic syndromes (see Table 1.3; Ries et al. 1999), but in total contribute to less than 5% of cases. Down syndrome is the most common genetic syndrome in children with leukemia. It is estimated that about 1 in 100 children with Down syndrome develop leukemia, which represents a 10–20-fold higher risk than children without Down syndrome; these odds increase to 500-fold for the AML-M7 megakaryocytic subtype (Zipursky et al. 1992). Trisomy 21, the hallmark of Down syndrome, is also found in the leukemia cells of children without Down syndrome. Further, as noted above, recurring translocations involving the *AML1* gene on chromosome 21, including t(12;21) in ALL, and t(8;21) in AML, have been characterized in children with leukemia. While candidate genes on chromosome 21 have been suggested to be etiologically relevant (Malinge et al. 2009), as well as other genes such as *GATA1* on the X chromosome (Cabelof et al. 2009), only a small minority of children with Down syndrome eventually develop leukemia. Thus, leukemia in children with Down syndrome is likely a multi-step process that involves additional genes, environmental exposures, or a combination of both.

Table 1.3 Major genetic syndromes associated with childhood leukemia

Leukemiat ype	Inheritedc ondition[a]
ALL and AML	Down syndrome, neurofibromatosis, Schwachman syndrome, Bloom syndrome, ataxia telangiectasia
ALL	Klinefelter syndrome, Langerhans cell histiocytosis
AML	Familial monosomy 7, Kostmann granulocytopenia, Fanconi anemia

[a]Summarizedi nR iese ta l. (1999)

Other syndromes which dramatically raise the risk of childhood leukemia are neurofibromatosis, Schwachman syndrome, Bloom syndrome, and ataxia telangiectasia (for both ALL and AML), Klinefelter syndrome, and Langerhans cell histiocytosis (for ALL), familial monosomy 7, Kostmann granulocytopenia, and Fanconi anemia (for AML).

1.3.2 Environmental and Other Risk Factors for Childhood Leukemia

Despite the large number of epidemiologic studies, few risk factors for childhood leukemia other than genetic syndromes have been identified. Many studies have been hampered by relatively small sample sizes, diagnostic heterogeneity (e.g., combining ALL and AML together, lack of consideration of additional molecular data (translocations, etc.)), and the limitations that accompany a case-control study design. Case-control studies are the standard epidemiological study design for rare diseases, but can be affected by potential biases that are difficult to quantify and correct. For example, for case-control studies of childhood leukemia, parents of children with leukemia and parents of healthy children (selected via various methods) are often interviewed about exposures and events that may have occurred years ago. Parents of children with leukemia may recall an event as being more noteworthy to report (e.g., a single pesticide exposure during pregnancy) than a parent of a healthy child, which can lead to spurious, inflated associations. Unless these parental reports can be validated, or replicated in other settings using different study designs, it can be difficult to draw definitive conclusions. Nonetheless, there are some associations of risk factors with childhood leukemia reported in the literature with fair consistency, which increase their credence. Some of the major risk factors that have been examined in leukemia epidemiology are summarized here.

1.3.2.1 Ionizing Radiation

Ionizing radiation exposure through in utero diagnostic x-rays is an established risk factor for childhood ALL and AML but it likely contributes to very few if any cases presently due to a decline in dosage and frequency of use during pregnancy (Doll and Wakeford 1997). Other sources of ionizing radiation, including radon (Raaschou-Nielsen 2008), fallout from atomic bombs (Delongchamp et al. 1997) and the Chernobyl nuclear power accident (Davis et al. 2006), postnatal x-rays (Little 1999; Meinert et al. 1999; Shu et al. 2002a; Infante-Rivard 2003), and parental occupation (Gardner et al. 1990; Urquhart et al. 1991; Draper et al. 1993; Kinlen et al. 1993; McLaughlin et al. 1993; Roman et al. 1993; Roman et al. 1996; Draper et al. 1997; Pobel and Viel 1997; Meinert et al. 1999; Dickinson et al. 2002; Johnson et al. 2008), have also been explored, but are, on the whole, equivocal. Exposure to electromagnetic fields (EMF), a non-ionizing radiation source, has been explored in relation to childhood leukemia in several studies, many of which used actual measurements rather than estimates based on proximity to voltage lines (Calvente et al, 2010). While there does not appear to be an overall association with EMF exposure and childhood leukemia, a recent review indicated that the highest level of EMF exposure, to which very few children are exposed, may increase the risk of leukemia (Schuz and Ahlbom 2008). However, the authors also thoughtfully noted that there is no biologic causal mechanism identified to explain the association between high levels of EMF and childhood leukemia, nor can chance or bias be ruled out. Lastly, it has been of interest to determine whether low-dose exposure to natural background radiation (e.g., cosmic rays, terrestrial radiation) in the range of 0.5–2.5 mSV/year contributes to the development of leukemia. Using statistical models developed by the U.S. Committee on the Biological Effects of Ionizing Radiation (BEIR VII) and the United Nations Scientific Committee on the Effects of Atomic Radiation (UNSCEAR), Wakeford et al. (2009) estimated that between 8% and 30% of childhood leukemia cases diagnosed in children younger than 14 years can be attributed to natural background radiation.

1.3.2.2 Prior Chemotherapy

Children who are treated for a prior malignancy, especially with treatments that include alkylating agents or epipodophyllotoxins, are at an increased risk of developing leukemia, particularly AML (Hijiya et al. 2009). The increased risk appears to be associated with dosing schedule, host factors (e.g., genetic susceptibility), and concurrent use of radiation and/or other treatments. While the overall proportion of children who subsequently develop leukemia following therapy for a primary cancer is quite small (Hawkins et al. 1992), there is recent evidence that an elevated risk continues long after therapy has ceased (Haddy et al. 2006).

1.3.2.3 Reproductive History

Maternal age greater than 35 years at the time of the child's birth appears to be associated with an increased risk of childhood leukemia, which is apparent even after controlling for Down syndrome, parity, and paternal age. A recent study analyzed data obtained from five states (Minnesota, New York, California, Washington, and Texas) that had linked their cancer and birth registries. Of 4,476 and 804 cases of ALL and AML, respectively, and ~54,000 controls, the risk of both types of leukemia increased by ~8% (95% CI 1.05–1.11) for every 5 year increase in maternal age (Johnson et al. 2009). Two other large studies have also reported increased risks of childhood leukemia with older maternal ages (Dockerty et al. 2001; Yip et al. 2006). It is not clear why advanced maternal age is associated with an increased risk of leukemia, but it could involve epigenetic mechanisms, since oocyte genetic mutations are not thought to increase substantially with maternal age (Crow 2000). Although the data are not entirely consistent, there is also a suggestion that history of maternal fetal loss (stillbirth, miscarriage) is associated with a slightly increased risk of childhood leukemia (van Steensel-Moll et al. 1985; Kaye et al. 1991; Yeazel et al. 1995; Ross et al. 1997). This association may reflect either a chronic exposure or an underlying genetic susceptibility that results in a range of effects from fetal death to leukemia.

1.3.3 Lifestyle Factors

1.3.3.1 Cigarette Smoking

Infante-Rivard (2008) recently reviewed 12 published reports since 1988 that evaluated maternal (or in some cases, paternal) cigarette smoking around the time of conception, during pregnancy, or postnatally in the etiology of childhood leukemia. While there was at least one case-control study published since this review that suggested a positive association for paternal but not maternal cigarette smoking (Rudant et al. 2008), the evidence by and large suggests little positive association (Infante-Rivard 2008). This lack of association is striking, given the known carcinogenicity of tobacco, and the identification of metabolites of a tobacco-specific carcinogen, 4-(methylnitrosamino)-1-(3-pyridyl)-1-butanone (NNK) in the urine of neonates of mothers who smoked cigarettes during pregnancy (Lackmann et al. 1999). However, since childhood leukemia is heterogeneous, it is possible that only a small subset would be at risk, and thus previous studies have been underpowered to detect such an association.

1.3.3.2 Alcohol Consumption

Maternal alcohol consumption during pregnancy has also been explored in relation to childhood leukemia overall as well as to ALL and/or AML (reviewed in Infante-Rivard and El-Zein (2007)). For childhood ALL, the data are equivocal; at least three studies have reported no association, two studies reported an increased risk, and two reported a decreased risk (Infante-Rivard and El-Zein 2007; Menegaux et al. 2007). For childhood AML, the evidence is more compelling for a positive association. At least three studies have reported an increased risk (Severson et al. 1993; van Duijn et al. 1994; Shu et al. 1996), which appeared to be more apparent in younger age groups and/or specific morphologic subtypes.

1.3.3.3 Occupational Exposures

There have been several studies that have evaluated parental job classifications and/or occupational exposures around the time of pregnancy in relation to childhood leukemia. While there are some suggestions of positive associations (e.g., pesticides, radiation, solvents), the data are largely inconsistent (reviewed in Belson et al. (2007)). It is difficult to compare findings across studies especially with the different methodologies used to measure occupational exposures (e.g., dosimetry, workplace records, job title, recall, etc.), various study designs employed, and lack of statistical power for specific exposures. In addition, some studies have used parental occupation as a proxy measure of exposure to infections, rather than to chemicals of interest (Roman et al. 1994; Fear et al. 1999, 2005). In a case-control study of occupational exposures and childhood leukemia in Germany, Schuz (Schuz et al. 2003) provided strong evidence of recall bias, with over-reporting of occupational exposures in the prenatal period, particularly when the time period between exposure and interview was short. Thus, for future interview studies, it will be important to consider methods to validate reported exposures.

1.3.3.4 Maternal/Child Diet

Dietary exposures have been infrequently studied in childhood leukemia. This lack of investigation is likely due to the difficulty in incorporating an extensive food frequency questionnaire into an already lengthy interview. Nevertheless, there are some intriguing findings regarding maternal dietary exposures. As noted above, the vast majority of infants with leukemia have translocations involving the *MLL* gene. Identical *MLL* translocations have been observed in patients who develop secondary leukemias (primarily AML) following chemotherapy with drugs that inhibit DNA topoisomerase II (Felix 1998). Thus, it was hypothesized that maternal exposure to DNA topoisomerase II inhibitors during pregnancy may contribute to the risk of infant leukemia with *MLL* translocations (Ross et al. 1994). Diet is a major source of DNA topoisomerase II inhibitors. Foods such as canned and dried legumes, onions, apples, berries, soy products, coffee and other caffeinated beverages, green and black tea, cocoa, and red wine are all rich sources of various chemicals that inhibit DNA topoisomerase II (Ross et al. 1994; Spector et al. 2005). A preliminary case-control study (84 infant cases, 97 infant controls) found a statistically significant increased risk of infant AML with increasing maternal consumption of foods that inhibited DNA topoisomerase II (Ross et al. 1996b). No association was found with infant ALL. Unfortunately, no data were available on *MLL* status. A subsequent larger study (240 cases, 255 controls) reported an increased risk of infant AML with *MLL* rearrangements with increasing maternal consumption of foods that inhibited DNA topoisomerase II (Spector et al. 2005). There was little evidence of an association with the other three infant groups (ALL/*MLL*–, ALL/*MLL*+, AML/*MLL*–). Additionally, indirect evidence of a potential association between DNA topoisomerase II inhibitors and infant leukemia has been investigated with regard to polymorphism in a gene, NAD(P)H: quinione oxidoreductase 1 (NQ01), which metabolizes some of the relevant biochemicals (see Sect. 1.3.4).

For childhood leukemia overall, analyses conducted in the Northern California Childhood Leukemia Study found an inverse association with a maternal diet high in fruits and vegetables (Jensen et al. 2004), which was also reported in a study from Greece (Petridou et al. 2005). These data coincide with reports of an inverse association with maternal vitamin supplementation described below. Child diet was investigated in one study (Kwan et al. 2004), also noting an inverse association with fruit and vegetable consumption. Finally, there were a few past reports that suggested a possible association with parental or child consumption of cured meats (Peters et al. 1994; Sarasua and Savitz 1994).

1.3.3.5 VitaminSup plementation

Growing evidence suggests maternal vitamin supplementation during pregnancy, especially folic acid, to be associated with a decreased risk of childhood ALL (Thompson et al. 2001; Wen et al. 2002; Ross et al. 2005), although at least one study found no association (Dockerty et al. 2007). There is no evidence of an inverse relation with childhood AML (Ross et al. 2005), but this has not been studied to any great extent. Unfortunately, these are isolated studies that have not taken into account individual genetic variation in vitamin metabolizing enzymes (discussed further in Sect. 1.3.4), which may influence the risk in association with the level of vitamin intake. For example, little data exists on whether single nucleotide polymorphisms (SNPs) in the *MTHFR* gene in combination with low maternal or childhood dietary folic acid intake influence the leukemia risk.

1.3.3.6 Pesticides

In addition to occupational exposure, studies have investigated in utero and child exposure to pesticides through household and garden use. Two comprehensive reviews of pesticides and childhood cancer, including leukemia, have been recently published (Infante-Rivard and Weichenthal 2007; Nasterlack 2007), to which the reader is directed for more detailed information. By and large, no firm conclusions can be drawn regarding household pesticide exposure, primarily because of concerns regarding bias and misclassification. Nevertheless, recent studies that have incorporated more comprehensive assessment of exposure are supportive of an increased risk of childhood leukemia (both ALL and AML). These positive associations appear most striking with reported exposure during pregnancy (Infante-Rivard and Weichenthal 2007). Again, as with vitamins, few studies have investigated these environmental toxins in the context of biomarkers of exposure or gene–environment interactions.

1.3.3.7 Infections

As noted above (in International incidence rates section), ALL occurs much more frequently in developed than in developing nations (Parkin et al. 1998). Moreover, the early childhood peak in ALL incidence has been noted to have emerged in populations experiencing economic growth (Fraumeni and Miller 1967; Hrusak et al. 2002). The fact that pre-B-cell ALL alone, and not other types of leukemia, comprises most of the childhood peak (Greaves et al. 1993) suggests that higher rates of ALL in industrialized countries are not due to improved reporting, and that it is this form of ALL, specifically, that is associated with some factor related to economic growth. Though there are many such factors, infection has been the focus of research since ALL is a malignancy of immune cell progenitors and the infectious burden clearly declines in nations with more developed economies. There are two prominent hypotheses that regard infection as explaining the international variation in childhood leukemia incidence. Kinlen suggests that childhood leukemia in general is a rare response of immune cells to infection by an as yet unrecognized pathogen, posited to be, most likely, a virus (Kinlen 1988). Greaves suggests that pre-B cell ALL, specifically, results from the proliferation of lymphoblasts, and the attendant acquisition of "second hit" mutations, following infections in general (Greaves 1988). Both theories postulate that delayed exposure to infection early in infancy, such as is seen in developed nations, will increase risk of developing leukemia in childhood.

Data in support of these related hypotheses include a weak but significant spatio–temporal clustering (Alexander et al. 1998) and seasonality of leukemia cases (Westerbeek et al. 1998; Ross et al. 1999), both of which are suggestive of a role for infections, though not exclusively. Several ecologic studies have consistently found that emigration to previously isolated areas is followed by a spike in leukemia incidence; such "population mixing" may indicate conditions that facilitate the transmission of infections (Kinlen 1995). More recent studies using more precise demographic measures of population mixing have, in general, found an increased risk of leukemia with greater population growth and diversity of immigrants, but have not established whether this increase was modified by urbanization (Langford 1991; Stiller and Boyle 1996; Dickinson and Parker 1999; Koushik et al. 2001; Boutou et al. 2002; Dickinson and Parker 2002; Parslow et al. 2002).

Unfortunately, history of infection as established by questionnaire or record abstraction is subject to recall bias and misclassification of asymptomatic individuals (McKinney et al. 1987; Shu et al. 1988; Buckley et al. 1994; Dockerty et al. 1999; McKinney et al. 1999; Schuz et al. 1999; Neglia et al. 2000; Chan et al. 2002; Naumburg et al. 2002; Perrillat et al. 2002). Evidence in support of infection is mainly through proxy measures, since serum taken at the time of leukemia diagnosis cannot assess whether infection preceded leukemia (Gahrton et al. 1971; Heegaard et al. 1999; MacKenzie et al. 1999; Groves et al. 2001; MacKenzie et al. 2001; Salonen et al. 2002). Rather, proxy measures of infection may be more readily recalled and less prone to misclassification. For instance, time in attendance at day care and birth order, both of which can be proxy measures of exposure to infection, have demonstrated inverse associations with leukemia with some consistency (Zack et al. 1991; Westergaard et al. 1997; Infante-Rivard et al. 2000a; Neglia et al. 2000; Rosenbaum et al. 2000; Dockerty et al. 2001; Chan et al. 2002; Ma et al. 2002; Perrillat et al. 2002; Shu et al. 2002b; Vineis et al. 2003). Lengthy breast feeding has also been inversely associated with leukemia (Parker 2001; Lancashire and Sorahan 2003) and may signify either early exposure to common viruses and bacteria or nutritional and immunologic benefits (Dworsky et al. 1983). The use of proxy measure of infection, while useful, still requires validation in a more controlled clinical research setting.

1.3.3.8 BirthW eight

High birth weight (variously defined, but usually >4,000 g) is associated with an increased risk of acute leukemia in most large studies (increased risks range from 25–75%) (Hjalgrim et al. 2003). A more recent study points to accelerated fetal growth, rather than high birth weight per se, as being important (Milne et al. 2007). The pathways or mechanisms underlying the association between fetal growth, birth weight, and subsequent development of cancer are largely unknown. It is possible that the increased risk of childhood leukemia may be due to increased levels of growth factors in heavier babies, such as insulin-like growth factor-1 (IGF1) (Ross et al. 1996a). As follow-up, others examined IGF1 levels in leukemia cells (Petridou et al. 2000). Further, correlations between growth factors (including IGF1) and stem cell potential have been reported in cord blood analyses (Baik et al. 2005). Associations with accelerated fetal growth and birth weight may also be due to disruptions in imprinting of growth factor-related genes (such as IGF2) through methylation. However, much remains to explore, including understanding temporal relationships and underlyingme chanisms.

1.3.4 Genetic Susceptibility

While certain inherited genetic mutations strongly increase the risk of leukemia as summarized in Table 1.3, the contribution of SNPs to leukemia risk is not well understood. Chokkalingam and Buffler (Chokkalingam and Buffler 2008) recently reviewed studies that have examined associations between SNPs and childhood leukemia. SNPs in genes hypothesized to modulate cancer risk were commonly examined, including those involved in folate metabolism, xenobiotic transport and metabolism, DNA repair, and immune function. Most genes have been examined in single studies that have neither taken into account gene–gene or gene–environment interactions nor examined comprehensive genetic pathways. Associations between childhood ALL and SNPs in the methylenetetrahydrofolate reductase (*MTHFR*) gene, the glutathione-S-transferase (*GST*) genes, the *CYP1A1* gene, and the *NQO1* gene have been reported most frequently (>6 studies); the key findings are summarized briefly here.

The *MTHFR* gene encodes the enzyme methylenetetrahydrofolate reductase, an enzyme that plays a critical role in the regulation of intracellular folate homeostasis. Two SNPs in *MTHFR* have been identified, C677T and A1298C, both of which have been linked to reduced enzymatic activity (Kim 2005). Two meta-analyses have recently reported pooled risk estimates from recessive random effects models for associations between childhood ALL and *MTHFR* polymorphisms (Pereira et al. 2006; Zintzaras et al. 2006). The first meta-analysis, based on four studies, reported a significant pooled odds ratio (OR) of 0.70 (0.51–0.94) for the 677TT genotype versus the 677CC/677TC genotypes, while the second meta-analysis, based on ten studies, reported a nonsignificant pooled OR of 0.88 (95% CI 0.73–1.06). Neither study reported a significant association between ALL and the 1298CC versus 1298AA/1297AC genotype. Although both studies used similar methods, they differed with respect to the studies included, with the larger meta-analysis including all studies included in the smaller meta-analysis. Three studies (Reddy and Jamil 2006; Kamel et al. 2007; Petra et al. 2007) published since these meta-analyses have reported inconsistent data with respect to *MTHFR* genotype and ALL risk. These data indicate that *MTHFR* genotype does not have a substantial influence on ALL risk.

GSTs encode for Phase II enzymes that are involved in the metabolism of several xenobiotics, including polycyclic aromatic hydrocarbons. Three enzymes from this family have been examined in >6 studies (*GSTM1*, *GSTT1*, and *GSTP1*) (Chokkalingam and Buffler 2008). Genotypes that have been frequently studied with regard to ALL risk are the null variants of the *GSTM1* and *GSTT1* genes and the A1578G variant of the *GSTP1* gene. The null variants result in complete loss of enzymatic activity, while the A1578G *GSTP1* polymorphism results in reduced enzymatic activity. A meta-analysis of studies published between 1/1997 and 7/2004 reported no significant associations between childhood ALL and the *GSTM1* null genotype (OR = 1.21; 95% CI 0.94 –1.55, $n = 9$ studies), the *GSTP1* A1578G allele (OR = 1.07; 95% CI 0.97–1.19, $n = 4$ studies), or the *GSTT1* null genotype (OR = 0.93; 95% CI 0.86–1.03, $n = 7$ studies) (Ye and Song 2005). Several studies published since the meta-analysis have been inconsistent, reporting no association or an increased risk for *GSTM1* (Chokkalingam and Buffler 2008; Rimando et al. 2008), and no significant associations for *GSTT1* (Chokkalingam and Buffler 2008; Rimando et al. 2008) or *GSTP1* with ALL (Chokkalingam and Buffler 2008).

CYP1A1 is the most frequently studied enzyme of the cytochrome P450 family whose members also function in xenobiotic metabolism. *CYP1A1* expression is upregulated in response to polycyclic aromatic hydrocarbons, including benzo[a]pyrene, a carcinogen in cigarette smoke (Nebert and Dalton 2006). The most frequently studied *CYP1A1* variant with respect to childhood ALL is termed “m1” (6235T>C, *CYP1A1*2A*). Seven studies reviewed by Chokkalingam and Buffler (Chokkalingam and Buffler 2008) reported inconsistent results, with four studies showing increased risks and three showing no association. One recently published study did not find an association between this variant and ALL (Lee et al. 2009).

The *NQO1* gene is a member of the NAD(P)H dehydrogenase (quinone) family that encodes for a Phase II enzyme that functions in the detoxification of quinones, including some that are known carcinogens. Over 93 SNPs have been reported in the *NQO1* gene, of which rs1800566 (*NQO1*2*) has been most commonly studied. The rs1800566 variant denotes a change from a C to a T at nucleotide position 609 and has been linked to reduced enzyme activity (Guha et al. 2008). A meta-analysis that included seven case-control studies reported no overall significant association between *NQO1*2* (≥1 allele) and ALL. Interestingly, in a subset of studies ($n = 4$) that examined the association between this SNP and *MLL* leukemia, a marginally significant increased OR of 1.39 (95% CI 0.98–1.97) was reported (Guha et al. 2008), a finding that emphasizes that distinct etiologies may exist for different molecular leukemia subtypes.

Although the data are largely null to date with respect to ALL risk for the most frequently examined candidate genes, it is possible that an individual's genotype is only relevant to leukemia risk in the presence of certain exposures. For example, three studies have provided varying degrees of evidence for the existence of a gene–environment interaction between *CYP1A1* genotype and parental smoking (Infante-Rivard et al. 2000b; Clavel et al. 2005; Lee et al. 2009). Thus, much further exploration is needed.

In contrast to the candidate gene approach described above that examines associations between SNPs and leukemia a few genes or variants at a time, genome-wide association (GWA) studies test associations of SNPs across the entire genome simultaneously. A key strength of a GWA study is that it does not require an a priori hypothesis about a gene–disease relationship. However, GWA studies have the main limitation of a large sample size requirement (estimated by one study to be >1,000 case and control subjects needed to detect significant relative risks in the range of 1.5 for risk allele frequencies of >0.05 with >60% power on commercially available platforms (Spencer et al. 2009)). A sample size of this magnitude is difficult to achieve in childhood leukemia studies, especially if heterogeneity is considered. Despite this limitation, two ALL GWA studies that included 503 and 317 cases, respectively, have been conducted and have reported the first unequivocal evidence that germline genetic variation contributes to ALL risk (Papaemmanuil et al. 2009; Trevino et al. 2009). Both studies reported the strongest associations with ORs ranging from 1.65–1.91 between ALL and SNPs in the *ARID5B* and *IKZF1* genes. Both of these genes have biologically plausible relationships to ALL due to their role in lymphoid differentiation and reported *IKZF1* deletions in childhood ALL (Mullighan et al. 2007; Mullighan et al. 2009). Interestingly, SNPs in some of the candidate genes described above were not reported to be significantly different between cases and controls in these GWA studies. For example, in one of the GWA studies, the authors specifically noted no significant associations with *MTHFR*, *CYP1A1*, and *NQO1* polymorphisms (Trevino et al. 2009).

1.4 Challenges and Future Directions

It is unfortunate that even with several large, well-designed epidemiological studies having been conducted, we still do not know what causes leukemia in most children. One of the difficulties in conducting studies is assembling a sufficient number of cases to have the ability to detect statistically significant associations. Further, there is concern regarding recruiting an appropriate comparison group, which is presenting more of a challenge today than years ago. Recently, there have been developments to help overcome some of the challenges involving identification of cases and controls (described below).

Another difficulty is that the primary exposure assessment tool in epidemiologic case-control studies is the questionnaire. As noted above, questionnaires can be fraught with misclassification (e.g., difficulty accurately remembering past events) and biases (e.g., over- or underreporting a specific exposure differently among cases and controls). Cohort studies, in which people are followed prior to development of the disease, minimizes or eliminates recall bias; however, it is practically very difficult to conduct a large enough study of pregnant women to accumulate enough cases of childhood leukemia among their offspring. Nevertheless, the International Childhood Cancer Cohort Consortium represents an opportunity to combine data from large cohort studies of pregnant women across nations to evaluate childhood cancer outcomes (Brown et al. 2007). The results of this ambitious effort will be of interest given the challenges in combining data across studies that used different questionnaires, sampling methods, etc.

In addition to the best study design possible, it may be wise to focus on biomarkers of exposure that could be exploited from currently available resources (e.g., NBS) as well as to incorporate gene–environment interaction when feasible. Lastly, it would be fruitful to consider utilization of animal models to test some of the strongest epidemiological observations. Examples are provided below.

1.4.1 Improvements in Identification of Cases and Controls for Studies in the United States

1.4.1.1 Cases

The Children's Oncology Group (COG) is a network of over 200 institutions and hospitals in the United States, Canada, Mexico, Australia, New Zealand, and Western Europe that treat the vast majority of childhood cancer, including leukemia (Ross et al. 1996c; Liu et al. 2003).

Since the 1980s, there have been a number of epidemiological studies of childhood leukemia. However, in addition to being approved by the institutional review board (IRB) at the investigator(s)' institution, epidemiological (as well as other nontherapeutic) studies were increasingly required to be approved by the IRB of every COG institution prior to implementation at a given site. This requirement often resulted in substantial delays, and thus subsequent loss of potential participants for study, which could contribute to bias. In order to address this issue, the Childhood Cancer Research Network (CCRN) protocol was recently developed in the COG (Steele et al. 2006). The CCRN protocol, administered around the time of diagnosis, requests written consent from parents (and children if they are age eligible) for release of information related to the cancer and some demographic information. Second, it requests written consent for possible future contact to consider taking part in a nontherapeutic study. Any future COG-approved study using CCRN data would be separately explained and consented to potential participants by the investigator(s) conducting the study following IRB approval at the institution overseeing the study.

Since implementation in December 2007, nearly all COG institutions have obtained IRB approval for the CCRN protocol and several thousand patients have been enrolled to date; over 93% have agreed to a future contact. Based on this outstanding institutional and parental participation, we expect that the CCRN will transform epidemiological research in COG by significantly diminishing administrative hurdles and providing approved COG investigators nearly real-time access to potential participants. New epidemiological studies are already underway for osteosarcoma and neuroblastoma, and a large leukemia study is planned.

1.4.1.2 Controls

One of the biggest challenges for conducting national case-control studies is the identification of an appropriate control group. Random-digit dialing (RDD) used to be the method of choice for selecting controls nationally in pediatric cancer studies (Robison and Daigle 1984). However, with the increasing use of answering machines, caller identification, and cell phones, along with the persistent annoyance of telemarketers, RDD is no longer viable on a national scale (Ross et al. 2004; Bunin et al. 2007; Spector et al. 2007b). One potential alternative to RDD may be birth records (Ross et al. 2004). In 2003, a survey of all vital statistics registrars was conducted in 32 states, representing close to 75% of young children in the United States; this survey indicated that obtaining birth certificate controls for recruitment with appropriate approvals is feasible (Spector et al. 2007b). Two recent COG epidemiology studies have utilized this method to recruit controls under the age of 6. In one of these studies, RDD and birth certificate controls were compared and the controls were similar to each other, which was reassuring, but still differed from the underlying population (Puumala et al. 2009). A clear advantage to birth registry controls, however, is that non-responders can be characterized through information on the birth certificates (not possible with RDD) as well as through geocoding.

1.4.2 Opportunities for Validation

1.4.2.1 NeonatalB loodSp ots

Screening tests for inborn errors of metabolism (e.g., galactosemia, phenylketonuria) are performed on virtually every child born in the United States through a NBS obtained shortly after birth. This testing involves lancing of a heel and collection of ensuing blood drops on a Guthrie card by medical personnel; the card is subsequently sent for testing at the respective state health department. Some NBS are stored after testing, but states have varying rules regarding length of storage and access (Olney et al. 2006; Therrell et al. 2006). Further, since laws are continually changing, it is difficult to predict how easily NBS will be able to be accessed in the future. Nevertheless, NBS represent an invaluable source of biological samples that could be used to evaluate in utero exposures. In addition to being a source of DNA, several research groups have developed (or are developing) methods to measure various biomarkers such as cytokines, nutrients, viruses, metals, and tobacco metabolites (Olshan 2007; Spector et al. 2007a). It will be of great interest to incorporate acquisition of NBS into national case-control studies of childhood leukemia for study of specific biomarkers, although there will need to be specific biomarker validation studies conducted before this could be implemented nationwide.

1.4.2.2 Maternal-FetalC ohortSt udies

It will also be important to utilize pregnancy cohort studies for the consideration of specific methodological issues. Women could be identified early in their pregnancies (or immediately prior to conception), administered questionnaires, and followed through pregnancy to evaluate issues related to recall. In addition, biospecimens could be collected from both the mother and infant for exposure validation and the exploration of gene–environment interactions. Some examples of the possibilities include the following:

Recall: As noted above, it is difficult to determine how well parents recall exposures during pregnancy. Maternal-fetal cohorts can provide insight into the reliability of parental recall by comparing responses to questionnaires given during pregnancy and repeated some time after birth. For instance, a study that gave a food frequency questionnaire to women during pregnancy and again 3–7 years later found fairly high correlations, of up to 80%, between surveys (Bunin et al. 2001). It should be noted that the ability of a questionnaire to elicit similar responses (i.e., reliability) is different than its ability to elicit an accurate measurement of exposure (i.e., validity). For those exposures that are not easily determined other than by questionnaire, it is only possible to determine reliability. Nevertheless, the validity of questionnaires for those exposures documented in medical records or elsewhere, which constitute gold standards, may be assessed in maternal–fetal cohorts.

Exposure validation: With the incorporation of detailed questionnaires, there is also the opportunity to validate specific exposures of interest that can be readily measured in biological samples. For example, using a food-frequency questionnaire along with an assessment of vitamin supplement use, a variable can be created with regard to folic acid intake during pregnancy. This variable in turn can be validated against maternal and cord blood levels of folate, along with an assessment of the influence of various polymorphisms in the folic acid pathway (Molloy et al. 2002; Torres-Sanchez et al. 2006; Barbosa et al. 2008).

Biomarkers of carcinogen exposure and effect: Many environmental mutagens (including pesticides, cigarette smoke metabolites, etc.) have only a short half-life *in vivo*. It has, therefore, been necessary to find more persistent surrogate markers of biological effect for clinical research studies, such as DNA adducts, glycophorin A (*GPA*) mutations and hypoxanthine-guanine phosphoribosyl transferase (*HPRT*) mutations. The frequency of *HPRT* mutations serves as a marker for mutations that occur through more direct mechanisms (point mutations, gross structural alterations), while the *GPA* assay can detect mutations resulting from chromosome–chromosome interactions (Bigbee et al. 1998). Both mechanisms are implicated in carcinogenesis. A few maternal-infant studies have explored environmental exposures such as cigarette smoking or pesticides and *GPA* or *HPRT* mutations in cord blood (Lunn et al. 1999; Yoshioka et al. 2001). Others have evaluated tobacco-related carcinogens (e.g., NNK) in infant urine (Lackmann et al. 1999). However, none takes into account a comprehensive assessment of exposures relevant to childhood leukemia risk. Further, few have considered genetic polymorphism pathways that may modify risk. A well-designed maternal-infant cohort could evaluate measures of exposure, biological effect, and potential modification by SNPs.

1.4.3 Comprehensive Use of Animal Models to Assess Exposure/ Cancer Relationships

Although animal models have been used for decades in the study of risk assessment and molecular pathogenesis, there has been minimal study relevant to the perinatal period (Anderson 2006), during which many leukemia cases have been shown to be initiated (Greaves 2005). Moreover, this period of development may be particularly pertinent to etiologic studies, as evidence from animal models that shows that the fetus is especially vulnerable to the genotoxic effects of carcinogens (Anderson 2004). A major limitation of the use of conventional animal models that develop hematological malignancies is their lack of genetic similarity to human childhood leukemia (McCormick and Kavet 2004). Given this limitation, genetically engineered murine models may be more relevant for childhood leukemia etiology research. A few of these models are reviewed briefly below.

Murine and other animal models have been developed to elucidate the role of cooperating genetic and environmental factors in leukemia etiology. Murine models now exist for several of the translocations found in childhood ALL. These include *ETV6-RUNX1*, found in the most common form of childhood ALL, and several of the *MLL* fusion genes, including *MLL-AF9* (present in AML), and *MLL-AF4* (found in B or mixed lineage ALL). *ETV6-RUNX1* and the *MLL* fusion genes are of special interest because they frequently develop prenatally. Data from *ETV6-RUNX1* murine and zebrafish models is generally consistent with the human epidemiological data showing that *ETV6-RUNX1* functions as a "first-hit" (Andreasson et al. 2001; Bernardin et al. 2002; Fischer et al. 2005; Sabaawy et al. 2006; Schindler et al. 2009) that requires additional cooperating oncogenic events and a prolonged period of time for the development of overt leukemia (Bernardin et al. 2002; Schindler et al. 2009).

The human *MLL* fusion gene leukemias differ from *ETV6-RUNX1,* in that the latency period is frequently shorter. Murine knock-in models of *MLL-AF4* and *MLL-AF9* have been developed in which the fusion gene is expressed under the control of endogenous regulatory mechanisms and thus expressed at physiologic levels (Corral et al. 1996; Johnson et al. 2003; Chen et al. 2006; Chen et al. 2008; Krivtsov et al. 2008). The constitutive expression murine models for the *MLL* fusion genes all suggest that, while latency is shorter than in the *ETV6-RUNX1* leukemia, additional cooperating events are important in the formation of overt leukemia.

The murine models for these and other fusion genes, including *AML1-ETO*, could be used for etiology studies (McCormick and Kavet 2004). These models can potentially be used to explore genetic variation in putative cancer susceptibility genes and environmental exposures (e.g., benzene, pesticides, high birth weight) that may influence leukemia development. We note, however, that the genetic differences between human and mouse provide constraints in fully modeling the etiology of human childhood leukemias.

1.5 Conclusion

In conclusion, it will be important for epidemiologists, clinicians, basic scientists, geneticists, and other disciplines to work together to develop a comprehensive interdisciplinary study of childhood leukemia, which includes bidirectional sharing of information across disciplines. An illustration of how such a study might be conducted in the United States is presented in Fig. 1.9. The COG CCRN would be used for the usual case-control study approach. For childhood leukemia, focus would be centered on exposures that are mainly important during the in utero/neonatal period, including high birth weight, vitamin supplements, infections, and chemicals. Once the case-control study is established, NBS could be obtained on some of the children through work with various health departments. The NBS could be used to evaluate translocations as well

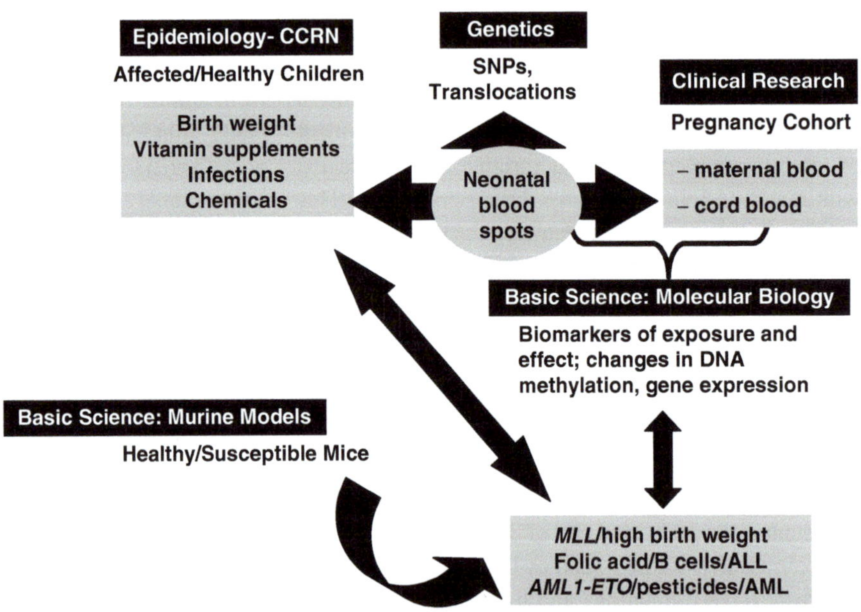

Fig. 1.9 Proposal for an interdisciplinary study of childhood leukemia

as biomarkers of exposure and effect. Further, a complementary maternal-fetal cohort could be conducted that includes collection of questionnaires and biological specimens. These data could be used to provide additional support for or against the interpretation of the case-control study. For example, do polymorphisms in the folic acid pathway influence cord blood levels of folate, and if so, how well does folate measured in NBS correlate with cord blood levels? Finally, in collaboration with basic science colleagues, high risk and normal risk murine models could be used to determine potential associations with the exposures. All of these studies would be intertwined in the sense that they provide additional data for or against the original hypothesesfromthe c ase-controls tudy.

Acknowledgements This work was supported by the National Cancer Institute (R01CA79940, T32CA099967, R01CA75169, U10CA13539, U10CA98543, and U10CA98413) and by the Children's Cancer Research Fund, Minneapolis, Minnesota.

References

Alexander FE, Boyle P et al (1998) Spatial temporal patterns in childhood leukaemia: further evidence for an infectious origin. EUROCLUS project. Br J Cancer 77(5):812–817

Anderson LM (2004) Predictive values of traditional animal bioassay studies for human perinatal carcinogenesis risk determination. Toxicol Appl Pharmacol 199(2):162–174

Anderson LM (2006) Environmental genotoxicants/carcinogens and childhood cancer: bridgeable gaps in scientific knowledge. Mutat Res 608(2):136–156

Andreasson P, Schwaller J et al (2001) The expression of ETV6/CBFA2 (TEL/AML1) is not sufficient for the transformation of hematopoietic cell lines *in vitro* or the induction of hematologic disease *in vivo*. Cancer Genet Cytogenet 130(2): 93–104

Armstrong SA, Look AT (2005) Molecular genetics of acute lymphoblastic leukemia. J Clin Oncol 23(26):6306–6315

Armstrong SA, Staunton JE et al (2002) MLL translocations specify a distinct gene expression profile that distinguishes a unique leukemia. Nat Genet 30(1):41–47

Baik I, Devito WJ et al (2005) Association of fetal hormone levels with stem cell potential: evidence for early life roots of human cancer. Cancer Res 65(1):358–363

Balgobind BV, Raimondi SC et al (2009) Novel prognostic subgroups in childhood 11q23/MLL-rearranged acute myeloid leukemia: results of an international retrospective study. Blood114(12):2489–2496

Bao PP, Zheng Y et al (2009) Time trends and characteristics of childhood cancer among children age 0–14 in Shanghai. Pediatr Blood Cancer 53(1):13–16

Barbosa PR, Stabler SP et al (2008) Association between decreased vitamin levels and MTHFR, MTR and MTRR gene polymorphisms as determinants for elevated total homocysteine concentrations in pregnant women. Eur J Clin Nutr62(8):1010–1021

Belson M, Kingsley B et al (2007) Risk factors for acute leukemia in children: a review. Environ Health Perspect 115(1): 138–145

Bennett JM, Catovsky D et al (1976) Proposals for the classification of the acute leukaemias. French-American-British (FAB) co-operative group. Br J Haematol 33(4):451–458

Bennett JM, Catovsky D et al (1985) Criteria for the diagnosis of acute leukemia of megakaryocyte lineage (M7). A report of the French-American-British Cooperative Group. Ann Intern Med103(3):460–462

Bennett JM, Catovsky D et al (1991) Proposal for the recognition of minimally differentiated acute myeloid leukaemia (AML-MO). Br J Haematol 78(3):325–329

Bernardin F, Yang Y et al (2002) TEL-AML1, expressed from t(12;21) in human acute lymphocytic leukemia, induces acute leukemia in mice. Cancer Res 62(14):3904–3908

Bigbee WL, Fuscoe JC et al (1998) Human *in vivo* somatic mutation measured at two loci: individuals with stably elevated background erythrocyte glycophorin A (gpa) variant frequencies exhibit normal T-lymphocyte hprt mutant frequencies. Mutat Res 397(2):119–136

Boutou O, Guizard A-V et al (2002) Population mixing and leukaemia in young people around the La Hague nuclear waste reprocessing plant. Br J Cancer 87:740–745

Brown RC, Dwyer T et al (2007) Cohort profile: the International Childhood Cancer Cohort Consortium (I4C). Int J Epidemiol 36(4):724–730

Buckley JD, Buckley CM et al (1994) Epidemiological characteristics of childhood acute lymphocytic leukemia. Analysis by immunophenotype. The Childrens Cancer Group. Leukemia8(5):856–864

Bunin GR, Gyllstrom ME et al (2001) Recall of diet during a past pregnancy. Am J Epidemiol 154(12):1136–1142

Bunin GR, Spector LG et al (2007) Secular trends in response rates for controls selected by random digit dialing in childhood cancer studies: a report from the Children's Oncology Group. Am J Epidemiol 166(1):109–116

Cabelof DC, Patel HV et al (2009) Mutational spectrum at GATA1 provides insights into mutagenesis and leukemogenesis in down syndrome. Blood 114(13):2753–2763

Calvente I, Fernandez MF et al (2010) Exposure to electromagnetic fields (non-ionizing radiation) and its relationship with childhood leukemia: a systematic review. Sci Total Environ 408(16):3062–9

Ceredig R, Rolink AG et al (2009) Models of haematopoiesis: seeing the wood for the trees. Nat Rev Immunol 9(4): 293–300

Chan LC, Lam TH et al (2002) Is the timing of exposure to infection a major determinant of acute lymphoblastic leukaemia in Hong Kong? Paediatr Perinat Epidemiol 16(2):154–165

Chen W, Li Q et al (2006) A murine Mll-AF4 knock-in model results in lymphoid and myeloid deregulation and hematologic malignancy. Blood 108(2):669–677

Chen W, Kumar AR et al (2008) Malignant transformation initiated by Mll-AF9: gene dosage and critical target cells. Cancer Cell 13(5):432–440

International Incidence of Childhood Cancer (1998) International incidence of childhood cancer, vol II. IARC Sci Publ 144: 1–391

Chokkalingam AP, Buffler PA (2008) Genetic susceptibility to childhood leukaemia. Radiat Prot Dosimetry 132(2): 119–129

Chowdhury T, Brady HJ (2008) Insights from clinical studies into the role of the MLL gene in infant and childhood leukemia. Blood Cells Mol Dis 40(2):192–199

Clavel J, Bellec S et al (2005) Childhood leukaemia, polymorphisms of metabolism enzyme genes, and interactions with maternal tobacco, coffee and alcohol consumption during pregnancy. Eur J Cancer Prev 14(6):531–540

Coebergh JW, Reedijk AM et al (2006) Leukaemia incidence and survival in children and adolescents in Europe during 1978–1997. Report from the Automated Childhood Cancer Information System project. Eur J Cancer 42(13):2019–2036

Corral J, Lavenir I et al (1996) An Mll-AF9 fusion gene made by homologous recombination causes acute leukemia in chimeric mice: a method to create fusion oncogenes. Cell 85(6):853–861

Crow JF (2000) The origins, patterns and implications of human spontaneous mutation. Nat Rev Genet 1(1):40–47

Davis S, Day RW et al (2006) Childhood leukaemia in Belarus, Russia, and Ukraine following the Chernobyl power station accident: results from an international collaborative population-based case-control study. Int J Epidemiol 35(2):386–396

Delongchamp RR, Mabuchi K et al (1997) Cancer mortality among atomic bomb survivors exposed in utero or as young children, October 1950-May 1992. Radiat Res 147(3): 385–395

Dickinson HO, Parker L (1999) Quantifying the effect of population mixing on childhood leukaemia risk: the Seascale cluster. Br J Cancer 81(1):144–151

Dickinson and Parker (2002) Leukaemia and non-Hodgkin's lymphoma in children of Sellafield male radiation workers. Int J Cancer 101(1):100

Dickinson HO, Hammal DM et al (2002) Population mixing and childhood leukaemia and non-Hodgkin's lymphoma in census wards in England and Wales, 1966–87. Br J Cancer 86(9):1411–1413

Dockerty JD, Skegg DC et al (1999) Infections, vaccinations, and the risk of childhood leukaemia. Br J Cancer 80(9):1483–1489

Dockerty JD, Herbison P et al (2007) Vitamin and mineral supplements in pregnancy and the risk of childhood acute lymphoblastic leukaemia: a case-control study. BMC Public Health7:136

Doll R, Wakeford R (1997) Risk of childhood cancer from fetal irradiation. Br J Radiol 70:130–139

Draper GJ, Stiller CA et al (1993) Cancer in Cumbria and in the vicinity of the Sellafield nuclear installation, 1963–90. BMJ 306(6870):89–94

Draper GJ, Little MP et al (1997) Cancer in the offspring of radiation workers: a record linkage study. BMJ 315(7117): 1181–1188

Dworsky M, Yow M et al (1983) Cytomegalovirus infection of breast milk and transmission in infancy. Pediatrics 72(3):295–299

Eguchi-Ishimae M, Eguchi M et al (2008) NOTCH1 mutation can be an early, prenatal genetic event in T-ALL. Blood 111(1):376–378

Fajardo-Gutierrez A, Juarez-Ocana S et al (2007) Incidence of cancer in children residing in ten jurisdictions of the Mexican Republic: importance of the Cancer registry (a population-based study). BMC Cancer 7:68

Fasching K, Panzer S et al (2000) Presence of clone-specific antigen receptor gene rearrangements at birth indicates an in utero origin of diverse types of early childhood acute lymphoblastic leukemia. Blood 95(8):2722–2724

Fear NT, Roman E et al (1999) Are the children of fathers whose jobs involve contact with many people at an increased risk of leukaemia? Occup Environ Med 56(7):438–442

Fear NT, Simpson J et al (2005) Childhood cancer and social contact: the role of paternal occupation (United Kingdom). Cancer Causes Control 16(9):1091–1097

Felix CA (1998) Secondary leukemias induced by topoisomerase-targeted drugs. Biochim Biophys Acta 1400(1–3): 233–255

Fischer M, Schwieger M et al (2005) Defining the oncogenic function of the TEL/AML1 (ETV6/RUNX1) fusion protein in a mouse model. Oncogene 24(51):7579–7591

Fischer S, Mann G et al (2007) Screening for leukemia- and clone-specific markers at birth in children with T-cell precursor ALL suggests a predominantly postnatal origin. Blood110(8):3036–3038

Ford AM, Ridge SA et al (1993) In utero rearrangements in the trithorax-related oncogene in infant leukaemias. Nature 363(6427):358–360

Ford AM, Pombo-de-Oliveira MS et al (1997) Monoclonal origin of concordant T-cell malignancy in identical twins. Blood89(1):281–285

Fraumeni JF Jr, Miller RW (1967) Epidemiology of human leukemia: recent observations. J Natl Cancer Inst 38(4): 593–605

Gahrton G, Wahren B et al (1971) Epstein-Barr and other herpes virus antibodies in children with acute leukemia. Int J Cancer 8(2):242–249

Gale KB, Ford AM et al (1997) Backtracking leukemia to birth: identification of clonotypic gene fusion sequences in neonatal blood spots. Proc Natl Acad Sci USA 94(25): 13950–13954

Garcia-Manero G, Yang H et al (2009) Epigenetics of acute lymphocytic leukemia. Semin Hematol 46(1):24–32

Gardner MJ, Snee MP et al (1990) Results of case-control study of leukaemia and lymphoma among young people near Sellafield nuclear plant in West Cumbria. BMJ 300(6722): 423–429

Graux C, Cools J et al (2006) Cytogenetics and molecular genetics of T-cell acute lymphoblastic leukemia: from thymocyte to lymphoblast. Leukemia 20(9):1496–1510

Greaves MF (1988) Speculations on the cause of childhood acute lymphoblastic leukemia. Leukemia 2(2):120–125

Greaves M (2005) In utero origins of childhood leukaemia. Early Hum Dev 81(1):123–129

Greaves MF, Wiemels J (2003) Origins of chromosome translocations in childhood leukaemia. Nat Rev Cancer 3(9): 639–649

Greaves MF, Katz FE et al (1985) Selective expression of cell surface antigens on human haemopoietic progenitor cells. Prog Clin Biol Res 184:301–315

Greaves MF, Colman SM et al (1993) Geographical distribution of acute lymphoblastic leukaemia subtypes: second report of the collaborative group study. Leukemia 7(1):27–34

Greaves MF, Maia AT et al (2003) Leukemia in twins: lessons in natural history. Blood 102(7):2321–2333

Groves FD, Sinha D et al (2001) Haemophilus influenzae type b serology in childhood leukaemia: a case-control study. Br J Cancer85(3):337–3 40

Guha N, Chang JS et al (2008) NQO1 polymorphisms and *de novo* childhood leukemia: a HuGE review and meta-analysis. Am J Epidemiol 168(11):1221–1232

Haddy N, Le Deley MC et al (2006) Role of radiotherapy and chemotherapy in the risk of secondary leukaemia after a solid tumour in childhood. Eur J Cancer 42(16):2757–2764

Hawkins MM, Wilson LM et al (1992) Epipodophyllotoxins, alkylating agents, and radiation and risk of secondary leukaemia after childhood cancer. BMJ 304(6832):951–958

Heegaard ED, Jensen L et al (1999) The role of parvovirus B19 infection in childhood acute lymphoblastic leukemia. Pediatr Hematol Oncol 16(4):329–334

Heerema NA, Sather HN et al (2000) Prognostic impact of trisomies of chromosomes 10, 17, and 5 among children with acute lymphoblastic leukemia and high hyperdiploidy (> 50 chromosomes). J Clin Oncol 18(9):1876–87

Hjalgrim LL, Westergaard T et al (2003) Birth weight as a risk factor for childhood leukemia: a meta-analysis of 18 epidemiologic studies. Am J Epidemiol 158(8):724–35

Hijiya N, Ness KK et al (2009) Acute leukemia as a secondary malignancy in children and adolescents: current findings and issues. Cancer 115(1):23–35

Hrusak O, Trka J et al (2002) Acute lymphoblastic leukemia incidence during socioeconomic transition: selective increase in children from 1 to 4 years. Leukemia 16(4):720–725

Infante-Rivard C (2003) Diagnostic x rays, DNA repair genes and childhood acute lymphoblastic leukemia. Health Phys 85(1):60–64

Infante-Rivard C (2008) Chemical risk factors and childhood leukaemia: a review of recent studies. Radiat Prot Dosimetry 132(2):220–227

Infante-Rivard C, El-Zein M (2007) Parental alcohol consumption and childhood cancers: a review. J Toxicol Environ Health B Crit Rev 10(1–2):101–129

Infante-Rivard C, Weichenthal S (2007) Pesticides and childhood cancer: an update of Zahm and Ward's 1998 review. J Toxicol Environ Health B Crit Rev 10(1–2):81–99

Infante-Rivard C, Fortier I et al (2000a) Markers of infection, breast-feeding and childhood acute lymphoblastic leukaemia. Br J Cancer 83(11):1559–1564

Infante-Rivard C, Krajinovic M et al (2000b) Parental smoking, CYP1A1 genetic polymorphisms and childhood leukemia (Quebec, Canada). Cancer Causes Control 11(6): 547–553

Jensen CD, Block G et al (2004) Maternal dietary risk factors in childhood acute lymphoblastic leukemia (United States). Cancer Causes Control 15(6):559–570

Johnson JJ, Chen W et al (2003) Prenatal and postnatal myeloid cells demonstrate stepwise progression in the pathogenesis of MLL fusion gene leukemia. Blood 101(8):3229–3235

Johnson KJ, Alexander BH et al (2008) Childhood cancer in the offspring born in 1921–1984 to US radiologic technologists. Br J Cancer 99(3):545–550

Johnson KJ, Carozza SE et al (2009) Parental age and risk of childhood cancer: a pooled analysis. Epidemiology 20(4): 475–483

Kamel AM, Moussa HS et al (2007) Synergistic effect of methyltetrahydrofolate reductase (MTHFR) C677T and A1298C polymorphism as risk modifiers of pediatric acute lymphoblastic leukemia. J Egypt Natl Canc Inst 19(2): 96–105

Karrman K, Forestier E et al (2009) Clinical and cytogenetic features of a population-based consecutive series of 285 pediatric T-cell acute lymphoblastic leukemias: rare T-cell receptor gene rearrangements are associated with poor outcome. Genes Chromosomes Cancer 48(9):795–805

Kawamoto H, Katsura Y (2009) A new paradigm for hematopoietic cell lineages: revision of the classical concept of the myeloid-lymphoid dichotomy. Trends Immunol 30(5): 193–200

Kaye SA, Robison LL et al (1991) Maternal reproductive history and birth characteristics in childhood acute lymphoblastic leukemia. Cancer 68(6):1351–1355

Kersey J, Nesbit M et al (1975) Evidence for origin of certain childhood acute lymphoblastic leukemias and lymphomas in thymus-derived lymphocytes. Cancer 36(4):1348–1352

Kim YI (2005) 5, 10-Methylenetetrahydrofolate reductase polymorphisms and pharmacogenetics: a new role of single nucleotide polymorphisms in the folate metabolic pathway in human health and disease. Nutr Rev 63(11):398–407

Kinlen L (1988) Evidence for an infective cause of childhood leukaemia: comparison of a Scottish new town with nuclear reprocessing sites in Britain. Lancet 2(8624)):1323–1327

Kinlen LJ (1995) Epidemiological evidence for an infective basis in childhood leukaemia. Br J Cancer 71(1):1–5

Kinlen LJ, Clarke K et al (1993) Paternal preconceptional radiation exposure in the nuclear industry and leukaemia and non-Hodgkin's lymphoma in young people in Scotland. BMJ306(6886):1153–1158

Koushik A, King WD et al (2001) An ecologic study of childhood leukemia and population mixing in Ontario, Canada. Cancer Causes Control 12(6):483–490

Krivtsov AV, Feng Z et al (2008) H3K79 methylation profiles define murine and human MLL-AF4 leukemias. Cancer Cell 14(5):355–368

Kumar A, Soares H et al (2005) Are experimental treatments for cancer in children superior to established treatments? Observational study of randomised controlled trials by the Children's Oncology Group. BMJ 331(7528):1295

Kwan ML, Block G et al (2004) Food consumption by children and the risk of childhood acute leukemia. Am J Epidemiol 160(11):1098–1107

Lackmann GM, Salzberger U et al (1999) Metabolites of a tobacco-specific carcinogen in urine from newborns. J Natl Cancer Inst 91(5):459–465

Lancashire RJ, Sorahan T (2003) Breastfeeding and childhood cancer risks: OSCC data. Br J Cancer 88(7):1035–1037

Langford I (1991) Childhood leukaemia mortality and population change in England and Wales 1969–73. Soc Sci Med 33(4):435–440

Lee KM, Ward MH et al (2009) Paternal smoking, genetic polymorphisms in CYP1A1 and childhood leukemia risk. Leuk Res33(2):250–258

Linabery AM, Ross JA (2008a) Childhood and adolescent cancer survival in the US by race and ethnicity for the diagnostic period 1975–1999. Cancer 113(9):2575–2596

Linabery AM, Ross JA (2008b) Trends in childhood cancer incidence in the U.S. (1992–2004). Cancer 112(2): 416–432

Little J (ed) (1999) Epidemiology of Childhood Cancer. International Agency for Research on Cancer, Lyon

Liu L, Krailo M et al (2003) Childhood cancer patients' access to cooperative group cancer programs: a population-based study. Cancer 97(5):1339–1345

Lunn RM, Langlois RG et al (1999) XRCC1 polymorphisms: effects on aflatoxin B1-DNA adducts and glycophorin A variant frequency. Cancer Res 59(11):2557–2561

Ma X, Buffler PA et al (2002) Daycare attendance and risk of childhood acute lymphoblastic leukaemia. Br J Cancer 86(9):1419–1424

MacKenzie J, Perry J et al (1999) JC and BK virus sequences are not detectable in leukaemic samples from children with common acute lymphoblastic leukaemia. Br J Cancer 81(5):898–899

MacKenzie J, Gallagher A et al (2001) Screening for herpesvirus genomes in common acute lymphoblastic leukemia. Leukemia 15(3):415–421

Maia AT, Tussiwand R et al (2004) Identification of preleukemic precursors of hyperdiploid acute lymphoblastic leukemia in cord blood. Genes Chromosomes Cancer 40(1):38–43

Malinge S, Izraeli S et al (2009) Insights into the manifestations, outcomes, and mechanisms of leukemogenesis in Down syndrome. Blood 113(12):2619–2628

Martinez-Climent JA, Garcia-Conde J (1999) Chromosomal rearrangements in childhood acute myeloid leukemia and myelodysplastic syndromes. J Pediatr Hematol Oncol 21(2): 91–102

McCormick DL, Kavet R (2004) Animal models for the study of childhood leukemia: considerations for model identification and optimization to identify potential risk factors. Int J Toxicol23(3):149–161

McKenzie S (1996) Textbook of hematology. Williams & Wilkens,B altimore

McKinney PA, Cartwright RA et al (1987) The inter-regional epidemiological study of childhood cancer (IRESCC): a case control study of aetiological factors in leukaemia and lymphoma. Arch Dis Child 62(3):279–287

McKinney PA, Juszczak E et al (1999) Pre- and perinatal risk factors for childhood leukaemia and other malignancies: a Scottish case control study. Br J Cancer 80(11):1844–1851

McLaughlin JR, King WD et al (1993) Paternal radiation exposure and leukaemia in offspring: the Ontario case-control study. BMJ 307(6910):959–966

Meinert R, Kaletsch U et al (1999) Associations between childhood cancer and ionizing radiation: results of a population-based case-control study in Germany. Cancer Epidemiol Biomarkers Prev 8(9):793–799

Menegaux F, Ripert M et al (2007) Maternal alcohol and coffee drinking, parental smoking and childhood leukaemia: a French population-based case-control study. Paediatr Perinat Epidemiol21(4):29 3–299

Michel G, von der Weid NX et al (2007) The Swiss Childhood Cancer Registry: rationale, organisation and results for the years 2001–2005. Swiss Med Wkly 137(35–36):502–509

Milne E, Laurvick CL et al (2007) Fetal growth and acute childhood leukemia: looking beyond birth weight. Am J Epidemiol 166(2):151–159

Molloy AM, Mills JL et al (2002) Maternal and fetal plasma homocysteine concentrations at birth: the influence of folate, vitamin B12, and the 5, 10-methylenetetrahydrofolate reductase 677C–>T variant. Am J Obstet Gynecol 186(3):499–503

Mori H, Colman SM et al (2002) Chromosome translocations and covert leukemic clones are generated during normal fetal development. Proc Natl Acad Sci USA 99(12):8242–8247

Mrozek K, Heerema NA et al (2004) Cytogenetics in acute leukemia. Blood Rev 18(2):115–136

Mullighan CG, Goorha S et al (2007) Genome-wide analysis of genetic alterations in acute lymphoblastic leukaemia. Nature 446(7137):758–764

Mullighan CG, Su X et al (2009) Deletion of IKZF1 and prognosis in acute lymphoblastic leukemia. N Engl J Med 360(5):470–480

Nasterlack M (2007) Pesticides and childhood cancer: an update. Int J Hyg Environ Health 210(5):645–657

Naumburg E, Bellocco R et al (2002) Perinatal exposure to infection and risk of childhood leukemia. Med Pediatr Oncol 38(6):391–397

Nebert DW, Dalton TP (2006) The role of cytochrome P450 enzymes in endogenous signalling pathways and environmental carcinogenesis. Nat Rev Cancer 6(12):947–960

Olney RS, Moore CA et al (2006) Storage and use of residual dried blood spots from state newborn screening programs. J Pediatr 148(5):618–622

Olshan AF (2007) Meeting report: the use of newborn blood spots in environmental research: opportunities and challenges. Environ Health Perspect 115(12):1767–1779

Papaemmanuil E, Hosking FJ et al (2009) Loci on 7p12.2, 10q21.2 and 14q11.2 are associated with risk of childhood acute lymphoblastic leukemia. Nat Genet 41(9):1006–1010

Parker L (2001) Breast-feeding and cancer prevention. Eur J Cancer37(2):155–158

Parslow RC, Law GR et al (2002) Population mixing, childhood leukaemia, CNS tumours and other childhood cancers in Yorkshire. Eur J Cancer 38(15):2033–2040

Pereira TV, Rudnicki M et al (2006) 5, 10-Methylenetetrahydrofolate reductase polymorphisms and acute lymphoblastic leukemia risk: a meta-analysis. Cancer Epidemiol Biomarkers Prev 15(10):1956–1963

Perrillat F, Clavel J et al (2002) Day-care, early common infections and childhood acute leukaemia: a multicentre French case-control study. Br J Cancer 86(7):1064–1069

Peters JM, Preston-Martin S et al (1994) Processed meats and risk of childhood leukemia (California, USA). Cancer Causes Control 5(2):195–202

Petra BG, Janez J et al (2007) Gene-gene interactions in the folate metabolic pathway influence the risk for acute lymphoblastic leukemia in children. Leuk Lymphoma 48(4): 786–792

Petridou E, Skalkidou A et al (2000) Endogenous risk factors for childhood leukemia in relation to the IGF system (Greece). The Childhood Haematologists-Oncologists Group. Cancer Causes Control 11(8):765–771

Petridou E, Ntouvelis E et al (2005) Maternal diet and acute lymphoblastic leukemia in young children. Cancer Epidemiol Biomarkers Prev 14(8):1935–1939

Petridou ET, Pourtsidis A et al (2008) Childhood leukaemias and lymphomas in Greece (1996–2006): a nationwide registration study. Arch Dis Child 93(12):1027–1032

Plass C, Oakes C et al (2008) Epigenetics in acute myeloid leukemia. Semin Oncol 35(4):378–387

Pobel D, Viel JF (1997) Case-control study of leukaemia among young people near La Hague nuclear reprocessing plant:

the environmental hypothesis revisited. BMJ 314(7074): 101–106
Pui CH, Relling MV et al (2004) Acute lymphoblastic leukemia. N Engl J Med 350(15):1535–48
Pui CH, Boyett JM et al (1999) Sex differences in prognosis for children with acute lymphoblastic leukemia. J Clin Oncol 17(3):818–824
Puumala SE, Spector LG et al (2009) Comparability and representativeness of control groups in a case-control study of infant leukemia: a report from the Children's Oncology Group. Am J Epidemiol 170(3):379–387
Raaschou-Nielsen O (2008) Indoor radon and childhood leukaemia. Radiat Prot Dosimetry 132(2):175–181
Raimondi SC, Behm FG et al (1988) Cytogenetics of childhood T-cell leukemia. Blood 72(5):1560–1566
Reaman GH (2004) Pediatric cancer research from past successes through collaboration to future transdisciplinary research. J Pediatr Oncol Nurs 21(3):123–127
Reddy H, Jamil K (2006) Polymorphisms in the MTHFR gene and their possible association with susceptibility to childhood acute lymphocytic leukemia in an Indian population. Leuk Lymphoma 47(7):1333–1339
Rimando MG, Chua MN et al (2008) Prevalence of GSTT1, GSTM1 and NQO1 (609C>T) in Filipino children with ALL (acute lymphoblastic leukaemia). Biosci Rep 28(3): 117–124
Robison LL, Daigle A (1984) Control selection using random digit dialing for cases of childhood cancer. Am J Epidemiol 120(1):164–166
Roman E, Watson A et al (1993) Case-control study of leukaemia and non-Hodgkin's lymphoma among children aged 0–4 years living in west Berkshire and north Hampshire health districts. BMJ 306(6878):615–621
Roman E, Watson A et al (1994) Leukaemia risk and social contact in children aged 0–4 years in southern England. J Epidemiol Community Health 48(6):601–602
Roman E, Doyle P et al (1996) Health of children born to medical radiographers. Occup Environ Med 53(2):73–79
Rosenbaum PF, Buck GM et al (2000) Early child-care and preschool experiences and the risk of childhood acute lymphoblastic leukemia. Am J Epidemiol 152(12):1136–1144
Ross JA, Potter JD et al (1994) Infant leukemia, topoisomerase II inhibitors, and the MLL gene. J Natl Cancer Inst 86(22):1678–1680
Ross JA, Perentesis JP et al (1996a) Big babies and infant leukemia: a role for insulin-like growth factor-1? Cancer Causes Control7(5):553–559
Ross JA, Potter JD et al (1996b) Maternal exposure to potential inhibitors of DNA topoisomerase II and infant leukemia (United States): a report from the Children's Cancer Group. Cancer Causes Control 7(6):581–590
Ross JA, Severson RK et al (1996c) Childhood cancer in the United States. A geographical analysis of cases from the Pediatric Cooperative Clinical Trials groups. Cancer 77(1):201–207
Ross JA, Potter JD et al (1997) Evaluating the relationships among maternal reproductive history, birth characteristics, and infant leukemia: a report from the Children's Cancer Group. Ann Epidemiol 7(3):172–179
Ross JA, Severson RK et al (1999) Seasonal variations in the diagnosis of childhood cancer in the United States. Br J Cancer81(3):549–553
Ross JA, Spector LG et al (2004) Invited commentary: Birth certificates – a best control scenario? Am J Epidemiol 159(10): 922–924, discussion 925
Ross JA, Blair CK et al (2005) Periconceptional vitamin useand leukemia risk in children with Down syndrome: a Children's Oncology Group study. Cancer 104(2):405–410
Rudant J, Menegaux F et al (2008) Childhood hematopoietic malignancies and parental use of tobacco and alcohol: the ESCALE study (SFCE). Cancer Causes Control 19(10): 1277–1290
Sabaawy HE, Azuma M et al (2006) TEL-AML1 transgenic zebrafish model of precursor B cell acute lymphoblastic leukemia. Proc Natl Acad Sci USA 103(41):15166–15171
Salonen MJ, Siimes MA et al (2002) Antibody status to HHV-6 in children with leukaemia. Leukemia 16(4):716–719
Sarasua S, Savitz DA (1994) Cured and broiled meat consumption in relation to childhood cancer: Denver, Colorado (United States). Cancer Causes Control 5(2):141–148
Schindler JW, Van Buren D et al (2009) TEL-AML1 corrupts hematopoietic stem cells to persist in the bone marrow and initiate leukemia. Cell Stem Cell 5(1):43–53
Schuz J, Ahlbom A (2008) Exposure to electromagnetic fields and the risk of childhood leukaemia: a review. Radiat Prot Dosimetry132(2):202–211
Schuz J, Kaatsch P et al (1999) Association of childhood cancer with factors related to pregnancy and birth. Int J Epidemiol 28(4):631–639
Schuz J, Spector LG et al (2003) Bias in studies of parental self-reported occupational exposure and childhood cancer. Am J Epidemiol158(7):710–716
Severson RK, Buckley JD et al (1993) Cigarette smoking and alcohol consumption by parents of children with acute myeloid leukemia: an analysis within morphological subgroups – a report from the Childrens Cancer Group. Cancer Epidemiol Biomarkers Prev 2(5):433–439
Shu XO, Gao YT et al (1988) A population-based case-control study of childhood leukemia in Shanghai. Cancer 62(3): 635–644
Shu XO, Ross JA et al (1996) Parental alcohol consumption, cigarette smoking, and risk of infant leukemia: a Childrens Cancer Group study. J Natl Cancer Inst 88(1):24–31
Shu XO, Han D et al (2002a) Birth characteristics, maternal reproductive history, hormone use during pregnancy, and risk of childhood acute lymphocytic leukemia by immunophenotype (United States). Cancer Causes Control 13(1): 15–25
Shu XO, Potter JD et al (2002b) Diagnostic X-rays and ultrasound exposure and risk of childhood acute lymphoblastic leukemia by immunophenotype. Cancer Epidemiol Biomarkers Prev 11(2):177–185
Silverman LB (2007) Acute lymphoblastic leukemia in infancy. Pediatr Blood Cancer 49(7 Suppl):1070–1073
Smith AD, Kim YI et al (2008) Is folic acid good for everyone? Am J Clin Nutr 87(3):517–533
Spector LG, Xie Y et al (2005) Maternal diet and infant leukemia: the DNA topoisomerase II inhibitor hypothesis: a report from the children's oncology group. Cancer Epidemiol Biomarkers Prev 14(3):651–655
Spector LG, Hecht SS et al (2007a) Detection of cotinine in newborn dried blood spots. Cancer Epidemiol Biomarkers Prev 16(9):1902–1905

Spector LG, Ross JA et al (2007b) Feasibility of nationwide birth registry control selection in the United States. Am J Epidemiol166(7):852–856
Spencer CC, Su Z et al (2009) Designing genome-wide association studies: sample size, power, imputation, and the choice of genotyping chip. PLoS Genet 5(5):e1000477
Stack M, Walsh PM et al (2007) Childhood cancer in Ireland: a population-based study. Arch Dis Child 92(10):890–897
Steele JR, Wellemeyer AS et al (2006) Childhood cancer research network: a North American Pediatric Cancer Registry. Cancer Epidemiol Biomarkers Prev 15(7): 1241–1242
Stiller CA, Boyle PJ (1996) Effect of population mixing and socioeconomic status in England and Wales, 1979–85, on lymphoblastic leukaemia in children. BMJ 313(7068): 1297–1300
Surveillance, Epidemiology, and End Results (SEER) Program (www.seer.cancer.gov) SEER*Stat Database: Incidence – SEER 13 Regs Limited-Use, Nov 2008 Sub (1992–2006) <Single Ages to 85+ Katrina/Rita Population Adjustment> – Linked To County Attributes – Total U.S., 1969–2006 Counties, National Cancer Institute, DCCPS, Surveillance Research Program, Cancer Statistics Branch, released April 2009, based on the November 2008 submission.
Surveillance, Epidemiology, and End Results (SEER) Program (www.seer.cancer.gov) SEER*Stat Database: Incidence – SEER 9 Regs Limited-Use, Nov 2008 Sub (1973–2006) <Single Ages to 85+ Katrina/Rita Population Adjustment> – Linked To County Attributes – Total U.S., 1969–2006 Counties, National Cancer Institute, DCCPS, Surveillance Research Program, Cancer Statistics Branch, released April 2009, based on the November 2008 submission.
Teitell MA, Pandolfi PP (2009) Molecular genetics of acute lymphoblastic leukemia. Annu Rev Pathol 4:175–198
Therrell BL, Johnson A et al (2006) Status of newborn screening programs in the United States. Pediatrics 117(5 Pt 2): S212–S252
Thompson JR, Gerald PF et al (2001) Maternal folate supplementation in pregnancy and protection against acute lymphoblastic leukaemia in childhood: a case-control study. Lancet358(9297):1935–1940
Torres-Sanchez L, Chen J et al (2006) Dietary and genetic determinants of homocysteine levels among Mexican women of reproductive age. Eur J Clin Nutr 60(6):691–697
Trevino LR, Yang W et al (2009) Germline genomic variants associated with childhood acute lymphoblastic leukemia. Nat Genet 41:1001–1005
Urquhart JD, Black RJ et al (1991) Case-control study of leukaemia and non-Hodgkin's lymphoma in children in Caithness near the Dounreay nuclear installation. BMJ 302(6778):687–692
van Duijn CM, van Steensel-Moll HA et al (1994) Risk factors for childhood acute non-lymphocytic leukemia: an association with maternal alcohol consumption during pregnancy? Cancer Epidemiol Biomarkers Prev 3(6):457–460
van Steensel-Moll HA, Valkenburg HA et al (1985) Are maternal fertility problems related to childhood leukaemia? Int J Epidemiol14(4):555–559
Van Vlierberghe P, Pieters R et al (2008) Molecular-genetic insights in paediatric T-cell acute lymphoblastic leukaemia. Br J Haematol 143(2):153–168
Vardiman JW, Thiele J et al (2009) The 2008 revision of the World Health Organization (WHO) classification of myeloid neoplasms and acute leukemia: rationale and important changes. Blood 114(5):937–951
Vineis P, Miligi L et al (2003) Delayed infection, late tonsillectomy or adenoidectomy and adult leukaemia: a case-control study. Br J Cancer 88(1):47–49
Wakefield J (2008) Ecologic studies revisited. Annu Rev Public Health29: 75–90
Wakeford R, Kendall GM et al (2009) The proportion of childhood leukaemia incidence in Great Britain that may be caused by natural background ionizing radiation. Leukemia 23(4):770–776
Wen W, Shu XO et al (2002) Parental medication use and risk of childhood acute lymphoblastic leukemia. Cancer 95(8): 1786–1794
Westerbeek RM, Blair V et al (1998) Seasonal variations in the onset of childhood leukaemia and lymphoma. Br J Cancer 78(1):119–124
Westergaard T, Andersen PK et al (1997) Birth characteristics, sibling patterns, and acute leukemia risk in childhood: a population-based cohort study. J Natl Cancer Inst 89(13): 939–947
Ye Z, Song H (2005) Glutathione s-transferase polymorphisms (GSTM1, GSTP1 and GSTT1) and the risk of acute leukaemia: a systematic review and meta-analysis. Eur J Cancer 41(7):980–989
Yeazel MW, Buckley JD et al (1995) History of maternal fetal loss and increased risk of childhood acute leukemia at an early age. A report from the Childrens Cancer Group. Cancer 75(7):1718–1727
Yip BH, Pawitan Y et al (2006) Parental age and risk of childhood cancers: a population-based cohort study from Sweden. Int J Epidemiol 35(6):1495–1503
Yoshioka M, O'Neill JP et al (2001) Gestational age and gender-specific in utero V(D)J recombinase-mediated deletions. Cancer Res 61(8):3432–3438
Zack M, Adami HO et al (1991) Maternal and perinatal risk factors for childhood leukemia. Cancer Res 51(14):3696–3701
Zintzaras E, Koufakis T et al (2006) A meta-analysis of genotypes and haplotypes of methylenetetrahydrofolate reductase gene polymorphisms in acute lymphoblastic leukemia. Eur J Epidemiol21(7):501–510
Zipursky A, Poon A et al (1992) Leukemia in Down syndrome: a review. Pediatr Hematol Oncol 9(2):139–149

Part II

Biology of Pediatric Leukemia

The Biology of Acute LymphoblasticL eukemia

2

William L. Carroll, Mignon Loh, Andrea Biondi, and Cheryl Willman

Contents

2.1 Introduction

Discoveries of the underlying biological pathways that drive leukemogenesis in children have taken place at an astonishing pace. These findings have resulted in large part because of the evolution of technical developments in analyzing chromosome structure, the development of monoclonal antibodies capable of recognizing discrete cell surface proteins that correlate with cell lineage and differentiation state, recombinant DNA technology, and engineered mouse models (e.g., transgenic and "knock out" models). More recently, advances in high-throughput genomics and progress in stem cell biology have transformed the field of cancer biology in general and perhaps more so in hematological malignancies. A cohesive view of the stepwise process of transformation and the cellular heterogeneity of the leukemic clone is emerging and, importantly, leukemia-specific targets have been identified and novel therapeutic approaches have been directed at these lesions.

W.L.C arroll(✉)
NYU Medical Center Smilow Research Building,
522 1st Avenue, SML 1201,
NewY ork, NY10016 , USA
e-mail:w illiam.carroll@nyumc.org

M.Loh
Clinical Pediatrics, Hematology-Oncology, University of California,Sa nFra ncisco,
e-mail:lohm@ peds.ucsf.edu

A.B iondi
UniversitaM ilano,
OspedaleSa nG eraldo,
Monza

C.W illman
UMN Cancer Research Facility, School of Medicine,
Universityof N ewM exico, MSC08- 4630, USA
e-mail:c willman@salud.unm.edu

G.H. Reaman and F.O. Smith (eds.), *Childhood Leukemia*,
DOI: 10.1007/978-3-642-13781-5_2,

2.2 TheC ellularB iologyo fA cute Lymphoblastic Leukemia (ALL)

2.2.1 *Lymphoid Development and Immunophenotype of Acute Lymphoblastic Leukemia*

2.2.1.1 LymphoidDevel opment

The immune system in mammals includes three main lymphoid cell populations: B-cells, T-cells, and Natural Killer (NK) cells. They arise from progenitors located in central lymphoid organs such as fetal liver, bone marrow, and thymus. Lymphocyte subpopulations can be recognized by the expression of surface and intracellular markers, which can allow the dissection of different lineage-restricted maturation stages and/or functional subtypes. Blood cells, including lymphocytes, originate from a small number of self-renewing hematopoietic stem cells (HSCs) capable of producing all cell types in the blood (Bryder et al. 2006). Amplifications in cell numbers in concert with progressive restrictions in lineage potential lead HSCs to generate terminally differentiated cell progeny.

The understanding of lymphoid differentiation has arisen primarily from studying mouse models. The majority of the multipotent progenitor cells in the mouse bone marrow (BM) do not express high levels of classical lineage markers, but express SCA1 and KIT (Lin–/SCA+/Kit+ (LSK) cells) (Fig. 2.1). A primary event in HSC differentiation is loss of self-renewing potential, while retaining the capacity for multilineage differentiation to give rise to multipotent progenitors (MPPs). Subsequent differentiation processes can be demonstrated by the identification of lympho-myeloid-restricted multipotent progenitors (LMPP), with the capacity to produce granulocytes, macrophages (GM), and all the defined lymphoid cell types such as B-cells, T-cells, and NK-cells (Adolfsson et al. 2005). LMPP can differentiate into early lymphoid progenitors (ELPs) that start to express recombination activating gene 1 (*Rag1*) and *Rag2* and initiate rearrangement at the immunoglobulin heavy chain (*IGH*) locus. ELPs can further differentiate into thymic precursors of the T-cell lineage (early T-cell-lineage progenitors, ETPs) or into bone-marrow common lymphoid progenitors (CLPs), which are lymphoid restricted.

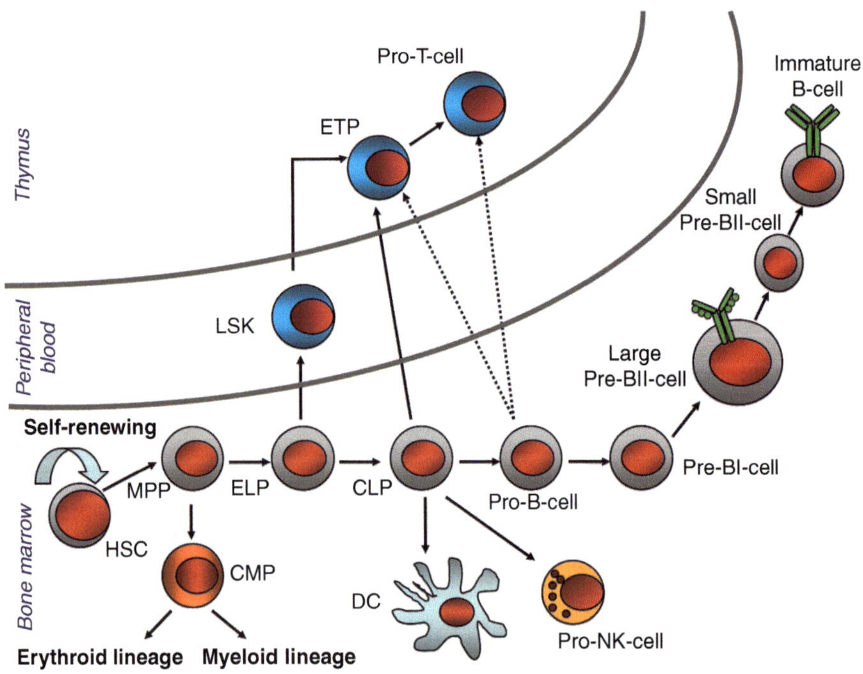

Fig. 2.1 MouseB -cell development from early hematopoietic progenitors. HSC, Hematopoietic stem cell; MPP, Multipotential progenitor; ELP, Early lymphoid progenitor; CMP, Common myeloid progenitor; CLP, Common lymphoid progenitor; DC, Dendritic cell; LSK, Lin-/SCA+/Kit+; ETP, Early T-cell-lineage progenitor; NK, Natural killer. (Modified from Czerny andB usslinger 1995)

2.2.1.2 B-CellDevel opment

Expression of the B-cell marker B220 by a subset of CLPs (known as pro-B cells) coincides with their entry into the B-cell-differentiation pathway. The next step can be identified by expression of CD19 and completion of *IGH* diversity (DH)-to-joining (JH) gene segment rearrangement by pre-BI cells. The *IGH* locus then continues to rearrange its variable (V)-region gene segments until productive VH–DJH alleles are generated in large pre-BII cells. These cells cease to express *Rag1* and *Rag2*, and they display the product of the rearranged *IGH* gene at the cell surface, where it assembles with the surrogate immunoglobulin light chains (IgLs), Vpre-B, and λ5, together with the signaling molecules IgA (which is encoded by the *MB-1* gene) and Igb (which is encoded by the *B29* gene) to form the pre-B-cell receptor (pre-BCR). Expression of the pre-BCR is a crucial check-point in early B-cell development, at which the functionality of the heavy chain is monitored. Signaling through the pre-BCR allows for allelic exclusion of the *IGH* locus and stimulates a burst of proliferative clonal expansion of large pre-BII cells, which is followed by reexpression of RAGs and rearrangement at the *IGL* locus in small pre-BII cells. During normal development, appearance of the assembled BCR at the cell surface defines the immature B-cell stage (Fig. 2.1) (Czerny and Busslinger 1995; Busslinger 2004).

Stages of human B-cell development seem to follow mechanisms similar to mouse, confirming the previous studies (reviewed in Ghia et al. (1998)). Although some differences in surface marker expression as well as differences in growth requirements remain, the strong resemblance of B-cell development in mouse to that in man allows for a comparison of the two systems. For the early multipotent progenitor to proceed in development into a lymphoid-restricted stage, an interplay between several concurrent mechanisms, including external signals, internal transcription factor networks, and epigenetic changes, have to take place (Bryder and Sigvardsson 2010; Ramirez et al. 2010). Differentiation processes of multipotent LSK cells into lymphoid-restricted progenitors is correlated with the expression of FLT3, the receptor for the FLT3 ligand (FL) and IL7R (Ramirez et al. 2010). The transcription factors essential for priming lineage-associated genes and restricting fates to the B-lineage within CLP compartment are Ikaros, Purine box factor 1 (PU.1), and E2A. Ikaros is encoded by Ikaros Family Zinc Finger 1 (*IKZF1*) and contains variable numbers of Kruppel-like zinc fingers in two domains that mediate DNA binding and formation of dimers and multimeric complexes (Yoshida et al. 2006). Following the expression of E2A and EBF1, Ikaros mediates chromatin accessibility necessary for V(D)J recombination, and it also modulates the expression of early B-cell-specific genes, including *IgLL1* (λ5) (Thompson et al. 2007).

2.2.1.3 T-CellDevel opment

Mammalian T-cells originate from pluripotent precursors in the bone marrow or fetal liver that migrate to the thymus, where T-cell differentiation is initiated and sustained. T-cell progenitors migrate into the thymus and then respond to the surrounding environment by proliferating extensively, and initiate the T-cell differentiation transcriptional program, gradually turning off genes that allow differentiation to non-T-cell lineages (Hayday and Pennington 2007). They then undergo T-cell receptor (*TCR*) gene rearrangements and assemble TcR complexes. These cells can mature into different T-cell lineages, including γδ T- and αβ T-cells. The αβ T-cells further diverge into different sublineages, such as CD4+ T-cells, CD8+ T-cells, natural killer T- (NKT) cells, and regulatory T-cells (TReg cells). The T-cell-lineage commitment process consists of a progression of distinct developmental stages, and particular regulatory changes that drive the cells from one stage to the next (Rothenberg et al. 2008) (Fig. 2.2). Clear changes in gene expression and developmental potential mark these transitions. Once they migrate from the thymus to the periphery, each of these cell subsets will have different functions. Genetic evidence, from germline and conditional knockout mouse models, emphasizes the requirements for a stable core group of transcription factors that act repeatedly at successives tages.

One major progenitor source in adult mice consists of LMPPs in the bone marrow or blood, which can give rise to macrophages, dendritic cells (DCs), NK-cells, B-cells, and T-cells, but not erythrocytes or megakaryocytes (Adolfsson et al. 2005; Yoshida et al. 2006). Within the mouse LMPP population, cells with the

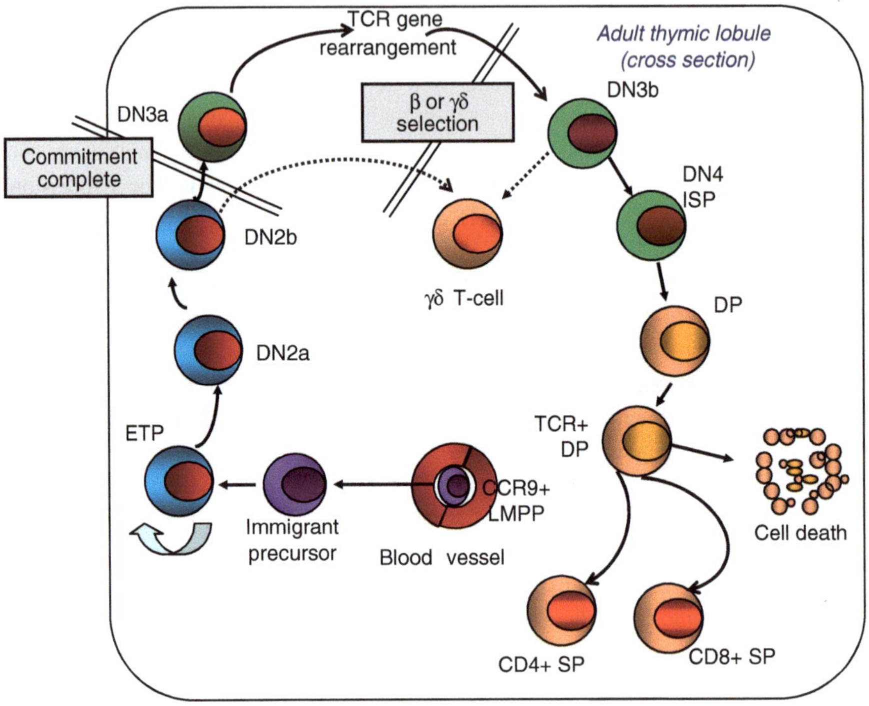

Fig.2.2 Stagesine arly T-cell development. LMPP, lymphoid primed multipotent progenitor; ETP, early T-cell-lineage progenitor; DN2a, double-negative 2a; DN2b, double-negative 2b; DN3a, double-negative 3a; TCR, T-cell receptor; DN3b, double-negative 3b; DN4 ISP, double negative 4 immature single positive; DP, double positive; SP, single positive. (see text). (Modified from Rothemberg VE et al., Nature Reviews Immunology 2008,8:9–21)

capacity to migrate to the thymus are probably distinguished by their expression of the CC-chemokine receptor 9 (CCR9), in addition to the stem- and progenitor-cell markers KIT, stem-cell antigen 1 (SCA1), and the growth-factor-receptor tyrosine kinase FLT3 (Schwarz et al. 2007). Development from the early T-cell-lineage progenitor (ETP) stage to the double-negative 3 (DN3) stage is independent of the TcR and is coordinated with migration through distinct thymic microenvironments. ETPs and DN2 cells proliferate extensively while acquiring their first T-cell characteristics. As the T-cells reach the DN3 stage, they stop proliferating, greatly increase *TCR* gene rearrangement, and generate the first fully rearranged *TCR* loci. DN3 T-cells that succeed in making in-frame *TCR* gene rearrangements become activated by TcR-dependent selection (these are referred to as DN3b cells); this distinguishes them from DN3 cells that are not yet selected (referred to as DN3a cells). Expression of TcRβ qualifies the cells to undergo β selection, turning on expression of CD4 and CD8 to become double positive (DP) cells, and eventually acquiring cell-surface TcRαβ complexes. This prepares them for positive selection and negative selection to generate mature CD4+ or CD8+ TcRαβ+ T-cells. Alternatively, DN3 T-cells that successfully rearrange *TCR* γ- and δ-chains instead of β-chains are selected as γδ T-cells (Rothenberg et al. 2008).

Several transcription factors are involved in expression during the progression of T-cell precursors from the ETP to the later stages, including most of the T-cell factors known to be essential for early T-cell development as well as most factors implicated in cell-lineage plasticity, those implicated in the regulation of *TCR* and other T-cell-lineage gene expression (reviewed in Rothenberge ta l. (2008)).

2.2.1.4 Immunophenotypeo fA cuteL eukemia

Cellular immunophenotype can be defined as the expression of leukocyte antigens (proteins or glycoproteins) either on the cell surface or in the cytoplasm, detectable by applying immunologic methods with the use of monoclonal antibodies. Many monoclonal antibodies available for such purposes have been grouped into Clusters of Differentiation (CD) based on their reactivity with identical antigens (Mason et al. 2002). Precursor cells and their malignant counterparts can be recognized on the basis of morphological and cytochemical characteristics. However, a more accurate characterization of the leukemic clone can be assessed by immunophenotyping (van Dongen et al. 1988). Modern immunophenotyping approaches are based on the use of flow cytometric technique (Carter and Meyer 1994). A typical flow cytometry consists of one or more laser-based light sources that provide monochromatic light beams (generally at 488 nm and at 635 nm). The cells, flowing through the laser beam, refract the light and, if present, fluorochromes are excited and emit fluorescence. Signals obtained by interaction of the cell with the light provide information about the cells including volume (Forward Side Scatter, FSC), nucleo-cytoplasmatic complexity (Orthogonal side light scatter, SSC), and presence of antigens due to their cross-link with fluorochrome-conjugated specific antibodies. By flow cytometry, it is possible to assess many biological features with potential impact on the diagnosis and management of acute leukemia including the detection of minimal residual disease (MRD). Systematic guidelines for immunological classification of acute lymphoblastic leukemias (ALLs) have been proposed by the European Group for the Immunological Characterization of Leukemia (EGIL) (Bene et al. 1995) (Table 2.1). More recently, correlation of immunophenotype with cytogenetic and molecular genetic characteristics has identified new biologically and clinically distinct subgroups of ALL. Details related to the immunological classification of ALL are provided in chapters dedicated to classification and treatment of ALL.

Table 2.1 Immunological classification of acute lymphoblastic leukemia according to EGIL proposal (Bene et al. 1995)

B-lineage ALL (CD19+ and/or CD79a+ and/or CD22+)	
Pro-B-ALL (B-I)	No expression of other differentiation of B-cell antigens
Common ALL (B-II)	CD10+
Pre-B- ALL (B-III)	Cytoplasmicl gM+
Mature B-ALL (B-IV)	Cytoplasmic ors urface kappa or lambda+
*T-lineage ALL (cytoplasmic/membrane*C D3+)	
Pro-T-ALL (T-I)	CD7+
Pre-T-ALL (T-II)	CD2+a nd/orC D5+ and/or CD8+
Cortical-T-ALL (T-III)	CD1a+
Mature T-ALL (T-IV)	Membrane CD3+,C D1a-

2.2.2 Antigen Receptor Genes and Clonality

2.2.2.1 Immunoglobulin(*Ig*) and T-Cell Receptor (*TCR*)G ene Rearrangements in ALL

Somatic rearrangement of *Ig* and *TCR* gene loci occurs during early differentiation of any B- and T-cell, by joining the germline variable (V), diversity (D), and joining (J) gene segments (reviewed in Janeway et al. (2001)). By this process, each lymphocyte gets a specific combination of V-(D-) J segments that encode the variable domains of Ig or TcR molecules. The uniqueness of each rearrangement further depends on random insertion and deletion of nucleotides at the junction sites of V, (D), and J gene segments, making the junctional regions of *Ig* and *TCR* genes "fingerprint-like" sequences for that particular clone. Due to the clonal origin of the neoplasm, each malignant lymphoid disease will represent the expansion of a clonal population with a specific *Ig/TCR* signature.

The frequencies and patterns of *Ig* and *TCR* gene rearrangements in ALL can be analyzed by Southern blot- and PCR-based methods (reviewed in Szczepanski et al. (2001)). Currently, PCR-based methodologies are more easily and frequently applied to the detection of clonal *Ig* and *TCR* gene rearrangements. Virtually all B-lineage ALL patients have rearranged Immunoglobulin heavy chain (*IGH*) genes (van Dongen and Wolvers-Tettero 1991). In addition, rearrangements of the Ig Kappa deleting element (*Kde*) occur at a relatively high frequency (approximately 60%) (Beishuizen et al. 1997). Cross-lineage incomplete TcR Delta (*TCRD*) rearrangements occur in more than 40% of all patients (40% Vd2-Dd3, 19% Dd2-Dd3, and 13% showed both) (van der Velden et al. 2003). Complete *TCRD* rearrangements (Vd-Jd) are very rare in B-lineage ALL. Detection of TcR Gamma (*TCRG*) rearrangements occurs in more than 50% of the B-lineage ALL patients (van der Velden et al. 2003). Cross-lineage TcR Beta (*TCRB*) recombination occurs in a small percentage (15–20%) of B-lineage ALL patients.

Most T-ALL patients have rearranged *TCRB*, *TCRG* and/or *TCRD* genes (van Dongen and Wolvers-Tettero 1991). Frequency analysis of the patterns of recombination in T-ALL patients showed that *TCRG* rearrangements represent the most frequent ones (identifiable in

84% of patients), followed by complete and incomplete *TCRD* joinings. In practice, *TCRG* and/or *TCRD* gene rearrangements occur in >95% of childhood T-ALL patients (Pongers-Willemse et al. 1999; van der Velden et al. 2003). Incomplete *IGH* rearrangements (DH-JH) could be identified in 12% of T-ALL cases, consistent with the finding that cross-lineage *Ig* gene rearrangements occurred at relatively low frequency in T-ALL (10–20%) and are virtually restricted to incomplete *IGH* rearrangements (Pongers-Willemse et al. 1999).

2.2.2.2 Assessmento fC lonality by PCR Amplification

The assessment of clonality by *Ig* and *TCR* gene relies on the PCR amplification of the different target gene recombinations. Primers and protocols have been standardized (van der Velden and van Dongen 2009). After PCR identification of *Ig/TCR* targets, the clonal origin of PCR products must be assessed by heteroduplex analysis or by gene scanning, to confirm their origin from the malignant cells and not from contaminating normal cells with similar *Ig* or *TCR* gene rearrangements. The homo-heteroduplex analysis takes advantage of the different migration properties in polyacrylamide gel of V-(D-) J rearrangements containing a few mismatches (heteroduplex) compared with fully matched V-(D-) J junctions (homoduplex). Fingerprint analysis consists of PCR amplification with a fluorescent primer and an electrophoretic run in polyacrylamide gels, where clonal amplification results in a single peak within a background of polyclonal, constitutional amplification products. After the clonal rearrangements are recognized, several methods can be applied to specifically detect the leukemia-derived PCR products, for example, during the follow-up of patients who have undergone therapy. The major variable lies in the sensitivity of the test, which can significantly interfere with interpretation of the assay results.

2.2.2.3 Useo f *Ig* and *TCR* Gene Rearrangements for the Detection of MRD

Sequential monitoring of MRD with specific and sensitive methods (capable of recognizing one leukemic cell among 10^{-4} or more normal BM cells, at least 100-fold more sensitive than morphologic examination), recently compelled the redefinition of complete remission in patients with ALL, and further improved the clinical utility of risk assessment. Several techniques have been developed over the past 10 to 15 years to complement morphology in assessing response to treatment, including immunologic and molecular methods, fluorescent in situ hybridization (FISH), *in vitro* drug response, and colony assays (reviewed in Szczepanski et al. (2001)). *Ig* and *TCR* genes are the most widely applicable genes and therefore can be considered a *universal* target for MRD detection in childhood ALL (Cazzaniga and Biondi 2005; van der Velden and van Dongen 2009). Its feasibility has been proved in a multicenter ALL trial (Flohr et al. 2008).

In the most sensitive assay so far available, clonal PCR products from homo-heteroduplex analysis are directly sequenced. V, D, and J gene segments are then identified, and randomly inserted nucleotides are recognized by comparison with germline sequences in databases (http://imgt.cines.fr; http://www.ncbi.nlm.nih.gov/igblast). The sequence information allows the design of junctional region-specific oligonucleotides, which can be used to detect malignant cells among normal lymphoid cells during follow-up of patients in two different ways. One uses the oligonucleotides as patient-specific junctional region probes in *semi-quantitative hybridization experiments* ("dot blot") to detect PCR products derived from the malignant cells. Alternatively, the junctional region-specific oligonucleotide can be used as a primer to *quantitatively amplify* the rearrangements of the malignant clone.

The applicability of the allele-specific oligonucleotide (ASO) primer approach depends on its sensitivity and specificity. The specificity of detection is checked for each probe on at least three different polyclonal samples. The sensitivity of each probe is assessed by testing serial dilutions of the patient's blasts in a mixture of polyclonal marrow mononuclear cells. In this way, PCR-based MRD detection via clone-specific junctional regions generally reaches a sensitivity of 10^{-4} to 10^{-5}. A less-sensitive assay consists of a modified *fingerprint analysis*, in which the patient- and clone-specific peak corresponding to PCR amplification from residual leukemic cells can be discriminated from normal background. Polyclonal background levels vary, but usually limit the sensitivity of this approach to the detection of one leukemic cell among 10^{-2} to 10^{-3} normal cells.

IGH rearrangements represented the most sensitive group of targets and usually reached sensitivities $\leq 10^{-4}$. However, despite excellent RT-PCR sensitivities, *IGH* gene loci are prone to oligoclonality in 30–40% of B-lineage ALL (for example, multiple rearrangements (subclones) within the same clone) owing to continuing and secondary rearrangement processes (Szczepanski et al. 2001). Therefore, the use of oligoclonal *Ig/TCR* targets in MRD PCR analysis can lead to an underestimation of the leukemic tumor load, because they might occur in a subclone of low frequency, hence leading to potentially false-negative results. In consequence, *IGH* targets should routinely be used in combination with *IGK-Kde* rearrangements (especially *Vk-Kde*), since these targets represent highly stable 'end-point rearrangements' suitable for sensitive MRD detection. Using incomplete *TCRD* rearrangements as a third priority further increases the number of applicable MRD targets as Vd2-Dd3 and Dd2-Dd3 recombinations show little clonal instability and also comprise a group of markers with sensitivity comparable to DH-JH rearrangements. In contrast, *TCRG* rearrangements in precursor B-lineage ALL have proven to be less applicable in MRD detection since their sensitivity is more frequently limited ($>10^{-4}$) due to small junctional regions and nonspecific amplification of *TCR* gene rearrangements in normal T-lymphocytes. Taking the published results on target availability and sensitivity into account, the following priority order using antigen receptor gene rearrangements for MRD PCR targets in B-lineage ALL can be deduced: *IGH* > *IGK* (Vk-Kde) > *TCRD* > *TCRG* and *IGK* (intron-Kde).

The success rate of detecting appropriate MRD-PCR targets is lower in T-ALL compared to precursor B-lineage cell ALL. The addition of *TCRB* gene rearrangements to MRD-PCR target identification increases the availability of targets in T-ALL. Moreover, the junctional regions of (complete) *TCRD* rearrangements, similar to *IGH* in B-lineage ALL, frequently include extensive N-nucleotide insertions, thus enabling the design of highly specific ASO primers. In contrast, the junctions of *TCRG* and incomplete *IGH* rearrangements are commonly smaller resulting in a significantly lower ratio of sensitive targets (about 75%). Taking results on target sensitivity in T-ALL together, the following conclusion on the preferential use of MRD PCR targets can be drawn: *TCRD/TCRB* > *IGH* (DH-JH) > *TCRG*.

2.2.3 Leukemia-Initiating Cells in ALL

Recent evidence supports the hypothesis that specific subsets of tumor cells retain features similar to stem cells and are capable of propagating clonal cancer cells. The presence of leukemia-initiating cells has important biologic and therapeutic implications. While there is generally broad acceptance about the identification of such a cell population in myeloid malignancies, which was first elegantly demonstrated by Dick and colleagues (Lapidot et al. 1994), the identification of a uniform lymphoblastic leukemia-initiating cell has been much more evasive. Indeed, it is also well recognized that murine xenograft modeling systems and different experimental methodologies can yield disparate results with respect to the engraftment of leukemia and the minimum number of cells required to propagate disease. These findings have undoubtedly made the field of ALL stem cell biology even more challenging.

While subtle differences in definitions have led to some confusion, for the purposes of this discussion, a cancer stem cell is a tumor-initiating cell. The definition of a cancer stem cell needs to be distinguished from a normal stem cell; while both share critical features of self-renewal and differentiation, it is important to realize that a tumor-initiating cell may in fact reflect a reprogrammed progenitor cell that acquires stem cell-like features (Krivtsov et al. 2006). There is general agreement, however, that one essential experimental property of any unique subpopulation of cancer initiating cells is its ability to produce leukemia in an immunocompromised mouse (Clarke et al. 2006). Recent advances in the identification of primitive stem cell markers have facilitated sorting methods to achieve very pure populations of normal stem cells, but it is not clear that cancer-initiating stem cells uniformly display only one set of these markers, and this is true for investigations of cancer stem cells in ALL.

In addition, the type and age of immunocompromised mouse, the level of radiation, and the mode of delivering the purified cancer initiating cells appear to greatly affect experimental results. In the earliest studies, Lapidot used intravenous injection of acute myeloid leukemia (AML) cells into severe combined immunodeficient (SCID) mice and determined that the cells required to confer leukemia were contained within the CD34+/CD38− cell fraction (Lapidot et al. 1994). Limiting dilution analysis in this system demonstrated that 1/250,000 cells were required. Since this seminal work was published, additional mouse models with progressive degrees of immunodeficiency have become available for study. Some of the more recent of these, the NK cell-depleted Non-Obese Diabetic/SCID (NOD/SCID) and the NOD/SCID gamma (NSG) mice have been recently used by le Viseur and colleagues to model ALL (le Viseur et al. 2008). Interestingly, these progressively more immunocompromised mouse models result in fewer and fewer cancer-initiating cell requirements. Intrafemoral injection has also been used by a number of investigators to maximize the "homing" of cancer initiating cells and limit the number of cells that get trapped in pulmonary capillaries, a potential requirement for engraftment of myeloid diseases, but ALL cells do not seem to absolutely require this additional step.

Identifying a single cancer initiating cell population for ALL has been elusive, not only in part due to the various strains of mice employed and the methodologies to engraft them, but also likely due to the genetic heterogeneity of human ALL. Recent genomic studies have firmly established that ALL is a disease requiring multiple genetic hits for full transformation (Mullighan et al. 2007a). Greaves and colleagues have further shown in elegant FISH studies that there is not always a linear hierarchy to acquiring these multiple mutations, but that, in fact, there is considerable complexity to the acquisition of these lesions that more resembles "a branching pattern," akin to Darwin's theories of evolution (Greaves 2009). In this manner, one can appreciate how difficult it would be to a priori identify a single population of leukemia-initiating cells for all subtypes of ALL.

Earlier data supported the ability of CD34+/CD38− or CD34+/CD19− human leukemia cells to engraft NOD-SCID mice (Cobaleda et al. 2000), while other studies have demonstrated the engraftment capability of several different lineages, including CD19+ cells. Indeed, it has been shown by several groups that *TEL/AML1 (ETV6/RunX1)*-positive leukemia cells able to confer disease are restricted to the CD34+/CD19+ population (Hotfilder et al. 2002; Castor et al. 2005; Hong et al. 2008) and are conspicuously absent from the CD19− fraction. Hong and colleagues were able to study a set of monochorionic twins, one of whom was diagnosed at the age of 2 years with *ETV6/RUNX1*-positive ALL, while the other remained healthy at the time of their report (Hong et al. 2008). A population of $CD34^{+}CD38^{-/low}CD19^{+}$ cells that was detected in the patient's bone marrow was also detected at extremely low levels in the healthy twin (0.002%) and harbored the identical fusion gene. However, further analysis of these cells revealed that a DJ recombination event had occurred in the healthy twin while a VDJ and DJ recombination event had occurred in the affected twin, suggesting that there was further clonal evolution from the same basic cell population shared by both siblings. Engineering healthy human cord blood to express *ETV6/RUNX1* alone resulted in a population of $CD34^{+}CD38^{-/low}CD19^{+}$ cells with significant self-renewal and differential potential, but did not confer acute leukemia, supporting that these cells exhibited at least some of the hallmark features of stem cells, but that additional events are required for full transformation. Indeed, the vast majority of children with *TEL/AML*-positive leukemia frequently display additional events at diagnosis, including loss of the normal *TEL* allele.

More recently, le Viseur and colleagues have reported that lymphoblasts displaying a wide spectrum of differentiation markers were able to engraft primary as well as successive immunocompromised recipients, using an intrafemoral injection strategy in NOD/SCID mice (le Viseur et al. 2008). One fascinating observation was that leukemia cells from patients with high-risk disease were more likely to yield multiple fractions (CD34+CD19−, CD34+CD19+, and CD34−CD19−) with stem cell potential and that only CD19+ cells from standard-risk patients were able to confer disease. While high-density single nucleotide polymorphism data was not available for sorted cell fractions, based on Greaves recent work showing the genetic heterogeneity within ALL cells by FISH analysis (Greaves 2009), one could hypothesize that these populations of high-risk leukemia cells might very well harbor a more complete compendium of genetic lesions required for full transformation as opposed to standard-risk leukemia cells.

In summary, recent data have yielded heterogeneous results about the identification of a unique leukemia-initiating cell population in B-lineage ALL, consistent with some variation in the phenotype within particular biological subtypes of ALL.

2.3 TheMo lecularB iologyo fA LL

2.3.1 Introduction to Cancer Genomics and New Technology

The development of new tools for high throughput evaluation of human genomes and detailed direct sequencing has ushered in a new field of personalized medicine.

This approach integrates clinical, genetic, and environmental information for treatment decisions on individual patients. "Genomic Medicine," defined as the use of information from the genome or its derivatives (mRNA, micro-RNA, protein, and metabolites), is already impacting the way childhood ALL is classified and treated.

The sequencing of the human genome was completed in 2003, 50 years after the landmark discovery by Drs. Watson and Crick of the structural basis of DNA. The human genome contains some 3.2 billion base pairs and it is estimated that only 2% of the genome encodes the 20,000 to 25,000 genes. The non-protein coding portion of the human genome contains regulatory sequences including regions that generate small noncoding RNAs that regulate transcription and translation of protein-coding elements. While the base sequence of individuals from different racial and ethnic backgrounds is 99.9% identical to one another, more subtle genomic variation exists between individuals with the most frequent difference being single nucleotide polymorphisms (SNPs). By definition, a SNP means that the frequency of the minor allele exceeds 1% in at least one population. In addition, many insertions and deletions occur and all such changes may lead to a change in protein structure, thereby influencing function and/or changes in regulatory regions that impact on expression.

The ability to analyze chromosome structure with new standard karyotyping techniques led to a molecular classification that correlated with outcome. However, karyotyping is limited by the need for fresh tumor, overgrowth of cultures by nonneoplastic cells, and generally low resolution. Many of these difficulties are overcome by FISH, which relies on the use of DNA probes that are hybridized to cells. While this technique requires preselection of possible lesions, it has refined the mapping of chromosome structure and led to the identification of new lesions such as the prognostically important *ETV6-RUNX1* (*TEL-AML1*), seen in 20% of B-precursor ALL that is not detected using standard karyotyping. Many subtypes of childhood ALL are characterized by sentinel translocations such as t(9;22)(q34;q11) that results in the chimeric *BCR-ABL1* fusion or the t(12;21)(p13;q21) *ETV6-RUNX1*. The well-defined structural elements of these fusions lend themselves to detection using PCR-based methods. The added value of these approaches is the greater sensitivity (1×10^5–10^6) compared to FISH (1 in 100) and the fact that they can be quantitative.

In recent years, high throughput hybridization array-based methods that are capable of detecting global mRNA and miRNA levels as well as DNA copy number changes (e.g., deletions and amplifications) have surfaced. In addition, the "SNP" arrays can survey the genome for the inheritance of SNPs that can also be used to discover predisposition loci (so-called genome-wide association studies (GWAS)).

2.3.2 Host Susceptibility to ALL

2.3.2.1 GeneticSyndr omesandDo wn Syndrome ALL

A number of genetic syndromes are linked to an increased incidence of leukemia. Many chromosomal breakage syndromes such as ataxia telangiectasia, Bloom syndrome, Fanconi anemia, and Shwachman syndrome are well known to be associated with ALL, but Down syndrome (DS) accounts for the overwhelming majority of ALL cases linked to a genetic condition (Malinge et al. 2009). The incidence of ALL and acute megakaryocytic leukemia in patients with DS is 20-fold and 500-fold, respectively, greater than the general population (Lange 2000). In fact, 97% of all cases of cancer in patients with DS are leukemia. What accounts for this predisposition is unknown, but the fact that trisomy 21 is a common acquired abnormality in ALL seems to indicate that a gene(s) on chromosome 21 influences hematopoiesis and predisposition to malignant transformation. Experiments using fetal liver cells show an increased number of erythroid, megakaryocytic, and other hematopoietic progenitors in culture. Analysis of children with partial trisomy 21 has led to definition of a "Down Syndrome Critical Region" that includes attractive candidates including *RUNX1*, *ERG*, and *ETS2*(K orenberge ta l. 1994).

The biological features of ALL in DS are unique from those that occur in non DS children. While children with DS who develop ALL do so at an age similar to other children with ALL, there are fewer cases of T-ALL, and among B-cell precursor cases (BCP), there are far fewer hyperdiploid (HD) and *ETV6-RUNX1* cases. In fact, the absence of HD and *ETV6-RUNX1* low-risk genotypes explains the relatively poor prognosis of ALL in DS (Whitlock et al. 2005).

A critical question is whether ALL in DS represents a unique biological subtype. Indeed, approximately 20%

of DS ALL samples harbor mutations in *JAK2* compared to 10% of very high risk non-DS ALL cases (Malinge et al. 2007). However, global gene expression profiling and copy number analysis using an unsupervised approach where samples are compared based on global genetic analysis indicates that ALL in DS is a very heterogeneous disease (Rabin et al. 2009). While molecular subtypes such as *BCR-ABL1* and *MLL* rearranged ALL cluster in relatively discrete subgroups indicating modulation of shared biological pathways, no such clustering is observed for ALL in DS. However, a more detailed supervised analysis to discovering unique changes shared by DS samples that are distinct from non-DS ALL reveals that approximately two-thirds of cases show increased expression of the cytokine receptor, cytokine receptor-like factor 2 (CRLF2) (Rabin et al. 2009). Deregulated expression of *CRLF2* seen in 5% of ALL can be caused by translocations into the *IGH* locus (Hertzberg et al. 2010). More commonly in ALL in DS, an interstitial deletion involving the pseudoautosomal region 1 of Xp22.3/Yp11.3 creates a fusion between the first noncoding exon of *P2RY8* with the coding region of *CRLF2* (Mullighan et al. 2009a). While *P2RY8-CRLF2* fusions are seen in 7% of patients with ALL, these lesions are observed in 53% of samples from patients with ALL in DS. CRLF2 is known to dimerize with IL7RA to form a receptor for thymic stromal lymphopoietin (TSLP) and this pathway has an important role in T-cell and dendritic cell development as well as B-cell proliferation. There is a strong association between activating *JAK2* mutations and the *P2RY8-CRLF2* fusion. In preclinical models, the two cooperate in transformation, while each alone fails to induce cytokine independence in Ba/F3 mouse B-progenitor cells. Since most cases of ALL with *CRLF2* overexpression lack *JAK2* mutations, it is suspected that other mutations in the JAK-STAT pathway exist. These findings are discussed in more detail below.

2.3.2.2 Germline Genetic Variation and ALL

The causes of most cases of ALL remain elusive and while a number of environmental exposures including infections have been proposed to be associated with ALL, many have not been substantiated in follow-up studies (Belson et al. 2007). Certain individuals may be predisposed to the multistep process of leukemogenesis based on differences in germline genetic variation possibly triggered by environmental exposures. The premise is that genetic variation in genes that affect the metabolism of environmental triggers, thereby heightening exposure and/or the response to infectious challenges, might prime lymphoid cells to second step molecular lesions (Greaves 2006). Indeed, studies in candidate genes like DNA mismatch repair, glutathione-S-transferase, cytochrome P450, and HLA genes have supported this hypothesis (Krajinovic et al. 2002a, b; Chen et al. 1997).

As mentioned, the sequencing of the human genome has identified individual variation such as SNPs and this variation can be used to determine the location of genes whose variation might be linked to the development of cancer (Dutt and Beroukhim 2007). These studies broadly compare variation between cancer and control populations in normal cells of the host (e.g., germline non cancer cells) and are called genome-wide association studies (GWAS). Two groups have now reported germline genetic variants that are associated with the risk of ALL. In one study, 10 SNPs representing three loci on 7p12.2, 10q21.2, and 14q11.2 were associated with the risk of ALL, while in the second study, 18 SNPS annotated to 12 unique genes were detected (Papaemmanuil et al. 2009; Trevino et al. 2009). In both studies, polymorphisms associated with *ARID5B*, a member of the AT-rich interaction domain of transcription factors, were linked to childhood ALL. This association was highly significant for B-cell hyperdiploid ALL. While the mechanism of the risk induced by SNPs located in *ARID5B* is unknown, homozygous knockout mice of *ARID5B* display disrupted B-cell development, indicating a role in differentiation of the B-cell lineage. A strong association with SNPs in *IKZF1* encoding the IKAROS transcription factor that plays a key role in B-cell differentiation was also observed. This finding is provocative since *IKZF1* deletions are observed in B-cell ALL and are associated with a poor prognosis (Papaemmanuil et al. 2009). It is noteworthy then that the risk alleles indentified are associated with decreased expression, thereby suggesting that the germline risk might be associated with less efficient B-cell differentiation.

2.3.3 Somatic Genetic Changes in ALL

2.3.3.1 Chromosomal Lesions and Karyotype

Successful treatment of ALL in the current era incorporates measures of modern risk classification that allow clinicians to allocate patients to specific therapies. Intensity of therapy has led to improvements in outcome; yet, it comes with added toxicity, so risk-based therapy optimally improves outcome and minimizes toxicity. One key determinant for allocating appropriate therapy includes the identification of specific somatic genetic risk factors that have been studied in cohorts of patients for prognostic significance and biological relevance. Indeed, the detection of somatic genetic events in human cancer remains a keen area of research as technologies have evolved to rapidly sequence the human genome with finer resolution.

The first insights into cancer genetics emerged with the ability to perform cytogenetic analysis on cultured bone marrow and peripheral blood (Tjio and Whang 1962), with subsequent mapping of chromosomes based on successful techniques to detect unique banding patterns. In 1960, Nowell and Hungerford first identified the Ph+ chromosome in human leukemias, characterized by a translocation between chromosome 9 and 22 detected by metaphase karyotype (Nowell and Hungerford 1960). Further molecular analysis in the 1970s revealed that the product of this balanced translocation was the *BCR/ABL* fusion gene, present in most cases of chronic myeloid leukemia, and in approximately 2–3% of childhood ALL. This seminal observation of cancer arising from a single clonal event is the subject of intense scrutiny today, and the complexity and heterogeneity of these somatic events across human disease is now astonishing.

Further refinement of karyotypic analysis has continued to evolve, and FISH allows clinicians to more accurately identify relatively large regions of gain, loss, disruption, and translocation, depending on the specific fluorescently labeled DNA probes utilized. Indeed, both traditional karyotype and FISH analysis are still able to more accurately identify translocations that are not detected by newer approaches such as high density SNP arrays. However, one complementary benefit to the copy number gain or loss information provided by SNP arrays is the identification of regions of copy neutral loss-of-heterozygosity, or acquired isodisomy, an increasingly frequent event detected in human cancer (Dutt and Beroukhim 2007). The spectrum of somatic abnormalities that can be detected using karyotypic or FISH analysis of ALL alone is powerful, but then, also somewhat limited in this era of high throughput genomic technologies. However, a discussion about ALL risk classification cannot proceed without a basic review of the most common and powerful cytogenetic predictors of outcome.

There are two main types of chromosomal lesions that can be detected using conventional karyotype: chromosomal number and structural abnormalities. Numerical abnormalities resulting in ploidy changes can be associated with dramatically different clinical outcomes. For instance, high hyperdiploidy (51–65 chromosomes) is generally associated with a favorable outcome in childhood ALL, especially when accompanied by trisomies of chromosomes 4, 10, and 17, while hypodiploidy (<44 chromosomes) is associated with inferior outcomes (Trueworthy et al. 1992; Heerema et al. 2000; Harrison et al. 2004; Nachman et al. 2007). Indeed, some of the most dismal outcomes with modern therapy occur amongst patients whose leukemia cells approach near haploidy (23–29 chromosomes) (Harrisone ta l. 2004).

Some of the most common structural abnormalities, such as balanced or unbalanced translocations, that carry variable prognostic significance in childhood ALL can be readily detected by metaphase analysis or FISH, including the t(4;11) (*MLL/AF4*), the t(12;21) (*TEL/AML1 or ETV6/RunX1*), the t(1;19) (*E2A/PBX1*), and the aforementioned t(9;22) (*BCR/ABL*) fusion genes. These alterations differ in incidence between children and adults with ALL. A brief discussion of each of the most significant translocations will ensue.

The t(4;11) or *MLL/AF4* translocation is most frequently found in infants with B-lineage ALL. Up to 93% of infants under the age of 90 days harbor *MLL* rearrangements (48% t(4;11), 32% (11;19), and 4% t(1;11)), and most of these children will die with currently available therapy (van der Linden et al. 2009). Beyond 90 days, the prognosis of infants with *MLL* rearrangements (alternative partners are myriad, but commonly include AF9 or ENL) is not as dismal, but event-free survival (EFS) remains at approximately 50% (Silverman et al. 1997; Pui et al. 2002; Silverman 2007; van der Linden et al. 2009). In older children with *MLL* rearrangements, early response to therapy seems to be an essential component to determine outcome, with patients exhibiting EFS ranging from 33 ± 16% (poor response to prednisone) to 80 ± 18% (favorable response to prednisone) (Pui et al. 2003).

Some controversy exists over the treatment of patients with high-risk *MLL* rearrangements; in infants, collective data does not support the automatic use of hematopoietic stem cell transplant (HSCT) for these children in first complete remission (CR1); and recent strategies in the Children's Oncology Group (COG) support this approach (Pui et al. 2003). However, novel approaches to therapy, including FLT3 inhibition, are being tested in these children based on data to suggest that overexpression (but not mutation) of *FLT3* is common in these children (Armstrong et al. 2001). Future analysis will determine if such targeted agents will be valuable in this disease.

The t(12;21) or *TEL/AML1 (ETV6/RUNX1)* fusion gene was initially identified using FISH strategies (Romana et al. 1995); it is a cryptic translocation that is not readily detectable by conventional karyotype. It is the most common translocation in childhood ALL, detected in up to 28% of B-lineage ALL patients (reviewed in Loh and Rubnitz (2002)). In multiple studies, it has been identified to confer a favorable prognosis, independent of presenting white blood cell count, age, or sex. It is most frequently found in younger children and is known to occur as a prenatal event in utero, leading to the hypothesis that it represents an initial somatic event, required but not sufficient for full leukemic transformation (Ford et al. 1998). Up to 1% of newborns harbor this fusion gene, but only a fraction of these children will subsequently develop ALL, supporting this hypothesis (Mori et al. 2002). At diagnosis, deletion of the wildtype TEL allele is found in approximately 80% of children with *TEL/AML1*-positive ALL, also supporting the idea that additional genetic "hits" are required (Romana et al. 1995). Experimentally, multiple established investigators have had difficulty modeling *TEL/AML1*-positive leukemia in transgenic mice. Taken together, this supports the multistep pathogenesis required for full transformation to leukemia.

The t(1;19) translocation results from a translocation of the *E2A* gene on chromosome 1 with the *PBX1* gene on chromosome 19. There are both balanced and unbalanced translocations, and the early data indicated that only the balanced translocation conferred an independent poor prognosis. However, this is a key example of the important component of therapy as a prognostic variable. Because of improvements in outcome related to the intensification of systemic chemotherapy over the years, most investigators no longer consider the t(1;19) as a higher risk leukemia. Indeed, through successive clinical trials, the St. Jude Children's Research Hospital studies have moved the t(1;19)-positive patients into a group with some of the best outcomes (Raimondi et al. 1990).

The t(9;22) or *BCR/ABL* translocation is also a very recent modern success story with the advent of tyrosine kinase inhibitor (TKI) therapy. Prior to the introduction of imatinib, cure rates for children with Ph+ ALL were 35% in the absence of HSCT (Arico et al. 2000; Schultz et al. 2007). The COG recently completed a clinical trial that combined TKI therapy with intensive chemotherapy (AALL0031) and reported EFS in patients continuously treated with imatinib and chemotherapy is 80% at a median follow-up time of 3 years (Schultz et al. 2009). Newer trials will test the contribution of dasatinib, a second generation of TKI, in combination with chemotherapy.

Additional, less common lesions with either prognostic significance or biological relevance that can be detected with karyotype or by FISH include deletion of 7p/monosomy 7, iamp21, or *CRLF2* translocations/deletions. The presence of monosomy 7 is frequently associated with a dismal prognosis in myeloid malignancies. Thus, Heerema and colleagues identified 75 children among 1880 (4%) who were treated on legacy Children's Cancer Group (CCG) clinical trials with a loss in chromosome 7, defined as either monosomy 7, del 7p, or del 7q (Heerema et al. 2004). Both monosomy 7 and del 7p were independently associated with a poorer EFS when adjusted for the presence of the Ph+ chromosome, National Cancer Institute (NCI) risk status, and ploidy. However, overall survival (OS) was not significant for monosomy 7 when Ph+ status was taken into account.

In children treated on Medical Research Council (MRC) UKALL trials, the presence of iAMP21 was significantly associated with a poorer EFS and OS at 5 years (Moorman et al. 2007). However, additional analyses published by the Berlin-Franfurt-Münster group (BFM) indicated that response to Induction therapy measured by minimal residual disease assays might allow further stratification of those patients with iAMP21 who require more intensive therapy (Attarbaschi et al. 2008). Indeed, in their series, only those patients with intermediate or high-risk MRD levels at the end of Induction experienced a relapse event (n=8), while those with low levels did not ($n = 9$) ($p = 0.02$).

2.3.3.2 CopyN umberA bnormalities

Over the past 3 years, using comprehensive genomic platforms and technologies such as gene expression profiling, genome-wide assessment of copy number variations in normal and leukemic DNA, targeted DNA resequencing of potential candidate genes, and the use of next generation sequencing methods that either sequence transcriptomes or whole genomes, many new genetic abnormalities have been discovered in pediatric ALL. Through these studies, a more comprehensive picture of the full spectrum and the unexpected and striking complexity of the cooperating somatic genetic lesions that promote lymphoid leukemogenesis has begun to emerge. New discoveries have emerged in particular through the work of several research teams around the world who have applied genomic approaches to the study of children with "high-risk" ALL, a clinical risk category largely defined by pretreatment clinical characteristics (age >10 years and presenting WBC count >50,000/μL) and the absence of genetic abnormalities associated with "low-risk" (hyperdiploidy, t(12;21)(*ETV6-RUNX1*)) or "very high-risk" (hypodiploidy, t(9;22)(*BCR-ABL1*)) disease. Over 25% of children diagnosed with ALL are initially classified as "high-risk," a risk category in which outcomes remain poor with high rates of relapse and relapse-free survivals (RFSs) of only 45–60%. As the underlying genetic features and recurring genetic mutations associated with this form of ALL had not been previously identified or characterized, this risk category was particularly ripe for discovery. As discussed herein, comprehensive molecular technologies focused on high-risk ALL have identified new genes and genetic differences that impact treatment response and molecular classifiers that are being rapidly translated to the clinical setting for improved risk classification. Therapeutic agents targeted to new genetic mutations are beginning to be tested in early phase clinical trials.

A landmark study published in 2007 (Mullighan et al. 2007c) first reported on the spectrum of genome-wide genetic abnormalities in pediatric ALL, focusing on DNA copy number variations and targeted sequencing of candidate genes in regions of copy number variation. Using relatively high resolution (500K) SNP arrays to detect copy number variations, these investigators studied a selected series of 242 pediatric ALL cases from St. Jude that represented a spectrum of B-precursor and T-cell ALL. They discovered that over 40% of pediatric B-precursor ALL cases had copy number variations (primarily deletions, but also regions of amplification), structural rearrangements, and point mutations in genes that primarily serve as transcriptional regulators of the B-cell development pathway. Strikingly, many of these copy number variations, deletions, and mutations occurred in concert with the established, frequently recurring cytogenetic abnormalities long known to be associated with ALL, such as t(12;21) (*ETV6-RUNX1*), t(1;19)(*TCF3-PBX1*), t(9;22)(*BCR-ABL1*), or translocations involving 11q23(*MLL*), highlighting the previously unappreciated genetic complexity of pediatric ALL (Table 2.2). *CDNK2* and *PAX5* deletions or mutations were the most frequent genetic abnormalities seen in the St. Jude ALL cohort, each occurring in approximately 32% of all cases studied. However the frequency of these mutations varied in specific cytogenetic subgroups. While PAX5 mutations were detected in 100% of ALL cases with hypodiploidy, only 50% of ALL cases with t(1;19)(*TCF3-PBX1*) or t(9;22)(*BCR-ABL1*), and only 33% of ALL cases with t(12;21)(*ETV6-RUNX1*) had *PAX5* mutations. These studies suggest that *PAX5* mutations, which result in reduced levels of the PAX5 protein or hypomorphic alleles, are an important secondary or cooperating mutation in the development of pediatric ALL. *PAX5* mutations were seen more rarely in ALL cases with 11q23 (*MLL*) abnormalities (18%), in hyperdiploid ALL (11%), and in T-cell ALL (10%) (Table 2.2) (Mullighan et al. 2007c).

Table 2.2 DNA copy number abnormalities detected in B-precursor ALL cases in a cohort from St. Jude Children's Research Hospital and the Children's Oncology Group 9906 Trial

Gene/copy number abnormality (deletion)	COG9906 B-ALL case cohort (*N* = 221) *N*(%)	St.J ude B-ALL case cohort (*N* = 232) *N*(%)	*P*(Fisher exact)
CDKN2A	101 (45.7)	77 (33.2)	0.007
PAX5	70(31.7)	72(31.0)	NS
IKZF1	55(24.9)	40(17.2)	0.05
ETV6	28(12.7)	52(22.4)	0.007
RB1	25(11.3)	14(6.0)	0.06
BTG1	23(10.4)	17(7.3)	NS
13q14.2 (miRNA)	21 (9.5)	16 (6.9)	NS
C20orf94	19(8.6)	18(7.8)	NS
EBF	18(8.1)	11(4.7)	NS
IL3RA	15(6.8)	15(6.5)	NS
DMD	15 (6.8)	9 (3.9)	NS
FHIT	2 (0.9)	12 (5.2)	0.012
B-Development Pathway Lesions	111(50.2)	98(42.2)	0.09

Other critical transcription factors regulating B-cell development were also found to be deleted in the St. Jude ALL cohort, including *ETV6* (in 22% of cases), *EBF1* (in 4% of cases), *IKZF1/IKAROS* (in 17% of cases), and *IKZF3* (*AIOLOS*). Deletions of *IKZF1/IKAROS* were noted to be particularly frequent in pediatric (75%) and adult (>90%) ALL cases with t(9;22)(*BCR-ABL1*). In a subsequent study, St. Jude investigators determined that *IKZF1/IKAROS* deletions were very frequently acquired with the transformation of chronic phase chronic myelogenous leukemia (CML) to ALL blast crisis in both children and adults (Mullighan et al. 2008a). These highly significant studies clearly demonstrated that, in addition to well-known recurring translocations, pediatric ALL is associated with a wide spectrum of cooperating mutations that arise by DNA deletion, amplification, or point mutation in transcription factors controlling B-cell development, implying that disruption of these development pathways is critical for the promotion of B-cell leukemogenesis.

As these studies by Charles Mullighan and James Downing were underway at St. Jude, other investigators, including Cheryl Willman and colleagues at the University of New Mexico Cancer Center, William L. Carroll at New York University Cancer Institute, Monique de Boer and Richard Pieters at Erasmus University, and Ursula Kees and colleagues in Australia were also focusing on the use of gene expression profiling platforms and computational and statistical modeling tools to identify genes and develop molecular classifiers for improved outcome prediction and risk classification in pediatric leukemias. A second, but equally important goal of many of these studies was to use these gene expression profiles to discover new therapeutic targets for ALL. Through the development of a collaboration with the COG, the Willman group focused on gene expression profiling in a uniformly treated group of approximately 200 high risk B-precursor ALL patients registered to COG trial P9906 testing an augmented BFM regimen. (Kang et al. 2010). Study of this high-risk ALL cohort by gene expression profiling, described in detail below, was ideal, as the majority of cases had no known recurring genetic abnormalities and had experienced a poor outcome to current therapies. As these studies progressed, it became clear that detailed investigation of this high-risk ALL cohort using multiple different comprehensive genomic platforms would be particularly fruitful for the identification of novel genetic abnormalities in leukemic cells and for the identification of germline genetic polymorphisms associated with risk, therapeutic response, and toxicity. Thus, a collaboration was born between the COG and investigators at the University of New Mexico Cancer Center, St. Jude Children's Research Hospital, the NCI, and the cancer genome sequencing efforts of the NCI Cancer Genome Atlas Project, and the first National Cancer Institute TARGET (Therapeutically Applicable Research to Generate Effective Treatments; www.target.cancer.gov) was launched. The goal of this project was to use multiple comprehensive genomic platforms (gene expression, copy number variation, and germline genetic polymorphisms) to derive large genomic data sets, and, to integrate the analysis of these datasets to identify candidate genes for targeted sequencing (and ultimately next generation sequencing) to identify new ALL-associated genetic abnormalities that could be exploited for the development of more effective therapies.

Using DNA samples from this same COG P9906 cohort of high-risk ALL cases, Mullighan and colleagues again assessed copy number variations in leukemic DNA with SNP arrays and found significant chromosome gains and losses (Mullighan et al. 2009b, c). In contrast to their initial studies in the St. Jude cohort, in which the majority of ALL cases were either low or standard/intermediate-risk, the spectrum and frequency of DNA deletions and amplifications were different in the COG high-risk ALL cohort (Table 2.2). In the high-risk cohort, in which the majority of cases lacked known recurring cytogenetic abnormalities, over 50% of the cases had deletions or amplifications in genes that serve as regulators of B cell development, with frequent deletions in *CDKN2A* (in 45% of cases), *PAX5* (in 32% of cases), and *IKZF1/IKAROS* (in 25% of cases). Though not statistically significant, deletions in *RB1* (11% of cases), *BTG1* (10%), the 13q14 region containing micro RNAs (9.5%), and *EBF* (8.1%) were also seen at a higher frequency in the high-risk ALL cohort when compared to the earlier St. Jude case series. However, as the COG P9906 high risk ALL cases had been uniformly treated, the prognostic significance of these copy number variations and mutations could be more readily determined. Strikingly, despite their frequency, *PAX5* mutations were not found to have any prognostic significance in either the St. Jude or the COG ALL cohorts. In contrast, deletion of *IKZFI/IKAROS*, *BTLA*, and *EBF1* were each individually associated with a significantly higher risk of

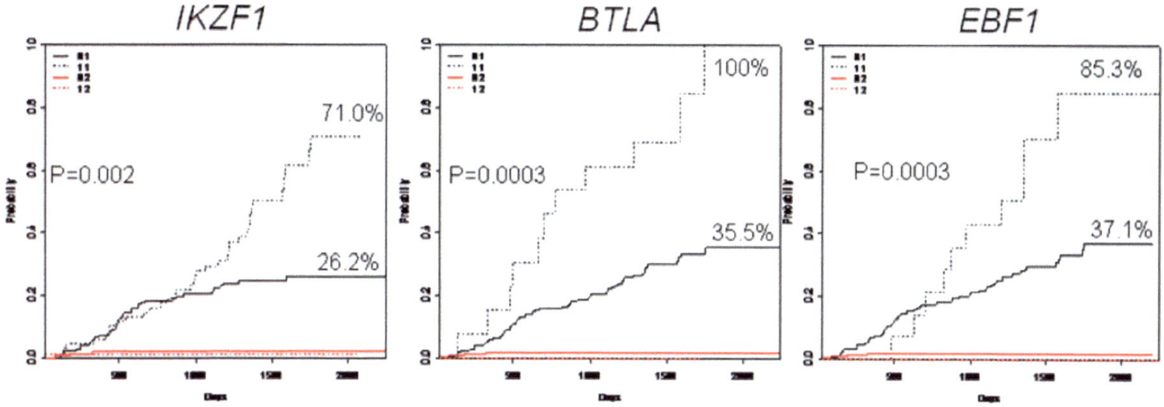

Fig. 2.3 Likelihood of relapse in high-risk B-precursor ALL patients from the COG 9906 cohort in children whose leukemic blasts contained (*dotted line*) or lacked (*solid line*) deletions of *IKZF1* (*left panel*), *BTLA* (*middle panel*), or *EBF1* (*right panel*). y-axis:pr obabilityof r elapse;x- axis:da ys

relapse (Fig. 2.3). Interestingly, all children whose ALL blasts contained a *BTLA* deletion experienced relapse. Yet, in multivariate analyses, only deletion of *IKZF1/IKAROS* was determined to have independent prognostic significance. In the COG high-risk cohort, 70% of the ALL cases containing *IKZF1/IKAROS* deletions relapsed, compared to only 26% in cases lacking *IKZF1/IKAROS* deletions (p = 0.002) (Mullighane ta l.2009b).

Through the integrated analysis of the copy number variation data and the gene expression profiling data performed on the same cohort, a second novel discovery was made: a significant fraction of the high-risk ALL cases containing *IKZF1/IKAROS* deletions shared a gene expression profile similar to or reflective of "activated" tyrosine kinase signaling pathways; these cases clustered similarly to, but distinct from, ALL cases containing a t(9;22)(*BCR-ABL1*) (Mullighan et al. 2009c; Harvey et al. 2010). Gene set enrichment analyses clearly demonstrated the similarity of these high-risk ALL cases that lacked a t(9;22)(*BCR-ABL1*) to true ALL cases with t(9;22)(*BCR-ABL1*), leading to the speculation that these cases might have an underlying mutation in a gene encoding a tyrosine kinase (Mullighan et al. 2009c). Den Boer and colleagues from the Netherlands published very similar results on an independent cohort of 190 newly diagnosed ALL cases (Den Boer et al. 2009). They reported that approximately 15% of cases had a gene expression signature that they termed "*BCR-ABL1*-like" and found that these cases were associated with a very poor outcome with a 5 year disease-free survival of 59.5% (95% CI: 37.1–81.9%); such cases were found to be particularly resistant to l-asparaginase (p = 0.001) and daunorubicin (p = 0.017). Interestingly, like Mullighan, Willman and colleagues, they reported that these "*BCR-ABL1*-like" ALL cases had frequent deletions of genes involved in the B-cell development pathway, including *IKAROS, E2A, EBF1, PAX5,* and *VPREB1*. Thus, parallel studies by these two teams of investigators not only demonstrated that pediatric ALL is a more genetically complex disease than previously appreciated, but also identified new genetic subtypes of ALL with prognostically important deletions of *IKZF1/IKAROS* and associated gene expression profiles reflective of activated or mutated tyrosine kinases. As discussed in subsequent sections, these and other studies laid the foundation for the discovery of novel tyrosine kinase mutations in pediatric ALL.

2.3.3.3 GeneExp ressionPr ofiling

Over the past 7 years since the technologic platform was first introduced, gene expression profiling microarrays have been used by several groups to identify gene expression "signatures" or profiles associated with recurrent cytogenetic abnormalities (Yeoh et al. 2002; Ross et al. 2003) and *in vitro* drug responsiveness in the acute leukemias (Cheok et al. 2003; Holleman et al. 2004; Lugthart et al. 2005; Sorich et al. 2008). Fewer studies have developed and reported gene expression signatures or have developed and modeled gene expression classifiers predictive of survival that could be validated on independent case cohorts or datasets generated by other laboratories. Using a selected cohort of approximately 90 children with high-risk ALL (a matched case: control series of failure vs. continuous complete remission), Bhowjani, Carroll, and colleagues developed a 24 probe set signature that predicted day 7 marrow status ($p = 0.0061$) and a 47 probe set signature predictive of long-term response (Bhojwani et al. 2006; Bhojwani et al. 2008). While these gene expression classifiers could be validated on other independent ALL cohorts, and while interesting candidate genes that are now being pursued as novel therapeutic targets (*SURVIVIN*) were identified, in multivariate analysis, these predictors did not retain independent prognostic significance beyond traditional prognostic features routinely used in risk classification, including age, WBC, and recurring cytogenetic abnormalities. Similarly, Hoffmann, Kees, and colleagues from the University of Western Australia profiled 55 ALL cases and identified 3 genes (*GLUL, AZIN,* and *IGJ*) whose signatures together were predictive of outcome in an independent test set; a multivariate analysis to determine whether these genes retained independent prognostic significance beyond traditional prognostic factors was not reported (Hoffmann et al. 2008).

Under the auspices of the NCI TARGET Project, using samples from the same COG P9990 high-risk ALL cohort used to discover *IKZF1/IKAROS* deletions and the activated tyrosine kinase signature or novel "*BCR-ABL1*-like" subset of ALL, Kang, Willman and colleagues performed gene expression profiling and employed supervised learning methods to develop a gene expression classifier highly predictive of outcome in high-risk ALL (Kang et al. 2010). From the gene expression profiles obtained using Affymetrix U133-Plus2 gene expression arrays with pretreatment leukemic samples from 207 uniformly treated children with high-risk ALL, supervised learning algorithms and extensive cross-validation techniques were used to build a 42 probe-set (38 gene) expression classifier predictive of RFS. This gene expression classifier was able to distinguish two groups with differing relapse risks at pretreatment: low (4 year RFS: 81%, $n = 109$) vs. high (4 year RFS: 50%, $n = 98$) ($p < 0.0001$). In multivariate analyses, only the gene expression classifier ($p = 0.001$) and flow cytometric measures of MRD ($p = 0.001$) retained prognostic significance and each provided independent prognostic information. Together, these measures could be used to classify children with high-risk ALL into low (87% RFS), intermediate (62% RFS), or high-risk (29% RFS) groups ($p < 0.0001$) (Fig. 2.4). A 21-gene expression classifier predictive of end-Induction MRD effectively substituted for flow cytometric measures of MRD, yielding a combined classifier that could distinguish these three risk groups at diagnosis ($P < 0.0001$). These classifiers were further validated on the independent high-risk ALL cohort ($P = 0.006$) studied by Carroll and colleagues (Bhojwani et al. 2008) and retained independent prognostic significance ($P < 0.0001$) in the presence of other recently described poor prognostic factors for high-risk ALL (*IKAROS*/*IKZF1* deletions, *JAK* mutations (discussed below), and the activated tyrosine kinase signature or novel "*BCR-ABL1*-like" signature). These studies thus demonstrated that gene expression classifiers could be used to improve ALL risk classification and for prospective identification of children who will respond to, or fail, current treatment regimens. The classifier developed by Kang and colleagues particularly identified a group of children most likely to fail current therapeutic approaches (whose 5 year RFS rate was essentially 0%). The ability to identify children at diagnosis who are likely to receive little to no benefit from therapeutic intensification allows one to prospectively target these children to alternative treatment regimens.

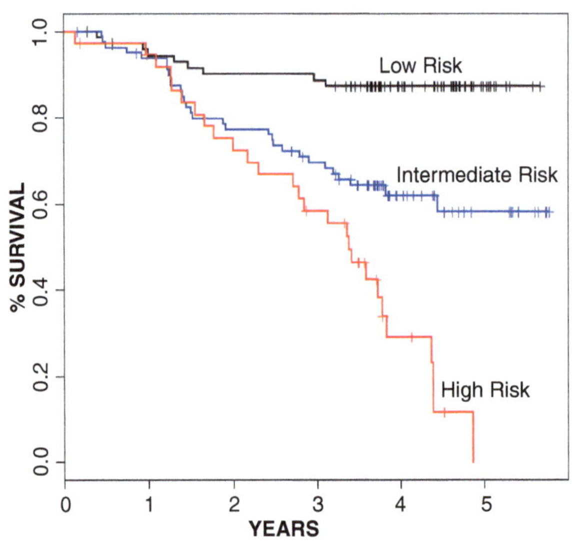

Fig. 2.4 Striking differences in relapse-free survival in the low, intermediate, and high-risk groups defined by the combined gene expression classifier for relapse-free survival and flow cytometric measures of minimal residual disease at end-Induction in a cohort of high-risk ALL patients from COG Trial 9906 (Modifiedf romK ange ta l. 2010)

Unexpectedly, 72/207 (38%) of the "high-risk" ALL patients studied in the COG 9906 ALL cohort were found by the combined gene expression classifier for RFS and flow MRD to have a significantly better survival (87% RFS at 4 years) when compared with the entire cohort (66% survival at 4 years). This group of patients, which included all 20 cases with t(1;19)(*TCF3-PBX1*) and an additional 52 cases whose underlying genetic abnormalities remain to be discovered, was characterized by high expression of the tumor suppressor genes and signaling proteins *RGS2, NFKBIB, NR4A3, DDX21,* and *BTG3*. Application of the combined classifier also identified 38/207 (20%) patients in the COG 9906 cohort who had a dismal 4 year RFS of 29% (approaching 0% at 5 years), as discussed above. Highly expressed in this group of patients with the worst outcome were genes (*BMPR1B, CRLF2, CTGF (CCN2), TTYH2, IGJ, PON2, CD73, CDC42EP3, TSPAN7, SEMA6A)* involved in adaptive cell signaling responses to TGFβ, stem cell function, B-cell development and differentiation, and the regulation of tumor growth. Not surprisingly, given that all cases with a "*BCR-ABL1*-like" or "activated tyrosine kinase" signature were assigned to the highest risk group with the combined classifier, six of the genes associated with the kinase signature (*BMPR1B, ECM1, IGJ, PON2, SEMA6A, and TSPAN7*), also found by Den Boer and colleagues (Den Boer et al. 2009), were contained within the gene expression classifier for RFS.

Perhaps most important among these findings, particularly in terms of the potential clinical utility of gene expression-based classifiers for risk classification, was the demonstration that the gene expression classifier for RFS and/or the combined classifier retained independent prognostic significance for outcome prediction in the presence of new genetic abnormalities associated with a poor outcome in pediatric ALL (*IKAROS/IKZF1* deletions, *JAK* mutations, and kinase signatures). Kang and colleagues found that the combined classifier further refined outcome prediction in the presence of each of these mutations or signatures, distinguishing which cases with *JAK* mutations, activated tyrosine kinase signatures, or *IKAROS/IKZF1* deletions would have a good ("low-risk"), intermediate, or poor ("high-risk") outcome. Thus, as discussed below, while *IKZF1* deletions and *JAK* mutations are exciting new targets for the development of novel therapeutic approaches in pediatric ALL, assessment of these genetic abnormalities alone may not be fully sufficient for risk classification or to predict overall outcome. As gene expression profiles reflect the full constellation and consequence of the multiple genetic abnormalities seen in each ALL patient and as measures of minimal residual disease are a functional biologic measure of residual or resistant leukemic cells, they may have an enhanced clinical utility for refinement of risk classification and outcome prediction.

Taking an alternative approach, Harvey, Willman, Mullighan, and colleagues also studied the gene expression profiles derived from the COG high-risk ALL cohort using unsupervised learning methods for "class discovery": the identification of distinct cluster groups of patients who shared common patterns of gene expression (Harvey et al. 2010a). Expression profiles were correlated with DNA copy number abnormalities and clinical and outcome features. Unsupervised clustering revealed eight unique patient cluster groups in the high-risk ALL cohort, two of which were associated with known chromosomal translocations (t(1;19) (*TCF3-PBX1*) or *MLL*), and six of which were novel, lacking known cytogenetic abnormalities. Harvey and colleagues developed a novel statistical method, termed ROSE (Recognition of Outliers by Sampling Ends), similar to COPA (Cancer Outlier Profile Analysis) (Tomlins et al. 2005) to define the "outlier" genes associated with each unique cluster group. Such "outlier" genes, frequently expressed several logs above or below the median in a subset of cases compared to levels of expression across all the samples, are often either directly involved in genetic lesions (e.g., translocations, deletions, insertions) or are present in pathways downstream of these activating events. Thus, methods such as COPA and ROSE allow one to potentially mine gene expression profiling data sets to identify potential target genes disrupted through novel genetic lesions. One of the unique clusters (termed R6) discovered by Harvey and colleagues was characterized by high expression of *AGAP1, CCNJ, CHST2/7, CLEC12A/B,* and *PTPRM; ERG* DNA deletions; and a 4-year RFS of 94.7±5.1%, compared to 63.5±3.7% for the remaining cohort ($p = 0.002$). A second unique cluster, termed R8, was characterized by high expression of distinct outlier genes *BMPR1B, CRLF2, GPR110, and MUC4;* frequent deletion of *EBF1, IKZF1, RAG1-2,* and *IL3RA-CSF2RA;* an activated tyrosine kinase or *BCR-ABL1-like* signature; Hispanic race/ethnicity ($p < .001$); and a very poor 4-year RFS (21.0 ± 9.5%; $p < .001$) (Harvey 2010b Fig. 2.5). These studies further revealed

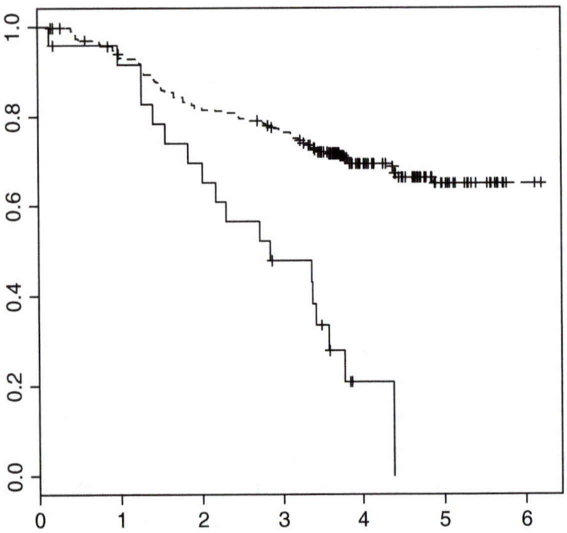

Fig. 2.5 Relapse-free survival in all high-risk B-precursor ALL patients accrued to COG Trial P9906 (*dotted line*) and in gene expression cluster group R8 (*solid line*), with the poorest overall survival. y-axis: survival; x-axis: years. (Modified from Harvey eta l., submittedf orpubl ication)

the striking clinical and genetic heterogeneity within high-risk B-precursor ALL and pointed to novel genes which may serve as new targets for diagnosis, risk classification, and therapy.

2.3.3.4 Discoveryo fN ovelT herapeutic Targets Through DNA Sequencing and Genomic Studies

The discovery of the subset of high-risk ALL cases with an "activated tyrosine kinase" or "*BCR-ABL1*-like" gene expression signature provided an important clue for targeted DNA resequencing. As part of the COG NCI TARGET Project, investigators selected 125 genes (based on recurrent copy number variations, gene expression profiles, genes involved in tyrosine kinase signaling pathways, and known cancer genes) and sequenced them in 187 cases in the COG high-risk B-precursor ALL cohort from COG P9906 (Zhang et al. 2009). The entire coding region and untranslated regions (UTRs) of each gene were sequenced. Somatic mutations were frequently found in genes that encode for proteins involved in signal transduction, B-cell development, and p53/RB signaling. A notable finding was the presence of somatic mutations resulting in constitutive activation of RAS signaling in at least 39% of the high-risk ALL cases. Seventy-three cases had at least one mutation in *NRAS* (30), *KRAS* (28), *PTPN11* (9), *FLT3* (7), and *NF1* (6), including seven patients with multiple mutations (*KRAS* and *NRAS* (3), *FLT3* and *NF1* (1), *PTPN11* and *FLT3* (1), *PTPN11* and *FLT3* (1), *PTPN11* and *NRAS* (1), *PTPN11* and *KRAS* (1)). While RAS may represent an important and previously unappreciated target in this form of ALL, *RAS* mutations were not predictive of event-free survival or relapse in this cohort. Notably, RAS pathway mutations occurred most frequently in ALL cases lacking known sentinel cytogenetic lesions (68/145 cases, 47%, $p <$ 0.0001). Sequence mutations that are known or predicted to impair normal B-cell development were observed in at least 14% of the cohort (*PAX5* (21), *IKZF1* (7)), while sequence mutations disrupting *TP53/RB1* signaling ((*TP53* (10), *RB1* (4), *CDKN2A* (4)) occurred in 10% of cases (Zhang et al. 2009).

In addition to the discovery of a high frequency of RAS pathway mutations in high-risk ALL, activating sequence mutations in members of the JAK family of tyrosine kinases were discovered in approximately 11% of the high-risk ALL cases (Mullighan et al. 2009c). Not unexpectedly, cases with *JAK* mutations were found nearly exclusively in the R8 gene expression cluster group, described above, where they were strongly associated with *IKZF1/IKAROS* deletions, the *BCR-ABL1*-like or activated tyrosine kinase gene expression signature, and the worst overall outcome. Activating mutations were found in *JAK1* ($n = 3$ cases), *JAK2* ($n = 16$, where the R683G mutation predominated), and *JAK3* ($n = 1$) in 20 of 187 (10.7%) cases (Fig. 2.6). Only two of the ALL cases in this high-risk

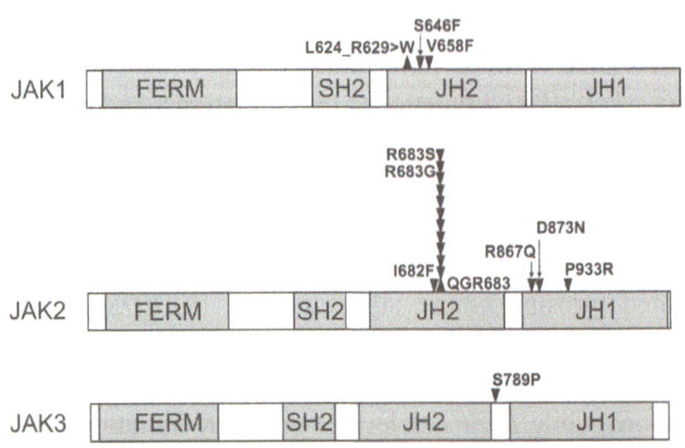

Fig. 2.6 The spectrum of mutations in the JAK family of tyrosine kinases in the COG 9006 High-Risk ALL cohort. Mutations in individual patients are shown in solid triangles. (FromM ullighane ta l.2009c)

cohort occurred in children with Down Syndrome. The *JAK1* and *JAK2* mutations involved highly conserved residues in the kinase and pseudokinase domains and resulted in constitutive JAK-STAT activation. These results first suggested that inhibition of *JAK* signaling is a logical target for therapeutic intervention in ALL cases harboring *JAK* mutations, and early phase clinical trials testing JAK inhibitors in pediatric malignancies are now underway in the COG. Interestingly, as these data developed, Bercovich, Izraeli, and colleagues also first reported the presence of *JAK2* mutations in nearly 20% of ALL cases arising in children with Down syndrome, with five different mutant alleles each affecting R683G (Bercovich et al. 2008), as mentioned in preceding sections. Thus, both ALL arising in Down Syndrome and cases of high-risk ALL were discovered to harbor novel mutations in the JAK family of kinases yielding a promising new target for therapeutic intervention in ALL.

While the discovery of *JAK* mutations in ALL was tantalizing and an important advance, the story continued to rapidly advance through parallel investigations by several teams of investigators. Examination of whole genome copy number variations in the COG high-risk ALL cohort, particularly focusing on cases with various gene mutations reported previously, led to the discovery of a subset of high-risk ALL cases, often with *JAK* mutations, who also had genomic deletions within the pseudoautosomal region (PAR1) of Xp22.3/Yp11.3, near the *IL3-RA* and a novel gene termed *CRLF2* (encoding cytokine receptor-like factor 2, or, the thymic stromal lymphopoietin receptor) (Mullighan et al. 2009a). Even more tantalizing was the finding that cases with these copy number variations frequently had very high levels of expression of *CRLF2*, which was previously discovered as an "outlier" gene associated with the gene expression cluster group that had the poorest overall outcome (R8), discussed above. Reexamination of the gene expression profiles within the COG high-risk ALL cohort revealed 29/207 cases (14%) with markedly elevated *CRLF2* expression. As these studies were underway, Christine Harrison and colleagues first reported two different *CRLF2* genomic rearrangements in ALL: a translocation of the immunoglobulin heavy chain locus (*IGH*) to *CRLF2* at Xp22.3 or Yp11.3, or deletion upstream of *CRLF2* in approximately 5% of patients with B-progenitor ALL (Russell et al. 2009). Investigators in the NCI TARGET Project then determined that the PAR1 deletion upstream (centromeric) of *CRLF2* juxtaposes the first noncoding exon of *P2RY8* to the entire coding region of *CRLF2*, resulting in a *P2RY8-CRLF2* fusion, and that this fusion occurs in over 50% of cases of childhood ALL associated with Down syndrome (DS) (Mullighan et al. 2009a). Similar results were rapidly reported by Izraeli and colleagues (Hertzberg et al. 2010). In each series of cases studied by each of these groups across the world, *CRLF2* rearrangements were also shown to be associated with concomitant mutation of *JAK1* and *JAK2* and these lesions together were shown to be transforming *in vitro* (Mullighan et al. 2009a; Harvey et al. 2010b; Hertzberg et al. 2010). Weinstock and colleagues also first reported interesting activating mutations of *CRLF2* in B-precursor ALL, particularly the Phe232Cys gain of function mutation (Yoda et al. 2010). *CRLF2* genetic abnormalities are particularly frequent in children with high-risk B-progenitor ALL, where they are very significantly associated with Hispanic/Latino ethnicity, *JAK1 or JAK2* mutations, *IKAROS/IKZF1* deletions, and a very poor outcome (Fisher exact test $P < .0001$ for each) (Harvey et al. 2010b). Within this cohort, ALL patients with *CRLF2* rearrangements had extremely poor treatment outcomes when compared to those without *CRLF2* rearrangements (35.3% vs. 71.3% relapse-free survival at 4 years; $p = .0001$). Together, these observations suggest that activation of *CRLF2* expression, mutation of *JAK* kinases, and alterations of *IKZF1* cooperate to promote B-cell leukemogenesis and identify these pathways as important new therapeutic targets in this disease (Fig. 2.7).

Continued discovery of novel genetic mutations in ALL are also resulting from the use of next generation sequencing techniques. As a complementary approach to identify novel genomic alterations, the NCI TARGET group of investigators is currently using Illumina next generation sequencing technology to sequence the tumor transcriptome of representative cases from the COG P9906 high-risk ALL cohort (Mulligan et al. 2009d). cDNA libraries were generated from poly-A enriched RNA, and 36–50 base paired-end sequencing was performed using the Illumina Genome Analyzer. Sequence alignment, variant detection, and fusion transcript identification were performed using custom scripts and multiple published reference alignment and *de novo* assembly algorithms. Interestingly, putative novel fusion transcripts were identified in several cases, including a novel transcript with an in-frame fusion of exon 9 of the striatin gene *STRN3* to exon 18 of *JAK2* (*STRN3-JAK2*) and a fusion of *NUP214* to *ABL1*. Both of these fusions occurred in ALLs with a

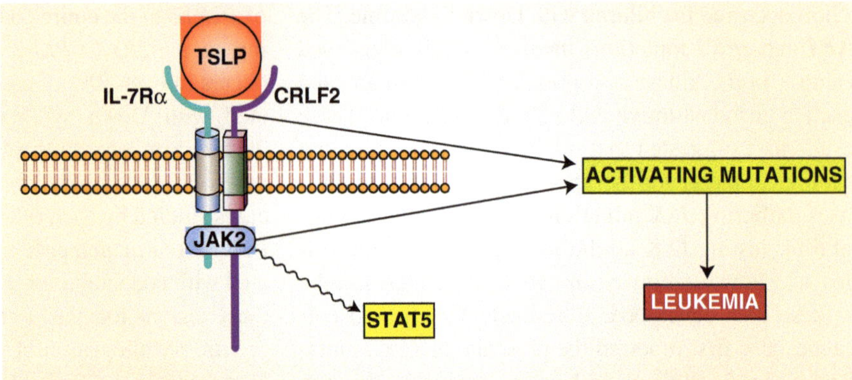

Fig. 2.7 Overexpression of CRLF2, which heterodimerizes with the IL-7a receptor, through genomic rearrangements or activating mutations in concert with activating mutations of the JAK kinase (*blue circle*) promote B-cell leukemogenesis

BCR-ABL1-like gene expression signature that lacked known *JAK* mutations, suggesting that additional novel activating kinase mutations can be discovered via detailed sequence analysis of the 50% of *BCR-ABL1*-like ALLs that have high levels of *CRLF2* expression and *CRLF2* genomic rearrangements but lack *JAK* mutations. In addition, these data identified over 400 candidate nonsynonymous single nucleotide and insertion/deletion variations in each patient. Whole genome sequencing of matched normal DNA is underway to remove germline variation from the putative variants, and transcriptomic sequencing of additional cases of high-risk childhood ALL are being performed. Together, these data indicate that transcriptomic sequencing is a powerful method to identify novel genetic alterations in ALL and may be used to identify novel targets for therapeutic intervention.

2.3.3.5 EpigeneticMo difications and Posttranscriptional Regulation by microRNAs

The structure of the genome, as it is packaged in the cell nucleus, comprises the helical DNA associated with multiple proteins to form a complex structure called chromatin. DNA strands are wrapped around histone proteins, forming disc-shaped nucleosomes that are arranged in arrays, like beads on a string. The tails of histone proteins protrude from the nucleosomes and can be chemically modified. Epigenetics is the study of biochemical modifications of chromatin. These modifications do not alter the primary sequence of DNA, but have an impact on gene expression regulation, most frequently gene suppression. The field of epigenetics is rapidly expanding from DNA methylation to include histone modifications and, more recently, to the discovery of microRNAs as having a role in DNA methylation control (Robertson and Wolffe 2000; Jones and Baylin 2007). Another relevant reason for the increased interest in epigenetic lesions in cancer lies in the possibility to reverse the epigenetic marks to a physiological gene expression by using several chemotherapeutics agents, including DNA hypomethylating agents and histone deacetylase inhibitors (Garcia-Manero and Issa 2005; Muller and Florek 2010).

Most current techniques use bisulfite treatment of DNA to detect regions of methylation (Clark et al. 1994). Sodium bisulfite is used to convert cytosine residues to uracil residues in single-stranded DNA, under conditions in which 5-methylcytosine remains nonreactive. The converted DNA is amplified with specific primers and sequenced. All the cytosine residues remaining in the sequence represent previously methylated cytosines in the genome. These concepts have been further developed by the combination of bisulfite PCR and pyrosequencing that allows assessment of allele-specific DNA methylation. In this method, DNA is first treated with sodium bisulfite and then genes of interest are subsequently amplified using PCR. Allele-specific methylation can then be determined by pyrosequencing each allele individually using sequencing primers that incorporate SNPs that allow differentiation between the two parental alleles (Wong et al. 2006). More recently, in order to overcome the limitations of analyses restricted to specific loci, a genome-scale and entire methylomes can now be performed and can be characterized at single-base-pair resolution. Several methods of DNA methylation profiling techniques are currently available with different relative merits and limitations, especially for data analysis and comparison (Laird 2010).

Aberrant DNA methylation of multiple promoter CpG islands is a common feature of adult ALL (reviewed in Garcia-Manero et al. (2009)). The results in pediatric ALL are far more limited. When selected genes were analyzed (i.e., the estrogen receptor gene (*ER*), multidrug resistance gene 1 (*MDR1*), *p15*, *c-ABL*, CD10, *p16*, and *p73*), most of the pediatric ALL patients had methylation of >/= 1 gene, and 4 patients (25%) had methylation of 3–4 genes. By contrast, methylation of the same genes was <2% (or methylation-specific polymerase chain reaction negative) in nonneoplastic tissues (Garcia-Manero et al. 2003). When aberrant methylation of multiple genes was correlated with standard prognostic factors, including immunophenotype, age, sex, WBC count, and presence of specific translocations (*ETV6/RunX1*, *BCR-ABL*, *E2A-PBX1*, or *MLL-AF4*), only age (≥10 years) and WBC count at diagnosis (≥50 × 10^9/L) were found associated with a higher frequency of methylation (Garcia-Manero et al. 2003). T-ALLs have a lower frequency of methylation than B-precursor ALLs. Among the different molecular subgroups, *MLL*-positive ALLs demonstrate the highest frequency of methylation, while ALLs carrying the t(1;19) have the lowest (Gutierrez et al. 2003). The most common epigenetic lesion in childhood ALL is the methylation of E-cadherin (72%) independent of the molecular subtype or other clinicopathological factors. Distinct promoter CpG island methylation patterns separate different genetic subtypes of *MLL*-rearranged ALL in infants. *MLL* translocations t(4;11) and t(11;19) characterize extensively hypermethylated leukemia, whereas t(9;11)-positive infant ALL and infant ALL carrying wild-type *MLL* genes epigenetically resemble normal bone marrow (Stumpel et al. 2009). The combination of gene expression and the analysis of methylation of the 5′CpG region of selected genes can provide new insights into leukemogenesis. In 100% of the infant *MLL* cases, methylation of the *FHIT* 5′CpG region occurs, resulting in strongly reduced mRNA and protein expression. *FHIT* expression can be restored upon exposing leukemic cells to the demethylating agent decitabine, which induces apoptosis. Likewise and more specifically, leukemic cell death is induced by transfecting *MLL* rearranged leukemic cells with expression vectors encoding wild-type *FHIT*, confirming tumor suppressor activity of this gene (Stam et al. 2006). The degree of aberrant methylation may portend a poor prognosis (Roman-Gomez et al. 2007). Among infant ALL patients carrying t(4;11) or t(11;19) translocations, methylation influences relapse-free survival, with patients displaying accentuated methylation being at high relapse risk (Stam et al. 2006).

Finally, whether inhibition of aberrant DNA methylation may be an important novel therapeutic strategy for childhood ALL is still uncertain. DNA methyltransferase inhibitors prevent hypermethylation of promoter CpG islands and rescue normal expression of tumor suppressor genes. Promising preclinical data in *MLL*-rearranged leukemia showed that demethylating agent zebularine reverses aberrant DNA methylation and effectively induces apoptosis (Stam et al. 2006). Clinical trials of the DNA methyltransferase inhibitor 5-azacytadine (azacitidine) has been assessed in adult malignancies (Muller and Florek 2010), but not in pediatric ALL. The more potent 5-aza-2′-deoxycytidine (decitabine) is currently being evaluated in several early phase studies in pediatric ALL, and has been associated with successful remission status in a case report of a pediatric patient with multiply relapsed ALL(Y aneze ta l. 2009).

MicroRNAs are small (19 to 22 nucleotide) RNA molecules that are capable of regulating genes at the posttranscriptional level (Iorio and Croce 2009). It is estimated that 1% of the genome is made up of miRNA genes and that up to 30% of genes may be regulated by miRNAs (Bartel 2004). MicroRNAs are first produced in the nucleus as longer transcripts with hairpin regions. They are subsequently processed by RNAase III Drosha into 70 to 100 nucleotide (nts) precursor molecules that are further processed in the cytoplasm by the RNAase III Dicer to generate a mature double stranded miRNA. miRNAs usually bind to the 3′ untranslated regions of transcripts where they lead to degradation and/or inhibition of translation.

Not surprisingly, miRNA dysregulation has been implicated in cancer development and progression. Indeed, two miRNAs, *miR-15a* and *miR-16-1*, were first shown to reside in an area of frequent deletion in chronic lymphocytic leukemia and subsequent experiments established that underexpression of these miRNAs resulted in downstream up-regulation of Bcl-2 and Mcl-1 (see below) (Calin et al. 2005). Many additional examples of how altered miRNA expression alters tumor suppressors and oncogenes have been discovered.

The contribution of miRNAs in the pathogenesis of childhood ALL is just being elucidated. Investigators have demonstrated that miRNA expression signatures correlate with biological subtype in childhood ALL (Fulci et al. 2009; Schotte et al. 2009). Kotani et al showed that miR – 128b and miR-221 are down regulated in MLL-AF4 ALL and that restoration of levels restores glucocorticoid sensitivity (Kotani et al. 2009). On the other hand, the miR-17–92 cluster may be amplified and overexpression has been shown to increase proliferation and replating capacity of normal bone marrow cells, thereby underscoring their importance as oncogenes (Mi et al. 2007). These observations underscore the therapeutic potential of such approaches. Antisense oligonucleotides to oncogenic miRNAs and the reintroduction of tumor suppressor miRNAs can reverse some aspects of the leukemia phenotype.

2.4 SignalingP athways in Childhood ALL

Although the majority of patients with ALL respond well to current therapies, some patients necessitate intensified chemotherapy regimens because of high-risk features. These patients are unlikely to benefit from further adjustments to the dosing or timing of the same chemotherapy. Research in the past years clearly demonstrated that childhood ALL is a heterogeneous group of cancers, containing different genotypic and phenotypic signatures. This progress has implicated signaling pathways in the pathogenesis of the disease, to which novel therapies can be directed, such as treating *MLL*-rearranged leukemia with FLT-3 inhibitors, or *Notch1*-mutated T-cell ALL with a gamma-secretase inhibitor. High throughput sequencing and array technology will continue to discover aberrant signaling pathways in childhood ALL that will lead to more refined targeting of leukemia-specific signaling pathways.

In lymphoid leukemias, several signaling pathways are pathologically altered to provide a survival advantage for uncontrolled malignant growth, and thus potentially serve as excellent targets for cancer treatment. Although tyrosine kinases represented the initial model of targeted therapy in CML, it is now known that a wide variety of biochemical intracellular pathways, gene expression patterns, and cell surface markers might be deregulated and thus contribute to a cell's malignant phenotype, and additional potential targets are likely to be discovered in the near future by new technologies. A number of relevant signaling pathways aberrantly regulated in pediatric ALL represent targets for novel therapeutic approaches.

2.4.1 BCR-ABL Tyrosine Kinase

The t(9;22) translocation, occurring in about 2–3% of childhood ALL, generates the Philadelphia chromosome (Ph+). As a consequence, the cytoplasmic tyrosine kinase *ABL* on chromosome 9 is linked with the *BCR* gene on chromosome 22, resulting in a constitutively active kinase protein (reviewed in Quintas-Cardama and Cortes (2009)). The dysregulated ABL tyrosine kinase (TK) leads to cellular proliferation by activating the phosphoinositide 3-kinase (PI3K) and the downstream prosurvival proteins AKT and mTOR, therefore inducing the transformation process. A small molecule, imatinib mesylate, has been developed to compete for the *BCR-ABL* tyrosine kinase ATP binding site, stabilizing it in its inactive conformation. In clinical trials in CML, it successfully halted the aberrant TK constitutive activity, leading to sustained clinical remissions (Druker et al. 2001). More recently, imatinib has been used in combination with chemotherapy in a small subset of pediatric patients with Ph+ ALL, with excellent results without any additional toxicity (Schultz et al. 2009) although long-term survival data are not yet known.

Despite initial successes with imatinib, *de novo* mutations involving the ATP binding pocket have been found in cases resistant to this first generation of ABL inhibitor. New generations of ABL TK inhibitors (i.e., dasatinib) have been developed in an attempt to overcome this resistance (reviewed in Quintas-Cardama andC ortes (2009)).

2.4.2 FLT-3 Receptor Tyrosine Kinase

Point mutations, overexpression or internal tandem duplications (ITD) of the Fms-like tyrosine kinase (FLT-3) are found in *MLL*-rearranged (MLL-R) ALL, some T-cell ALLs, and high hyperdiploid ALL, as well as acute myelogenous leukemia and other malignancies (reviewed in Meshinchi and Appelbaum (2009)).

These mutations constitutively activate the FLT-3 tyrosine kinase, which in turn activates the RAS/RAF/ERK, PI3K/AKT/mTOR and signal transducer and activator of transcription-5 (STAT5) pathways, resulting in uncontrolled cell proliferation and loss of normal apoptotic control. Therefore, the presence of *FLT-3* aberrancies is associated with a prosurvival phenotype, high resistance to multiple chemotherapeutic agents, and poor prognosis. Several drugs have been developed to target this signaling pathway, including lestaurtinib (CEP-701), midostaurin (PKC-412), and several others, and are currently being tested in clinical studies to improve selectivity and efficacy of targeting this receptor (reviewed in Meshinchi and Appelbaum (2009)).

2.4.3 JAK Tyrosine Kinase

The Janus kinase (JAK) family of tyrosine kinases is activated by cytokine binding to a Type I cytokine receptor. Activation of JAK leads to phosphorylation of STAT, and subsequent activation of both the RAS/RAF and PI3K/AKT pathways, ultimately leading to the leukemic phenotype. As noted previously, several activating *JAK* mutations have been identified, freq-uently associated with other gene abnormalities, including deletion or mutation of I*KZF1* and overexpression the *CRLF2* gene as a consequence of genomic rearrangements, both of which confer poor prognosis (Bercovich et al. 2008; Mullighan et al. 2009b,c; Harvey et al. 2010; Hertzberg et al. 2010b). Interestingly, two mutations affecting the same domain of the JAK2 gene are associated with two completely different hematological diseases, polycythemia vera (617 mutation) and ALL (683 mutation). An explanation for this unusual genotype-phenotype association may be due to differences in protein binding with crucial lineage-specific signaling molecules mediated by the two sites.

The *IKZF1* gene codes for the IKAROS transcription factor, necessary for normal lymphocyte development. *IKAROS* deletion is present in up to 30% of ALL cases depending on the clinical and biological subtype (for example, it is more frequent in Ph+ ALL) and is associated with poor prognosis (Mullighan et al. 2008a; Mullighan et al. 2009b). CRLF2 is a subunit of the type I cytokine receptor, which forms a heterodimer with IL7R; cytokine binding to this receptor is known to stimulate B-cell proliferation. Rearrangements involving CRLF2 have been found to cause constitutive dimerization with *IL7R*, resulting in cytokine-independent activation of JAK2 and STAT5, B-cell proliferation and cell transformation, especially in the presence of a constitutively activated *JAK* mutation. Several JAK inhibitors are being clinically tested in adult trials, and in the future, they might lead to improved prognosis for pediatric patients with *IKAROS* mutations and CRLF2 overexpression, particularly in Down syndrome ALL cases and Latino/Hispanic patients in whom those rearrangements are more prevalent (Harvey et al. 2010b).

2.4.4 Pre-B Cell Receptor

The pre-B cell receptor in normal early B cell development has the dual function to promote survival and proliferation of pre-B cells and subsequently to induce differentiation. It consists of an immunoglobulin μ heavy chain (*IGHM*) coupled to the surrogate light chain with its two components VpreB (*VPREB1*) and λ5 (*IGLL1*) (Nahar and Muschen 2009). B cell precursor-ALL is characterized by cells arrested at early stages of B cell development. Interestingly, a defective expression of *IGLL1, CD79B, IGHM,* and *SLP65* was shown as a frequent feature in Ph+ ALL; in addition, recent genomic studies in various subtypes of ALL identified multiple genetic lesions within the pre-B-cell receptor signaling pathway (Mullighan et al. 2007), indicating that the developmental arrest in B-cell lineage ALL may predominantly reflect aberrant pre-B cell receptor function, although this hypothesis needs to be functionally tested.

2.4.5 RAS Pathway

Activating mutations of the *RAS* gene have been observed in several pediatric leukemias. The intracellular protein RAS is associated with prosurvival cytokine receptor signaling via RAF, MEK, and ERK 1/2 (Case et al. 2008). Because the addition of a farnesyl isoprene group by farnesyltransferase is a posttranslational modification of the RAS protein required for its localization to the cellular membrane and subsequent cell transformation, farnesyltransferase inhibitors are currently tested as target therapies for multiple intercellular proteins, including RAS, especially in T-ALL, which seems to be more sensitive to this drug than precursor B-cell leukemias (Goemans et al. 2005).

2.4.6 NOTCH1 Pathway

NOTCH is a transmembrane heterodimeric receptor that, after activation by ligands and cleavage by the γ-secretase, releases the intracellular domain Notch1, which translocates to the nucleus and acts as a transcription factor regulating T-cell development in normal cells. The fundamental components of the NOTCH pathway include the Delta and Serrate family of ligands, four distinct NOTCH receptors (NOTCH1-4), and the RBPJ/CSL (CBF1/Su(H)/LAG-1) DNA-binding protein (reviewed in Ferrando (2009)). Mutations in the NOTCH receptor have been found in more than 50% of pediatric T-cell ALL; they result in ligand-independent cleavage and activation of Notch1, and are leukemogenic in *in vivo* studies (Ferrando 2009). The prognostic significance of NOTCH activation in T-ALL is still uncertain, because differences in therapy seem to influence the effect of *NOTCH1* mutations on prognosis (Ferrando 2009). Currently, γ-secretase inhibitors are under testing, with the aim to prevent release of Notch1 from the transmembrane receptor, thereby decreasing viability of T-cell ALL. Although severe gastrointestinal toxicity has been observed, this could be prevented by concomitant use of glucocorticoids, which also seem to increase their antileukemic effects. Moreover, second generation γ- secretase inhibitors, with decreased toxicity, are being evaluated (Real and Ferrando 2009).

2.4.7 Therapy Targeted to Signaling Pathways

Although a better comprehension of the signaling pathways can direct several selected and promising therapies, many challenges still need to be overcome, including definition of resistance pathways, either intrinsic to the leukemic cell or induced by the treatment. In addition, considering the complexity of the biological system, inhibition of a single protein might be compensated by related pathways. Moreover, all therapies have a certain degree of potential side effects due to their relative activity on normal somatic cells. In the future, increasing recognition that childhood ALL is a heterogeneous group of cancers, composed by different genotypic and phenotypic signatures, each of which requires development of novel specific treatments based on the exact specifications of the disease, such as treating MLL-rearranged leukemia with a FLT-3 inhibitor, or treating T-cell ALL with a gamma-secretase inhibitor is likely. Moreover, this specificity will require ongoing editing based on new knowledge coming from high throughput sequencing and array technologies. The overarching goal is that application of targeted therapy will allow improvement and/or maintenance of the cure rate by reducing or eliminating the use of pan-cytotoxic chemotherapeutic agents, thereby decreasing both short and long-term side effects of current ALL treatment.

2.5 TheA poptoticPat hwayandA LL

Apoptosis is an evolutionarily conserved intrinsic cell death mechanism required for the maintenance of cell and tissue homeostasis. In contrast to necrosis, apoptotic cells display a distinct morphology characterized by membrane blebbing, cell shrinkage, nuclear condensation, DNA cleavage, and phagocytosis by neighboring mononuclear cells (Fulda 2009a). Progress in this field greatly accelerated with the first discovery of the antiapoptotic Bcl-2 protein family, whose expression is upregulated as a result of the t(14; 18) in follicular lymphoma (Reed and Pellecchia 2005). Many agents used in anticancer therapy eradicate cancer cells by initiating apoptosis. Apoptosis in hematological malignancies is initiated by two major pathways (Fulda 2009b); both pathways converge terminally to activate "effector" caspases including caspases -6, -7, and -3 (Schimmer et al. 2001). These cysteine proteases mediate the dismantling of essential structural and biochemical elements of the cell. The intrinsic pathway is activated by DNA damage, among other stimuli, that leads to changes in mitochondrial permeability, usually through elevation of p53. This leads to the release of proapoptotic factors from the intermembrane space into the cytoplasm: cytochrome c, second mitochondria-derived activator of caspase (Smac)/direct inhibitor of apoptosis binding protein with low pI (DIABLO), apoptosis inducing factor (AIF) and Omi/high temperature requirement protein A2 (HtrA2) (Kroemer and Blomgren 2007). Cytochrome c interacts with Apaf-1 and procaspase 9 within the apoptosome to activate caspase 9, an "initiator" caspase that in turn activates downstream effector caspases. The extrinsic pathway is activated by the engagement of death receptors of the tumor necrosis family such as the CD95 receptor and TNF-related apoptosis inducing ligand (TRAIL) receptor. Upon ligand binding Fas-associated death receptor domain (FADD) and caspase 8, another initiator caspase, form the death-induced signaling complex (DISC).

The Bcl-2 family of proteins is made up of individual members that modulate the apoptotic response (Adams and Cory 2007). The family is composed of antiapoptotic members such as Bcl-2, Bcl-X_L, and Mcl-1 and proapoptotic members like Bax and Bak. BH3 only proteins are important proapoptotic molecules such as Bim, Bid, Bad, Bik, Noxa, and Puma. While the exact mechanism of their interaction is controversial, the relative balance of family members appears to sensitize the cell to apoptosis. Activation of Bax and/or Bak leads to oligomerization on the mitochondrial membrane and loss of membrane integrity. Antiapoptotic proteins like Bcl-2, Bcl-XL, and Mcl-1 inhibit Bax/Bak activation. Certain BH-3 proteins like Bim, tBid (the activated form of Bid), and Puma bind all antiapoptotic Bcl-2 family members, whereas the others bind selected members. BH-3 proteins either directly activate Bax/Bak or indirectly activate them by interfering with antiapoptotic proteins.

Inhibitors of apoptosis (IAP) proteins are endogenous caspase inhibitors that provide another layer of modulation to the apoptotic pathway (Hunter et al. 2007). There are eight human homologs including X-linked inhibitor of apoptosis (XIAP), cellular IAP1 (cIAP1), surviving BIRC5 and living among others. IAP proteins prevent apoptosis through a variety of mechanisms depending on the individual family member, including direct inhibition of caspase enzymatic function, promotion of caspase protein degradation, stabilization of other IAPs, and inhibition of Smac/DIABLO.

Corruption of the basic apoptotic machinery allowing evasion of cell death is postulated to be one of the universal steps in the multistep process of cancer development. A key development in the field was the cloning of the t(14;18) characteristic of adult lymphomas, where juxtaposition of the *IGH* locus leads to overexpression of Bcl-2. However, the prognostic relevance of Bcl-2 family proteins in childhood ALL has not be shown conclusively. Bcl-2 levels were not predictive of outcome in the majority of studies published and levels are not elevated at relapse (Coustan-Smith et al. 1996). Paradoxically, in one study, a high Bcl-2/Bax ratio was associated with a good outcome, but in another study, a low Bax/Bcl-2 ratio was observed at relapse (Prokop et al. 2000). Conflicting results concerning the prognostic relevance of Bcl-2 family expression indicate a complex relationship that may be related to the relative balance of pro- and antiapoptotic members. Indeed, in looking at apoptotic protein expression *in vivo* following chemotherapy, Bcl-2 levels were stable, whereas, Bax levels either remained stable, increased, or decreased (Liu et al. 2002).

Other components of the apoptotic machinery have been examined for their role in childhood ALL especially as they may modulate therapeutic response. Many chemotherapeutic agents lead to increased p53 protein levels and activation of the intrinsic apoptotic pathway. p53 mutations are distinctly rare in childhood ALL, although elevated MDM-2, a protein that degrades p53, has been noted to be overexpressed at relapse (Marks et al. 1997). Certain drugs, like steroids and vincristine, initiate apoptosis via non-p53 dependent mechanisms and even p53-dependent drugs like anthracyclines can initiate apoptosis *in vivo* without up-regulation of p53. While mutations in *CD-95* were identified in T-ALL, they were not observed in B-precursor ALL, and levels of CD-95, not sensitivity to CD-95-induced apoptosis, correlated with response or outcome in childhood ALL (Beltinger et al. 1998). However, low levels of caspase 8-associated protein are associated with high levels of minimal residual disease, thus implicating participation of the extrinsic pathway in treatment response. The sensitivity of ALL cells to glucocorticoids appears in part to be related to up-regulation of the proapoptotic Bim protein while resistance in infants with *MLL* rearranged ALL is predicted based on higher levels of antiapoptotic *Mcl-1* transcripts (Stam et al. 2010; Bachmann et al. 2005). *Survivin* levels were prognostic of outcome of B-precursor ALL in one study, while others investigators have reported high levels at relapse (Bhojwani et al. 2006).

The elucidation of the apoptotic pathway has provided new opportunities for drug development to promote apoptosis in cancer cells with new agents alone or in combination with conventional chemotherapy and irradiation. The first agent targeting the apoptotic pathway focused on Bcl-2, since overexpression confers chemoresistance. Oblimersen sodium (G3139, Genasense) is a *BCL-2* antisense oligodeoxynucleotide that leads to degradation of *BCL-2* mRNA (O'Brien et al. 2005). Preclinical models show that oblimersen can induce apoptosis alone and is synergistic with conventional agents. There is data to indicate that its mechanism of action may also be due to nonantisense effects mediated by the CpG motifs present in the molecule (Kim et al. 2007). Oblimersen has been evaluated in a number of clinical trials including those involving patients with chronic lymphocytic leukemia, acute myelogenous leukemia, multiple myeloma, and small cell lung cancer among others (Kang and Reynolds 2009). While there was a suggestion in some of these trials that oblimersen might have added a survival advantage, the drug is yet to gain FDA approval.

More recently, a series of small molecules has been developed that interact directly with Bcl-2 proteins (e.g., Bcl-2, Bcl-XL, Mcl-1, and Bcl-w) at their hydrophobic binding groove in the place of BH3 only proteins. These "BH3 mimetics" include gossypol, ABT-737, ABT-263 (an oral version of ABT-737), GX15-070 (Obatoclax), and others. Each has differing affinities for Bcl-2 protein family members, and preclinical evaluation documents increased response to conventional radiation and chemotherapy. These agents are actively being explored in clinical trials for a wide variety of malignancies including ALL (Kang and Reynolds 2009).

Finally, since increased expression of IAPs has correlated with outcome in some hematological malignancies, multiple strategies have been developed to negate the antiapoptotic effect of these proteins (Fulda 2009b). Based on the structure of Smac binding to XIAP (Bir3) as well as cIAP 1 and cIAP2, small molecule antagonists of IAPs have been developed. Since the BIR2 domain of XIAP interacts with caspase-3, XIAP BIR2 antagonists have also been developed. Survivin is a particularly attractive target since expression is enhanced in tumor cells compared to normal cells. Gene expression profiling has also shown that *survivin* is upregulated in ALL blasts at relapse (Bhojwani et al. 2006). Many Phase II trials are now evaluating LY2813008, a *survivin* antisense oligonucleotide, and agents to repress *survivin* transcription (YM155 and EM-1421) are also in early phase protocols.

2.6 TheB iologyo fR elapsedA LL

A central question related to the biology of relapse is what is the origin of the relapsed clone? Does it emerge with therapy or was it present at diagnosis? Is relapse a completely new clone or did it surface from a reservoir of premalignant cancer stem cells? Many studies have confirmed that relapsed blasts demonstrate biological differences from those noted at diagnosis. (Lilleyman et al. 1995; Guglielmi et al. 1997) However, analysis of antigen receptor rearrangements confirms that, in almost all cases, relapsed blasts are clonally related to the original disease. As mentioned, rearrangements of the T-cell receptor (*TCR*) and immunoglobulin (*Ig*) genes are clonal markers that can be detected in 90% of B-precursor ALL and 95% of T-cell ALL cases. While 40–50% of all relapse samples display a new rearrangement, at least one stable clonal *Ig/TCR* rearrangement is almost always observed (>95%) at relapse. (Szczepanski et al. 2002; Germano et al. 2003) Furthermore, studies show that the relapsed sample almost always contains the same dominant karyotypic features observed at initial diagnosis (Heerema et al. 1992). Thus studies prove, with rare exceptions, that relapse is clonally related to the disease at diagnosis. Despite this, the only consistent genetic change characteristic of relapse involves frequent deletions involving 9p, consistent with $p16^{INK4a}$ deletion/inactivation (Germanoe ta l. 2003).

A number of studies examining antigen receptor rearrangements on a broader range of diagnosis/relapse samples have now shown that, in many cases, the relapsed clone existed at diagnosis, albeit making up a minor subset of the bulk leukemia population (Guggemos et al. 2003). These resistant cells showed a much lower rate of regression after application of initial chemotherapy and the greater their numerical contribution to the bulk leukemia at diagnosis, the shorter the duration of first remission (Choi et al. 2007). However, while the relapse clone could be detected at diagnosis in many cases, this was not a uniform finding, still suggesting that some relapses may be due to the genesis of additional mutations during therapy (Henderson et al. 2008). Finally, in a select number of relapse cases defined by the presence of the t(12;21) *ETV6/RUNX1* (*TEL-AML1*) fusion, there is evidence of a fetal preleukemic stem cell that acts as a reservoir for the re-emergence of a clonally related second leukemia (Seeger et al. 2001; Pine et al. 2003; Zuna et al. 2004).

The development of chemoresistance is another key issue in relapsed ALL, as evidenced by the lower remission re-Induction rate and event-free survival. Ex vivo analysis of chemosensitivity to individual agents demonstrates that relapsed samples are significantly more resistant to 6-thiogaunine, vincristine, prednisone, dexamethasone, cytarabine, doxorubicin, idarubicin, and steroids (Hongo and Fujii 1991; Klumper et al. 1995). Resistance to steroids is the most dramatic difference noted in relapsed blasts.

Global gene expression analysis correlating gene expression signatures with drug resistance provides for a nonbiased approach to identifying biological pathways responsible for drug resistance and relapse of the disease. Recent analysis of *in vitro* resistant vs. sensitive samples led to the definition of genes whose protein products play a role in drug resistance (Holleman et al. 2004). Differentially expressed genes were noted for cells resistant to four drugs commonly used in therapy. Notably, 121 of these 124 genes had previously never been implicated in resistance to the four agents studied. Furthermore, resistance genes were unique to each agent and no single cross-resistance gene was identified. In a follow-up study, 45 genes were identified for which expression correlated with cross-resistance to all four agents, as well as an unanticipated signature that was associated with sensitivity to asparaginase and resistance to vincristine (Lugthart et al. 2005).

Gene expression profiles of 35 matched diagnosis/relapse pairs (32 B-precursor cases) revealed 126 probe sets (48 high at diagnosis, 78 high at relapse) that were significantly different at relapse compared to diagnosis in B-precursor ALL (pair wise analysis: false discovery rate <10%). The most striking difference was the much greater representation of genes involved in proliferation, cell cycle control, and cellular metabolism in samples at early relapse (Bhojwani et al. 2006). Previous studies have also noted that relapsed blasts are in a higher proliferative state (Staber et al. 2004; Beesley et al. 2005). Genes that were identified, including those involved in DNA repair (e.g., *PTTG1, RAD51, POLE2*) and those that play a role in inhibiting apoptosis (e.g., *survivin (BIRC5), AATF, API5, AVEN*), may aid the cells in overcoming the toxic effects of DNA damaging chemotherapeutic agents. Importantly, many of these genes such as *survivin (BIRC5)* are attractive targets for therapeutic intervention.

While gene expression studies are informative, they are incapable of distinguishing "driver" vs. "passenger" pathways. To discover genes and pathways fundamentally involved in drug resistance, many investigators have performed copy number analysis, reasoning that the identification of unique copy number abnormalities (CNAs) at relapse could be associated with outgrowth of a clone that escaped chemotherapy. In a pilot cohort of 20 diagnosis/relapse leukemia pairs from B-precursor ALL patients, genome-wide copy number profiles were surveyed using Affymetrix 500K SNP arrays. (Yang et al. 2008) This analysis revealed a total of 758 somatic genetic lesions. The number of genetic lesions varied significantly among patients, ranging from 3 to 84 per sample. These CNAs included gross copy number changes indicated by conventional cytogenetic analysis, but were mostly cryptic. Thus, the median size of CNAs identified in this study was 353 Kb, with 22.7% < 100 Kb, and 66.4% < 1 Mb. The median copy number loss per sample was 9 at diagnosis and 9.5 at relapse. Copy number gains were less common ($p < 0.001$), with a median of only 3.5 amplification events per sample at diagnosis and 4 at relapse. Across patients, there was a modest increase of CNAs at relapse ($p = 0.035$). Systematic enumeration of CNA events in the matched diagnosis and relapse samples revealed features that are common and those that differ at these two time points. Of the 74 copy number gains observed at diagnosis, 71 (94.7%) persisted in the relapse sample from the same individual. Likewise, 256 of 288 (88.9%) copy number loss events at diagnosis remained at relapse. Conversely, 24 novel amplifications and 45 novel deletions arose at relapse, accounting for 25.0% and 14.9% of total copy number gains and losses at relapse, respectively. It should also be noted that the majority of the diagnosis or relapse-specific CNAs were focal, with a median size of 537 Kb. There was a significant correlation between the change in DNA copy number and change in gene expression from diagnosis to relapse ($p = 2.2 \times 10^{-16}$).

Although all 44 autosome arms showed one or more CNAs, a number of regions appeared to be affected more frequently. The most common CNA events were deletions at 9p21.3, occurring in 12 of 20 (60.0%) cases and persisting from diagnosis to relapse. Of these 12 cases, 11 exhibited deletion of both *CDKN2A* and *CDKN2B*, consistent with prior reports (Maloney et al.

1999; Graf Einsiedel et al. 2002). CNAs involving several transcription regulators essential in early lymphoid specification and B-lineage commitment (Nutt and Kee 2007) (*PAX5*, *EBF1*, and *IKZF1*) were also common in this relapsed ALL cohort. Somatically acquired deletions at these four loci (*CDKN2A/B*, *PAX5*, *EBF1*, and *IKZF1*) have been previously reported in childhood ALL. (Maloney et al. 1999; Graf Einsiedel et al. 2002; Mullighan et al. 2007; French et al. 2009) However, the frequencies of these lesions (except *PAX5*) appeared to be higher in the relapsed cases analyzed here relative to newly diagnosed B-precursor ALL (Mullighan et al. 2007) *CDKN2A*, 60.0% vs. 33.9% ($p = 0.038$); *EBF1*, 25.0% vs. 4.2% ($p = 0.0013$); and *IKZF1*: 35.0% vs. 8.9% ($p = 0.0016$). Overrepresentation of these genetic aberrations, especially *IKZF1* and *EBF1* in relapsed ALL cases indicate their potential prognostic value at diagnosis. The fact that numerous examples were identified in which *IKZF1* and *EBF1* deletions were seen only in the relapse clone indicates that such deletions may not be required for full transformation, but that they endow a subclone with drug resistance properties. Other investigators have published similar findings in 47 matched pairs of B-precursor ALL (Mullighan et al. 2008b). While many regions of interest were identical in the two studies, there were clear differences. Whether these differences are due to variations in therapeutic regimens can be answered only with a larger data set.

These results show clear differences in the genetic profile of blasts from patients who relapse early vs. late, consistent with the better (but still suboptimal) salvage rates for those patients who relapse off therapy. (Fig. 2.8) shows a model that incorporates findings from many laboratories. In this model, most cases of early relapse occur because an intrinsically drug-resistant (IDR) clone exists at diagnosis before therapy is initiated. Under the selective pressure of chemotherapy the clone emerges relatively soon in treatment. In another scenario, a subclone that may or may not represent a leukemic stem cell (LSC) and is relatively resistant to standard therapy undergoes additional genetic events that lead to drug resistance (acquired drug resistance, ADR). A version of this second model is represented by late relapsing *ETV6/RunX1* cases described to date, which represent a "new" but clonally related clone that is sensitive to retreatment since it emanates from a LSC. However, more commonly, the low salvage rates

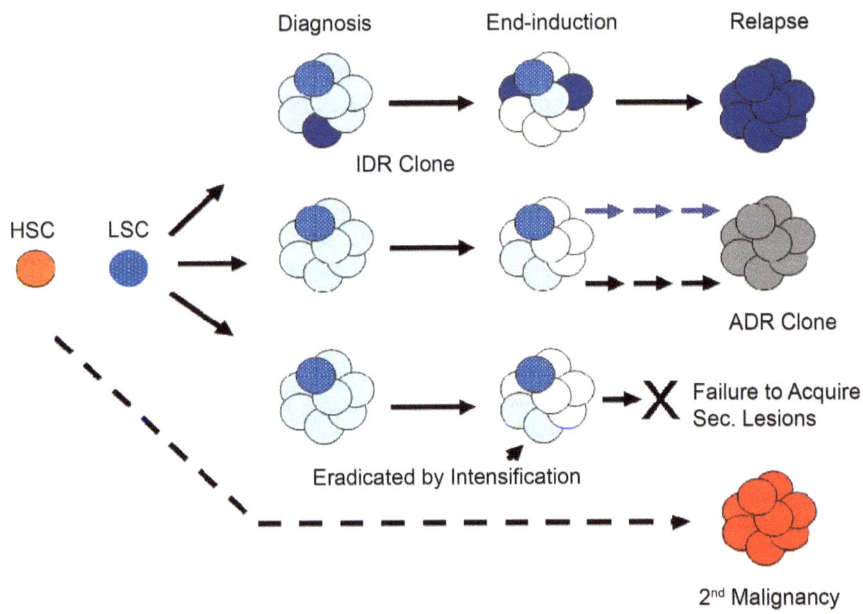

Fig. 2.8 Hypothetical Model of Relapsed ALL. A pre-leukemic stem cell (LSC, blue) gives rise to frank ALL (light blue cells). Intrinsically drug resistant (IDR) clones (dark blue) may be present at diagnosis. LSCs and other subclones may survive initial treatment and acquire additional lesions that result in acquired drug resistance (ADR). IDR clones are more likely to account for early relapse whereas more cases of late relapse are associatedw ithA DRc lones

seen in most cases of late relapse indicate that acquired drug resistance is operative (for example, not a "new leukemia"). In both models (IDR and ADR clones), residual blasts at end-Induction signify a greater likelihood of relapse. However, the remaining clones in these two cases are qualitatively different insofar as in the second scenario, additional mutations and or epigenetic lesions are needed to result in the drug-resistant phenotype. Early Intensification is capable of eradicating such clones, but failure to apply augmented therapy early allows a window for such changes to occur. Finally, in a small number of cases, relapse represents a true non-clonally related second malignancy.

2.7 Summary

ALL is a biologically heterogeneous disease represented by distinct clinical and biological subtypes. Recent data using genome-wide approaches indicates that certain individuals may be predisposed to the development of ALL and host differences are likely to account for some differences in response to therapy also. ALL is a multistep process requiring the acquisition of multiple somatic lesions, and the definition of such pathways are being elucidated, including those lesions directly associated with drug resistance. These pathways are now being used for treatment assignment and serve as targets for novel therapy.

References

Adams JM, Cory S (2007) The Bcl-2 apoptotic switch in cancer development and therapy. Oncogene 26(9):1324–1337

Adolfsson J, Mansson R et al (2005) Identification of Flt3+ lympho-myeloid stem cells lacking erythro-megakaryocytic potential a revised road map for adult blood lineage commitment. Cell 121(2):295–306

Arico M, Valsecchi MG et al (2000) Outcome of treatment in children with Philadelphia chromosome-positive acute lymphoblastic leukemia. N Engl J Med 342(14):998–1006

Armstrong SA, Staunton JE et al (2001) MLL translocations specify a distinct gene expression profile that distinguishes a unique leukemia. Nat Genet 30(1):41–47

Attarbaschi A, Mann G et al (2008) Minimal residual disease values discriminate between low and high relapse risk in children with B-cell precursor acute lymphoblastic leukemia and an intrachromosomal amplification of chromosome 21: the Austrian and German acute lymphoblastic leukemia Berlin-Frankfurt-Munster (ALL-BFM) trials. J Clin Oncol 26(18):3046–3050

Bachmann PS, Gorman R et al (2005) Dexamethasone resistance in B-cell precursor childhood acute lymphoblastic leukemia occurs downstream of ligand-induced nuclear translocation of the glucocorticoid receptor. Blood 105(6): 2519–2526

Bartel DP (2004) MicroRNAs: genomics, biogenesis, mechanism, and function. Cell 116(2):281–297

Beesley AH, Cummings AJ et al (2005) The gene expression signature of relapse in paediatric acute lymphoblastic leukaemia: implications for mechanisms of therapy failure. Br J Haematol131(4):447–456

Beishuizen A, de Bruijn MA et al (1997) Heterogeneity in junctional regions of immunoglobulin kappa deleting element rearrangements in B cell leukemias: a new molecular target for detection of minimal residual disease. Leukemia 11(12): 2200–2207

Belson M, Kingsley B et al (2007) Risk factors for acute leukemia in children: a review. Environ Health Perspect 115(1): 138–145

Beltinger C, Bohler T et al (1998) Mutation analysis of CD95 (APO-1/Fas) in childhood B-lineage acute lymphoblastic leukaemia. Br J Haematol 102(3):722–728

Bene MC, Castoldi G et al (1995) Proposals for the immunological classification of acute leukemias. European Group for the Immunological Characterization of Leukemias (EGIL). Leukemia 9(10):1783–1786

Bercovich D, Ganmore I et al (2008) Mutations of JAK2 in acute lymphoblastic leukaemias associated with Down's syndrome. Lancet 372(9648):1484–1492

Bhojwani D, Kang H et al (2008) Gene expression signatures predictive of early response and outcome in high-risk childhood acute lymphoblastic leukemia: A Children's Oncology Group Study [corrected]. J Clin Oncol 26(27): 4376–4384

Bhojwani D, Kang H et al (2006) Biologic pathways associated with relapse in childhood acute lymphoblastic leukemia: a Children's Oncology Group study. Blood 108(2): 711–717

Bryder D, Rossi DJ et al (2006) Hematopoietic stem cells: the paradigmatic tissue specific stem cell. Am J Pathol 169: 338–346

Bryder D, Sigvardsson M (2010) Shaping up a lineage – lessons from B lymphopoesis. Curr Opin Immunol 22(2):148–153

Busslinger M (2004) Transcriptional control of early B cell development. Annu Rev Immunol 22:55–79

Calin GA, Ferracin M et al (2005) A MicroRNA signature associated with prognosis and progression in chronic lymphocytic leukemia. N Engl J Med 353(17):1793–1801

Carter NP, Meyer EW (1994) Introduction to the principles of flow cytometry. In: Ormerod MG (ed) Flow cytometry: a practical approach. Oxford University Press, New York

Case M, Matheson E et al (2008) Mutation of genes affecting the RAS pathway is common in childhood acute lymphoblastic leukemia. Cancer Res 68(16):6803–6809

Castor A, Nilsson L et al (2005) Distinct patterns of hematopoietic stem cell involvement in acute lymphoblastic leukemia. Nat Med 11(6):630–637

Cazzaniga G, Biondi A (2005) Molecular monitoring of childhood acute lymphoblastic leukemia using antigen receptor

gene rearrangements and quantitative polymerase chain reactionte chnology.H aematologica90(3):382–390
Chen CL, Liu Q et al (1997) Higher frequency of glutathione S-transferase deletions in black children with acute lymphoblastic leukemia. Blood 89(5):1701–1707
Cheok MH, Yang W et al (2003) Treatment-specific changes in gene expression discriminate *in vivo* drug response in human leukemia cells. Nat Genet 34(1):85–90
Choi S, Henderson MJ et al (2007) Relapse in children with acute lymphoblastic leukemia involving selection of a preexisting drug-resistant subclone. Blood 110(2):632–639
Clark SJ, Harrison J et al (1994) High sensitivity mapping of methylated cytosines. Nucleic Acids Res 22(15): 2990–2997
Clarke MF, Dick JE et al (2006) Cancer stem cells–perspectives on current status and future directions: AACR Workshop on cancer stem cells. Cancer Res 66(19):9339–9344
Cobaleda C, Gutierrez-Cianca N et al (2000) A primitive hematopoietic cell is the target for the leukemic transformation in human philadelphia-positive acute lymphoblastic leukemia. Blood 95(3):1007–1013
Coustan-Smith E, Kitanaka A et al (1996) Clinical relevance of BCL-2 overexpression in childhood acute lymphoblastic leukemia. Blood 87(3):1140–1146
Czerny T, Busslinger M (1995) DNA-binding and transactivation properties of Pax-6: three amino acids in the paired domain are responsible for the different sequence recognition of Pax-6 and BSAP (Pax-5). Mol Cell Biol 15(5): 2858–2871
Den Boer ML, van Slegtenhorst M et al (2009) A subtype of childhood acute lymphoblastic leukaemia with poor treatment outcome: a genome-wide classification study. Lancet Oncol10(2):125–1 34
Druker BJ, Sawyers CL et al (2001) Activity of a specific inhibitor of the BCR-ABL tyrosine kinase in the blast crisis of chronic myeloid leukemia and acute lymphoblastic leukemia with the Philadelphia chromosome. N Engl J Med 344(14):1038–104 2
Dutt A, Beroukhim R (2007) Single nucleotide polymorphism array analysis of cancer. Curr Opin Oncol 19(1):43–49
Ferrando AA (2009) The role of NOTCH1 signaling in T-ALL. Hematology Am Soc Hematol Educ Program 353–361
Flohr T, Schrauder A et al (2008) Minimal residual disease-directed risk stratification using real-time quantitative PCR analysis of immunoglobulin and T-cell receptor gene rearrangements in the international multicenter trial AIEOP-BFM ALL 2000 for childhood acute lymphoblastic leukemia. Leukemia22(4):771–782
Ford AM, Bennett CA et al (1998) Fetal origins of the TEL-AML1 fusion gene in identical twins with leukemia. Proc Natl Acad Sci USA 95(8):4584–4588
French D, Yang W et al (2009) Acquired variation outweighs inherited variation in whole genome analysis of methotrexate polyglutamate accumulation in leukemia. Blood 113(19): 4512–4520
Fulci V, Colombo T et al (2009) Characterization of B- and T-lineage acute lymphoblastic leukemia by integrated analysis of MicroRNA and mRNA expression profiles. Genes Chromosomes Cancer 48(12):1069–1082
Fulda S (2009a) Apoptosis pathways and their therapeutic exploitation in pancreatic cancer. J Cell Mol Med 13(7): 1221–1227
Fulda S (2009b) Therapeutic opportunities for counteracting apoptosis resistance in childhood leukaemia. Br J Haematol 145(4):441–454
Garcia-Manero G, Issa JP (2005) Histone deacetylase inhibitors: a review of their clinical status as antineoplastic agents. Cancer Invest 23(7):635–642
Garcia-Manero G, Jeha S et al (2003) Aberrant DNA methylation in pediatric patients with acute lymphocytic leukemia. Cancer97(3):695–702
Garcia-Manero G, Yang H et al (2009) Epigenetics of acute lymphocytic leukemia. Semin Hematol 46(1):24–32
Germano G, del Giudice L et al (2003) Clonality profile in relapsed precursor-B-ALL children by GeneScan and sequencing analyses. Consequences on minimal residual disease monitoring. Leukemia 17(8):1573–1582
Ghia P, ten Boekel E et al (1998) B-cell development: a comparison between mouse and man. Immunol Today 19(10):480–485
Goemans BF, Zwaan CM et al (2005) *In vitro* profiling of the sensitivity of pediatric leukemia cells to tipifarnib: identification of T-cell ALL and FAB M5 AML as the most sensitive subsets. Blood 106(10):3532–3537
Graf Einsiedel H, Taube T et al (2002) Deletion analysis of p16(INKa) and p15(INKb) in relapsed childhood acute lymphoblastic leukemia. Blood 99(12):4629–4631
Greaves M (2006) Infection, immune responses and the aetiology of childhood leukaemia. Nat Rev Cancer 6(3):193–203
Greaves M (2009) Darwin and evolutionary tales in leukemia. American Society of Hematology, New Orleans
Guggemos A, Eckert C et al (2003) Assessment of clonal stability of minimal residual disease targets between 1st and 2nd relapse of childhood precursor B-cell acute lymphoblastic leukemia. Haematologica 88(7):737–746
Guglielmi C, Cordone I et al (1997) Immunophenotype of adult and childhood acute lymphoblastic leukemia: changes at first relapse and clinico-prognostic implications. Leukemia 11(9):1501–1507
Gutierrez MI, Siraj AK et al (2003) Concurrent methylation of multiple genes in childhood ALL: Correlation with phenotype and molecular subgroup. Leukemia 17(9): 1845–1850
Harrison CJ, Moorman AV et al (2004) Three distinct subgroups of hypodiploidy in acute lymphoblastic leukaemia. Br J Haematol125(5):552–559
Harvey R, Mulligan RC et al (2010a) Identification of novel cluster groups in pediatric high-risk B-precursor acute lymphoblastic leukemia with gene expression profiling: correlation with genomw wide copy mumber alterations, clinical charactersitics, and outcome
Harvey RC, Mullighan CG et al (2010b) Rearrangement of CRLF2 is associated with mutation of JAK kinases, alteration of IKZF1, Hispanic/Latino ethnicity, and a poor outcome in pediatric B-progenitor acute lymphoblastic leukemia. Blood 115 (26): 5312–5321
Hayday AC, Pennington DJ (2007) Key factors in the organized chaos of early T cell development. Nat Immunol 8(2): 137–144
Heerema NA, Nachman JB et al (2004) Deletion of 7p or monosomy 7 in pediatric acute lymphoblastic leukemia is an adverse prognostic factor: a report from the Children's Cancer Group. Leukemia 18(5):939–947
Heerema NA, Palmer CG et al (1992) Cytogenetic analysis in relapsed childhood acute lymphoblastic leukemia. Leukemia 6(3):185–192
Heerema NA, Sather HN et al (2000) Clinical significance of deletions of chromosome arm 6q in childhood acute

lymphoblastic leukemia: a report from the Children's Cancer Group. Leuk Lymphoma 36(5–6):467–478
Henderson MJ, Choi S et al (2008) Mechanism of relapse in pediatric acute lymphoblastic leukemia. Cell Cycle 7(10): 1315–1320
Hertzberg L, Vendramini E et al (2010) Down syndrome acute lymphoblastic leukemia, a highly heterogeneous disease in which aberrant expression of CRLF2 is associated with mutated JAK2: a report from the International BFM Study Group. Blood 115(5):1006–1017
Hoffmann K, Firth MJ et al (2008) Prediction of relapse in paediatric pre-B acute lymphoblastic leukaemia using a three-gene risk index. Br J Haematol 140(6):656–664
Holleman A, Cheok MH et al (2004) Gene-expression patterns in drug-resistant acute lymphoblastic leukemia cells and response to treatment. N Engl J Med 351(6):533–542
Hong D, Gupta R et al (2008) Initiating and cancer-propagating cells in TEL-AML1-associated childhood leukemia. Science 319(5861):336–339
Hongo T, Fujii Y (1991) *In vitro* chemosensitivity of lymphoblasts at relapse in childhood leukemia using the MTT assay. Int J Hematol 54(3):219–230
Hotfilder M, Rottgers S et al (2002) Immature CD34+CD19– progenitor/stem cells in TEL/AML1-positive acute lymphoblastic leukemia are genetically and functionally normal. Blood100(2):640–646
Hunter AM, LaCasse EC et al (2007) The inhibitors of apoptosis (IAPs) as cancer targets. Apoptosis 12(9):1543–1568
Iorio MV, Croce CM (2009) MicroRNAs in cancer: small molecules with a huge impact. J Clin Oncol 27(34):5848–5856
Janeway CA, Travers P et al (2001) Immunobiology. Garland, New York, London
Jones PA, Baylin SB (2007) The epigenomics of cancer. Cell 128(4):683–692
Kang H, Chen IM et al (2010) Gene expression classifiers for relapse-free survival and minimal residual disease improve risk classification and outcome prediction in pediatric B-precursor acute lymphoblastic leukemia. Blood 115(7):1394–1405
Kang MH, Reynolds CP (2009) Bcl-2 inhibitors: targeting mitochondrial apoptotic pathways in cancer therapy. Clin Cancer Res15(4):1126–11 32
Kim R, Emi M et al (2007) Antisense and nonantisense effects of antisense Bcl-2 on multiple roles of Bcl-2 as a chemosensitizer in cancer therapy. Cancer Gene Ther 14(1):1–11
Klumper E, Pieters R et al (1995) *In vitro* cellular drug resistance in children with relapsed/refractory acute lymphoblastic leukemia. Blood 86(10):3861–3868
Korenberg JR, Chen XN et al (1994) Down syndrome phenotypes: the consequences of chromosomal imbalance. Proc Natl Acad Sci USA 91(11):4997–5001
Kotani A, Ha D et al (2009) miR-128b is a potent glucocorticoid sensitizer in MLL-AF4 acute lymphocytic leukemia cells and exerts cooperative effects with miR-221. Blood 114(19):4169–4178
Krajinovic M, Labuda D et al (2002a) Polymorphisms in genes encoding drugs and xenobiotic metabolizing enzymes, DNA repair enzymes, and response to treatment of childhood acute lymphoblastic leukemia. Clin Cancer Res 8(3):802–810
Krajinovic M, Sinnett H et al (2002b) Role of NQO1, MPO and CYP2E1 genetic polymorphisms in the susceptibility to childhood acute lymphoblastic leukemia. Int J Cancer 97(2):230–236
Krivtsov AV, Twomey D et al (2006) Transformation from committed progenitor to leukaemia stem cell initiated by MLL-AF9. Nature 442(7104):818–822
Kroemer G, Blomgren K (2007) Mitochondrial cell death control in familial Parkinson disease. PLoS Biol 5(7):e206
Laird PW (2010) Principles and challenges of genome-wide DNA methylation analysis. Nat Rev Genet 11(3):191–203
Lange B (2000) The management of neoplastic disorders of haematopoiesis in children with Down's syndrome. Br J Haematol110(3):512–524
Lapidot T, Sirard C et al (1994) A cell initiating human acute myeloid leukaemia after transplantation into SCID mice. Nature367(6464):645–648
le Viseur C, Hotfilder M et al (2008) In childhood acute lymphoblastic leukemia, blasts at different stages of immunophenotypic maturation have stem cell properties. Cancer Cell 14(1):47–58
Lilleyman JS, Stevens RF et al (1995) Changes in cytomorphology of childhood lymphoblastic leukaemia at the time of disease relapse. Childhood Leukaemia Working Party of the United Kingdom Medical Research Council. J Clin Pathol 48(11):1051–1053
Liu T, Raetz E et al (2002) Diversity of the apoptotic response to chemotherapy in childhood leukemia. Leukemia 16(2): 223–232
Loh ML, Rubnitz JE (2002) TEL/AML1-positive pediatric leukemia: prognostic significance and therapeutic approaches. Curr Opin Hematol 9(4):345–352
Lugthart S, Cheok MH et al (2005) Identification of genes associated with chemotherapy crossresistance and treatment response in childhood acute lymphoblastic leukemia. Cancer Cell7(4):375–386
Malinge S, Ben-Abdelali R et al (2007) Novel activating JAK2 mutation in a patient with Down syndrome and B-cell precursor acute lymphoblastic leukemia. Blood 109(5): 2202–2204
Malinge S, Izraeli S et al (2009) Insights into the manifestations, outcomes, and mechanisms of leukemogenesis in Down syndrome. Blood 113(12):2619–2628
Maloney KW, McGavran L et al (1999) Acquisition of p16(INK4A) and p15(INK4B) gene abnormalities between initial diagnosis and relapse in children with acute lymphoblastic leukemia. Blood 93(7):2380–2385
Marks DI, Kurz BW et al (1997) Altered expression of p53 and mdm-2 proteins at diagnosis is associated with early treatment failure in childhood acute lymphoblastic leukemia. J Clin Oncol 15(3):1158–1162
Mason D, Andre P et al (2002) Leucocyte Typoing VII. Oxford University Press, Oxford
Meshinchi S, Appelbaum FR (2009) Structural and functional alterations of FLT3 in acute myeloid leukemia. Clin Cancer Res15(13):4263–4269
Mi S, Lu J et al (2007) MicroRNA expression signatures accurately discriminate acute lymphoblastic leukemia from acute myeloid leukemia. Proc Natl Acad Sci USA 104(50): 19971–19976
Moorman AV, Richards SM et al (2007) Prognosis of children with acute lymphoblastic leukemia (ALL) and intrachromosomal amplification of chromosome 21 (iAMP21). Blood 109(6):2327–2330
Mori H, Colman SM et al (2002) Chromosome translocations and covert leukemic clones are generated during normal

fetal development. Proc Natl Acad Sci USA 99(12): 8242–8247
Muller A, Florek M (2010) 5-Azacytidine/Azacitidine. Recent Results Cancer Res 184:159–170
Mullighan CG, Goorha S et al (2007a) Genome-wide analysis of genetic alterations in acute lymphoblastic leukaemia. Nature 446(7137):758–764
Mullighan CG, Miller CB et al (2008a) BCR-ABL1 lymphoblastic leukaemia is characterized by the deletion of Ikaros. Nature453(7191):1 10–114
Mullighan CG, Phillips LA et al (2008b) Genomic analysis of the clonal origins of relapsed acute lymphoblastic leukemia. Science322(5906): 1377–1380
Mullighan CG, Collins-Underwood JR et al (2009a) Rearrangement of CRLF2 in B-progenitor- and Down syndrome-associated acute lymphoblastic leukemia. Nat Genet 41: 1243–1246
Mullighan CG, Su X et al (2009b) Deletion of IKZF1 and prognosis in acute lymphoblastic leukemia. N Engl J Med 360(5):470–480
Mullighan CG, Zhang J et al (2009c) JAK mutations in high-risk childhood acute lymphoblastic leukemia. Proc Natl Acad Sci USA 106(23):9414–9418
Mullighan RC, Morin RD et al (2009d) Next generation transcriptomic resequencing identifies novel genetic alterations in high-risk (HR) childhood acute lymphoblastic leukemia (ALL): a report from the Children's Oncology group HR ALL TARGET Project. Blood 114:704
Nachman JB, Heerema NA et al (2007) Outcome of treatment in children with hypodiploid acute lymphoblastic leukemia. Blood110(4):1112–1115
Nahar R, Muschen M (2009) Pre-B cell receptor signaling in acute lymphoblastic leukemia. Cell Cycle 8(23): 3874–3877
Nowell PC, Hungerford DA (1960) Chromosome studies on normal and leukemic human leukocytes. J Natl Cancer Inst 25:85–109
Nutt SL, Kee BL (2007) The transcriptional regulation of B cell lineage commitment. Immunity 26(6):715–725
O'Brien SM, Cunningham CC et al (2005) Phase I to II multicenter study of oblimersen sodium, a Bcl-2 antisense oligonucleotide, in patients with advanced chronic lymphocytic leukemia. J Clin Oncol 23(30):7697–7702
Papaemmanuil E, Hosking FJ et al (2009) Loci on 7p12.2, 10q21.2 and 14q11.2 are associated with risk of childhood acute lymphoblastic leukemia. Nat Genet 41(9):1006–1010
Pine SR, Wiemels JL et al (2003) TEL-AML1 fusion precedes differentiation to pre-B cells in childhood acute lymphoblastic leukemia. Leuk Res 27(2):155–164
Pongers-Willemse MJ, Seriu T et al (1999) Primers and protocols for standardized detection of minimal residual disease in acute lymphoblastic leukemia using immunoglobulin and T cell receptor gene rearrangements and TAL1 deletions as PCR targets: report of the BIOMED-1 CONCERTED ACTION: investigation of minimal residual disease in acute leukemia. Leukemia 13(1):110–118
Prokop A, Wieder T et al (2000) Relapse in childhood acute lymphoblastic leukemia is associated with a decrease of the Bax/Bcl-2 ratio and loss of spontaneous caspase-3 processing *in vivo*. Leukemia 14(9):1606–1613
Pui CH, Chessells JM et al (2003) Clinical heterogeneity in childhood acute lymphoblastic leukemia with 11q23 rearrangements. Leukemia 17(4):700–706
Pui CH, Gaynon PS et al (2002) Outcome of treatment in childhood acute lymphoblastic leukaemia with rearrangements of the 11q23 chromosomal region. Lancet 359(9321): 1909–1915
Quintas-Cardama A, Cortes J (2009) Molecular biology of bcr-abl1-positive chronic myeloid leukemia. Blood 113(8): 1619–1630
Rabin KR, Wang J et al (2009) Gene expression profiling in Down Syndrome acute lymphoblastic leukemia identifies distinct profiles assocaited with CRLF2 expression. Blood 114:2389
Raimondi SC, Behm FG et al (1990) Cytogenetics of pre-B-cell acute lymphoblastic leukemia with emphasis on prognostic implications of the t(1;19). J Clin Oncol 8(8):1380–1388
Ramirez J, Lukin K et al (2010) From hematopoietic progenitors to B cells: mechanisms of lineage restriction and commitment. Curr Opin Immunol 22(2):177–184
Real PJ, Ferrando AA (2009) NOTCH inhibition and glucocorticoid therapy in T-cell acute lymphoblastic leukemia. Leukemia23(8):1374–1377
Reed JC, Pellecchia M (2005) Apoptosis-based therapies for hematologic malignancies. Blood 106(2):408–418
Robertson KD, Wolffe AP (2000) DNA methylation in health and disease. Nat Rev Genet 1(1):11–19
Roman-Gomez J, Jimenez-Velasco A et al (2007) Poor prognosis in acute lymphoblastic leukemia may relate to promoter hypermethylation of cancer-related genes. Leuk Lymphoma 48(7):1269–1282
Romana SP, Mauchauffe M et al (1995) The t(12;21) of acute lymphoblastic leukemia results in a tel-AML1 gene fusion. Blood85(12):3662–3670
Ross ME, Zhou X et al (2003) Classification of pediatric acute lymphoblastic leukemia by gene expression profiling. Blood 102(8):2951–2959
Rothenberg EV, Moore JE et al (2008) Launching the T-cell-lineage developmental programme. Nat Rev Immunol 8(1): 9–21
Russell LJ, Capasso M et al (2009) Deregulated expression of cytokine receptor gene, CRLF2, is involved in lymphoid transformation in B-cell precursor acute lymphoblastic leukemia. Blood 114(13):2688–2698
Schimmer AD, Hedley DW et al (2001) Receptor- and mitochondrial-mediated apoptosis in acute leukemia: a translational view. Blood 98(13):3541–3553
Schotte D, Chau JC et al (2009) Identification of new microRNA genes and aberrant microRNA profiles in childhood acute lymphoblastic leukemia. Leukemia 23(2):313–322
Schultz KR, Bowman WP et al (2009) Improved early event-free survival with imatinib in Philadelphia chromosome-positive acute lymphoblastic leukemia: a children's oncology group study. J Clin Oncol 27(31):5175–5181
Schultz KR, Pullen DJ et al (2007) Risk- and response-based classification of childhood B-precursor acute lymphoblastic leukemia: a combined analysis of prognostic markers from the Pediatric Oncology Group (POG) and Children's Cancer Group (CCG). Blood 109(3):926–935
Schwarz BA, Sambandam A et al (2007) Selective thymus settling regulated by cytokine and chemokine receptors. J Immunol 178(4):2008–2017
Seeger K, von Stackelberg A et al (2001) Relapse of TEL-AML1–positive acute lymphoblastic leukemia in childhood: a matched-pair analysis. J Clin Oncol 19(13):3188–3193

Silverman LB (2007) Acute lymphoblastic leukemia in infancy. Pediatr Blood Cancer 49(7 Suppl):1070–1073
Silverman LB, McLean TW et al (1997) Intensified therapy for infants with acute lymphoblastic leukemia: results from the Dana-Farber Cancer Institute Consortium. Cancer 80(12): 2285–2295
Sorich MJ, Pottier N et al (2008) *In vivo* response to methotrexate forecasts outcome of acute lymphoblastic leukemia and has a distinct gene expression profile. PLoS Med 5(4):e83
Staber PB, Linkesch W et al (2004) Common alterations in gene expression and increased proliferation in recurrent acute myeloid leukemia. Oncogene 23(4):894–904
Stam RW, den Boer ML et al (2006) Silencing of the tumor suppressor gene FHIT is highly characteristic for MLL gene rearranged infant acute lymphoblastic leukemia. Leukemia 20(2):264–271
Stam RW, Den Boer ML et al (2010) Association of high-level MCL-1 expression with *in vitro* and *in vivo* prednisone resistance in MLL-rearranged infant acute lymphoblastic leukemia. Blood 115(5):1018–1025
Stumpel DJ, Schneider P et al (2009) Specific promoter methylation identifies different subgroups of MLL-rearranged infant acute lymphoblastic leukemia, influences clinical outcome, and provides therapeutic options. Blood 114(27): 5490–5498
Szczepanski T, Orfao A et al (2001) Minimal residual disease in leukaemia patients. Lancet Oncol 2(7):409–417
Szczepanski T, Willemse MJ et al (2002) Comparative analysis of Ig and TCR gene rearrangements at diagnosis and at relapse of childhood precursor-B-ALL provides improved strategies for selection of stable PCR targets for monitoring of minimal residual disease. Blood 99(7):2315–2323
Thompson EC, Cobb BS et al (2007) Ikaros DNA-binding proteins as integral components of B cell developmental-stage-specific regulatory circuits. Immunity 26(3):335–344
Tjio JH, Whang J (1962) Chromosome preparations of bone marrow cells without prior *in vitro* culture or *in vitro* colchicine administration. Stain Technol 37:17–20
Tomlins SA, Rhodes DR et al (2005) Recurrent fusion of TMPRSS2 and ETS transcription factor genes in prostate cancer. Science 310(5748):644–648
Trevino LR, Yang W et al (2009) Germline genomic variants associated with childhood acute lymphoblastic leukemia. Nat Genet 41(9):1001–1005
Trueworthy R, Shuster J et al (1992) Ploidy of lymphoblasts is the strongest predictor of treatment outcome in B-progenitor cell acute lymphoblastic leukemia of childhood: a Pediatric Oncology Group study. J Clin Oncol 10(4):606–613
van der Linden MH, Valsecchi MG et al (2009) Outcome of congenital acute lymphoblastic leukemia treated on the Interfant-99 protocol. Blood 114(18):3764–3768
van der Velden VH, Szczepanski T et al (2003) Age-related patterns of immunoglobulin and T-cell receptor gene rearrangements in precursor-B-ALL: implications for detection of minimal residual disease. Leukemia 17(9):1834–1844
van der Velden VH, van Dongen JJ (2009) MRD detection in acute lymphoblastic leukemia patients using Ig/TCR gene rearrangements as targets for real-time quantitative PCR. Methods Mol Biol 538:115–150
van Dongen JJ, Adriaansen HJ et al (1988) Immunophenotyping of leukaemias and non-Hodgkin's lymphomas. Immunological markers and their CD codes. Neth J Med 33(5–6): 298–314
van Dongen JJ, Wolvers-Tettero IL (1991) Analysis of immunoglobulin and T cell receptor genes. Part I: Basic and technical aspects. Clin Chim Acta 198(1–2):1–91
Whitlock JA, Sather HN et al (2005) Clinical characteristics and outcome of children with Down syndrome and acute lymphoblastic leukemia: a Children's Cancer Group study. Blood106(13):4043–4049
Wong HL, Byun HM et al (2006) Rapid and quantitative method of allele-specific DNA methylation analysis. Biotechniques 41(6):734–739
Yanez L, Bermudez A et al (2009) Successful induction therapy with decitabine in refractory childhood acute lymphoblastic leukemia. Leukemia 23(7):1342–1343
Yang JJ, Bhojwani D et al (2008) Genome-wide copy number profiling reveals molecular evolution from diagnosis to relapse in childhood acute lymphoblastic leukemia. Blood 112(10):4178–4183
Yeoh EJ, Ross ME et al (2002) Classification, subtype discovery, and prediction of outcome in pediatric acute lymphoblastic leukemia by gene expression profiling. Cancer Cell 1(2):133–143
Yoda A, Yoda Y et al (2010) Functional screening identifies CRLF2 in precursor B-cell acute lymphoblastic leukemia. Proc Natl Acad Sci USA 107(1):252–257
Yoshida T, Ng SY et al (2006) Early hematopoietic lineage restrictions directed by Ikaros. Nat Immunol 7(4): 382–391
Zhang J, Mulligan RC et al (2009) Mutations in the RAS Signaling, B-cell development, TP53/RB1, and JAK signaling pathways are common in high risk B-precursor childhood acute lymphoblastic leukemia (ALl): A report from the Children's Oncology group High Risk TARGET Project. Blood114: 85
Zuna J, Ford AM et al (2004) TEL deletion analysis supports a novel view of relapse in childhood acute lymphoblastic leukemia.C linC ancerR es10(16):5355–5360

Biologyo fA cuteMyel oidL eukemia

3

Robert J. Arceci and Soheil Meshinchi

Contents

3.1 Introduction

AML is a heterogeneous and complex disease that is the culmination of the interaction between genetic and epigenetic alterations in the hematopoietic progenitors, leading to dysregulation of multiple critical signal transduction pathways, resulting in hematopoietic insufficiency due to the accumulation of immature myeloid progenitors. Despite identification of numerous cytogenetic, molecular and epigenetic alterations in AML, attempts at defining a unifying disease causing event in AML have failed. In contrast to chronic myeloid leukemia (CML), in which evolution of a single event (*BCR-ABL* translocation) is causally associated with disease pathogenesis, such a single step process does not appear to be responsible in AML pathogenesis. *In vivo* studies have demonstrated that common cytogenetic alterations such as t(8;21) or inv(16) that are highly associated with AML are not sufficient for the disease pathogenesis. These findings led to the hypothesis that evolution of AML may require multiple genetic changes and that the disease may require cooperation between two or more alterations.

One such model suggests that AML is the result of cooperation between two classes of genetic alterations, in which the initial event leads to maturation arrest (Dash and Gilliland 2001). The initial transforming events are genomic alterations such as core binding factor (*CBF*) translocations and mixed lineage leukemia (*MLL*)

R.J.A rceci(✉)
Johns Hopkins University, The Sidney Kimmel Comprehensive Cancer Center,
1650O rleansSt reet,2M 51 Baltimore, MD21231- 1000, USA
e-mail:a rcecro@jhmi.edu

S.M eshinchi
Seattle Children's Hospital Fred Hutchinson Cancer Research Center, Clinical Research Division, 1100 Fairview Avenue North,D 5-380 Seattle,
WA98109-1024, USA
e-mail:s meshinc@fhcrc.org

G.H. Reaman and F.O. Smith (eds.), *Childhood Leukemia*,
DOI: 10.1007/978-3-642-13781-5_3, © Springer-Verlag Berlin Heidelberg 2011

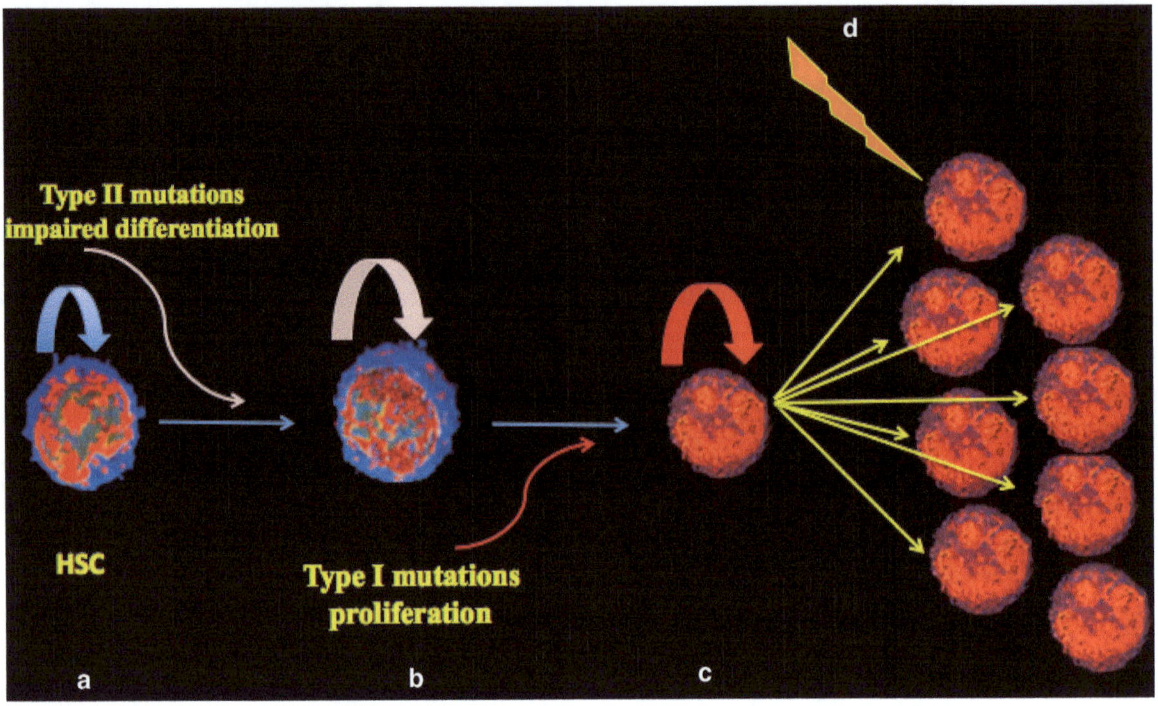

Fig. 3.1 Acquisition of type II mutations such as core binding factor (CBF) translocations in the hematopoietic stem/progenitor population (**a**) leads to the transformation of the progenitor cell by causing impaired differentiation (**b**). This transformed clone with impaired differentiation capacity may persist as a minor population for years or decades until such time as it acquires a second "hit" that imparts proliferative advantage to the arrested clone, leading to explosive expansion of the clone, and the leukemic phenotype (**c**). Acquisition of additional genomic or epigenomic events in the leukemic cells may lead to clonal evolution within the leukemic population (**d**)

translocations that are referred to as type II mutations and are thought to arise in the hematopoietic stem/progenitor cells (Fig. 3.1a). Cells which are transformed by such a mechanism would have self renewal properties, but lack proliferative potential and represent a minor clone in the hematopoietic progenitor population, and may potentially persist as a minor clone for extended periods of time.

Multiple studies have demonstrated that in teenage patients with t(8;21) AML, the fusion transcript was able to be detected in the patients' neonatal Guthrie card blood spots, demonstrating intrauterine origin of the transforming event and long latency of evolution of AML (Greaves 1993; Mahmoud et al. 1995; Wiemels et al. 2002). The arrested clone would persist as a subclinical population until a time when an additional genetic event occurs, providing a proliferative advantage to the arrested clone. The proliferative change referred to as type I mutation includes activating mutations such FLT3/ITD and *c-KIT* mutations (Fig. 3.1b). Hematopoietic cells with concomitant type I and type II mutations would have both self-renewal capacity and a significant proliferative advantage (Fig. 3.1c), thus outcompeting other hematopoietic cells, resulting in AML phenotype and the resultant hematopoietic insufficiency. *In vivo* studies have provided support for this cooperativity model, in which transduction of individual mutations did not result in AML phenotype; however, simultaneous introduction of the two mutations led to rapid evolution of leukemia (Schessl et al. 2005). Recent technologic advances have allowed more complete interrogation of the AML transcriptome, genome and epigenome, leading to the identification of an increasing number of alterations associated with AML and suggesting that the process that leads to AML pathogenesis may prove to be even more complex. Data suggest that additional genomic and epigenomic events in leukemic cells may lead to further alteration of the leukemic clone and introduce genomic heterogeneity and clonal evolution within the leukemic cell population (Fig. 3.1d).

Disease associated alterations in AML can be grouped into several broad categories as outlined below. Large structural alterations of the chromosomes identified in leukemic cells, including duplications, deletions and translocations, are identified by standard karyotype analysis in the majority of children with AML. Specific karyotypic abnormalities remain the most significant tools for diagnosis as well as for defining prognosis in AML. More recently, disease associated mutations of specific genes that mediate hematopoietic development have been identified that alter multiple signal transduction pathways and contribute to AML pathogenesis. Such mutations have come to define AML biology as they are prevalent, provide prognostic information and act as potential targets for directed therapy. Additional areas are emerging as major contributors to the pathogenesis of AML, including regulation of translation by non-coding RNA (miRNA) as well as epigenetic alterations due to aberrant DNA methylation and altered histone modifications.

3.2 CytogeneticA lterations

Nonrandom numerical and structural chromosome aberrations have been identified in approximately 80% of children with AML and are considered to be major contributors in an early stage of disease development. Karyotypic alterations of the leukemic blast are regarded as one of the most significant biological markers that define AML biology, and the presence of specific chromosomal abnormalities have significant prognostic implications. New WHO classification of AML has recognized this intimate association of cytogenetic alterations with diagnosis and prognosis in AML, by including the cytogenetic alterations as part of the classification schema of AML (Chap. 5). Informative cytogenetics are generally available in >80% of children with AML and clonal abnormalities are demonstrated in 80% of those with informative cytogenetics (Kalwinsky et al. 1990; Raimondi et al. 1999).

The number of chromosomal alterations identified in AML is in excess of 300, although >70% of pediatric AML cases fall into six specific cytogenetic categories, in which about 20% lack cytogenetic abnormalities, nearly 20% have CBF AML, 12% have t(15;17) and nearly 20% have rearrangements involving the *MLL* gene (Fig. 3.2) In addition to karyotypic alterations, disease associated mutations are identified in AML, with the highest prevalence in those with normal karyotype; >90% pediatric AML cases have at least one genomic alteration.

3.2.1 t(15;17) Translocation

Acute promyelocytic leukemia (APL), which is due to the abnormal accumulation of immature granulocytes (promyelocytes), is defined by a chromosomal translocation involving the retinoic acid receptor alpha (*RARα* or *RARA*) gene and is unique from other forms of AML in its biology as well as responsiveness to targeted therapy with retinoids. Retinoids are derivatives of Vitamin A, which upon binding and stimulation of their receptors (RAR and RXR receptors), regulate embryogenesis, cell differentiation and apoptosis. In the absence of ligand, RAR-RXR dimers create a complex with transcriptional repressors that cause transcriptional repression through

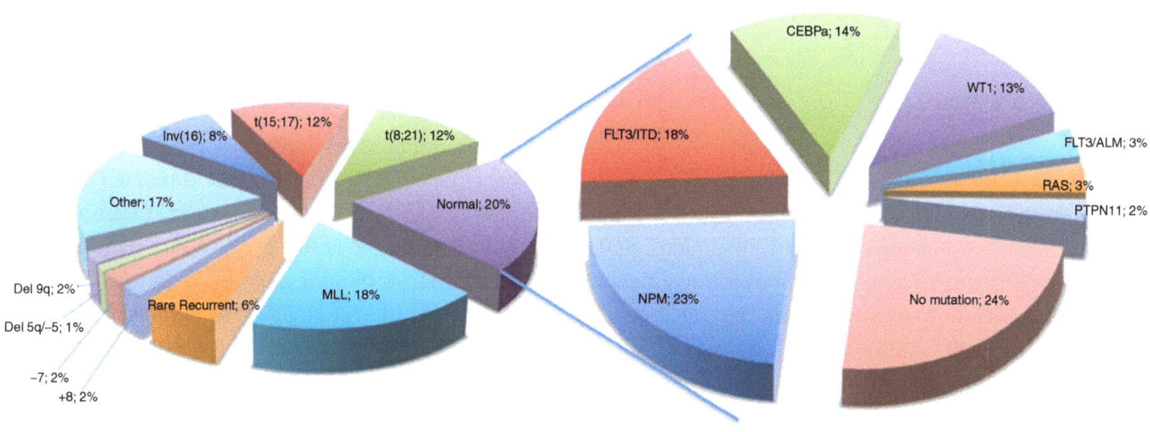

Fig. 3.2 Cytogenetic abnormalities identified in childhood AML. Panel to the left demonstrates the most common karyotypic alterations identified in childhood AML; 80% of all children have disease associated genomic structural alterations. Mutation profile in those without cytogenetic abnormalities (normal karyotype) is shown in the right panel, where 76% of those in the normal karyotype population have one of the known mutations; thus >95% of all children with AML have at least one genomic alteration

histone deacetylation (HDAC). Stimulation with retinoic acid (RA) causes conformational change of the complex, leading to the release of co-repressors and recruitment of co-activators, acetylation of histones associated with activation of transcription of target genes resulting in cellular differentiation. Translocations of chromosome 17 involving the *RARA* gene also usually involve the reciprocal translocation of *PML* zinc finger gene on chromosome 15. The t(15;17) translocation juxtaposes the *PML* and *RARA* gene and leads to the expression of a novel fusion product, which is a potent recruiter of transcriptional repressors that are resistant to de-repression by physiologic concentrations of RA. Leukemic cells with t(15;17) are arrested in the immature, promyelocyte stage. Identification of the underlying molecular biology of APL allowed for the utility of pharmacologic doses of RA to overcome the transcription repression induced by the *PML/RARA* fusion product, allowing for continued differentiation of the leukemic cells down granulocytic pathway; such findings led to APL being the first disease to be treated by a molecularly targeted therapy. With the incorporation of all trans retinoic acid (ATRA) into the therapeutic regimen, patients with APL have an excellent outcome with an overall survival of approximately 75–85% at 3 years; thus patients with APL are currently treated differently from those having other types of AML. Understanding the biologic basis of APL allowed for the development of a rational, targeted therapy for this subtype of AML. The resultant fusion transcript is also used for monitoring response to therapy and predicting relapse, as emergence of the fusion transcript can be detected in advance of morphologic relapse, allowing for initiation of treatment at the time of minimal disease, thus improving the survival for those with impending relapse.

3.2.2 CBF AML

Recurrent chromosome translocations, inversions, and deletions result in structural genomic rearrangements often involving genes that encode transcription factors (Caligiuri et al. 1997; Look 1997). CBF is an alpha/beta heterodimeric transcription factor involved in the transcriptional regulation of several genes important in hematopoiesis. They are characterized by a DNA binding subunit (CBF-alpha; encoded by *AML1* or *RUNX-1* gene) and a non-DNA binding subunit (CBF-beta; encoded by *CBFB*). Disruption of the *CBF* subunit alpha and beta genes is involved in t(8;21)(q22;q22) and inv(16)(p13q22), respectively (Ito 1996; Mrozek et al. 1997). The *RUNX1/AML1* gene, which is located on chromosome band 21q22, is disrupted in t(8;21) (q22;q22) translocation, which is present in nearly 12% of children with *de novo* AML. The CBF-*beta* subunit is encoded by *CBF-beta* on chromosome 16q22 and is disrupted by inv(16)(p13q22) and t(16;16)(p13;q22) rearrangements. The *CBF-alpha* subunit binds directly to the enhancer core DNA sequence of target genes, whereas the beta subunit, which lacks DNA binding capacity, increases the affinity and stabilizes the binding of the alpha subunit to the DNA. The precise mechanism through which the disruption of *AML1* and *CBF beta* in the t(8;21)(q22;q22) and inv(16)(p13q22), respectively, contribute to leukemogenesis is unclear. Data from *in vitro* studies and transgenic animal models suggest a dominant negative role for the fusion genes created by these rearrangements that lead to the expression of a leukemic phenotype through a possible common pathway.

3.2.3 t(8;21); AML1/ETO

This balanced translocation between chromosomes 8 and 21 results in the creation of a novel fusion transcript that juxtaposes the *AML1* gene on chromosome 21 to the *ETO* gene on chromosome 8. The *AML1* N-terminus contains the DNA binding motif, whereas the C-terminus contains a transcriptional activation domain (Ito 1996). The *ETO* gene on chromosome 8 encodes a protein that functions as a transcription factor. The functional domains of the protein include two zinc finger domains as well as a proline rich region (Miyoshi et al. 1993). The chimeric *AML1/ETO* fusion gene that is created as a result of t(8;21) translocation contains virtually the entire *ETO* coding region that is fused to the DNA binding domain of the AML1 gene minus the activation domain. Over-expression of this AML1/ETO chimeric protein, which retains the DNA binding function of the *AML1* gene but without its activation function, acts as a dominant negative regulator of *AML1* function, thus preventing trans-activation of CBF targets and contributing to leukemic transformation.

3.2.4 Inv(16)

Two distinct translocations, inv(16)(p13q22) and t(16;16)(p13;q22), collectively referred to as inv(16), result in the fusion of the *CBF-beta* gene from chromosome 16q22 with the *MYH11* gene from chromosome 16p13. The *MYH11* gene encodes a myosin heavy chain (van der Reijden et al. 1993). A number of variants of the *CBFbeta/MYH11* fusion transcripts have been identified in those with inv(16) AML, with the most common variant detected in approximately 85% of patients with inv(16). It is not known whether the different fusion transcripts have any clinical or biological significance.

The exact mechanism whereby the *CBFbeta/MYH11* fusion gene contributes to malignant transformation is unclear; however, data from murine models suggest that *CBFbeta/MYH11* interferes with normal hematopoiesis in a dominant-negative manner, resulting from the N-terminal portion of the *CBF-beta* fusing to the C-terminal domain of the *MYH11*. Such an interaction directly represses the AML1-mediated transcriptional activation by sequestering *AML1* into a functionally inactive complex, resulting in a similar leukemogenic paradigm as in t(8;21).

Cumulatively, CBF AML (inv(16) and t(8;21)) account for nearly a quarter of all childhood AML cases, and the prevalence of these translocations declines with age; in contrast, the prevalence is 10–15% in adults and <5% in AML patients older than 60 years. The presence of t(8;21) or inv(16) is associated with clinical outcome. Patients with either of these mutations appear to have a more rapid response to chemotherapy, a lower rate of relapse and improved survival compared to those without these translocations (Lange et al. 2008). Although the exact mechanism of responsiveness in this subtype is not clear, there are data that support the conclusion that patients with CBF AML benefit from intensification of cytarabine arabinoside as part of their Consolidation therapy.

3.2.5 AML with MLL Rearrangement

MLL is a large protein with multiple functional domains that is ubiquitously expressed in hematopoietic cells and is involved in the regulation of hematopoietic differentiation and proliferation. The *MLL* gene is located on chromosome 11, band 23; it is a methyltransferase that is involved in the regulation of *Hox* gene expression and methylation of histone residue H3K4. *In vitro* data have demonstrated that MLL fusion proteins can transform hematopoietic precursors to leukemia initiating cells, implicating this gene in stem cell maintenance and hematopoietic regulation. (Krivtsov et al. 2006; Krivtsov et al. 2009). Structural alterations involving the *MLL* gene are common in AML and appear to have an age dependent prevalence. There is a high prevalence of *MLL* rearrangements in AML patients less than 2 years of age (Chessells et al. 1995), and this prevalence decreases with increasing age (Balgobind et al. 2009); the prevalence of *MLL* rearrangements in adults with AML is <5% (Fig. 3.3a)

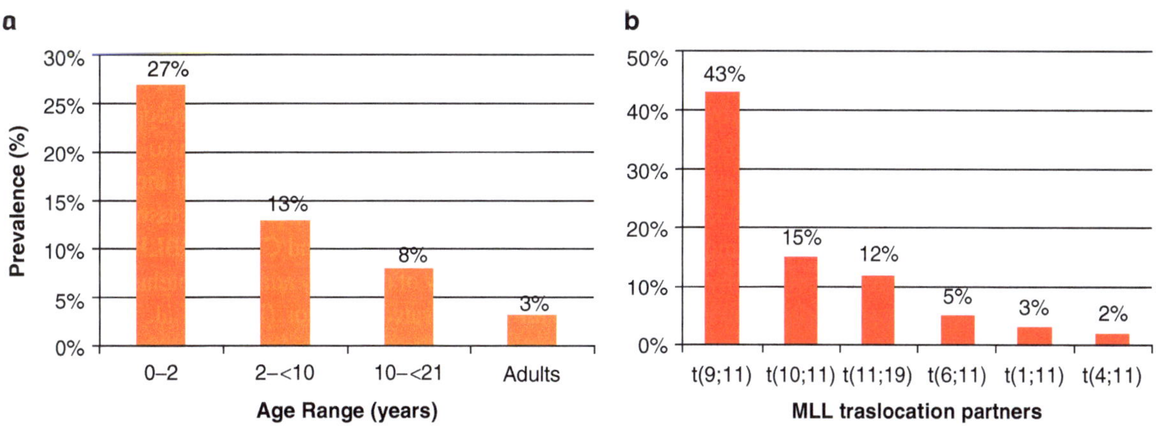

Fig. 3.3 (**a**) Prevalence of mixed lineage leukemia (MLL) translocations in different age groups. MLL is highly prevalent (27%) in children < 2 years of age. The prevalence decreases to 13% and 8% in those 2–10 and >10, respectively. Prevalence of MLL in adults is 3%. (**b**) Prevalence of most common MLL translocationpa rtners

(Grimwade et al. 1998; Balgobind et al. 2009). In *MLL* rearrangements, the N terminus of *MLL* can be juxtaposed to the C terminus of over 50 different partners (Fig. 3.3b), resulting in the loss of the methyltransferase domain. A major group of *MLL* fusion partners appears to interact with the methyltransferase that positively regulates transcription by methylation of specific histone lysine residues. Studies using gene expression profiling in *MLL* patients with AML, ALL or biphenotypic leukemia have demonstrated that those with *MLL* translocations have a unique gene expression profile regardless of the morphologic diagnosis of their disease, suggesting a common set of regulated pathways that could be therapeutically exploited.

In addition to the above mentioned alterations that are present in nearly 70% of all childhood AML, less common structural alterations are described with variable biology and prognostic significance. Notable examples are monosomy 7 (−7), monosomy 5 and deletion 5q. These alterations cumulatively account for 2–4% of cases of childhood AML, and >10% of adult AML. Although specific genes in these chromosomal regions that contribute to disease pathogenesis have not been identified, the presence of these alterations is associated with resistance to chemotherapy and extremely poor survival (Hasle et al. 2007).

3.2.6 Sub-karyotypic (Cryptic) Chromosomal Abnormalities

Gross cytogenetic abnormalities involving large chromosomal regions can be detected by conventional cytogenetics, and the frequency and implication of these changes have been described above. Karyotypic analysis in AML is limited by the ability to grow leukemic cells *in vitro* prior to analysis as well as the size of the region involved. Small structural alterations, including deletions or duplications, can escape detection by conventional cytogenetics and may require more specialized techniques such as fluorescence in situ hybridization (FISH). Loss of heterozygosity (LOH) that is generally associated with deletions leads to haplo-insufficiency that may contribute to malignant transformation. New technology using single nucleotide polymorphism (SNP) genotyping and copy number evaluation of the leukemic DNA can identify genomic alterations not amenable to detection by conventional means. The new techniques have identified regions of copy-neutral LOH (CN-LOH), also referred to as acquired uniparental disomy (aUPD) (Raghavan et al. 2005, 2008; Gupta et al. 2008). aUPD is a homologous recombination mediated process by which a homozygous state is achieved after an initial acquisition of a heterozygous mutation. In this DNA repair process, a mutant allele is used as a template, and the wild-type allele is converted to that of the mutant one, resulting in a homozygous state. Such an event leading to acquisition of LOH can alter the gene dosage of a particular mutation and may have significant clinical implications. aUPD has been described in specific populations of AML including FLT3/ITD and *CEBPA* mutations with varying prevalence in different studies (Radtke et al. 2009; Walter et al. 2009).

3.3 DiseaseA ssociatedMut ations in Signal Transduction Pathways

Chromosomal translocations described above are considered to cause differentiation arrest. A broad body of data has demonstrated that such alterations are not sufficient for frank leukemic transformation, and additional events are required for the evolution of leukemic phenotype. Activating mutations of the kinase-mediated RAS/MAP signal transduction pathways have been demonstrated to provide the proliferative signal for the arrested clone and lead to leukemic progression. Regulation of cellular processes is initiated by extracellular signals (cytokines) whose actions are mediated through various signal transduction pathways, resulting in cellular differentiation, proliferation and survival. Stimulation of specific membrane bound receptors by their native ligand leads to the activation of their intracellular kinase moieties. The activated receptor recruits a number of proteins in the cytoplasm to form a complex of protein–protein interactions in the intracellular domain. SHC proteins, GRB2, GRB2-associated binder 2 (GAB2), SHIP, CBL, and CBLB (CBLB-related protein) are a few of the many adaptor proteins that interact with the activated receptor (Dosil et al. 1993; Zhang et al. 2000; Lavagna-Sevenier et al. 1998a, b). As each protein binds to the complex, it becomes activated in turn, resulting in a cascade of phosphorylation reactions that culminates in activation of a number of secondary mediators, including MAP kinase, STAT, and AKT/PI3 kinase signal transduction pathways.

These activated mediators are chaperoned to the nuclear interphase by heat shock protein 90 (HSP90), in which the message is translocated to the nucleus. In the nucleus, these transcriptional mediators trigger a series of events culminating in regulation of cell differentiation, proliferation, apoptosis, and cell survival. As integrity of cellular processes are highly dependent on regulation of signal transduction pathways, alterations of pathway stimulation, either upstream (by receptor mutations) or downstream (by signal transducers), can alter the balance of proliferation, differentiation and apoptosis. Mutations in the above mentioned signaling cascades are common in AML and their prevalence and biologic significance is described below.

3.3.1 FLT3 Mutations

FMS-like tyrosine kinase 3 (FLT3), a receptor tyrosine kinase (RTK), is a membrane-bound receptor with an intrinsic tyrosine kinase activity that is highly expressed in hematopoietic stem/progenitor cells and regulates hematopoietic differentiation and proliferation. FLT3 is expressed at variable levels in all myeloid malignancies. Mutations in the *FLT3* gene have been identified in AML that lead to constitutive activation of the receptor kinase activity. Internal tandem duplication of the juxtamembrane domain coding sequence in *FLT3* (FLT3/ITD) was initially identified in a high proportion of patients with AML (Nakao et al. 1996). Additional studies identified missense mutations in the activation loop domain of the tyrosine kinase moiety of the FLT3 receptor (*FLT3* Activation loop mutation, FLT3/ALM)(Y amamotoe ta l. 2001).

3.3.2 FLT3 Internal Tandem Duplications (FLT3/ITD)

These mutations are the result of a segmental duplication of a fragment of the juxtamembrane domain coding region (encoded by exons 14 and 15) of *FLT3* and are highly prevalent in hematologic malignancies, occurring in CML (5–10%), MDS (5–10%), and AML (15–35%) patients (Nakao et al. 1996; Stirewalt et al. 2001; Meshinchi et al. 2006; Kottaridis et al. 2001; Gale et al. 2007). Prevalence of FLT3/ITD is highly age dependent; it is rare in infant AML and the prevalence increases in a step-wise manner to 5–10% in age 5–10, 20% in young adults and >35% in AML patients older than 55 years (Meshinchi et al. 2006). There is also considerable variability in the size of the duplicated segment (ranging from 3 to >400 base pairs) and this variability may have biologic and clinical significance (Nakao et al. 1996; Stirewalt et al. 2001; Meshinchi et al. 2006). FLT3/ITDs lead to constitutive activation of the FLT3 receptor and promote cellular proliferation *via* the activation of multiple signaling pathways including RAS/MAPK, STAT and the AKT/PI3 kinase pathways. Studies have demonstrated that cytokine independent cellular proliferation of FLT3/ITD-transduced cells was mediated by RAS and STAT5 pathways (Mizuki et al. 2000). Demonstration of STAT5 activation in FLT3/ITD highlighted that some of the effects of FLT3/ITDs are unique to the mutated receptor, where in contrast to FLT3/ITD, ligand-induced *FLT3*-WT activation does not lead to STAT5 activation and no STAT5 DNA binding (Mizuki et al. 2000). Other studies have demonstrated that in addition to RAS and STAT pathways, FLT3/ITDs constitutively phosphorylate and activate AKT, and that ligand independent growth requires this aberrant AKT activation by FLT3/ITDs, such that the ligand independent growth is reversed if AKT activation is blocked. Presence of FLT3/ITD is associated with laboratory and clinical characteristics and outcome. Patients with FLT3/ITD have higher diagnostic white blood count, higher marrow blast percentage and more likely to have normal karyotypes. Furthermore, presence of FLT3/ITD is highly associated with clinical outcome, where those with FLT3/ITD have a higher relapse rate and poor outcome. Large studies have demonstrated the prognostic significance of FLT3/ITD in adult and pediatric AML trials (Thiede et al. 2002; Meshinchi et al. 2006). In these studies, survival of patients with FLT3/ITD was 20–30% compared to 50% for those without FLT3/ITD. In addition, it was demonstrated that the mutant to wild type allelic ratio observed in patients with FLT3/ITD appeared to influence outcome (Meshinchi et al. 2006; Thiede et al. 2002) Evaluation of various thresholds of FLT3/ITD allelic ratio (ITD-AR) established an allelic ratio threshold that demarcates patients with FLT3/ITD at high risk of relapse from those expected to have a more favorable outcome, demonstrating that it is not merely the presence of FLT3/ITD, but the level of mutant allele that determines clinical outcome (Meshinchi et al. 2006). Additional reports have demonstrated similar difference in clinical outcome for patients with AML having different mutant to wild type allelic ratios (Thiede et al. 2007). Currently, AML trials conducted by the Children's Oncology Group (COG) utilize a FLT3/ITD allelic ratio of ≥0.4 to identify FLT3/ITD positive patients who are at high risk of relapse; these patients are referred for stem cell transplantation using the most suitable available donor.

3.3.3 FLT3 Activation Loop Mutation (FLT3/ALM)

FLT3/ALM are missense point mutations within the activation loop of the *FLT3* kinase domain that promote autonomous and constitutive activation of the receptor kinase, similar to that of FLT3/ITD (Yamamoto et al. 2001; Thiede et al. 2002). However, there are significant biological differences between the two types of *FLT3* mutations (Choudhary et al. 2005; Grundler et al. 2005; Rocnik et al. 2006; Vempati et al. 2007), as FLT3/ITDs and FLT3/ALMs appear to promote activation of different downstream effectors (Choudhary et al. 2005) and different biological responses. Animal studies have demonstrated that mice harboring FLT3/ITDs primarily develop an oligoclonal myeloproliferative disorder, while mice harboring FLT3/ALM are more likely to develop oligoclonal lymphoid disorders (Grundler et al. 2005). In addition, despite their biologic similarity, patients who harbor the two different mutations appear to have drastically different clinical outcome; those with FLT3/ALM differ from those with FLT3/ITD as their outcome is not different from those without *FLT3* mutations. Prevalence of FLT3/ALM is 6–8%, regardless of age, and the presence of FLT3/ALM and FLT3/ITD appears to be mutually exclusive (Meshinchi et al. 2006). These studies further demonstrated that the presence of FLT3/ALM is not associated with leukocytosis, and in contrast to FLT3/ITD, patients with FLT3/ALM AML do not have adverse outcomes.

3.3.4 c-KIT Mutations

c-KIT is a proto-oncogene located on chromosome band 4q11–12 which, similar to *FLT3*, encodes a transmembrane protein that is a member of the type III receptor tyrosine kinase family (Paschka et al. 2006; Renneville et al. 2008). Ligand induced activation leads to *c-KIT* dimerization and transphosphorylation, thereby activating downstream signaling pathways (Renneville et al. 2008). Preferential activation of alternative pathways leading to cytokine independent growth and increased drug resistance have been reported to be linked to specific *c-KIT* mutations (Ning et al. 2001a, b, c). Mutations of *c-KIT* are infrequent in adult AML (2–8%) and tend to cluster within the activation loop (exon 17) and a region of the extracellular domain integral to receptor dimerization (exon 8) (Renneville et al. 2008). Their prevalence is higher, however, in CBF AML patients (6–48%) and may be associated with worse clinical outcome in adults (Care et al. 2003; Cairoli et al. 2005; Nanri et al. 2005; Schnittger et al. 2005; Paschka et al. 2006). Although adult data suggested that the presence of *KIT* mutations are associated with worse clinical outcome, a study conducted in pediatric cooperative trials demonstrated a prevalence of *c-KIT* mutations of nearly 20% but lack of clinical significance in pediatric CBF AML (Pollard et al. 2010).

3.3.5 Other Receptor Tyrosine Kinase Mutations

FMS and PDGFR are other members of class III RTK receptors that function in hematopoietic development. Activating point mutations in the kinase domains of *FMS* have been described in 5–10% of selected AML cases in adults (Ridge et al. 1990; Padua et al. 1998), although mutations in *FMS* were not identified in pediatric patients with AML (Meshinchi et al. 2003). Although expression and translocations involving *PDGFR* have been demonstrated in hematopoietic disorders, mutations in this gene have not been reported inA ML(Y amadae ta l. 2006).

3.4 OtherFr equentMut ationsi nA ML

3.4.1 RAS Mutations

Mutations in *N-RAS* gene occur in approximately 10–30% of adult AML cases (Radich et al. 1990; Stirewalt et al. 2001) and 10% of pediatric AML

(Berman et al. 2009). Point mutations frequently occur in codons 12, 13, and 61 (Byrne and Marshall 1998), and prevent the hydrolysis of RAS-GTP, keeping RAS in the "on" or activated state. The coincident occurrence of both a *FLT3* and *RAS* mutation in the same case is very rare, as might be expected, since there may be no *a priori* selective advantage to two mutations affecting the same pathway. However unlike *FLT3-ITD* mutations, *RAS* mutations are not prognostically important (Berman et al. 2009). With both *FLT3* and *RAS* mutations, there may be discordance between diagnostic and relapse specimens. Thus, a patient with either a *RAS* or *FLT3* mutation at diagnosis may relapse without the mutation (or vice versa). This suggests that these mutations are not the primary oncogenic events.

3.4.2 Nucleophosmin (NPM1) Mutations

NPM1 encodes a ubiquitously expressed and highly conserved phosphoprotein that is primarily localized to the nucleolus, but shuttles rapidly between the nucleus and cytoplasm in its role as a molecular chaperone. The NPM1 protein has been shown to contribute to many basic cellular processes, including biosynthesis of ribosomes, prevention of protein aggregation in the nucleolus, and regulation of centrosome duplication through cyclin E/cyclin-dependent kinase 2 phosphorylation. Abnormalities in *NPM1* have been implicated in the pathogenesis of various hematopoietic malignancies, including anaplastic large cell lymphoma with t(2;5) translocation, resulting in expression of the NPM1-ALK fusion protein. Mutations in *NPM1* are common in AML, with a prevalence of 30% in adult and 8–10% in pediatric AML (Dohner et al. 2005; Brown et al. 2007; Gale et al. 2007; Hollink et al. 2007). *NPM1* mutations appear to be more prevalent in AML with normal karyotype, with a prevalence of nearly 40–50% in adults and 20% in pediatric AML. Disease associated mutations, characterized by four base insertions in exon 12 of the *NPM* gene, lead to impaired nuclear localization of the nucleophosmin protein. Presence of *NPM* mutations portends favorable outcome with reduced relapse risk and improved survival; those with *NPM* mutations have an outcome similar to those with CBF AML. There is significant overlap between *NPM* mutations and FLT3/ITD, as nearly one third of those with *NPM* mutations also have FLT3/ITD. In adult AML, it has been shown that FLT3/ITD retains its high-risk status in the presence of *NPM* mutations. In pediatric AML, the presence of *NPM1* mutations in the presence of FLT3/ITD has been reported to partially ameliorate the poor prognosis conferred by FLT3/ITD alone (Hollink et al. 2007).

3.4.3 CEBPA Mutations

CCAAT/enhancer binding protein-alpha (C/EBPa) is encoded by the *CEBPA* gene and functions as a transcription factor that regulates proliferation and terminal granulocytic differentiation. It is a member of the basic region leucine zipper class of transcription factors, and is expressed in a variety of tissues, including adipocytes, hepatocytes, and Type II alveolar cells. In the hematopoietic system, C/EBPa is expressed in cells of myelomonocytic origin and regulates the expression of genes that regulate granulocyte differentiation. CEBPa has been shown to inhibit E2F pathways, downregulate *C-MYC* and thus allow myeloid differentiation. Mutations in the *CEBPA* occur in 4% of childhood AML cases and the overwhelming majority of cases with these mutations occur in a bi-allelic manner, in which two distinct mutations occur, one in the N-terminal domain (NTD) and the second in the opposite allele affecting the bZip domain (Ho et al. 2008). *NTD* mutation results in an early termination codon, which truncates the p42 protein, allowing intact translation of only the p30 protein. In a bi-allelic model, the bZip mutation in the opposite allele disrupts the bZip domains of its protein products, resulting in loss of function. Such a bi-allelic mutation would result in the expression of p30 as the only functional protein. Kirstetter et al. demonstrated that sole expression of p30 may be sufficient for the development of AML; in their mouse model, expression of the p30 isoform in the absence of p42 resulted in a fully-penetrant AML phenotype (Kirstetter et al. 2008). This model would argue that both types of mutations are required for AML pathogenesis. COG studies have demonstrated that *CEBPA* mutations tend to occur in patients with normal cytogenetics and are associated with decreased relapse risk as well as improved survival compared to patients without a mutation (Ho et al. 2009).

3.4.4 Wilms Tumor-1 (WT1) Gene Expression and Mutation

The *WT1* gene, located on chromosome 11p13, encodes a zinc-finger protein that exists in multiple isoforms and functions as a transcription factor. *WT1* is expressed primarily in tissues of the developing genitourinary and hematopoietic systems, and mutations in *WT1* occur in both syndrome-associated and sporadic cases of nephroblastoma (Wilms Tumor), the most common childhood renal malignancy. *WT1* is also expressed in CD34+ hematopoietic progenitors, and is over-expressed in a subset of acute leukemias, including AML, ALL, and CML in blast crisis (Bergmann et al. 1997). Somatic mutations of *WT1* gene have been reported to have variable prognostic significance (Paschka et al. 2007). Initial studies in adults suggested that the presence of *WT1* mutations was an independent prognostic factor for poor outcome. However, recent studies, including a comprehensive evaluation of pediatric AML, have identified *WT* mutations in 8–10% of patients; further, it was demonstrated that a strong association between *WT1* mutations and FLT3/ITD existed. In that study, although the presence of *WT1* mutation was associated with worse outcome, it was shown that the prognostic significance of *WT1* mutation was due to FLT3/ITD; however, in patients without FLT3/ITD, the presence of a *WT1* mutation did not portend poor outcome (Pollard et al. 2008). In contrast, Hollink et al. have reported that *WT1* mutations represent an independent poor risk factor (Hollink et al. 2009). Furthermore, although expression of *WT1* has been used as a marker of disease response and emergence of MRD (Bergmann et al. 1997; Lapillonne et al. 2006), no significant association of *WT1* expression was observed in a pediatric trial study (Noronha et al. 2009). Comprehensive evaluation of *WT1* expression within specific risk groups has not been performed in childhood AML and currently is not utilized in risk group stratification.

3.4.5 TET2 Mutations

Disease associated genomic alterations in *TET2* gene (4q24) have recently been demonstrated in myeloid malignancies in adults. The prevalence of these mutations appears to be 20% in MDS, 10–20% in myeloproliferative disease and 12% in adult AML (Delhommeau et al. 2009; Tefferi et al. 2009). Although the prevalence of *TET2* mutations is not well defined in childhood AML, early data from COG suggest that these mutations are uncommon, with a prevalence of 3% and unclear prognostic significance (Fig. 3.4).

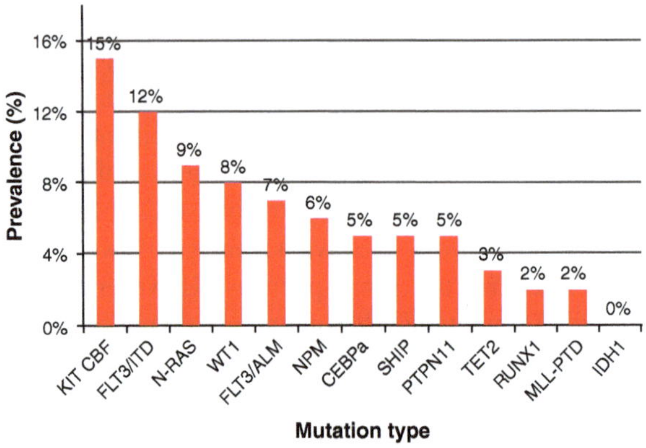

Fig. 3.4 Prevalence of disease-associated mutations in pediatric AML

Recent advances in whole genome sequencing have enabled interrogation of the entire leukemic genome for identification of novel disease associated mutations. Initial evaluation of a patient with AML, identified numerous previously undescribed mutations; however, screening of an additional 200 patients failed to demonstrate any of these mutations in a larger cohort (Ley et al. 2008). This study highlights the need to separate the mutations that promote the leukemic process from "passenger" mutations that do not contribute to AML initiation or progression. Whole exome sequencing and whole transcriptome sequencing allow sequencing of the entire exonic and the transcribed sequences, respectively, allowing additional means of evaluating disease profile. Application of these new technologies to AML will enable identification of genomic alterations that would be impractical to identify on a gene by gene basis.

3.5 EpigeneticDys regulation in Myeloid Leukemogenesis

As described above, AML is characterized by genomic alterations that are crucial to disease pathogenesis. An increasing body of evidence demonstrates that epigenetic modifications may contribute to the pathogenesis of leukemia. The term epigenetics refers to heritable changes in phenotype or gene expression caused by mechanisms other than alterations in the genome (DNA). Epigenetic changes that underlie the development of leukemia can be in one of two major categories: changes in the DNA methylation state and alterations in histone modification patterns. These two processes work in concert to lead to the activation or repression of gene expression. Emerging evidence shows that altered methylation and changes in histone modifications may be involved in normal and malignant hematopoiesis and contribute to myeloid leukemia and outcome (Chen et al. 2010).

3.5.1 Altered Methylation Pattern in AML

Evidence linking alterations in DNA methylation and malignancies has prompted comprehensive evaluations of DNA methylation patterns in AML in an attempt to identify specific methylation "signatures" that can be used for risk identification as well as identification of potential targets for epigenetically directed therapies. One study in adult AML used DNA methylation patterns to group patients into 16 different cohorts based on their methylation pattern (Figueroa et al. 2010). The methylation pattern segregated patients with specific mutations and cytogenetic groups. This study also identified a 15 gene methylation classifier predictive of overall survival. The contribution of alterations in DNA methylation patterning and its clinical significance is not yet well defined in childhood AML, but such evaluations are currently underway. Histone acetylation is associated with transcriptionally active chromatin (euchromatin) and is catalyzed by histone acetyltransferases (HATs). Several transcriptional co-activators, including CREB binding protein (CBP), have been shown to possess HAT activity. Conversely, transcriptional co-repressor complexes such as nuclear co-repressor 1 (NCOR1) have been shown to contain subunits with histone deacetylase (HDAC) activity. As acetylation and methylation status of the histone lysine residues help to determine whether chromatin is in the transcriptionally active or repressed state, altered histone modification patterns could mediate malignant transformation by altering expression of oncogenes. As alterations in methylation and acetylation status have significant contributions to myeloid transformation and proliferation, they are attractive targets for epigenetic therapy by DNA methyltransferase (DNMT), as well as histone deacetylase (HDAC) or methylase inhibitors.

3.5.2 MicroRNA Dysregulation in AML

MicroRNAs (miRNAs) are evolutionarily conserved non-coding RNAs that contain 19–25 nucleotides and arise by cleavage from 70 to 100 nucleotide hairpin precursors (Bartel 2004, 2009; Bartel and Chen 2004; Chen et al. 2010). They hybridize to complementary messenger RNA (mRNA) targets and most commonly function by inhibiting translation of specific mRNAs. miRNAs have provided a new dimension to our understanding of complex gene regulatory networks. miRNAs can function as oncogenes or as tumor suppressor genes in leukemias, although the data for the latter are more limited. Specific miRNAs have been shown to be highly expressed in MLL leukemias (Mi et al. 2007), and miRNA expression signatures have been defined for AML cases with specific mutations or translocations. Common oncogene and tumor suppressor mutations also appear to be associated with unique miRNA signatures. For example, miR155 is up-regulated in cases with *FLT3*-ITD mutations (Garzon and Croce 2008). miRNA deregulation, specifically the expression pattern of 12 miRNAs, has also been associated with clinical outcome (Marcucci et al. 2008). As miRNAs can contribute to leukemogenesis by functioning as oncogenes or tumor suppressor genes, miRNAs also have the potential to be therapeutic targets or tools. They can be targeted by modulating expression level of the miRNA, or using miRNA-based cancer gene therapy to target multiple gene networks that are controlled by a single, aberrantly expressed miRNA. Increased understanding of epigenetic regulation of myeloid leukemogenesis may provide new understanding of AML biology and identify new tools for more accurate diagnosis, risk stratificationa ndtre atment.

3.6 Conclusions

Acute myeloid leukemia is an enormously complex disease characterized by a myriad of genomic and epigenomic alterations that interact to create a wide variety of different AML subtypes having significantly different outcomes. Knowledge of the genomic alterations, whether karyotypic abnormalities or specific disease associated mutations, provides a great deal of information for clinical decision making. Patients with CBF AML (t(8;21) and inv(16)) are expected to have a favorable outcome and these patients can be spared more intensive post-Induction therapy such as hematopoietic cell transplantation. Given the growing body of evidence on the prognostic significance of *CEBPA* and *NPM* mutations, patients with these mutations are considered low-risk and are treated similar to those with CBF AML. In contrast, patients with monosomy 7 or with monosomy 5/del5q are considered to have an extremely high risk of relapse and although these alterations are rare in childhood AML, there have been no improvements in the outcome of patients with these alterations in the last decade.

More complete understanding of the underlying mechanisms and the genes linked to disease pathogenesis is needed. Patients with FLT3/ITD are at high risk of relapse. As *FLT3* mutation causes constitutive activation of the FLT3 receptor kinase, specific kinase inhibitors are being clinically tested. Patients with high mutant FLT3/ITD to normal allelic ratios also have high risk disease and are thus usually considered for stem cell transplantation in first complete remission. Although the presence of *c-KIT* mutations have not been definitively shown to be associated with adverse outcome in children, such mutant receptors may be inhibited by kinase inhibitors; these patients would be candidates for directed therapy with specific kinase inhibitors. Despite the increasing breadth of information about the genetic and epigenetic alterations in AML, a specific risk status can be identified for only 30–40% of the patients and the ability to assign risk status or specific therapy for the remaining cohort, with a survival rate of near 50%, is lacking. With the increase in the number of tools for interrogation of AML genomic and epigenomic changes, the ability to allocate patients to individualized therapy directed by the underlying biology of their disease is anticipated.

References

Balgobind BV, Raimondi SC et al (2009) Novel prognostic subgroups in childhood 11q23/MLL-rearranged acute myeloid leukemia: results of an international retrospective study. Blood114(12):248 9–2496

Bartel DP (2004) MicroRNAs: genomics, biogenesis, mechanism, and function. Cell 116(2):281–297

Bartel DP (2009) MicroRNAs: target recognition and regulatory functions. Cell 136(2):215–233

Bartel DP, Chen CZ (2004) Micromanagers of gene expression: the potentially widespread influence of metazoan microRNAs. Nat Rev Genet 5(5):396–400

Bergmann L, Miething C et al (1997) High levels of Wilms' tumor gene (wt1) mRNA in acute myeloid leukemias are associated with a worse long-term outcome. Blood 90(3):1217–1225

Berman JN, Gerbing RB et al (2009) Prevalence and clinical implications of N-RAS mutations in childhood AML – a report from the Children's Oncology Group. ASH Annu Meet Abstr 114(22):3115

Brown P, McIntyre E et al (2007) The incidence and clinical significance of nucleophosmin mutations in childhood AML. Blood110(3):979–985

Byrne JL, Marshall CJ (1998) The molecular pathophysiology of myeloid leukaemias: Ras revisited. Br J Haematol 100(2):256–264

Cairoli R, Beghini A et al (2005) Prognostic impact of c-KIT mutations in core binding factor leukemias. an Italian retrospective study. Blood 107:3463–3468

Caligiuri MA, Strout MP et al (1997) Molecular biology of acute myeloid leukemia. Semin Oncol 24(1):32–44

Care RS, Valk PJM et al (2003) Incidence and prognosis of c-KIT and FLT3 mutations in core binding factor (CBF) acute myeloid leukaemias. Br J Haematol 121:775–777

Chen J, Odenike O et al (2010) Leukaemogenesis: more than mutant genes. Nat Rev Cancer 10(1):23–36

Chessells JM, Bailey C et al (1995) Intensification of treatment and survival in all children with lymphoblastic leukaemia: results of UK Medical Research Council trial UKALL X. Medical Research Council Working Party on Childhood Leukaemia [see comments]. Lancet 345(8943):143–148

Choudhary C, Schwable J et al (2005) AML-associated Flt3 kinase domain mutations show signal transduction differences compared with Flt3 ITD mutations. Blood 106(1): 265–273

Dash A, Gilliland DG (2001) Molecular genetics of acute myeloid leukaemia. Best Pract Res Clin Haematol 14(1):49–64

Delhommeau F, Dupont S et al (2009) Mutation in TET2 in myeloid cancers. N Engl J Med 360(22):2289–2301

Dohner K, Schlenk RF et al (2005) Mutant nucleophosmin (NPM1) predicts favorable prognosis in younger adults with acute myeloid leukemia and normal cytogenetics: interaction with other gene mutations. Blood 106(12):3740–3746

Dosil M, Wang S et al (1993) Mitogenic signalling and substrate specificity of the Flk2/Flt3 receptor tyrosine kinase in fibroblasts and interleukin 3-dependent hematopoietic cells. Mol Cell Biol 13(10):6572–6585

Figueroa ME, Lugthart S et al (2010) DNA methylation signatures identify biologically distinct subtypes in acute myeloid leukemia. Cancer Cell 17(1):13–27

Gale RE, Green C et al (2007) The impact of FLT3 internal tandem duplication mutant level, number, size and interaction with NPM1 mutations in a large cohort of young adult patients with acute myeloid leukemia. Blood 111: 2776–2784

Garzon R, Croce CM (2008) MicroRNAs in normal and malignant hematopoiesis. Curr Opin Hematol 15(4):352–358

Greaves M (1993) A natural history for pediatric acute leukemia. Blood 82(4):1043–1051

Grimwade D, Walker H et al (1998) The importance of diagnostic cytogenetics on outcome in AML: analysis of 1, 612 patients entered into the MRC AML 10 trial. The Medical Research Council Adult and Children's Leukaemia Working Parties. Blood 92(7):2322–2333

Grundler R, Miething C et al (2005) FLT3-ITD and tyrosine kinase domain mutants induce 2 distinct phenotypes in a murine bone marrow transplantation model. Blood 105(12):4792–4799

Gupta M, Raghavan M et al (2008) Novel regions of acquired uniparental disomy discovered in acute myeloid leukemia. Gene Chromosome Cancer 47(9):729–739

Hasle H, Alonzo TA et al (2007) Monosomy 7 and deletion 7q in children and adolescents with acute myeloid leukemia: an international retrospective study. Blood 109(11): 4641–4647

Ho P, Alonzo TA et al (2008) CEBPA mutations predict favorable prognosis in pediatric AML. ASH Annu Meet Abstr 112(11):142

Ho PA, Alonzo TA et al (2009) Prevalence and prognostic implications of CEBPA mutations in pediatric acute myeloid leukemia (AML): a report from the Children's Oncology Group. Blood113(26):655 8–6566

Hollink IH, Zwaan CM et al (2007) Nucleophosmin gene mutations identify a favorable risk group in childhood acute myeloid leukemia with a normal karyotype. ASH Annu Meet Abstr 110(11):366

Hollink IH, van den Heuvel-Eibrink MM et al (2009) Clinical relevance of Wilms tumor 1 gene mutations in childhood acute myeloid leukemia. Blood 113(23):5951–5960

Ito Y (1996) Structural alterations in the transcription factor PEBP2/CBF linked to four different types of leukemia. J Cancer Res Clin Oncol 122(5):266–274

Kalwinsky DK, Raimondi SC et al (1990) Prognostic importance of cytogenetic subgroups in *de novo* pediatric acute nonlymphocytic leukemia. J Clin Oncol 8(1):75–83

Kirstetter P, Schuster MB et al (2008) Modeling of C/EBPalpha mutant acute myeloid leukemia reveals a common expression signature of committed myeloid leukemia-initiating cells. Cancer Cell 13(4):299–310

Kottaridis PD, Gale RE et al (2001) The presence of a FLT3 internal tandem duplication in patients with acute myeloid leukemia (AML) adds important prognostic information to cytogenetic risk group and response to the first cycle of chemotherapy: analysis of 854 patients from the United Kingdom Medical Research Council AML 10 and 12 trials. Blood98(6):1752– 1759

Krivtsov AV, Twomey D et al (2006) Transformation from committed progenitor to leukaemia stem cell initiated by MLL-AF9. Nature 442(7104):818–822

Krivtsov AV, Feng Z et al (2009) Transformation from committed progenitor to leukemia stem cells. Ann N Y Acad Sci. 1176:144–149

Lange BJ, Smith FO et al (2008) Outcomes in CCG-2961, a Children's Oncology Group phase 3 trial for untreated pediatric acute myeloid leukemia: a report from the Children's Oncology Group. Blood 111(3):1044–1053

Lapillonne H, Renneville A et al (2006) High WT1 expression after induction therapy predicts high risk of relapse and death in pediatric acute myeloid leukemia. J Clin Oncol 24(10):1507–1515

Lavagna-Sevenier C, Marchetto S et al (1998a) The CBL-related protein CBLB participates in FLT3 and interleukin-7 receptor signal transduction in pro-B cells. J Biol Chem 273(24):14962–14967

Lavagna-Sevenier C, Marchetto S et al (1998b) FLT3 signaling in hematopoietic cells involves CBL, SHC and an unknown P115 as prominent tyrosine-phosphorylated substrates. Leukemia 12(3):301–310

Ley TJ, Mardis ER et al (2008) DNA sequencing of a cytogenetically normal acute myeloid leukaemia genome. Nature 456(7218):66–72

Look A (1997) Oncogenic transcription factors in the human acute leukemias. Science 278:1059

Mahmoud HH, Ridge SA et al (1995) Intrauterine monoclonal origin of neonatal concordant acute lymphoblastic leukemia in monozygotic twins. Med Pediatr Oncol 24(2):77–81

Marcucci G, Radmacher MD et al (2008) MicroRNA expression in cytogenetically normal acute myeloid leukemia. N Engl J Med358(18):1919–1928

Meshinchi S, Stirewalt DL et al (2003) Activating mutations of RTK/ras signal transduction pathway in pediatric acute myeloid leukemia. Blood 102:1474–1479

Meshinchi S, Alonzo TA et al (2006) Clinical implications of FLT3 mutations in pediatric AML. Blood 108(12):3654–3661

Mi S, Lu J et al (2007) MicroRNA expression signatures accurately discriminate acute lymphoblastic leukemia from acute myeloid leukemia. Proc Natl Acad Sci USA 104(50): 19971–19976

Miyoshi H, Kozu T et al (1993) The t(8;21) translocation in acute myeloid leukemia results in production of an AML1-MTG8 fusion transcript. EMBO J 12(7):2715–2721

Mizuki M, Fenski R et al (2000) Flt3 mutations from patients with acute myeloid leukemia induce transformation of 32D cells mediated by the Ras and STAT5 pathways. Blood 96(12):3907–3914

Mrozek K, Heinonen K et al (1997) Clinical significance of cytogenetics in acute myeloid leukemia. Semin Oncol 24:17

Nakao M, Yokota S et al (1996) Internal tandem duplication of the flt3 gene found in acute myeloid leukemia. Leukemia 10(12):1911–1918

Nanri T, Matsuno N et al (2005) Mutations in the receptor tyrosine kinase pathway are associated with clinical outcome in patients with acute myeloblastic leukemia harboring t(8;21)(q22;q22). Leukemia 19(8):1361–1366

Ning ZQ, Li J et al (2001a) Activating mutations of c-kit at codon 816 confer drug resistance in human leukemia cells. Leuk Lymphoma 41(5–6):513–522

Ning ZQ, Li J et al (2001b) Signal transducer and activator of transcription 3 activation is required for Asp(816) mutant c-Kit-mediated cytokine-independent survival and proliferation in human leukemia cells. Blood 97(11):3559–3567

Ning ZQ, Li J et al (2001c) STAT3 activation is required for Asp(816) mutant c-Kit induced tumorigenicity. Oncogene 20(33):4528–4536

Noronha SA, Farrar JE et al (2009) WT1 expression at diagnosis does not predict survival in pediatric AML: a report from the Children's Oncology Group. Pediatr Blood Cancer 53(6): 1136–1139

Padua RA, Guinn BA et al (1998) RAS, FMS and p53 mutations and poor clinical outcome in myelodysplasias: a 10-year follow-up. Leukemia 12(6):887–892

Paschka P, Marcucci G et al (2006) Adverse prognostic significance of KIT mutations in adult acute myeloid leukemia with inv(16) and t(8;21): a Cancer and Leukemia Group B Study. J Clin Oncol 24(24):3904–3911

Paschka P, Marcucci G et al (2007) Wilms tumor 1 (WT1) gene mutations predict poor outcome in adults with cytogenetically normal (CN) acute myeloid leukemia (AML): a cancer and leukemia group B (CALGB) Study. ASH Annu Meet Abstr110(11):362

Pollard JA, Zeng R et al (2008) Prevalence and prognostic implications of WT1 mutations in pediatric AML A: report from Children's Oncology Group. ASH Annu Meet Abstr 112(11):143

Pollard JA, Alonzo TA et al (2010) Prevalence and prognostic significance of KIT mutations in pediatric patients with core binding factor AML enrolled on serial pediatric cooperative trials for *de novo* AML. Blood 115(12):2372–2379

Radich JP, Kopecky KJ et al (1990) N-Ras mutations in adult *de novo* acute myelogenous leukemia: prevalence and clinical significance. Blood 76:801

Radtke I, Mullighan CG et al (2009) Genomic analysis reveals few genetic alterations in pediatric acute myeloid leukemia. Proc Natl Acad Sci USA 106(31):12944–12949

Raghavan M, Lillington DM et al (2005) Genome-wide single nucleotide polymorphism analysis reveals frequent partial uniparental disomy due to somatic recombination in acute myeloid leukemias. Cancer Res 65(2):375–378

Raghavan M, Smith LL et al (2008) Segmental uniparental disomy is a commonly acquired genetic event in relapsed acute myeloid leukemia. Blood 112(3):814–821

Raimondi SC, Chang MN et al (1999) Chromosomal abnormalities in 478 children with acute myeloid leukemia: clinical characteristics and treatment outcome in a cooperative pediatric oncology group study-POG 8821. Blood 94(11): 3707–3716

Renneville A, Roumier C et al (2008) Cooperating gene mutations in acute myeloid leukemia: a review of the literature. Leukemia22(5):915–931

Ridge SA, Worwood M et al (1990) FMS mutations in myelodysplastic, leukemic, and normal subjects. Proc Natl Acad Sci USA 87(4):1377–1380

Rocnik JL, Okabe R et al (2006) Roles of tyrosine 589 and 591 in STAT5 activation and transformation mediated by FLT3-ITD. Blood 108(4):1339–1345

Schessl C, Rawat VP et al (2005) The AML1-ETO fusion gene and the FLT3 length mutation collaborate in inducing acute leukemia in mice. J Clin Invest 115(8):2159–2168

Schnittger S, Kohl TM et al (2005) KIT-D816 mutations in AML1-ETO positive AML are associated with impaired event-free and overall survival. Blood 105(8):3319–3321

Stirewalt DL, Kopecky KJ et al (2001) FLT3, RAS, and TP53 mutations in elderly patients with acute myeloid leukemia. Blood97(11):3589–3595

Tefferi A, Pardanani A et al (2009) TET2 mutations and their clinical correlates in polycythemia vera, essential thrombocythemia and myelofibrosis. Leukemia 23(5):905–911

Thiede C, Steudel C et al (2002) Analysis of FLT3-activating mutations in 979 patients with acute myelogenous leukemia: association with FAB subtypes and identification of subgroups with poor prognosis. Blood 99(12):4326–4335

Thiede C, Bloomfield CD et al (2007) The high prevalence of FLT3-ITD mutations is associated with the poor outcome in adult patients with t(6;9)(p23;q34) positive AML – results of an international metaanalysis. ASH Annu Meet Abstr 110(11):761

van der Reijden BA, Dauwerse JG et al (1993) A gene for a myosin peptide is disrupted by the inv(16)(p13q22) in acute nonlymphocytic leukemia M4Eo. Blood 82(10):2948–2952

Vempati S, Reindl C et al (2007) Arginine 595 is duplicated in patients with acute leukemias carrying internal tandem duplications of FLT3 and modulates its transforming potential. Blood 110(2):686–694

Walter MJ, Payton JE et al (2009) Acquired copy number alterations in adult acute myeloid leukemia genomes. Proc Natl Acad Sci USA 106(31):12950–12955

Wiemels JL, Xiao Z et al (2002) In utero origin of t(8;21) AML1-ETO translocations in childhood acute myeloid leukemia. Blood 99(10):3801–3805

Yamada Y, Rothenberg ME et al (2006) The FIP1L1-PDGFRA fusion gene cooperates with IL-5 to induce murine hypereosinophilic syndrome (HES)/chronic eosinophilic leukemia (CEL)-like disease. Blood 107(10):4071–4079

Yamamoto Y, Kiyoi H et al (2001) Activating mutation of D835 within the activation loop of FLT3 in human hematologic malignancies. Blood 97(8):2434–2439

Zhang S, Fukuda S et al (2000) Essential role of signal transducer and activator of transcription (Stat)5a but not Stat5b for Flt3-dependent signaling. J Exp Med 192(5):719–728

Part III

Treatment Considerations in Childhood Leukemia

Classification and Treatment of Acute Lymphoblastic Leukemia

4

Stephen P. Hunger, Valentino Conter, Elizabeth A. Raetz, Maria Grazia Valsecchi, and Guenter Henze

Contents

S.P. Hunger (✉)
The Children's Hospital Denver and the Department of Pediatrics, University of Colorado School of Medicine, Aurora, CO, USA
e-mail: hunger.stephen@tchden.org

V. Conter
Pediatric Hematology Oncology, San Gerardo Hospital, Monza, Italy

E.A. Raetz
Division of Pediatric Hematology/Oncology, New York University Cancer Institute, New York University School of Medicine, New York, NY 10016, USA

M.G. Valsecchi
Medical Statistics Unit, University of Milano-Bicocca, Milan, Italy

G. Henze
Department of Pediatric Oncology/Hematology, Charité, Universitätsmedizin Berlin, Berlin, Germany

G.H. Reaman and F.O. Smith (eds.), *Childhood Leukemia*,
DOI: 10.1007/978-3-642-13781-5_4, © Springer-Verlag Berlin Heidelberg 2011

4.1 IntroductionandOver view

Acute lymphoblastic leukemia (ALL) is the most common pediatric malignancy and accounts for 25% of cancers that occur before 15 years of age and 19% among persons less than 20 years of age (Ries et al. 1999). Based on the most recent estimates from the Surveillance, Epidemiology and End Results (SEER) Program of the National Cancer Institute (NCI), there are about 3,000 cases of ALL diagnosed in the United States each year among persons less than 20 years of age. The incidence peaks at 80–90 cases/million at 2–3 years of age, begins to drop abruptly at age 5–6 years reaching a rate of about 20 cases/million at 8–11 years of age, and then gradually decreases to an annual rate of about 10 cases/million by 20 years of age.

Cure rates for ALL have improved dramatically over time, with 5-year overall survival (OS) rates increasing from less than 10% in the late 1960s to 80% in the period 1990–1994 and 87.5% in 2000–2004 (Pulte et al. 2008). Many individual institutions and cooperative groups have reported continued improvements in outcome in the past 10–15 years, and it is anticipated that 85–90% of children and adolescents diagnosed with ALL in the current era will be long-term survivors (Moricke et al. 2008, 2010; Pulte et al. 2008; Pui et al. 2009; Conter et al. 2010; Gaynon et al. 2010; Pui et al. 2010; Salzer et al. 2010; Silverman et al. 2010). Incidence and survival rates for ALL are similar in high income countries in North American and Western Europe, but are generally much lower in developing and/or low income countries (Hunger et al. 2009).

While lymphoblasts from patients with ALL generally have a similar appearance, the disease is clinically and biologically heterogeneous, and is more accurately considered as a constellation of different disorders. There are major clinical, epidemiological, biological and outcome differences between B-precursor cell (about 85% of cases) and T-cell (about 15% of cases) ALL. Immunophenotypic classes can be further subclassified into groups characterized by recurrent sentinel chromosome abnormalities, particularly translocations that are early, perhaps even initiating, events in leukemogenesis (Pui et al. 2008). Translocations activate cellular proto-oncogenes by one of two general mechanisms (Harrison 2009). The first, which is common in both precursor B- and T-ALL, joins an oncogene to one of the immunoglobulin (*Ig*) heavy or light chain loci (chromosome 14q32: heavy chain gene, *IgH*; chromosome 2q12: light chain gene, *Igκ*; chromosome 22q11: light chain gene, *Igλ*), or to one of the T-cell receptor (*TCR*) loci (chromosome 14q11: *TCRδ* or *TCRα* chromosome 7q35: *TCRβ*). This juxtaposition leads to dysregulated expression of structurally intact proteins whose expression is normally tightly regulated. An example of this class of translocations is the t(8;14)(q24;q32) and variant translocations that occur in essentially all cases of Burkitt lymphoma/leukemia and result in dysregulated high-level expression of c-MYC (Thorley-Lawson and Allday 2008). The second type of chromosome translocation occurs much more frequently in B-precursor as compared to T-cell ALL and creates fusion genes that encode for chimeric proteins possessing novel structural and functional properties not present in the parental wild type proteins (Hunger 1996). This class of translocation typically affects transcription factors, often fusing a DNA binding and/or protein oligomerization domain from one protein with effector domains, such as a transcriptional activation domain, from another protein. Translocations of this class typically occur in introns of each gene; exons of the two genes are then joined together during mRNA splicing. Creation of a functional chimera generally requires that the joined exons from each gene are in the same reading frame (Hunger et al. 1994). A prototypic example is the cryptic t(12;21)(p13;q22) that occurs in about 25% of B-precursor ALL cases and leads to production of an ETV6-RUNX1 (TEL-AML1) fusion protein (Loh and Rubnitz 2002). When gene expression profiles of ALL lymphoblasts are analyzed using unsupervised methods, leukemias that share specific common recurrent sentinel chromosome translocations cluster together with one another, suggesting that these sentinel lesions drive the phenotype (Yeoh et al. 2002; Ross et al. 2003).

4.2 HistoricalDevel opment of Treatment Regimens for Newly Diagnosed Childhood ALL

4.2.1 Early Events Leading to First Cures of Childhood ALL

The development of effective treatments for childhood ALL was one of the major successes of twentieth century medicine. The first demonstration of effective use of chemotherapy in any cancer occurred in 1948 when

Sidney Farber reported that children with ALL treated with aminopterin could enter remission (Farber and Diamond 1948). Despite the identification of other effective chemotherapy agents (methotrexate [MTX], cyclophosphamide, prednisone, 6-mercaptopurine [6-MP]) for ALL during the next 15 years, few children with ALL were cured until the early 1960s. During the 1960s, parallel developments at several centers and cooperative groups showed that childhood ALL could be cured. These early groups included many of the centers and cooperative groups that play major roles in contemporary childhood ALL therapy: the "total therapy" trials at St. Jude Children's Research Hospital (SJCRH), the pilot studies in West Berlin that evolved into the Berlin-Frankfurt-Münster (BFM) group, the Cancer Chemotherapy Group A that evolved into the Children's Cancer Group (CCG) and subsequently merged with the Pediatric Oncology Group (POG, which started as the Pediatric divisions of the Cancer and Leukemia Group B and the Southwest Oncology Group) to form the Children's Oncology Group (COG), and the Dana Farber Cancer Institute (DFCI) and later the DFCI consortium (Riehm et al. 1980; Rivera et al. 1993; Gaynon et al. 2000; Maloney et al. 2000; Silverman et al. 2000).

Studies performed at SJCRH in the 1960s were summarized by Pinkel in a 1971 publication describing experience treating 37 children with ALL, eight of whom were alive 5 years later; seven of these eight remained in remission after stopping chemotherapy (Pinkel 1971). This was the first demonstration that a significant number of children with ALL could be *cured*. The introduction of routine presymptomatic central nervous system (CNS) therapy led to further improvements in outcome for childhood ALL. The therapy utilized was quite limited by today's standards: Induction with vincristine and prednisone, followed by long-term use of daily 6-MP, weekly MTX, vincristine and cyclophosphamide every 1–2 weeks, and craniospinal irradiation (500 cGy initially, later increased to 1,200c Gy)(R iverae ta l. 1993).

4.2.2 Phases of Multi-agent Chemotherapy

By the 1980s, the basic structure of contemporary ALL treatment regimens was recognizable and consisted of four phases: Induction, CNS preventative therapy or Consolidation, Intensification, and Maintenance or Continuation. Induction therapy in ALL typically lasts 4–6 weeks and includes 3–5 systemic agents. Almost all regimens include a corticosteroid (either prednisone or dexamethasone), vincristine, and L-asparaginase, which comprise the "3-drug" Induction (Ortega et al. 1977). An anthracycline, typically daunorubicin, is also included in many regimens ("4 drug" Induction) (Sallan et al. 1978), with other agents such as cyclophosphamide used in a small minority of protocols. Over 98% of children with ALL will enter remission by the end of 4 weeks of Induction therapy, and the mortality rate from toxicity during Induction therapy is generally less than 2–3% in industrialized countries (Puie ta l. 2008).

The idea that the CNS served as a "sanctuary site" for lymphoblasts emerged in the mid-1960s when the introduction of effective systemic chemotherapy led to high remission rates, but a majority of patients experienced relapse within 6–12 months, with many of these relapses involving only the spinal fluid. Based on these observations, presymptomatic CNS radiation was introduced in the late 1960s and early 1970s and led to substantial increases in cure rates (Aur et al. 1972). Modern CNS preventative therapy includes periodic administration of intrathecal (IT) chemotherapy (usually MTX, but sometimes "triple IT therapy" that also includes cytarabine and hydrocortisone) starting at the time of the first diagnostic lumbar puncture (Pui and Howard 2008). Systemic agents with improved CNS penetration (dexamethasone rather than prednisone, intravenous MTX) may also play an important role in CNS control (Bostrom et al. 2003; Pui et al. 2008). Most groups now administer cranial irradiation to only a minority (15–25%) of ALL patients, and some have completely eliminated this treatment modality (see below) (Pui et al. 2009; Veerman et al. 2009).

Following the induction of remission, patients receive additional chemotherapy designed to "consolidate" the remission that lasts about 6 months. The intensity and duration of the Consolidation or Intensification phase differs between regimens. Alternating cycles of non-cross resistant chemotherapy drugs are commonly employed, and almost all regimens include a re-Induction/re-Consolidation phase based on the BFM protocol II (see below) (Schrappe 2004). The Maintenance phase of treatment generally continues until 2–3 years from the time of diagnosis and consists of daily oral 6-MP and weekly oral MTX, with variable administration of IT chemotherapy. Some centers or groups also employ periodic doses of vincristine and corticosteroid "pulses" lasting 5–7 days.

4.2.3 Evolution of BFM Therapy

One of the major developments in childhood ALL therapy was the report by Riehm and colleagues in 1977 of their experience with an intensive 8-week, 8-drug Induction protocol (the BFM Protocol I) (Riehm et al. 1977). In the second 4 weeks of Protocol I, four doses of IT MTX and cranial radiotherapy (18 Gy) were given. Protocol I was followed by Maintenance therapy that consisted of daily 6-MP, weekly MTX, and three prednisone-vincristine pulses. Patients treated with this regimen in the original West Berlin pilot study obtained a 55% 5-year EFS (Riehm et al. 1977, 1980). Once a significant percentage of children with ALL could be cured, it became possible to identify prognostic factors (see below for a more detailed discussion of prognostic factors). One of the first recognized prognostic factors was the initial white blood cell count (WBC), with children with a higher WBC having inferior cure rates as compared to those with a lower WBC (Henze et al. 1981a, b). The BFM 76/79 study showed that outcome, especially of those with a high WBC, could be improved by repeating Protocol I (with minor modifications) (Henze et al. 1981a). This second 7-week block became known as Protocol II (delayed Intensification (DI) in the COG studies) and was administered either immediately after Protocol I or after a 4-month interim Maintenance (IM) phase. Overall, patients treated in the BFM 76/79 study had a 10-year disease-free survival (DFS) rate of 67%, with the best results obtained when the IM phase was given between Protocols I and II (Henze et al. 1981a).

Another major development in BFM-based therapy was the introduction of the prednisone prophase in ALL-BFM 83 (Riehm et al. 1990). This 1-week course of prednisone (60 mg/m^2/day × 7 days) with a single dose of IT MTX given on day 1 was designed to decrease complications related to tumor lysis syndrome. The prednisone prophase became highly predictive of outcome as an indicator of rapid response to therapy (Riehm et al. 1990). In ALL-BFM-86, protocol M was introduced (Reiter et al. 1994). This 8-week phase occurs between Protocol I and Protocol II (substituting for the IM phase used in prior studies) and consists of four courses of high-dose (HD; 5 g/m^2) MTX infused over 24 h with leucovorin rescue. In parallel to the introduction of protocol M, the indications for cranial radiotherapy were progressively restricted.

The German BFM group expanded to include the Austrian (1980s) and Swiss (1990s) groups. Other European groups began to cooperate with the BFM group in this time frame, forming the so-called "BFM-family." In the 1990s, other groups from Europe and other continents joined the BFM-family, which in 1995 was named the International BFM Study Group (I-BFM-SG) (Schrappe et al. 2000a, b). The BFM, AEIOP (Italy), GATLA (Argentina), PINDA (Chile), CPH (Czech Republic), Hungarian, and EORTC-CLCG (Belgium, France and Portugal) study groups began the first I-BFM-SG trial in 1995, which was designed as a prospective meta-analysis to evaluate the role of vincristine/dexamethasone pulses during Maintenance in the context of contemporary BFM therapy (see below) (Conter et al. 2007).

In 2000, the AIEOP and BFM groups started a common study (AIEOP-BFM ALL 2000) in which patients were stratified according to early response based on measurement of minimal residual disease (MRD) by PCR of *Ig/TCR* gene rearrangements (Flohr et al. 2008). The treatment schedules used by the two groups were, however, slightly different. A major development in BFM regimens over the past several decades has been the use of different post-Induction treatment strategies for patients at high risk of treatment failure (Moricke et al. 2008). Three different therapeutic strategies were evaluated in the AIEOP-BFM ALL 2000 study for very high-risk patients following completion of protocol: (1) six high-risk blocks of myelosuppressive therapy and one Protocol II; (2) three high-risk blocks and Protocol II given twice; (3) three high-risk blocks and Protocol III (a 4-week reduced intensity version of Protocol II) given three times.

The AIEOP-BFM ALL 2009 study has recently begun to accrue patients and additional groups including the CPH, INS (Israel) and SW (Sydney, Australia) will participate in this trial. Patients at high risk of relapse, defined on the basis of early response (poor prednisone response or high levels of MRD) or adverse cytogenetic features will receive three polychemotherapy blocks followed by three delayed Intensifications as post-Induction treatment. Indications for hematopoietic stem cell transplantation (HSCT) will depend largely on MRD response; treatment tailoring will also be implemented for patients with persistent high MRD levels.

4.2.4 COG Adaptation and Modification of BFM-Based Therapy

In the early to mid-1980s, the CCG recognized that reported outcomes with BFM therapy appeared superior to those obtained by the CCG with less intensive treatment. Based on this, two pivotal trials were conducted to compare BFM-based therapy to CCG regimens of the time. The CCG trials used BFM-76 therapy and so never included the prednisone prophase introduced in BFM-83, or HD MTX as given in protocol M introduced in BFM-86. Children with ALL and unfavorable presenting factors were randomized in CCG 106 (1983–1987) to receive either the CCG standard regimen, a regimen based on BFM-76 that included slightly modified versions of Protocol I (referred to as Induction and Consolidation) and Protocol II (DI, which included re-Induction and re-Consolidation phases), or the "New York" regimen (Gaynon et al. 1993). Both experimental regimens produced outcomes that were substantially better than those obtained with the control CCG regimen, but the BFM-76-based regimen was associated with less toxicity, fewer inpatient hospital days, and lower cumulative anthracycline and cyclophosphamide doses than the New York regimen. Because of these factors, the BFM-76-based regimen became the backbone for subsequent CCG high-risk (HR) ALL trials, which therefore have included a 4-drug Induction (Protocol Ia), a cyclophosphamide and cytarabine-based Consolidation (Protocol Ib), 2 months of IM consisting of daily oral 6-MP and weekly oral MTX, and a DI that included re-Induction and re-Consolidation phases.

In parallel, the CCG 105 trial (1983–1989) randomized children with intermediate-risk (similar, but not identical, to NCI standard-risk) ALL to receive either the baseline CCG regimen, the BFM-76-based regimen with both Protocols I and II, or intermediate BFM-76-based arms that included either Protocol I but not Protocol II, or Protocol II but not Protocol I. All three BFM-76-based arms were better than the CCG arm, but there was little difference between the BFM arms (Tubergen et al. 1993; Hunger et al. 2005). As a consequence of these results, the CCG adopted the regimen that included Protocol II but not Protocol I, so that subsequent CCG (and COG) trials for standard-risk (SR) ALL utilized a 3-drug Induction without anthracyclines, a 4-week Consolidation with oral 6-MP and weekly IT MTX, 2 months of IM with daily oral 6-MP and weekly oral MTX, followed by a DI phase analogous to the BFM Protocol II. Earlier CCG studies that included a less intensive (and less effective) chemotherapy backbone had shown that monthly 5-day pulses of prednisone with one intravenous (IV) dose of vincristine given during Maintenance therapy improved outcome (Bleyer et al. 1991). These pulses have remained a component of all subsequent CCG/COG treatment regimens, although their importance in the context of contemporary treatment regimens has never been proven (see below) (Richards et al. 1996; Conter et al. 2007).

Several subsequent clinical trials established the framework of contemporary COG ALL treatment regimens. Trials were typically stratified to include patients at either lower or higher risk of relapse. Starting in the late 1980s and early 1990s, this stratification was generally based on the "NCI/Rome" criteria, with standard-risk patients being those 1–9.99 years of age with an initial WBC less than 50,000/μL, and high-risk patients being those age 10+ years and/or with an initial WBC greater than or equal to 50,000/μL (Smith et al. 1996). The CCG also showed that early response was an important predictor of outcome, analogous to the prednisone response used in BFM trials (Gaynon et al. 1997). However, the CCG focused on the bone marrow (BM) blast count after 7 or 14 days of multi-agent systemic therapy. In children with HR ALL, an M3 (>25% blasts) day 8 BM response was the strongest predictor of poor outcome (Gaynon et al. 1990; Steinherz et al. 1996). Based on this, CCG 1882 randomized HR-ALL patients with slow early response (M3 BM at day 8 of Induction) to receive the standard CCG BFM-76-based regimen or an "augmented" regimen that included multiple changes (Nachman et al. 1998). The major changes included: (1) lengthening the Consolidation phase to 2 months and adding doses of non-myelosuppressive agents (vincristine and asparaginase) during periods of myelosuppression that occur 2 weeks after cyclophosphamide and cytarabine pulses; (2) utilizing the Capizzi I regimen of escalating IV MTX without leucovorin rescue plus asparaginase, rather than an oral MTX and 6-MP based IM phase; and (3) administering two rather than one IM and DI phases. This "augmented BFM (ABFM)" regimen resulted in significant improvements in 5-year EFS (75% vs 55%; $p < 0.001$) and OS (78 vs 67%; $p = 0.02$) for these slow responder patients (Nachman et al. 1998). The subsequent CCG 1961 trial showed that the ABFM regimen also improved outcome for HR-ALL patients with a rapid early response

(25% or fewer BM blasts at day 8 of Induction), and that the key components of ABFM were the augmented post-Induction therapy rather than second IM/DI phases (Seibel et al. 2008).

For children with intermediate-risk ALL (most of whom met current SR-ALL definitions), CCG 1891 showed that, in the context of a prednisone-based Induction, administering two DI courses was better than one (Lange et al. 2002). The successor CCG 1922 SR-ALL trial showed that dexamethasone (6 mg/m^2) was superior to prednisone (40 mg/m^2) when given during Induction and Maintenance therapy in a treatment backbone that had a single DI phase (Bostrom et al. 2003). Interestingly, outcomes in CCG 1891 with a prednisone backbone and two DI phases appeared quite similar to those obtained in CCG 1922 with a dexamethasone backbone and one DI phase. CCG 1991 was conducted in parallel to CCG 1961 and randomized SR-ALL patients in a 2 × 2 manner to compare, on a dexamethasone backbone, one versus two DI phases and the standard oral MTX and 6-MP based IM phase to a regimen of escalating intravenous (IV) MTX without leucovorin rescue, in this case without any additional doses of asparaginase. The IV MTX based IM phase proved superior to the oral regimen, almost entirely due to a reduction in the rate of extramedullary relapses, and nearly identical outcomes were obtained with one or two DI phases (Matloub eta l. 2006, 2008).

These studies established the foundation of contemporary COG B-precursor ALL trials, which enroll approximately 1,800 patients/year. The baseline regimen for children with NCI SR-ALL (AALL0331 trial) includes a 3-drug Induction, a 4-week oral Consolidation, an 8-week IV MTX based IM phase, an 8-week DI phase, and Maintenance therapy with monthly dexamethasone and vincristine pulses. A low risk group, that includes patients with *ETV6-RUNX1* fusion or simultaneous trisomies of chromosomes 4, 10 and 17, is randomized to receive this baseline regimen with or without four additional doses of PEG-asparaginase given every 3 weeks following Induction therapy. Standard-risk ALL patients without favorable genetic features are randomized to receive the 4-week oral Consolidation or the 8-week augmented Consolidation from the ABFM regimen. Those standard risk patients with a poor initial response (>5% BM blasts at day 15 or >0.1% MRD at day 29 of Induction) are non-randomly assigned to receive the full ABFM therapy with two IM and DI phases. The AALL0331 trial completed accrual in May 2010.

In parallel, the COG AALL0232 trial for children, adolescents and young adults with HR B-precursor ALL uses the so-called hemi-ABFM (hABFM) baseline regimen that consists of a 4-drug induction, augmented 8-week Consolidation, an 8-week Capizzi IV MTX with PEG asparaginase-based IM phase, a single 8-week DI phase, followed by Maintenance therapy with monthly corticosteroid and vincristine pulses. All patients are randomized to receive the Capizzi MTX IM phase or four courses of HD MTX given as administered in BFM trials. When AALL0232 began in 2003, all patients were randomized to receive 14 days of dexamethasone (10 mg/m^2) or 28 days of prednisone (60 mg/m^2) during Induction. However, patients older than 10 years experienced excess rates of osteonecrosis (ON) with dexamethasone during induction, so the steroid randomization was subsequently limited to patients <10 years of age. High-risk patients with a poor initial response (>5% BM blasts at day 15 or >0.1% MRD at day 29 of Induction) are non-randomly assigned to receive the full ABFM therapy with two IM and DI phases. This study will complete accrual in late 2010.

The COG now treats children with T-cell ALL on a separate clinical trial (AALL0434, accrual about 200 patients/year), which uses the same baseline hABFM regimen as is used for those with high-risk B-precursor ALL. The AALL0434 trial, which will continue to accrue patients until 2013, asks two randomized questions. The first is a Capizzi MTX vs. HD MTX question during IM, identical to that asked in the high-risk B-precursor ALL trial. The second question involves the randomized administration of six 5-day courses of nelarabine integrated into the hABFM backbone. Nelarabine, a prodrug of Ara-G, is uniquely cytotoxic to T-lymphoblasts and demonstrated very promising efficacy in patients with relapsed/refractory T-ALL (Berg et al. 2005). However, significant neurotoxicity was encountered when this agent was administered to heavily pre-treated patients with relapsed T-ALL. Prior to starting the current Phase III trial, the COG conducted a pilot study in newly diagnosed T-ALL patients and showed minimal toxicity and encouraging signs of efficacy in patients with a poor initial response to therapy (Dunsmore et al. 2008). The current AALL0434 study will establish whether or not this promising agent improves the outcome of newly diagnosed T-ALLpa tients.

4.2.5 Development and Evolution of DFCI Consortium ALL Regimens

The DFCI consortium trials have evolved independently of BFM and COG regimens. A key component of DFCI therapy has been the use of weekly high doses of asparaginase during the Consolidation or Intensification phase of therapy. This approach was first shown to be beneficial in the DFCI 77-01 trial (1977–1979) (Sallan et al. 1983). In more recent DFCI trials, high-dose (25,000 IU/m^2) weekly asparaginase treatment begins immediately after the conclusion of Induction therapy. The DFCI 91-01 trial utilized 30 weeks of high-dose asparaginase and found that patients that tolerated 25 or fewer doses had an inferior outcome to that obtained by patients who tolerated 26 or more doses (Silverman et al. 2001). The manner in which asparaginase is used in DFCI trials is quite different from that employed by most other groups, and the excellent outcome of DFCI trials has prompted others to explore whether intensified asparaginase treatment might improve outcomes when added to different chemotherapy backbones.

The DFCI trials have also included frequent vincristine/steroid pulses during all phases of post-Induction therapy, and relatively high cumulative doses of anthracyclines in higher risk patients. Significant cardiotoxicity was encountered early in the evolution of DFCI studies in the 77–01 trial, after which the total anthracycline dose was limited and a lower cumulative dose was used for non-high-risk patients (Sallan et al. 1983). The DFCI group has tested several interventions to limit cardiotoxicity, including different schedules of anthracycline administration and the use of the cardioprotectant dexrazoxane, with the latter showing very promising early reductions in cardiac injury as measured by less elevation in troponin T levels (Lipshultz et al. 2004). Long-term studies currently in progress will determine whether changes in this biomarker are reflective of reductions in the incidence of late clinical cardiotoxicity.

4.2.6 Development and Evolution of SJCRH ALL Regimens

Therapy used in SJCRH trials has evolved considerably from the early Total Therapy trials (Rivera et al. 1993; Pui et al. 2000, 2010). A major focus of recent SJCRH trials has been the reduction, and now complete elimination, of presymptomatic cranial irradiation along with the use of up-front windows to explore new therapies and detailed correlative biology studies (Pui and Howard 2008; Pui et al. 2009). The initial 7 weeks of therapy on SJCRH trials is an intensive Induction/Consolidation phase similar to the BFM Protocol I, but with the second block of therapy starting earlier (Pui et al. 2009); this is followed by an 8-week block analogous to the BFM Protocol M, but with doses of MTX individualized to obtain pre-specified target blood concentrations. Patients then receive a 6-month early Continuation/re-Induction phase, during which all patients (low, standard and high-risk) receive two re-Induction treatments. Standard and high-risk patients also received 20 weekly doses of asparaginase during this phase. Maintenance therapy for low-risk patients consists of oral 6-MP and MTX with periodic dexamethasone/vincristine pulses, while the remaining patients are treated with rotating pairs of agents (6-MP plus MTX, cyclophosphamide plus cytarabine, dexamethasone plus vincristine). Intrathecal triple therapy rather than IT MTX alone is used throughout treatment. This approach produced outstanding results in the Total XV study conducted from 2000 to 2007, with no signs of increased CNS failures after the elimination of cranial irradiation (see below) (Puie ta l.2009).

4.2.7 Treatments Used by Other ALL Cooperative Groups

A number of other cooperative groups have made significant contributions to ALL therapy; outcomes of trials from most of these groups have recently been published (Conter et al. 2010; Kamps et al. 2010; Liang et al. 2010; Mitchell et al. 2010). The outcomes obtained with the different regimens are relatively similar to one another and the minor differences that exist may be due to the different number and size of centers included, the different age ranges of treated patients, and the differences in genetic composition of patients treated by different groups.

4.3 UniqueSu bsetso fA LL

4.3.1 Infants

Only 2–3% of ALL cases occur in infants less than 1 year old (approximately 100 cases/year in the United States), but this is a biologically unique subset of ALL with a poor outcome. While outcome for infants with ALL has improved significantly over the past 10–15 years, the 4-year EFS was only 47% in the Interfant-99 trial, which was the largest infant ALL study ever conducted, but which still only enrolled 482 patients from 1999 to 2005 (Pieters et al. 2007). Infant ALL is biologically distinct from acute leukemia that occurs in older children, with translocations of the 11q23 *MLL* (mixed lineage leukemia) gene present in 70–80% of infant ALLs (Rubnitz et al. 1994; Pieters et al. 2007). Infants with *MLL*-rearranged ALL have a significantly worse outcome than do the 20–30% with germline *MLL*, but the outcome of the latter group is still significantly worse than obtained among older children with ALL. Approximately 50% of the 11q23 translocations join *MLL* to *AF-4* (chromosome 4q21), 20% to *ENL* (chromosome 19p13.3) and 10% to *AF9* (chromosome 9p22). Several dozen other *MLL* translocation partners have been described, with most occurring in a small percentage of cases. While some controversy exists, the outcome of infants with different *MLL* translocation partners is generally similar.

New therapies are needed for infant ALL, as only about half of patients (and even fewer of the patients with *MLL* translocations) are cured despite the use of extremely intensive chemotherapy regimens that approach, or in some cases cross, the bounds of acceptable toxicity (Dreyer et al. 2007a). HSCT has been explored by both US and European groups with marginal impact on outcome. The Interfant group found that HSCT was modestly superior to chemotherapy for a high risk subgroup (*MLL*-rearranged with age < 6 months or initial WBC > 300,000/μL), but did not benefit most patients (Pieters et al. 2007). The COG found no benefit for HSCT in infant ALL (Dreyer et al. 2007b). Further improvements in outcome for this group will likely require integration of more targeted non-cytotoxic therapies; both the COG and Interfant are currently testing, or planning to test, FLT3 inhibitors in infant ALL (Brown et al. 2006).

4.3.2 Young Adults

Young adults (YA) 16–21 years of age with ALL have historically had significantly lower EFS and OS compared to children and younger adolescents (Chessells et al. 1998; Pulte et al. 2009). The inferior outcome in older adolescents may be partially attributable to the differences in biology between YA and younger children, with the YA showing a lower rate of favorable biological subsets (*ETV6-RUNX1* fusion or hyperdiploidy with favorable chromosome trisomies) and a modestly higher rate of unfavorable biological subsets such as Philadelphia chromosome-positive (Ph+) ALL. However, these differences do not completely account for the differences observed in outcome between YA and young children with ALL.

One important factor that influences outcome is the setting in which treatment is delivered to YA ALL patients. There have now been several retrospective studies that have demonstrated dramatically better outcomes for YA ALL patients enrolled and treated on pediatric as compared to adult cooperative group protocols. The first and largest was a comparison of ALL patients 16–20 years of age treated on CCG or Cancer and Leukemia Group B (CALGB) (adult) clinical trials from 1988 to 2001 (Stock et al. 2008). Despite having similar percentages of patients with favorable or unfavorable biological features in the two groups, the YA patients treated on CCG trials had a dramatically better outcome than those treated on CALGB trials (7-EFS 63% vs 34%; $p < 0.001$). Similar differences were seen when the outcome of YA patients 15–20 years old with ALL treated on the pediatric FRALLE-93 protocol was compared to outcome of patients of the same age treated on the adult LALA-94 protocol (5-year EFS of 67% vs 41%; $p < 0.0001$) (Boissel et al. 2003). Analogous differences in the outcome of YA ALL patients treated in different environments were seen in the Netherlands (de Bont et al. 2004). Outcomes for YAs with ALL treated on pediatric cooperative group trials continue to improve. Nachman et al. reported the largest series to date; 262 YAs with ALL treated on CCG 1961 between 1996 and 2002 attained a 5-year EFS of 71.5% and OS of 77.5%, with rapid responder patients randomized to the ABFM therapy having a 5-year EFS of 81.8% (Nachman et al. 2009). While the adult cooperative groups have tested routine use of HSCT in ALL patients older than 15 years of age (Goldstone et al. 2008), the results of CCG 1961 establish that there is no role for the routine use of HSCT in first remission for YAs with ALL.

While the reason(s) behind the dramatically better outcome of YA patients treated on pediatric rather than adult ALL trials are uncertain, clearly the outcome differential suggests that it should be considered standard of care for YAs with ALL to be treated at a pediatric center on a pediatric ALL regimen, or at an adult center that is testing such a regimen as part of a clinical trial. It also seems logical to test pediatric ALL regimens in adults older than 21–22 years of age. Indeed, the COG has extended the age of eligibility on its ALL trials to 30 years of age, but very few patients older than 23–24 years old have been enrolled. A number of adult cooperative groups and centers have begun to use pediatric ALL regimens for YAs and to test these regimens in adults older than 22 years of age. The US adult cooperative groups are conducting a joint study (C10403) of COG ALL therapy in patients 16–29 years of age. Ribera and colleagues recently reported outcomes of the Spanish Program Espanol de Tratamiento en Hematologia pediatric based protocol ALL-96 regimen in patients 15–30 years of age (Ribera et al. 2008). Outcomes were similar for patients 15–18 vs 19–30 years of age, with 6-year EFS 61% and OS 69%. The DFCI group has been treating adults with ALL who are 18–50 years of age with a regimen identical to their pediatric protocol, with very promising early results and an acceptable toxicity profile (DeAngelo et al. 2007). Similarly, the French extended pediatric ALL regimens to patients up to 60 years of age on the GRAAL2 study with encouraging results, but they did encounter increased rates of morbidity and mortality in patients older than 45 years of age (Huget et al. 2008). These emerging data establish that is feasible to use pediatric ALL regimens for patients up to 45–50 years of age, and suggest that this approach leads to major improvements in cure rates.

4.3.3 Philadelphia Chromosome-Positive ALL

Historically, one of the worst prognostic factors in pediatric ALL has been the t(9;22)(q34;q11.2) or Philadelphia chromosome. Although Ph+ ALL accounts for only about 3% of children with ALL, this group has had an extremely poor outcome, with the largest study of patients treated from 1986 to 1996 showing a 7-year EFS of 25% and OS of 36% (Arico et al. 2000). Optimizing chemotherapy and HSCT regimens produced only a modest improvement in outcome with a subsequent retrospective review of over 600 Ph+ ALL patients treated by 14 cooperative groups from 1995 to 2005 showing 7-year EFS of 31.2% and OS of 44.2% (Aricoe ta l. 2008).

However, the development of imatinib, a tyrosine kinase inhibitor (TKI) targeted at the BCR-ABL1 kinase produced by the t(9;22), has revolutionized treatment of chronic myeloid leukemia and serves as a paradigm for the potential benefit of targeted therapies in high-risk ALL subtypes defined by sentinel molecular lesions (Druker 2009). Imatinib is active as a single agent in patients with Ph+ ALL, but responses are transient. A number of groups have incorporated imatinib into multi-agent chemotherapy regimens. The COG AALL0031 trial (2002–2006) incorporated imatinib, starting after completion of Induction therapy, into a very intensive chemotherapy regimen in a stepwise fashion (Schultz et al. 2009). Patients in the last cohort of this study (#5) received continuous treatment with imatinib 340 mg/m^2/day from the start of Consolidation, with the drug administered on a 2 week on/2 week off schedule for the last year of Maintenance therapy. Addition of imatinib did not increase toxicities and the regimen was well tolerated. The patients treated in Cohort 5 attained a 3-year EFS of 80%, which was more than double that seen in historical controls (35 ± 4%; $p < 0.0001$). There was no advantage for HSCT, with 3-year EFS similar for patients in Cohort 5 treated with chemotherapy plus imatinib or sibling donor HSCT. While these results require longer follow-up, they suggest that active molecularly targeted therapies can dramatically improve the outcome of ALL patients with specific sentinel chromosome lesions. One can anticipate that this paradigm will be extended to other patient subgroups in the next 5–10 years as new high-risk genetic lesions are identified and new targeted therapies are developed (Mullighan et al. 2009 a, b).

4.3.4 Down Syndrome

Acute lymphoblastic leukemia occurs much more frequently in children with Down syndrome (DS-ALL) as compared to those without DS (1 in 300 children with DS vs 1 in 3,500 children without DS) (Whitlock 2006). The subgroup of DS patients, which accounts for about 3% of children with ALL, presents unique challenges, since DS patients have increased treatment-related morbidity and mortality. Many groups have reported that children with DS-ALL have inferior outcomes to those without DS, with both an increased risk of relapse and higher rates of non-relapse death. The distribution of ALL subtypes that occurs in children with DS differs from that seen in non-DS ALL. For example, T-ALL is almost never seen in children with DS (Forestier et al. 2008). Among B-precursor ALL patients there also appears to be a different frequency of sentinel cytogenetic lesions in children with DS-ALL. An analysis of 2,811 consecutive children with B-precursor ALL enrolled in COG protocols who underwent comprehensive analysis to detect the common recurrent sentinel genetic lesions, provided important insights into these differences (Maloney et al. 2010). While there was no difference in common clinical risk factors (age, gender, WBC, and NCI risk group) between patients with (80) and without (2,731) DS, the DS-ALL patients had significantly lower rates of the favorable cytogenetic lesions *ETV6-RUNX1* (2.5% vs 24%, $p < 0.0001$) and trisomies of chromosomes 4 and 10 (7.7% vs 24%, $p = 0.0009$). Without correcting for these sentinel genetic lesions, the outcome of DS-ALL patients was inferior to that of the non-DS patients with 5-year EFS of 69.9% versus 78.1±% ($p = 0.078$), and 5-year OS of 85.8% versus 90.0% ($p = 0.033$). However, when children with the unfavorable (*MLL*, *BCR-ABL1*) or favorable (*ETV6-RUNX1* and trisomies 4 and 10) genetic lesions were excluded, the EFS and OS were similar for children with and without DS. Recent identification of genetic lesions that lead to over-expression of the cytokine receptor homologue CRLF2 and *JAK2* mutations in DS-ALL further underscore the unique genetic features of this ALL subtype (Bercovich et al. 2008; Mulligan et al. 2009c Nature Genetic; Russell et al. 2009). These differences and the increased rates of non-relapse mortality in children with DS-ALL suggest that this subgroup might be treated differently from children without DS, with more attention to supportive care and perhaps incorporation of targeted therapies in the future.

4.4 TreatmentC ontroversiesand Critical Questions in Childhood ALL

4.4.1 The Role of Cranial Radiotherapy

The addition of presymptomatic cranial or craniospinal irradiation to ALL treatment regimens produced dramatic improvements in cure rates of childhood ALL in the late 1960s and early 1970s (Aur et al. 1972; Pui and Howard 2008). However, irradiation also resulted in development of secondary brain tumors and caused significant long-term deleterious effects on growth, endocrine and neurocognitive function (Pui and Howard 2008). With improvements in systemic therapy it has become possible to progressively decrease the percentage of patients that receive cranial irradiation as well as the dose. However, 15–30% of patients still receive cranial irradiation (1,200–1,800 cGy for selected patients that do not have CNS disease and 1,800–2,400 cGy for patients with overt CNS disease) with most ALL treatment protocols (Pui and Howard 2008). Patients in whom presymptomatic cranial irradiation is employed include those with poor early responses to therapy, adverse genetic features, high WBC, and T-cell ALL. Two recent reports have described very encouraging early outcomes with treatment regimens in which no patients received cranial irradiation (Pui et al. 2009; Veerman et al. 2009). Both studies were relatively small compared to large cooperative BFM and COG trials, but the findings are provocative and challenge other groups to consider ways in which the use of presymptomatic cranial irradiation can be further reduced or eliminated. Pui has also suggested other approaches that may help to decrease the rate of CNS relapse, including having highly experienced clinicians perform diagnostic lumbar punctures with platelet transfusions used to bring the platelet count above 100,000/μL, optimal choice of equipment and positioning of the patient post lumbar puncture (Pui and Howard 2008).

4.4.2 Pulses of Steroids and Vincristine During Maintenance Therapy

There are significant differences in how different cooperative groups use pulses of vincristine and steroids during Maintenance therapy. The pulses were first shown to improve outcome in studies conducted in the 1970s and early 1980s that used relatively non-intensive chemotherapy backbones. For example, CCG 161 (1978–1983) randomized low-risk patients to receive or not receive monthly pulses of vincristine 1.5 mg/m^2 and 5 days of prednisone 40 mg/m^2; they showed a significant EFS advantage in the patients that received pulses (Bleyer et al. 1991). However, patients treated in this study received only a 3-drug prednisone-based Induction and no post-Induction DI phase or other form of Intensification. A meta-analysis of randomized ALL trials showed a statistically significant advantage of vincristine/prednisone pulses on EFS, but there was no effect on OS (Richards et al. 1996). However, this analysis was limited to trials that began before 1987, which are not reflective of contemporary therapy. None of the regimens used a dexamethasone-based Induction and none included a DI phase; the overall EFS was less than 70%.

More recently, the I-BFM SG IR-95 group conducted a prospective meta-analysis trial that randomized almost 3,000 patients treated with BFM-based therapy to receive or not receive six pulses of dexamethasone 6 mg/m^2/day × 7 and vincristine 1.5 mg/m^2 on days 1 and 8 during Maintenance therapy (Conter et al. 2007). The outcomes of the two groups were virtually identical with 7-year DFS rates of 77.5% with pulses and 78.4% without pulses, showing no benefit to pulses in the context of intensive BFM-based therapy. Thus, while maintenance steroid/vincristine pulses may be beneficial in the context of low intensity therapy, pulses (as administered in the BFM trial) have little effect on outcome when modern intensive treatment backbones are used. The groups (COG, DFCI, SJCRH) that currently use significant amounts of steroid/vincristine pulses administer them somewhat differently than given in the I-BFM trial and the routine use of such pulses may need to be reconsidered. The COG plans to conduct a randomized trial to examine this question starting in 2010.

4.4.3 Identification of the Optimum Corticosteroid for Induction Therapy

CCG 1922 established that dexamethasone 6 mg/m^2 was superior to prednisone 40 mg/m^2 for children with SR-ALL (Bostrom et al. 2003). Similarly, the United Kingdom MRC97 trial found that dexamethasone 6.5 mg/m^2 was superior to prednisone 40 mg/m^2 among all children with ALL (Mitchell et al. 2005). Other groups have asked analogous randomized questions, but different prednisone to dexamethasone conversion factors have been used. A major confounding factor has been the occurrence of increased infectious morbidity and mortality when dexamethasone was incorporated into a 4-drug Induction regimen, making it challenging to balance the improvements in outcome obtained with dexamethasone with the increased occurrence of major morbidities and toxic deaths. A prime example of this dilemma is provided by recent results of the AIEOP-BFM ALL 2000 study that randomized patients to receive a 4-drug Induction containing 10 mg/m^2/day of dexamethasone or 60 mg/m^2/day of prednisone (Schrappe et al. 2008). Patients randomized to receive dexamethasone had a significant improvement in 6-year EFS, a significant reduction in risk of relapse, but also a significant increase in infectious death during Induction. However, at the time the results were presented there was no effect of steroid preparation on survival. The beneficial effects of dexamethasone were seen particularly in patients with poor prednisone response and those with T-ALL. Trying to strike a balance between the relative advantages and disadvantages of dexamethasone, the AEIOP-BFM group has decided to use dexamethasone in Induction for T-ALL patients, but to continue to use prednisone for patients with B-precursor ALL.

4.4.4 Identification and Treatment of Low-Risk Subsets of Childhood ALL

Subsets of patients with ALL can be identified that have an outstanding outcome with contemporary treatment regimens. It is tempting to try to minimize morbidity and long-term toxicity by identifying patients for whom treatment might be de-escalated. Hunger and colleagues have advocated that reductions in therapy and/or not including patients in randomized trials designed to improve EFS should only be considered for patients with an expected long-term EFS of at least 95% (Hunger et al. 2005). It can be challenging to consider what to do with patient groups that attained an outstanding EFS with intensive therapies. For example, the SJCRH Total XV trial attained a 5-year EFS of 97.6% and OS of 98.9% for patients with *ETV6-RUNX1* fusion, but all patients received an intensive Induction/Consolidation similar to the BFM Protocol Ia and Ib, followed by four courses of HD MTX (Pui et al. 2009; NEJM). Could this outstanding result be maintained with less therapy? If so, which components of therapy should be eliminated? In contrast, other cooperative groups have treated lower risk patients less intensively, potentially providing a mechanism to identify an effective therapy that provides a high cure rate to lower risk patients that could be defined as the "standard" therapy for future trials. The POG had a large experience with using a 3-drug Induction regimen and six courses of intermediate dose MTX (1 gm/m^2 over 24 h) as the only post-Induction Consolidation therapy, with no anthracyclines or alkylating agents. While this regimen does not yield cure rates that are as high as obtained with BFM-type regimens for most patients, the 12% of B-precursor ALL patients with SR-ALL, *ETV6-RUNX1* fusion or trisomies of both chromosomes 4 and 10, and Induction day 8 peripheral blood and day 29 BM MRD <0.01%, had a 97% 5-year EFS with this therapy (Borowitz et al. 2008). This excellent outcome has been maintained with longer follow-up and this therapy will be one of two regimens recommended for these low risk patients in the next generation of COG ALL trials.

4.4.5 The Role of Hematopoietic Stem Cell Transplant in First Remission

The indications for HSCT in children with ALL in first remission (CR1) have evolved as chemotherapy outcomes have improved, and will continue to evolve in the future (Mehta and Davies 2008). There are no randomized trials that directly address the question of when HSCT is appropriate for ALL in CR1, so most recommendations have been based on historical control comparisons and/or parallel clinical experiences. Distinctions are sometimes, but not always, made between matched sibling HSCT and unrelated donor HSCT, although more and more agreement is being reached that unrelated donor transplant using a highly matched donor will yield equivalent outcomes to HSCT with a matched sibling donor.

With these caveats in mind, there are currently only two widely agreed upon indications for HSCT in CR1: low hypodiploidy (modal chromosome number less than 44) and classic Induction failure (M3 marrow at the end of primary Induction therapy). The consensus on the use of HSCT in CR1 for patients with hypodiploidy is based more upon universally poor outcomes obtained with chemotherapy than on definitive proof that HSCT results in improved outcomes, although there are some encouraging unpublished data with HSCT in hypodiploid ALL (Nachman et al. 2007; Mehta and Davies 2008). Most clinicians also consider primary Induction failure to be an indication for HSCT in CR1 based on the very poor outcomes seen in these patients, and there are data from non-randomized trials suggesting that outcomes are better with HSCT than with chemotherapy (Silverman et al. 1999; Balduzzi et al. 2005; Oudot et al. 2008). A nearly-completed large international collaborative review of over 1,000 patients with ALL and Induction failure will provide more insight into clinical features associated with outcome following Induction failure and the relative role of HSCT in different patient subsets (Biondi et al. 2009).

Until recently, HSCT was considered the treatment of choice for children with Ph+ ALL in CR1. A large collaborative review of 326 children with Ph+ ALL published in 2000 showed a clear advantage for matched sibling HSCT vs. chemotherapy, but no advantage for unrelated donor HSCT (Arico et al. 2000). Preliminary results from a follow-up study of 762 children with Ph+ ALL treated between 1995 and 2005 without tyrosine kinase inhibitors showed similar outcomes of matched sibling and unrelated donor HSCT in CR1, with both yielding significantly better DFS than chemotherapy, but this did not translate into an advantage in OS (Arico et al. 2008). The early results of intensive chemotherapy plus imatinib from COG AALL0031 call for a reconsideration of the role of HSCT in CR1 for children and adolescents with Ph+ ALL (see above) (Schultz et al. 2009).

There is much less agreement on the role of HSCT in CR1 for other high-risk subsets of childhood ALL. As discussed earlier, the COG and European Inter-fant groups are currently taking different approaches regarding the role of HSCT in infants with ALL in CR1. Older children with ALL and *MLL* translocations, particularly the t(4;11)(q21;q23) have classically had poor outcomes with chemotherapy and are often considered to be candidates for HSCT in CR1, especially if they have also had a poor early response to chemotherapy. A large retrospective review failed to show benefit to HSCT in patients over 1 year of age with the t(4;11), but was limited to patients diagnosed between 1983 and 1995 (Pui et al. 2003). More recent experience showed an EFS advantage, but no OS advantage, for matched sibling HSCT in CR1 for HR-ALL patients including those with the t(4;11) (Balduzzie ta l. 2005).

Another group that has often been considered as candidates for HSCT in CR1 are patients with T-cell ALL and either a poor early response or high WBC count (Balduzzi et al. 2005). However, results of CCG 1961 showed nearly identical results with chemotherapy for children with T-cell ALL and an initial WBC above or below 200,000/μL, suggesting that HSCT in CR1 is not warranted in such patients (Hastings et al. 2006). Early results from a COG pilot study of Nelarabine plus BFM-based chemotherapy were very promising for T-ALL patients with a poor prednisone response or high levels of MRD at end-Induction, suggesting that these may not be appropriate indications for HSCT in patients with T-ALL in CR1 (Dunsmore et al. 2008). In contrast, Coustan-Smith and colleagues have recently identified a subset of T-ALL patients with "early T-cell precursor (ETP)" ALL that have a very poor outcome with chemotherapy and might be appropriate candidates for HSCT in CR1 (Coustan-Smith et al. 2009).

4.5 PrognosticFac torsandR isk Stratification Approaches

A number of prognostic factors have been defined in childhood ALL and are used by many treatment groups to guide the selection of treatment regimens. The factors of critical importance are those which have been predictive of outcome over time, regardless of the nature of treatment administered. Collectively, prognostic factors are assessed in individual patients at diagnosis and during early phases of treatment and used to predict risk for disease recurrence. The term "risk stratification" is used to describe the selection of a treatment regimen whose intensity is modulated according to the risk for relapse, such that those children who are predicted to have favorable outcomes receive lesser intensity regimens, sparing unwanted toxicity, while those at a higher risk for treatment failure receive more intensified therapy. Several clinical parameters (e.g., age, gender, extramedullary disease), routine laboratory tests (WBC), blast cytogenetic features (e.g., presence or absence of specific translocations and ploidy) and initial response to therapy as assessed by reduction in tumor burden during early phases of therapy are now used routinely for risk stratification and are described below. As additional prognostic markers are defined and the interrelationship of variables such as blast cytogenetics and early treatment response are better understood, treatment will evolve to become more individually tailored. While there is general agreement between different cooperative groups about important risk factors, the groups have taken very different approaches to treatment stratification.

Despite the contribution of risk stratification to overall improvements in ALL outcomes, further refinements are needed, as the majority of children who relapse lack known adverse prognostic markers.

4.5.1 Clinical Features

The two most important clinical prognostic features in childhood ALL are age and initial WBC. Infants and adolescents with ALL have inferior outcomes (Crist et al. 1986; Sather 1986) and a high presenting WBC was one of the first recognized adverse prognostic markers in BFM studies (Henze et al. 1981b). The prognostic importance of these variables was solidified at a NCI sponsored workshop in the US in 1993, where the impact of age and WBC was analyzed across several cooperative group protocols (Smith et al. 1996). This led to the so-called NCI/Rome definitions of standard and high-risk ALL summarized earlier, which have allowed a common framework and context within which to assess the importance of additional and evolving prognostic features, such as blast cytogenetics and early treatment response.

Gender has also been prognostic of outcome in many studies, with boys having a higher rate of relapse than girls; because of this, some cooperative groups administer Maintenance therapy longer in males than in females (Shuster et al. 1998; Pui et al. 1999). The presence of CNS leukemia is also an adverse prognostic factor (Mahmoud et al. 1993; Schultz et al. 2007), prompting some groups to classify patients with CNS leukemia (at least 5 WBCs/μl with blasts) as high-risk and to intensify CNS-directed therapy for those with CNS-2 disease (less than 5 WBCs/μlw ithbla sts).

4.5.2 Blast Immunophenotype and Genotype

Blast immunophenotype is also prognostic of outcome and T-ALL, which represents approximately 15% of cases of newly diagnosed ALL in children, has historically been linked with a poorer prognosis. In comparison to B-precursor ALL, T-ALL is more frequently associated with unfavorable clinical features such as older age, a high WBC count, male gender, bulky adenopathy and CNS involvement (Crist et al. 1986; Pui et al. 1990; Uckun et al. 1997a). The difference in prognosis may in part also relate to intrinsic differences in the chemosensitivity of lymphoblasts. For example, T-ALL blasts are less sensitive than B-precursor ALL blasts to MTX (Kager et al. 2005). However, despite these features, the outcome for T-ALL has improved markedly in recent years due to the application of intensive chemotherapy and now mirrors that seen in B-precursor ALL (Goldberg et al. 2003; Pui et al. 2008). An exception to this is the recently defined ETP subset of T-ALL discussed earlier (Coustan-Smith et al. 2009).

Early studies suggested that antigen promiscuity in B-precursor ALL, most commonly with coexpression of the CD13 and CD33 myeloid antigens, was also associated with inferior outcomes (Wiersma et al. 1991). Subsequent studies (Uckun et al. 1997b; Putti et al. 1998) did not support this conclusion and at the present time therapy is generally not intensified or altered for myeloid antigen positive ALL.

The leukemia karyotype has emerged as one of the most important prognostic variables across multiple cooperative group trials, regardless of the therapy administered. Blast ploidy is one of the most significant prognostic indicators in B-precursor ALL. Patients with high hyperdiploid blasts (>50 chromosomes), which is commonly associated with simultaneous trisomies of specific chromosomes, have a very favorable prognosis with a 5-year EFS rate likely exceeding 90% (Harris et al. 1992; Trueworthy et al. 1992; Heerema et al. 2000; Sutcliffe et al. 2005; Schultz et al. 2007).

In contrast, hypodiploidy portends a poor outcome. Hypodiploidy occurs in 6–9% of childhood ALL cases, with the vast majority having 45 chromosomes. Approximately 1% of children with ALL have extreme hypodiploidy, which is defined as blasts with <44 chromosomes, or a DNA index < 0.81. While the outcomes for children with a modal chromosome number of 44–45 is intermediate, and similar to that observed with pseudodiploid and low-hyperdiploid ALL (47–50 chromosomes), outcomes for children with extreme hypodiploidy are particularly poor, and this group is now classified as very high-risk by most groups (Chessels et al. 1997; Heerema et al. 1999; Nachman et al. 2007; Schultz et al. 2007). As a part of clonal evolution, doubling of the hypodiploid clone can occur, mimicking hyperdiploid ALL (Nachman et al. 2007). Care should be taken to identify these cases so that appropriate therapy can be administered.

In addition to alterations in chromosome number, certain sentinel chromosome translocations have major prognostic importance in childhood ALL. The most common chromosomal translocation is t(12;21), which results in the *ETV6-RUNX1* fusion gene. This alteration occurs in approximately 25% of cases of childhood B-precursor ALL and is associated with favorable outcomes (Loh et al. 2006; Schultz et al. 2007; Rubnitz et al. 2008). The favorable chromosome trisomy and *ETV6-RUNX1* positive cases together account for up to 50% of standard-risk B-cell precursor ALL cases (Loh et al. 2006; Schultz et al. 2007; Rubnitz et al. 2008), and when associated with a favorable early response to treatment as described below, they constitute the "low-risk" group of patients on COG therapeutic studies with outcomes exceeding 95% with less intensive therapy, lacking alkylating agents or anthracyclines (Borowitz et al. 2008).

In contrast to the favorable outcomes observed in *ETV6-RUNX1* positive ALL, the t(9;22) translocation, producing the *BCR-ABL1* fusion transcript, and translocations involving the *MLL* gene portend poor outcomes (Arico et al. 2000; Pui et al. 2002). Treatment of Ph+ ALL was discussed earlier. *MLL* translocations lead to production of chimeric transcription factors consisting of the amino-terminal portion of *MLL* fused to one of more than 40 partner genes (Hunger et al. 1993; Daser and Rabbitts 2005), and are another unfavorable risk cytogenetic subgroup (Behm et al. 1996).

These translocations are observed in more than 80% of infant ALL cases. *MLL* translocations can also be seen in older children, and while they have a negative prognostic impact with EFS of 40–60%, outcomes of older children with these rearrangements are superior to those seen in infants, who have long-term EFS ranging from 20% to 40% (Rubnitz et al. 1994; Chessells et al. 2002; Pui et al. 2002). *MLL* translocations in non-infant patients confer a particularly poor prognosis in those with slow initial responses to chemotherapy (Schultze ta l. 2007).

While the biological basis for differential treatment responses among the cytogenetic subtypes of ALL is often unclear, *in vitro* drug sensitivity studies have linked sensitivity to particular classes of drugs to certain cytogenetic subtypes. For example, *ETV6-RUNX1* positive lymphoblasts show particular sensitivity to L-asparaginase (Ramakers-van Woerden et al. 2000; Loh et al. 2006). Similarly, hyperdiploid ALL blasts have been shown to accumulate very high levels of MTX polyglutamates, making them particularly sensitive to MTX cytotoxicity (Whitehead et al. 1992). These differences in drug sensitivity *in vitro* may offer an explanation for the excellent outcomes achieved in these subsets of patients when treated with regimens in which MTX and asparaginase are essential components of therapy.

With the advent of new technologies for genome-wide analyses, several new cytogenetic alterations of potential prognostic importance are emerging. A gene expression signature was recently identified among children with high-risk B-precursor ALL treated on the COG 9906 study, which was highly predictive of relapse free survival, identifying a group of patients with a 50% likelihood of relapse (Kang et al. 2010). The "molecular risk classifier" was validated in an independent high-risk cohort and further prospective validation is presently underway.

Several other novel genetic aberrations of prognostic significance have been identified from genome-wide single-nucleotide polymorphism (SNP) array analyses in children with high-risk ALL, including alterations of *PAX5*, *IKZF1* (Ikaros) and the *JAK* family of tyrosine kinase (Mullighan et al. 2007, 2009a, b). Genomic alterations of the gene encoding the cytokine receptor CRLF2 are also emerging as a high-risk cytogenetic feature (Mullighan et al. 2009c Native Genetic; Russell et al. 2009). Future risk algorithms will likely incorporate some of these new genetic alterations, if their prognostic significance is confirmed in ongoing prospective trials.

4.5.3 Early Treatment Response

Early response to therapy is one of the most important prognostic variables in childhood ALL, as it encompasses aspects of the host, disease and therapy. Early response can be measured in many ways, including reduction of blasts in the blood or bone marrow, or by more sensitive measures such as the detection of MRD using flow-cytometry or molecular techniques. Numerous studies have shown the favorable prognostic impact of rapid responses to treatment, regardless of the measure used.

The BFM group established the prognostic importance of early treatment response by demonstrating that the rate and magnitude of disappearance of lymphoblasts from the peripheral blood after a 1-week prednisone prophase was highly predictive of outcome (Riehm et al. 1990). Patients with ≥1,000/μL blasts in the blood on day 8 after an initial 7-day prednisone prophase combined with a single dose of intrathecal MTX defined a group of poor-responders at very high risk for subsequent relapse (Schrappe et al. 2000a, b). Investigators at SJCRH have also confirmed the negative prognostic significance of residual peripheral blasts after an initial week of multi-agent Induction therapy; patients who were blast negative on day 8 had a 5-year EFS of 77% compared to 34% among those with residual circulating blasts (Gajjar et al. 1995).

Using morphological measurement of residual marrow blasts after 7 or 14 days of multi-agent Induction chemotherapy, the Children's Cancer Group (CCG) also demonstrated that early treatment response was highly associated with favorable long-term outcomes (Gaynon et al. 1990, 1997). In CCG studies conducted from 1989 to 1995, day 8 marrow status was routinely determined by conventional morphology. Among non-infant patients who achieved remission at end-Induction, 52%, 23%, and 25% of children had an M1 (<5% blasts), M2 (5–25% blasts) and M3 (>25% blasts) day 8 marrow status, respectively. Their EFS was 80 ± 1%, 74 ± 2% and 68 ± 2%, respectively (Gaynon et al. 2000). Similarly, the combined impact of the day 8 and 15 marrow response on outcome was investigated in CCG studies for NCI standard-risk and high-risk ALL conducted from 1996 to 2002. The outcomes for both standard-risk and high-risk patients who achieved an M1 marrow by day 15 were superior to those with M2/3 marrows, with a 5-year EFS of 84.4% versus 66.6% for NCI standard-risk patients and 77% versus

59% for NCI high-risk patients, despite intensification of therapy for those with slow early responses (Schultz eta l. 2007).

Despite the demonstrated value of early morphological response in predicting outcome, the majority of relapses still occur among those with favorable kinetic responses. For example, 70% of events on ALL-BFM 90 occurred in patients with prednisone good response (Schrappe 2004). Thus, more sensitive measures to monitor the tempo and depth of remission were sought. Over the past 20 years, technological advances have allowed for the detection of residual leukemia cells below the threshold detected by conventional morphology, and MRD can now be identified with lower limits of sensitivity of 1 in 10^4 to 1 in 10^6 cells (Roberts et al. 1997; Cave et al. 1998; Evans et al. 1998; Goulden et al. 1998; van Dongen et al. 1998; Biondi et al. 2000; Coustan-Smith et al. 2000; Panzer-Grumayer et al. 2000; Uckun et al. 2000; Schmiegelow et al. 2001; Borowitz et al. 2008). A number of strategies have been developed to monitor MRD including flow cytometry, PCR techniques to identify *Ig/TCR* rearrangements, and PCR detection of fusion gene transcripts.

Several prospective studies (Cave et al. 1998; van Dongen et al. 1998; Coustan-Smith et al. 2000) provided initial strong evidence that quantitative measures of MRD identify patients at high risk for relapse (Cave et al. 1998; van Dongen et al. 1998; Coustan-Smith et al. 2000). Recent data from the COG protocol P9900 have also demonstrated the powerful prognostic impact of end-Induction MRD in almost 2,000 patients (Borowitz et al. 2008). Day 8 peripheral blood and end-Induction (day 29) BM MRD was measured by flow cytometry in a single central reference laboratory; however, the results were not provided to treating physicians or used to alter therapy on the linked series of therapeutic trials. Informative end-Induction flow cytometry MRD results with sensitivity of at least 0.01% were available for 92% of patients within 24–48 h of specimen receipt. End-Induction MRD was highly prognostic, with 5-year EFS of 88 ± 1%, 59 ± 5%, 49 ± 6% and 30 ± 8% for those patients who were MRD negative, or MRD positive in the ranges of 0.01–0.1%, 0.1–1%, and >1%, respectively. This study also defined 0.01% an optimal cutoff for risk stratification given the differences in outcome between those patients who were MRD negative compared to those with end-Induction MRD in the range of 0.01–0.1%. End-Induction marrow MRD was the most important prognostic variable in multivariate analysis in this study. However, 50% of relapses still occurred in the patients that had MRD <0.01% at end-Induction. Day 8 peripheral blood MRD further identified a group of patients with excellent outcomes. When used in conjunction with favorable clinical and cytogenetic features, along with negative day 29 MRD, the absence of peripheral blood MRD on day 8 identified a subgroup of 12% of patients that had a 97 ± 1% 5-year EFS with minimal therapy.

Given the prognostic significance of MRD, it has become a critical determinant for risk stratification within the COG and other cooperative groups. On the AIEOP-BFM ALL2000 trial, PCR-based MRD at two time points (day 33 and day 78) was feasible in 78% of patients and was used for risk stratification and selection of post-Consolidation treatment intensity, replacing many other risk variables (Flohr et al. 2008). Within the COG, risk algorithms are used initially to assign children with newly diagnosed ALL to a standard-risk (3-drug) or high-risk (4-drug) Induction based on NCI risk group and clinical features. At the end of Induction, blast cytogenetics, as well as early morphological response and end-Induction MRD, are used to refine classification into one of four risk groups: low, standard, high, and very high-risk. Future risk algorithms in the COG will use the combination of favorable cytogenetics and negative day 8 peripheral blood MRD and day 29 BM MRD to define a low-risk group of patients with B-precursor ALL who will receive minimal therapy with a predicted EFS exceeding 95%.

Given the powerful predictive value of early MRD response, MRD may be a useful surrogate marker to assess the potential utility of novel treatment interventions. Although it may never replace randomized trials with EFS as a primary endpoint, it can allow investigators to prioritize the many new agents among patient groups where novel approaches are urgently needed.

4.6 RelapsedA LL

4.6.1 Overview

Relapse of ALL is defined as the reappearance of leukemia in bone marrow, blood or any other anatomic compartment following achievement of complete remission with first-line therapy. Relapses have become less frequent during the past 10–20 years as frontline therapies have been improved by tailoring treatment intensity based on patient clinical and response characteristics. Moreover, molecular genetic techniques enabled us to identify patients with poor response to therapy early by measuring MRD and to allocate them to allogeneic stem cell transplantation. With contemporary frontline treatment regimens, the probability of EFS is now above 80%, and relapse rates have been reduced to about 15%. Because of the high frequency of childhood ALL, relapses nevertheless still constitute a substantially frequent diagnosis in pediatric oncology and have still been reported to be the most common cause for death from cancer in children under 15 years of age (Henze 1997; Roy et al. 2005b; Nguyen et al. 2008).

The success of treatment for relapse is limited by various factors. In general, leukemia cells that have survived frontline therapy are more resistant than those present in newly diagnosed patients. In addition, patients have a worse tolerance of treatment, particularly when relapse occurs, while the patient is still receiving primary therapy. Because of the already accumulated toxicity of chemotherapy and/or radiation therapy, doses of certain drugs and irradiation must be restricted in order to avoid severe and unacceptable late effects.

Thus, treatment for relapsed ALL is associated with specific problems that must be considered and addressed for each individual patient, and the chances for success are significantly worse than in newly diagnosed ALL.

4.6.2 Diagnostic Procedures at Relapse

It is essential that a diagnosis of relapsed ALL be absolutely certain. Thus, the diagnostic procedures should follow the same rules as applied at first diagnosis: following careful physical examination, BM, cerebrospinal fluid (CSF) and, if applicable, biopsy material from additional involved sites have to be obtained and investigated morphologically as well as by immunophenotyping, cytogenetic and molecular genetic methods.

A relapse is considered to be an isolated BM relapse if the BM contains at least 25% leukemia cells without evidence of leukemia at other sites. Isolated extramedullary relapse is diagnosed when there is proven leukemia at sites other than the BM, and there are less than 5% blasts in the BM. Combined relapses are those with extramedullary involvement and ≥5% BM blasts.

The most frequent sites of extramedullary relapses are the CNS and the testicles. Clinical signs of a CNS relapse may be headaches, vomiting, blurred vision or polyphagia. Usually, the CSF contains a clearly elevated number of leukemic cells. The standard criteria for CNS relapse are the presence of at least 5 WBC/μL of CSF with blasts identified on a cytospin preparation. Mere pleocytosis with single suspicious cells is not proof of a CNS relapse, and the lumbar puncture should be repeated after 1 or 2 weeks. Rarely, leukemic infiltrates may be detected by MRI scan.

The second most common site of extramedullary relapse of ALL is in the testicle(s). Testicular relapses may be uni- or bilateral and are usually diagnosed following detection of painless testicular enlargement. Definitive diagnosis requires biopsy or orchiectomy of the involved testis and biopsy of the other, clinically uninvolved testis. Other far less frequent extramedullary relapse sites of leukemia include the mediastinum, skin, bone and muscle, prostate or other abdominal organs, or the eye.

At relapse, immunophenotyping and (molecular) genetic testing should be performed as was done at initial presentation. Translocations (e.g., t(9;22), t(12;21), and t(4;11)) can provide important prognostic information. Clone-specific rearrangements of *Ig*/*TCR* genes can be used as MRD markers to assess the quality of second remission (CR2) and for monitoring therapy (Steward et al. 1994). Sentinel cytogenetic lesions and clone-specific *Ig*/*TCR* rearrangements can also be used to distinguish a relapse from a second leukemia (Vora et al. 1998; Lo Nigro et al. 1999).

4.6.3 Risk Factors in Relapsed ALL

Relapse of ALL should be regarded as a new condition, i.e., almost all previously relevant prognostic factors lose their significance. There are several very important prognostic factors that can be used to assess the possibility of cure after relapse, and to select the appropriate treatment for a patient who has relapsed.

4.6.3.1 Timet oR elapse

As shown in Fig. 4.1, the most important risk factor at relapse is the duration of first CR, with lower cure rates

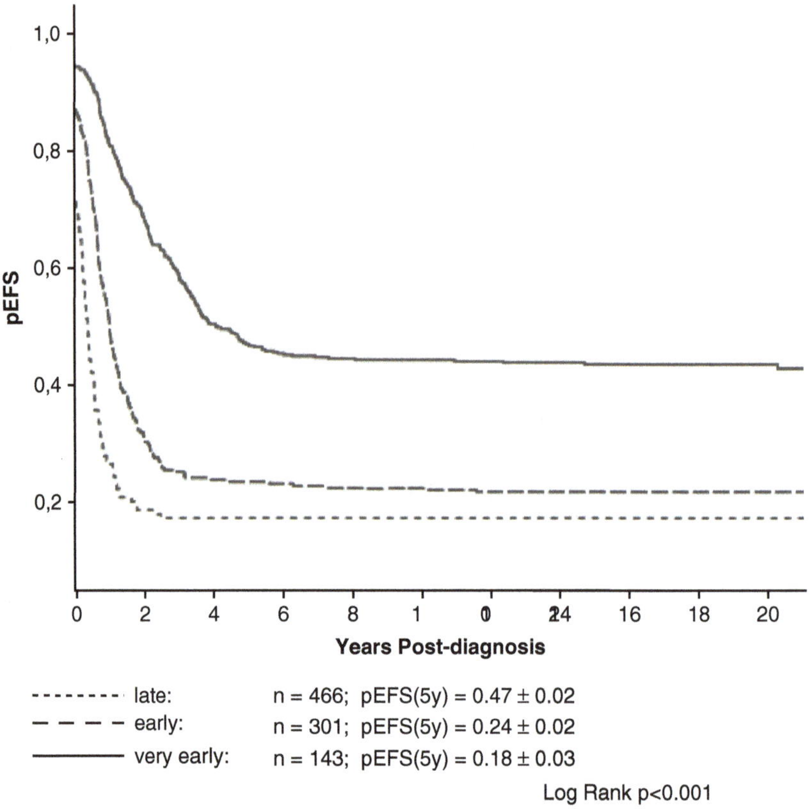

Fig. 4.1 Event-frees urvival(EFS) by time to relapse in BFM REZ trials (late: later than 6 months after cessation of frontline therapy; early: earlier than 6 months after cessation of frontline therapy and later than 18 months after initial ALL diagnosis; very early: earlier than 18 months after initial ALL diagnosis). *pEFS* probability of event-free survival, *cens*.c ensored

for those that relapse earlier following initial diagnosis (Chessells et al. 1994; Gaynon et al. 1998; Nguyen et al. 2008). Different cooperative groups use slightly different definitions of early, intermediate, and late relapse. In the BFM trials for treatment of children with relapsed ALL, late relapses are defined as those occurring more than 6 months after cessation of frontline therapy. Very early relapses occur within 18 months after the initial diagnosis, and early relapses are all others between very early and late. These definitions allow a very clear discrimination concerning the second CR rate as well as the probability of EFS (Fig. 4.1).

Similar results have been reported by other groups, although the relevant points of reference for the definition of early or late relapse are somewhat different (Schroeder et al. 1995; Gaynon et al. 1998; Wheeler et al. 1998; Nguyen et al. 2008). Some groups use the duration of remission after elective cessation of frontline treatment (Miniero et al. 1995) and some others the duration of first CR not related to the duration of frontline therapy. For example, the COG uses the following definitions for time from initial diagnosis to relapse: early: <18 months; intermediate: 18–36 months; and late: >36 months (Nguyen et al. 2008). These different definitions used by different groups make it complicated to compare outcomes of studies for relapsed ALL.

4.6.3.2 Siteo fR elapse

As shown in Fig. 4.2, the site of relapse is also highly predictive of outcome following relapse. Children with BM relapses have a worse outcome compared to those with extramedullary relapses, particularly in the case of late relapses. Surprisingly, the prognosis of patients with combined BM relapses is superior to those with isolated BM relapses (Buhrer et al. 1993; Chessells 1998; Jahnukainen et al. 1998; Nguyen et al. 2008). Although this has been a constant finding in BFM relapse trials and also been confirmed by multivariate Cox regression analysis, the reason for this observation is uncertain. A possible explanation would be that, in part, extramedullary relapses originate from leukemia cells that have survived in a protected environment, such as CNS or testis that has lower exposure to chemotherapy. As a consequence, these cells might be less drug-resistant and more

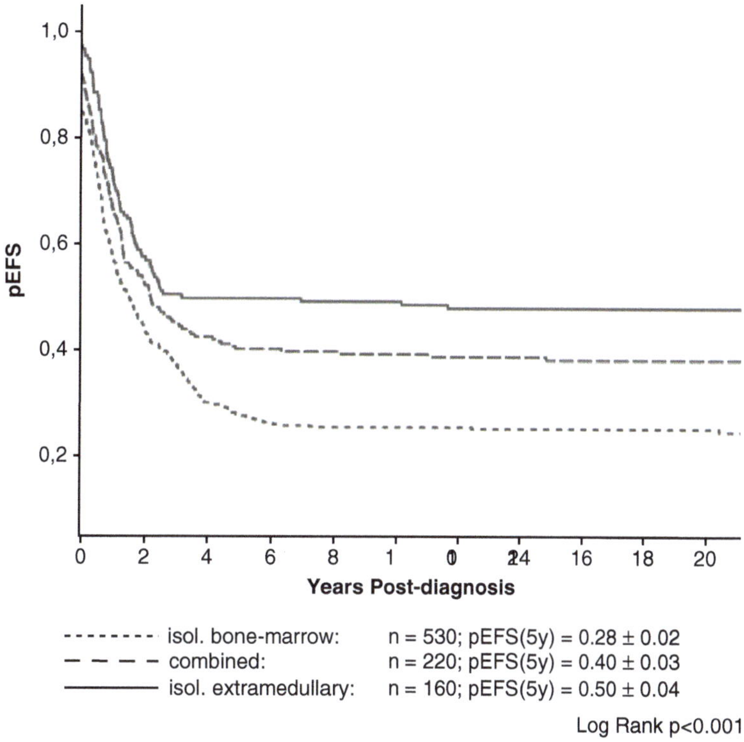

Fig. 4.2 Event-frees urvival(EFS) by site of relapse in BFM REZ trials. *pEFS* probability of event-free survival, *cens.*c ensored

responsive to chemotherapy even after they have reseeded the BM and then appeared as a combined relapse.

Less exposure to chemotherapy may therefore be the explanation for the better prognosis of extramedullary relapses in general. In the CNS, leukemic cells are partially protected by the blood brain barrier; in the testes, the lower temperature might play a role in modulating of the effect of chemotherapy. In case of relapse at these sites, however, it has to be assumed that the leukemic cell burden is so high that chemotherapy alone is not sufficient to eliminate these cells completely. Additional local therapy is necessary to control the leukemia at the extramedullary site and to prevent subsequent hematological relapses which occur as second events at about the same frequency as local relapses. This gives impressive evidence that leukemia is always a systemic disease and the term "isolated" relapse is, at best, descriptive. Local therapy is never sufficient to treat relapse and additional systemic therapy is always necessary, even for "isolated" extramedullary relapses (Buchanan et al. 1991; Henze et al. 1991; Winick et al. 1993; Ribeiro et al. 1995; Gaynon et al. 1998). Consistent with this clinical observation, a significant majority of patients with clinically "isolated" extramedullary relapse are found to have clear evidence of BM involvement with high sensitivity molecular techniques (Neale et al. 1994; Lal et al. 1998;Uckun et al. 1999; Hagedorn et al. 2007).

4.6.3.3 Immunophenotype

The distribution of immunophenotypes in relapse patients is generally similar to that seen at initial presentation. In ALL-REZ BFM trials 90–96, about 14.7% of children with relapsed ALL had T-cell ALL. In a multivariate Cox regression analysis, T-cell immunophenotype was found to be a statistically significant adverse prognostic factor, a finding confirmed by other groups (Henze et al. 1989; Abshire et al. 1992; Chessells et al. 1994). The vast majority of T-cell ALL relapses are very early and early relapses, and late relapses are extremely rare. The response to re-Induction treatment is typically poor, even worse than in otherwise comparable patients with B-precursor ALL. Therefore, T-cell immunophenotype constitutes an independent adverse prognostic feature at relapse.

4.6.3.4 Genotype

Even more than in newly diagnosed ALL, the presence of the Philadelphia chromosome at relapse predicts a poor outcome. In the pre-imatinib era, up to 10% of relapsed pediatric ALL cases were Ph+, with particularly increased rates among those with early or very early relapses. After relapse, the prognosis of these patients was dismal due to a high rate of nonresponse to therapy or subsequent relapses (Fletcher et al. 1991; Beyermann et al. 1997). With the availability of imatinib, the percentage of relapses that are Ph+ is decreasing(Sc hultze ta l. 2009).

As discussed earlier, the most common chromosome translocation in newly diagnosed childhood ALL is the cryptic t(12;21)(p13;q22) that produces *ETV6-RUNX1* fusion. This fusion gene is associated with a favorable prognosis (Borkhardt et al. 1997; Takahashi et al. 1998; Rubnitz et al. 2008). After the first description of this genetic abnormality, a low incidence in relapsed ALL was reported (Rubnitz et al. 1997, 1999; Loh et al. 1998). Surprisingly, in patients enrolled in the BFM relapse trials the frequency of *ETV6-RUNX1*-positivity was not much different than that observed in children with newly diagnosed ALL. However, the median time to relapse was about 4 years, markedly longer than in other patients and the prognosis of successful salvage therapy for these patients was significantly better compared with *ETV6-RUNX1* negative children(Se egere t al. 1998).

Evidence of *ETV6-RUNX1* fusion has been detected in 1–2% of normal cord blood samples. This oncogene can induce a preleukemic phenotype but is insufficient for overt leukemogenesis. Remarkably, the *ETV6-RUNX1* fusion generated during fetal hematopoiesis has been shown to produce a clinically covert preleukemic clone that can persist postnatally for at least 15 years (Greaves and Wiemels 2003). Therefore, evidence exists that some *ETV6-RUNX1* positive "relapses" may be second leukemias caused by an accumulation of additional genetic lesions in cells of a persisting preleukemic clone (Konrad et al. 2003). This could also be an explanation for the better prognosis after "relapse" in this ALL subtype.

Intrachromosomal amplification of chromosome 21 (iAMP21) is a recently described sentinel genetic lesion in childhood ALL that was present in 2% of 1,630 children treated on the UK MRC ALL97 protocol. The abnormality was found in common or pre-B ALL; the children were significantly older (median 9 years vs 5 years), and had a lower WBC count (median 3.9 vs 12.4) compared with children without this abnormality. Patients with iAMP21 had a significantly worse outcome compared with other patients (Strefford et al. 2006; Moorman et al. 2007). The same incidence of this abnormality with slightly better outcomes was reported for patients having been treated according to BFM protocols (Attarbaschi et al. 2008). Thus far, there is no data about the potential impact of iAMP21 in relapse patients.

4.6.3.5 Summary of Risk Factors in Relapsed ALL

Time to relapse, site of relapse and immunophenotype of leukemic cells have been identified as independent prognostic factors determining the risk for subsequent relapse. In addition, the presence of the Philadelphia chromosome has, at least in the pre-imatinib era, been a strong independent adverse prognostic feature at relapse. Taking these factors together, the BFM relapse group has proposed a risk stratification system that includes four groups, S1–S4 (Table 4.1, Fig. 4.3a). Within this system, patients of group S2 with an intermediate prognosis can be split into subgroups based on peripheral blast cell count, site, and Ph+ positivity, leading to subsets with probabilities of post-relapse EFS between 24% and 53% (Table 4.2 and Fig. 4.3b).

Table4.1 BFM ALL relapse risk groups by immunophenotype, timepoint and site of relapse

Site	Immunophenotypenon- T			Immunophenotype(pre-)T		
	IsolatedE M	CombinedB M	IsolatedB M	IsolatedE M	CombinedB M	IsolatedB M
Time						
Verye arly	S2	S4	S4	S2	S4	S4
Early	S2	S2	S3	S2	S4	S4
Late	S1	S2	S2	S1	S4	S4

EM extramedullary, *BM* bone marrow

Fig.4.3 (**a**) Event-free survival of different post-relapse risk groups (ALL-REZ BFM 83–90). *pEFSpr* obability of event-free survival; *cens.*c ensored, *S1-S4* BFM ALL relapse risk groups. (**b**) Event-free survival for subgroups of risk group S2 (ALL-REZ BFM 83–90). *pEFS* probability of event-free survival; *cens.* censored, *S2A-S2D* BFM strategic groupS2s ubsets

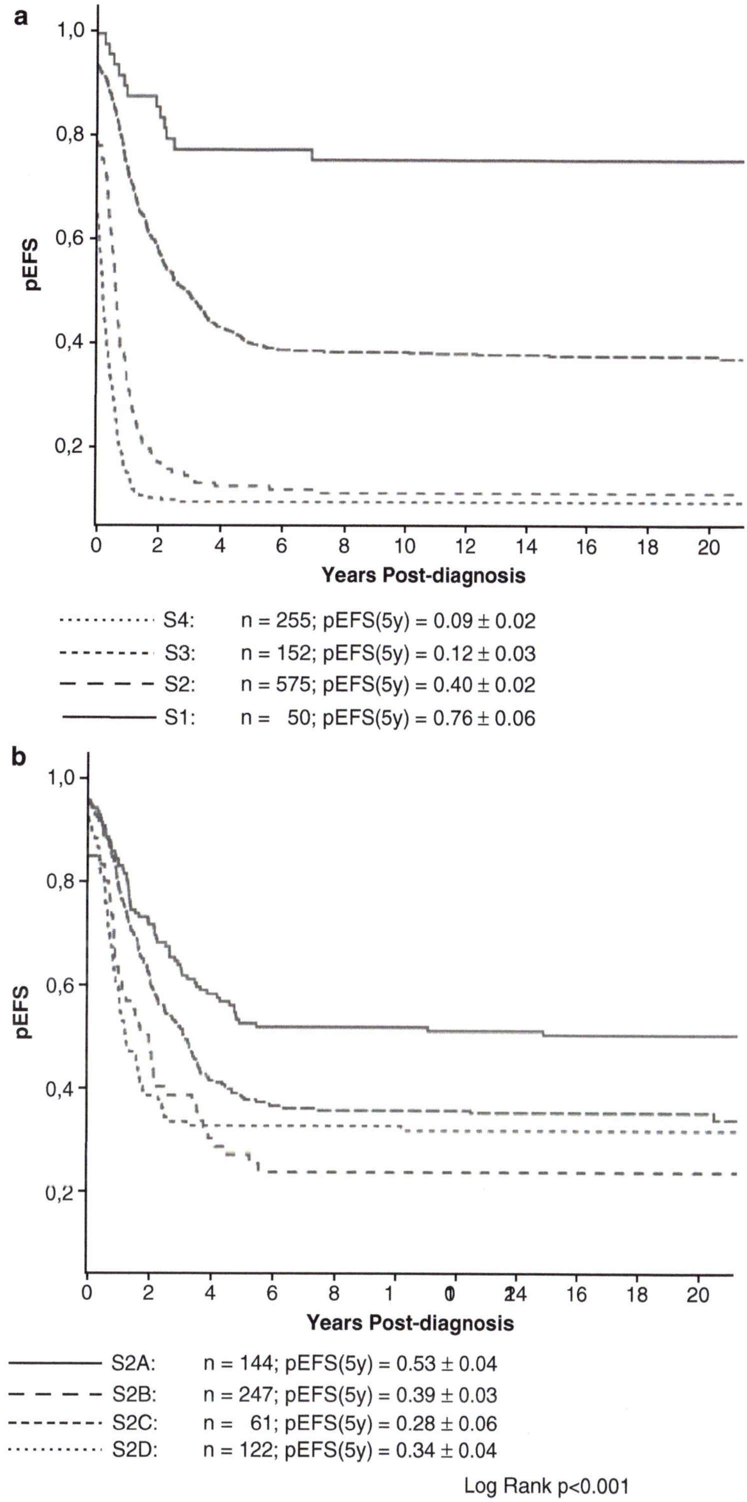

For this group, the indications for HSCT in CR2 have been controversial. Recently, response to relapse therapy, as measured by MRD, has helped to better define the chances of treatment success and refine the indications for HSCT in CR2. Children with a systemic relapse in the S2 group that responded rapidly to re-Induction therapy had a better prognosis with continuing chemotherapy than those children with slow or

Table 4.2 Subsets of ALL strategic group S2 by peripheral blast cell count (PBC), BCR-ABL1 status, timepoint and site of relapse

Site	Isolated BM	Combined BM		Isolated EM
Time	Late	Late	Early	Early/very early
PBC < 1/μL	A	A	B	D
PBC 1–10,000/ μL	B			
PBC ≥10,000/ μL	C			
BCR-ABL positive	C	C	C	

EM extramedullary, *BM* bone marrow

insufficient response (Eckert et al. 2001). Based on these results, the ALL-REZ BFM 2002 trial, which continues to accrue patients, uses MRD response to stratify treatment and identify patients for whom HSCT is indicated in CR2.

4.6.4 Treatment of Relapsed ALL

4.6.4.1 Remission Induction Chemotherapy

Chemotherapy is always required in order to obtain a second remission. In general, the probability of success is high in children with late relapses, whereas second CR rates are lower in early relapses and much lower in children with very early systemic recurrences or with T-cell or Ph+ ALL. The lower CR rates in relapse patients are presumably due to drug resistance. Resistance may be due to subclones already existing at initial diagnosis or may be acquired (Langlands et al. 1993; Klumper et al. 1995). Several mechanisms of resistance (e.g., *MDR1* gene related multiple drug resistance, *p53* mutations, increased activity of dihydrofolate reductase, or reduced expression and/or function of the glucocorticoid receptor and postreceptor pathways) have been described (Kaspers et al. 1994; Kawamura et al. 1995). However, in spite of the clinical significance of resistance to glucocorticoids, the molecular mechanism is not yet defined, and there is no clear general pattern of clinically relevant resistance mechanisms in childhood ALL.

Attempts have been made to measure the sensitivity of ALL blasts to chemotherapy *in vitro* using the methyl-thiazol-tetrazolium assay. Such studies have typically shown that blasts obtained at relapse were much more resistant to a variety of chemotherapy agents including glucocorticoids, L-asparaginase, anthracyclines and thiopurines as compared with samples obtained at first diagnosis of childhood ALL (Klumper et al. 1995). However, the results of these measurements could not successfully be transferred into clinical practice by attempting to "tailor" therapy according to the resistance profile.

Systematic prospective and structured trials for relapsed ALL have been developed on a broader basis since the 1980s. Consecutive trials including patients on a nation-wide basis with stratified treatment have been performed by the ALL-REZ BFM study group since 1983 and in the United Kingdom starting in the early 1990s. The general assumption was that treatment for relapse had to be more intensive than frontline therapy because the cells were likely to be resistant to the conventionally used drugs. In fact, this is not always the case; relatively high remission rates of over 90% could be achieved using a 4-drug Induction regimen with vincristine, prednisone, asparaginase and daunorubicin. However, the quality and duration of these remissions were poor and were followed by frequent and rapid subsequent relapses.

In general, patients with late relapses may be treated with chemotherapy regimens using drugs similar to frontline therapy. Late relapses occur more frequently in patients who were standard or low-risk patients at first manifestation of ALL, and the long time to relapse is a biologic feature of the leukemia. Usually, in these children high second CR rates can be obtained and maintained by re-Induction/Consolidation courses followed by Maintenance therapy or HSCT. Different Induction regimens have been used, consisting either of conventional 4-drug regimens or multi-drug combination chemotherapy (Culbert et al. 1991; Sadowitz et al. 1993; Morland and Shaw 1996; Rivera et al. 2005; Roy et al. 2005a, b). In the ALL-REZ BFM protocols, the short R1 and R2 courses have been the backbone of Induction and post-Induction therapy, as shown in Fig. 4.4 and Table 4.3, and resulted in remission rates of about 95% in patients with late BM relapse (Einsiedel et al. 2005; von Stackelberg et al. 2008).

In contrast, re-Induction rates are much lower in patients with very early and early relapses (Raetz et al. 2008a). Early relapses occur most frequently in patients with high-risk features at first manifestation, and the poor response rates have in part to be attributed to the more aggressive biology of the leukemia cells, but may

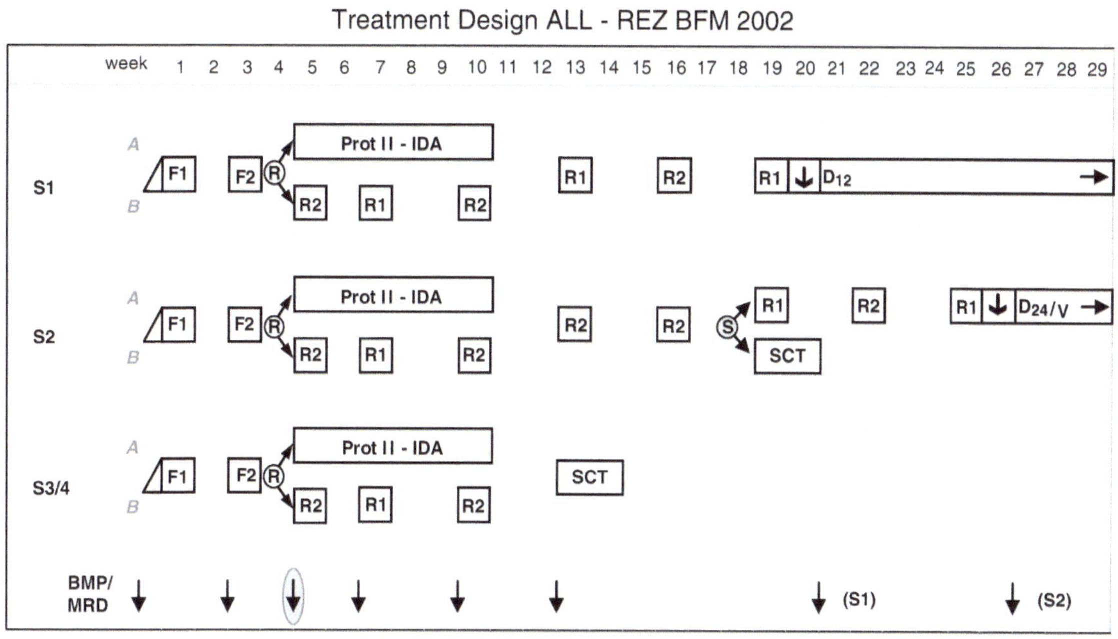

D_{12}/D_{24}, 12/24 months maintenance therapy; Ⓡ, randomization; Ⓢ, stratification; V, VP16-reinduction pulses, ↓ local irradiation; ↓ BMP-time-point for postremission-stratification in S2; SCT, stem-cell transplantation; BMP, bone marrow puncture; MRD, minimal residual disease; chemotherapy courses: F1, F2, R2, R1, protocol II-IDA.

Fig.4.4 Overview of treatment regimens in the ALL-REZ BFM 2002 study

also be a consequence of the more intensive frontline therapy that has been given to these patients. Thus, treatment after relapse has to be more intensive, but even with intensive regimens second CR rates are only about 70%, which is still quite unsatisfactory. There is an urgent need for new and alternative drugs for these children(R aetze ta l. 2008a, b).

As frontline therapies have changed and are different in various study groups and the definitions of relapse characteristics are not uniform, data on treatment results for relapsed ALL are not easy to compare. Interestingly, evidence was found in trial ALL-REZ BFM 95/96 that increased dose intensity during early Induction therapy might be beneficial. Both remission rate and EFS were significantly better in patients with short time intervals between the first two courses of chemotherapy administered for relapse than in children with delayed administration of therapy (Herold et al. 2004).

4.6.4.2 Post-remissionT herapy

For many years, allogeneic stem cell transplantation was believed to be necessary and the treatment of choice for all children with BM relapses. Post-remission chemotherapy, as well as autologous HSCT, were only utilized for patients in whom no suitable stem cell donor could be found. Because of this, there are relatively few published results on long-term outcome of treatment with relapsed ALL using chemotherapy alone. The POG reported results using alternating drug pairs combined with re-Induction courses consisting of weekly cytarabine/teniposide alternating with weekly vincristine/cyclophosphamide for children with early BM relapse (Buchanan et al. 2000; Rivera et al. 2005). Maintenance therapy with standard doses of 6-MP/MTX plus vincristine/cyclophosphamide, prednisone/doxorubicin or teniposide/cytarabine re-Induction pulses has been administered to children with late BM relapse (Sadowitz et al. 1993). In the UK, 4-drug remission Induction therapy was followed by etoposide, cytarabine, dexamethasone, asparaginase, epirubicin, vincristine, thioguanine and cyclophosphamide for children allocated to chemotherapy. Stem cell transplantation was recommended for children who relapsed on frontline treatment and those with a relapse in the marrow (isolated or combined) within 24 months of

Table 4.3 Drugs and dosing of alternating chemotherapy: courses R1 and R2, backbone of ALL-REZ BFM trials

Drug	Dose	Route	Daysdr ug given
Course R1			
Dexamethasone	20m g/m^2	PO	1–5
6-Mercaptopurine	100m g/m^2	PO	1–5
Vincristine	1.5m g/m^2	IV	1,6
Methotrexate	1g/ m^2	IV	1
Methotrexate	12m g	IT	1
Cytarabine	30m g	IT	1
Prednisone	10m g	IT	1
Cytarabine	2g/ m^2	q 12 h IV	5
L-asparaginase	25,000U /m^2	IM/IV	6
CourseR 2			
Dexamethasone	20m g/m^2	PO	1–5
6-Thioguanine	100m g/m^2	PO	1–5
Vindesine	3m g/m^2	IV	1
Methotrexate	1g/ m^2	IV	1
Methotrexate	12m g	IT	1(and5) [a]
Cytarabine	30m g	IT	1(and5) [a]
Prednisone	10m g	IT	1(and5) [a]
Daunorubicin	50m g/m^2	IV	5
Ifosfamide	400m g/m^2	IV	1–5
L-asparaginase	25,000U /m^2	IM/IV	6

PO by mouth, *IV* intravenously, *IT* intrathecally, *q* every, *IM*intra muscularly

[a]Children with overt meningeal leukemia

stopping treatment. However, acceptance of these recommendations varied with treatment centers and availability of donors (Lawson et al. 2000; Roy et al. 2005a, b). In BFM relapse trials, alternating multidrug courses, R1 and R2, followed by standard-dose MTX/6-thioguanine Maintenance therapy up to a total duration of 2 years, has been used as post-remission treatment for children with early or late BM relapse (Henze et al. 1991). Preventive cranial irradiation has been administered to all children with isolated bone marrow relapse in ALL-REZ BFM 87 and subsequent ALL-REZ trials because an excess of CNS relapses following isolated BM relapse was observed in earlier trials. This approach led to a significant reduction of CNS relapses and an improved overall outcome (Buhrer et al. 1994).

In summary, results with chemotherapy have been poor in patients with early systemic relapses, mostly below 10% EFS, in all published trials. However, long-term EFS of approximately 40% can be achieved with chemotherapy in children with late BM relapse (Pui et al. 1988; Sadowitz et al. 1993; Lawson et al. 2000; Einsiedel et al. 2005; Roy et al. 2005a, b).

4.6.5 Treatment of Extramedullary Relapses

4.6.5.1 CNSR elapse

Even though the use of cranial irradiation has been progressively decreased, and in some cases eliminated, in the treatment of newly diagnosed ALL, the rate of CNS relapse has continued to decrease over time. As this has happened, new factors have been identified that define patients at increased risk of CNS relapse. For example, presence of the t(1;19) has emerged as a risk factor for CNS relapse in SJCRH trials (Jeha et al. 2009). Once a CNS relapse occurs, cranial irradiation, in the context of systemic chemotherapy, is a critical component of treatment. The question of whether or not craniospinal irradiation is necessary is still an issue of some debate. Although craniospinal irradiation was reported to be superior to cranial irradiation in an early trial (Land et al. 1985), many contemporary protocols for treatment of CNS relapse do not employ spinal irradiation (Barredo et al. 2006). When CNS irradiation is used in combination with intensive chemotherapy, high rates of long-term neurotoxicity, in particular leukoencephalopathy, can occur. In POG trial 8304, the observed rate of leukoencephalopathy after 24 Gy cranial irradiation was 17% (Winick et al. 1993). In particular, intrathecal and/or high-dose IV MTX should be avoided following CNS irradiation therapy. Because of this, most trials defer radiation therapy until after high-dose systemic chemotherapy has been completed.

Exceptionally good results, with about 70% EFS accompanied with acceptable neurotoxicity, were achieved in POG trial 9061 with delayed craniospinal irradiation following intensive systemic chemotherapy for CNS relapse (Ritchey et al. 1999). No specific factors could be identified that would explain the excellent outcome compared with other published approaches. In a subsequent POG trial for children with a first isolated CNS relapse occurring after at least 18 months of first CR, favorable results were achieved with 12 months of intensive systemic chemotherapy followed by 18 Gy cranial radiation and Maintenance chemotherapy (Barredo et al. 2006). Building on this, the current COG trial for children with late (>18 months after initial diagnosis) isolated CNS relapse intensifies systemic chemotherapy and decreases the cranial irradiation dose to 12 Gy. In two other large series of patients with isolated CNS relapse, DFS rates were 37 ± 3% (CCG; $n = 220$), or ranged from 24% to 64% (UKALL; $n = 98$), depending on the duration of first remission (Gaynon et al. 1998; Wheeler et al. 1998). BFM relapse trials, in which patients with isolated CNS relapse were treated with the same chemotherapy regimens used for systemic relapse, supplemented by CNS irradiation, have achieved similar results (Henze 1997).

The role of HSCT in the treatment of CNS relapses is unclear, in particular because there is probably no graft-versus-leukemia effect in the CNS. However, about half of the relapses following CNS relapses are systemic relapses. Thus, HSCT might well have a beneficial effect. In a retrospective analysis, favorable results were observed with HSCT in patients with early CNS relapses (Harker-Murray et al. 2008). Similar 8-year probabilities of leukemia-free survival were reported after chemotherapy with irradiation and transplantation (66% and 58%, respectively) when patients were adjusted for age and duration of first remission (Eapen et al. 2008). No advantage of HSCT was found in study Cooprall-97 (Domenech et al. 2008), and similar outcomes with HSCT as reported for chemotherapy were also observed in a retrospective analysis from Japan (Tsurusawa et al. 2007).

4.6.5.2 Testicular Relapse

Like CNS relapses, testicular relapses have also become rare. In part, this is a consequence of the introduction of high or intermediate dose MTX into frontline trials. However, in trials not using these elements, the frequency of testicular relapses has also been reduced compared with earlier reports. Whereas the majority of CNS relapses are early relapses occurring during the first 2 years after diagnosis of ALL, testicular relapses tend to occur later, frequently only after the end of Maintenance therapy. The better prognosis after testicular relapse as compared with CNS relapse is therefore at least in part explained by the late time point of relapse.

A frequently discussed question is the choice of local therapy. Most study groups in the U.S. recommend bilateral irradiation of the testes, and most authors recommend radiation doses above 22 Gy (Atkinson et al. 1976; Nachman et al. 1990; Buchanan et al. 1991; Wofford et al. 1992; Grundy et al. 1997). However, the optimum dose of testicular irradiation is not clear, and second relapses have been observed after doses of 20–26 Gy in about 5% of patients (Uderzo et al. 1990; Buchanan et al. 1991; Wofford et al. 1992).

A significant negative consequence of testicular irradiation is that reproductive gonadal function is not preserved after doses of 24 Gy (Freeman et al. 1983; Brecher et al. 1986; Leiper et al. 1986). In contrast, with 12 or 15 Gy testicular irradiation, Leydig cell function is sufficiently preserved to allow spontaneous puberty (Castillo et al. 1990). Therefore, orchiectomy of a clinically involved testis is recommended for patients treated in BFM relapse trials with biopsy of a clinically uninvolved testis. If biopsy shows no histologic evidence of involvement with leukemia, irradiation at a reduced dose of 15 Gy is performed (Henze 1997). With this approach, the incidence of relapse in the contralateral uninvolved testicle was very low, and most boys with unilateral relapse experienced spontaneous puberty.

Adverse prognostic factors in patients with testicular relapse are short duration of first CR and T-cell immunophenotype. In addition, in BFM trials, boys with bilateral testicular involvement at relapse had a clearly inferior outcome when compared to those who only had unilateral involvement at relapse (G. Henze, unpublished observations).

4.6.6 Role of Allogeneic Stem Cell Transplantation

While HSCT is rarely indicated for children in first CR, salvage therapy after relapse remains the major indication for HSCT in childhood ALL. Large donor registries have been established such that suitable donors can be found for about 80% of patients (MacMillan et al. 2008). Furthermore, banked unrelated donor cord blood as a source of stem cells has become an important option for children with leukemia, particularly smaller children with weight less than about 50 kg (Lori et al. 2007; Gluckman and Rocha 2008). In recent years, there has been renewed interest in HSCT using haploidentical related donors (Handgretinger et al. 2007; Aversa et al. 2008; Lang and Handgretinger 2008). As the options for allogeneic HSCT donors have increased, autologous HSCT has been largely abandoned for patients with relapsed ALL.

During the past 10 years, the number of alternative donor HSCT performed on children in Europe has increased significantly and has reached 61% of the allografts (Lanino et al. 2008). Guidelines have been developed to facilitate identification of a suitable donor for children with relapsed ALL who lack a matched sibling donor. It is recommended that a simultaneous search for an unrelated donor and for a cord blood unit should be started. To maximize the chance of success of an unrelated donor HSCT, the patient and the donor should be matched at the HLA-A, -B, -C and -DRB1 alleles. A single HLA class I or II allele mismatch is accepted. However, multiple mismatching for more than one class I allele and simultaneous disparities in class I and II alleles increase mortality. The impact of additional mismatches for HLA-DQ and -DP loci is still under investigation. Optimally, a 10/10 allele-matched donor should be used. Whereas in a matched pair analysis, persistently high rates of treatment-related mortality (TRM) were observed in earlier years (Borgmann et al. 2003), current transplant results with well-matched unrelated donors appear to be no different than those obtained following HSCT with matched sibling donor (Dahlke et al. 2006; Eapen et al. 2006b; Gassas et al. 2007). If a suitable donor or a cord blood unit cannot be found within an acceptable time span, haploidentical HSCT should be offered. The outcomes of children with acute leukemia transplanted with unrelated donor BM, cord blood, and also with haploidentical stem cells have improved markedly in the past 5–10 years, largely attributable to lower TRM.

In general, HSCT provides better control of leukemia, particularly for those children with early relapse, and, as long as TRM is minimized, leads to a higher relapse-free survival rate than chemotherapy. Very high-dose chemotherapy can be administered in combination with total body irradiation (TBI) in order to destroy remaining resistant leukemia cells. In addition, the anti-leukemic effect of allogeneic HSCT is enforced by the immunologically mediated and actually desired graft-versus-leukemia (GVL) effect, which is, however, associated with graft-versus-host disease (GVHD), the latter and infection still being responsible for most of the transplant-related deaths. Nevertheless, subsequent relapse remains the most common cause of failure after allogeneic HSCT. Despite the better anti-leukemic effect of HSCT as compared with chemotherapy, the risks of a subsequent relapse have to be carefully balanced against the hazards of the still substantial acute and long-term toxicity. Therefore, outcomes after HSCT should continue to be tracked in prospective and controlled clinical trials (Schrauder et al. 2008).

For ALL, most data indicate that transplants using preparative regimens that include TBI in conjunction with chemotherapy lead to better results than those that do not include TBI. Various chemotherapy/TBI preparative regimens have been reported and are used widely in pediatrics (Brochstein et al. 1987; Dopfer et al. 1991; Weyman et al. 1993; Moussalem et al. 1995; Uderzo et al. 1995). A retrospective analysis of the BFM Study Group showed that best results were achieved with TBI plus etoposide (Dopfer et al. 1991). In a more recent publication, however, no significant difference in outcome could be found comparing TBI/etoposide and TBI/cyclophosphamide (Gassas et al. 2006).

Attempts to compare results of chemotherapy with HSCT for treatment of relapsed ALL are very difficult because of the numerous confounders, such as type of donor, stem cell source, time to transplant, conditioning regimen, experience and size of the transplant center and others. Therefore, most published data are based on retrospective analyses. In a matched pair analysis, results of allogeneic HSCT and chemotherapy were compared. The two patient groups were matched for sex, age, immunophenotype, initial leukocyte count and duration of first remission (Barrett et al. 1994). The EFS obtained with HSCT was 40 ± 3%, which was significantly better than the 17 ± 3% EFS in patients treated with chemotherapy alone. The probability of treatment-related death, however, was almost twice as high after HSCT (27 ± 4% for HSCT vs 14 ± 4% after chemotherapy). In contrast, no advantage of allogeneic HSCT over chemotherapy or autologous HSCT was found in the PETHEMA ALL 93 trial (Ribera et al. 2007).

In general, HSCT is more effective than chemotherapy in controlling leukemia in patients with BM relapse, particularly those with early BM relapse. Thus, early BM relapse represents a clear and established indication for HSCT. For patients with late BM relapses, the indication for HSCT has been a long-lasting subject of debate. Subsequent relapses occur more frequently after chemotherapy, but the final outcome was not significantly different than after HSCT. Similarly, no advantage of HSCT over chemotherapy was observed for late relapsing patients in a collaborative study of the COG and the Center for International Blood and Marrow Transplant Research (Eapen et al. 2006a, b). Therefore, many investigators prefer to defer allogeneic bone marrow transplantation at the time of first (late) BM relapse, and reserve it for use in third CR (Borgmann et al. 1997). As already mentioned above, the data supporting the use of HSCT for patients with isolated extramedullary relapses are much more limited.

The BFM relapse study group aimed to identify more accurately the group of patients with late BM relapses who would benefit from allogeneic HSCT in CR2. As shown in Fig. 4.3b, the S2 group can be split into subgroups with a better or worse prognosis. However, this was not sufficiently precise to identify clearly which patients should undergo HSCT in CR2. Much better discrimination was achieved using MRD response to chemotherapy administered for relapse as a criterion (Eckert et al. 2001). Rapid and early response as defined by MRD $<10^{-3}$ after the first two courses of Induction therapy was capable of distinguishing two subsets of group S2 with a markedly different prognosis (probability of EFS 0.86 in children with MRD $<10^{-3}$ vs 0 in children with MRD $> 10^{-3}$, $p < 0.001$). In the current ALL-REZ BFM 2002 trial, MRD forms the basis of allocation of children of group S2 to either chemotherapy or HSCT in CR2.

The burden of MRD immediately prior to the time of transplant has also been shown to be a predictor of outcome post-HSCT (Bader et al. 2009). Patients with a low leukemic cell burden before HSCT (MRD $< 10^{-4}$) had a much better prognosis than patients with MRD $\geq 10^{-4}$. Detectable MRD prior to HSCT was also reported to be an adverse prognostic factor by others (Sramkova et al. 2007). Thus, there is now evidence that MRD has become an important tool to assess the quality of remission, to guide selection of treatment strategies, and to predict the outcome of children with relapsed ALL (Szczepanski 2007; Kreyenberg et al. 2009).

In summary, allogeneic HSCT is an important component in the treatment of children with relapsed ALL. HSCT is clearly indicated in patients with high-risk features, such as early and very early BM relapses, as well as with T-cell ALL. MRD has become a reliable and helpful method to discriminate between patients with late BM relapse who will benefit from HSCT and others who will not. Potential benefits always have to be balanced against transplant-related early toxicity and late sequelae.

4.6.7 Study of New Agents in Relapsed ALL

One of the top priorities in pediatric ALL is the identification of new agents to improve outcomes for patients with recurrent ALL, particularly those with early marrow relapses and T-cell disease. Responses to single agent therapy have been poor in patients with refractory and recurrent leukemia, so most contemporary regimens combine new agents with an established chemotherapy platform. This presents a challenge as the baseline toxicity with chemotherapy alone is often significant(R aetze ta l. 2008a, b).

Ideal new agent candidates are those that uniquely target blasts and have favorable toxicity profiles. One class of agents that is currently under investigation in relapsed ALL is monoclonal antibodies. This class of drugs has unique mechanisms of action and generally has limited and non overlapping toxicities when compared with cytotoxic agents, making them attractive candidates for combined therapy. Campath-1H, a monoclonal antibody directed against CD52, has been combined with chemotherapy (Angiolillo et al. 2009) and a COG study using epratuzumab, an anti-CD22 IgG1 monoclonal antibody (Carnahan et al. 2007) that is expressed in >90% of cases of B-precursor ALL, is presently under way (Raetz et al. 2008a, b).

Other agents of potential promise that are being investigated in relapsed ALL include clofarabine and bortezomib. Clofarabine is a new-generation nucleoside analog. After promising 30% overall response rates were observed in heavily pretreated pediatric patients with refractory or relapsed ALL (Jeha et al. 2004), this agent was granted accelerated approval by the US Food and Drug Administration in 2004 for the treatment of children with relapsed or refractory ALL after at least two prior regimens. Clofarabine is presently being investigated in combination with cytarabine, and also with etoposide and cyclophosphamide; favorable early outcomes have been observed (Hijiya et al. 2009; Locatelli et al. 2009).

Bortezomib, which selectively inhibits the 26S proteasome, stabilizes many cell cycle-regulatory proteins and appears to sensitize malignant cells to apoptosis (Horton et al. 2006). Single-agent Phase I studies of bortezomib in relapsed/refractory pediatric leukemia (Horton et al. 2007) and solid tumors (Blaney et al. 2004) have been completed, and this agent is currently being studied in combination with chemotherapy for children with relapsed B-precursor and T-ALL (Messinger 2010).

The COG is using CR2 rates and MRD levels at the end of Induction therapy as well as 4-month EFS to measure the activity of combinations containing new agents in patients with early first relapse of ALL in order to prioritize and identify agents and regimens of promise for further study in the future. If these or other agents prove effective in the relapse setting, they also may be suitable candidates for incorporation into frontline therapies in the future.

4.6.8 Summary and Perspectives on Relapsed ALL

Relapses have become relatively rare events in ALL although, because of the frequency of ALL, they are still a significant cause of death. With currently available treatment modalities, cure rates after relapse are in the range of 50% and contribute to the overall increased survival of children with ALL to approximately 90% in the modern era. Remission rates are still unsatisfactory in children with high-risk features; novel drugs and approaches are urgently needed for these patients. Candidate agents include small molecules or other targeted immunological or pharmacological therapies using individual immunological or genetic characteristics of leukemia cells. If such distinctive features can be detected in relapse patients, they will probably also have consequences for newly diagnosed patients and contribute to further reduction of relapses, higher cure rates and hopefully to the development of better and less harmful therapies. Therefore, careful and comprehensive diagnostic procedures have to be performed in relapse patients in order to improve insight into the biology of ALL and to use the newly acquired knowledge for future patients.

4.7 Clinical Trial Design Considerations and Endpoints

4.7.1 Trial Design

Randomized clinical trials have been conducted in pediatric ALL for almost 50 years, and these trials have had significant influence on clinical trial design for other types of pediatric and adult cancer. Data from a randomized trial conducted in the early 1960s in childhood ALL, likely the first ever conducted in this disease, have been used in survival analysis books (ACUTE LEUKEMIA GROUP B et al. 1963; Marubini and Valsecchi 1995). This trial had a sophisticated sequential design and tested, in a randomized fashion, the use of 6-MP versus placebo as Maintenance therapy for children with ALL who had achieved partial/complete remission at the end of a corticosteroid Induction. The trial was stopped due to superiority of the experimental 6-MP arm in preventing relapses (9/21 relapses in the experimental group vs 21/21 relapses in the control group). The authors presented the study as "a model for evaluation of other potentially useful therapy." Since that time, remarkable progress has been made in the development of effective treatments in childhood ALL. Critical to these advances has been the conduct of many clinical trials, randomized or not, and national and international cooperation.

A clinical trial is an experiment testing a medical treatment on human subjects. During trial design, the experiment must be structured so that a clinical question on the relative merits of different therapies can be answered. The design and conduct of a clinical trial is subject to ethical constraints, to protect the subject safety and well being, and to scientific constraints, to guarantee its integrity. Rigorous methodologies and procedures are necessary to ensure that biases are minimized (*validity*), so to avoid systematic errors that can cause the estimate of interest to deviate from its "true" unknown value. Moreover, trial design and conduct must aim to maximize *precision* (i.e., accuracy of estimates, through control of random errors with appropriate sample size) and the *applicability* of trial results to future patients. *Randomization* (when done properly) is the best approach to ensure validity, and characterizes Phase III studies. Phase II studies can also utilize randomized trial designs, for instance to select one drug from between two or more promising drugs to be considered for the comparison with best standard treatment in a subsequent Phase III trial. Classification into *Phase I-IV* studies has evolved into a more general classification in order to describe the development of medical products, like biologically targeted therapies, other than traditional pharmaceuticals (Piantadosi 2005). This classification distinguishes studies based on their principal aim as follows: (I) *early-development* studies (translational or treatment-mechanism testing studies); (II) *middle-development* studies (assessing treatment tolerability); (III) *late-development* studies (including comparative studies as well as expanded safety or post-marketing studies). Broadly speaking, whichever classification is adopted, different phases are characterized by different designs simply because they have different objectives. A complete review of the methodologies of these trials is beyond the scope of the current section, which will focus on highlighting specific aspects of trial design that have recently drawn the attention of childhood ALL researchers. One important distinction in Phase III trials is between trials that seek to establish *superiority* (or *difference*) as compared to those designed to test for *non-inferiority*. This latter type of trial design has a useful application in the context of intensive frontline chemotherapy regimens, for addressing questions on de-intensification. Non-inferiority trials are designed to answer the question "Does the experimental treatment produce cure rates that are as good as the established therapy, while being preferable on other grounds such as increased safety, improved patient convenience, lower costs, etc.?"

Typically, non-inferiority trials are considered for patients that are projected to have an excellent outcome with an established therapy, for example at least 90–95% 5-year EFS. The trial is designed to optimize therapy under controlled conditions, de-intensifying certain therapy elements with known short or long-term side effects, without compromising the excellent expected EFS. Up to 30% of children with ALL treated in current protocols in North America and Western Europe may be candidates for this type of trial.

Most commonly, however, the type of question that is of interest in clinical trials is whether or not a new treatment, obtained by adding novel drugs or modifying how existing drugs are administered, improves outcome. A prudent approach is that of designing the trial to test whether the new treatment differs from the established therapy using a two-sided test of hypothesis rather than a one-sided test, as in a pure superiority design. This approach is recommended especially in the context of comparing two different treatment strategies, where the experimental arm is not an "add-on" arm that involves a novel promising drug with regard to the standard control arm but, for instance, uses the same drugs with increased intensity. *Superiority (difference)* trials lead the way to building scientific evidence on new therapeutic options in two different scenarios in childhood ALL.

The first scenario consists of Phase III trials that are designed to achieve modest, but clinically important, outcome improvements (efficacy), with more efficient definitions of therapeutic strategies that use existing chemotherapeutic agents. These studies are generally powered to detect less than 10% absolute increase (or difference) in EFS in the subpopulation of patients, usually of relevant size, who have a relatively good prognosis. In childhood ALL, these studies typically address the so called intermediate-risk patients, accounting for approximately 50% of the ALL population, who have a 70–80% 5-year EFS. These studies may ask a randomized question on intensification or on the inclusion of new formulations of existing drugs such as, for example, using the pegylated form of L-asparaginase instead of the native product.

The second scenario focuses on subgroups of patients at high risk of failure, for example, those with persistent disease, either at the molecular or morphological level, following completion of Induction or Consolidation frontline therapies. In these relatively rare ALL subpopulations, characterized by less than 50% 5-year EFS, there is hopefully room for marked improvement in outcome with treatment alterations such as intensification of conventional cytotoxic chemotherapy, use of HSCT, or addition of novel agents, as in the case of tyrosine kinase inhibitors in Ph+ ALL patients. Studies that evaluate the role of HSCT in high-risk patients are challenging both in the design and analysis phase. Transplant is administered based on donor availability and clinical judgement rather than on random assignment and the comparison with outcome of non-transplanted patients may be seriously biased. Basic principles which should be kept in mind when designing such trials include the precise definition of the target population and donor search (e.g., criteria of eligibility for HSCT and of donor selection) and the recruitment of all eligible patients in the trial, regardless of clinical course and result of the donor search. An unbiased evaluation can be obtained by a design based on donor availability, rather than on the treatment actually performed, the so-called evaluation by "genetic randomization," which mimics the intention-to-treat principle in this context (Balduzzi et al. 2005). When this approach is not reasonable or feasible, efforts should be made to ensure that statistical analysis properly adjusts for potential sources of bias (e.g., waiting time to transplant, confounding factors) and/or by using novel statistical approaches (Galimberti et al. 2002).

Superiority (difference) trials also include those that test new drugs or HSCT in patients with relapsed ALL. Such patients, especially those with an early first relapse or a second relapse, may also be candidates for Phase I and II studies on the pharmacokinetics, safety and activity of new drugs. In recent years, new regulations have been introduced in Europe that may facilitate the evaluation of new drugs (Pritchard-Jones et al. 2008). These regulations mandate submission of pediatric investigational plans for new drugs that have potential benefit for children's diseases. Optimization of the design of Phase I and II studies is particularly important in ALL in view of the limited number of high-risk patients available and the growing number of new drugs that must be assessed for toxicity, activity and efficacy. The development of adaptive designs or of Bayesian designs is an area of increasing interest in this context (Thall 2008; Schoenfeld et al. 2009).

Much progress has been made in the treatment of childhood ALL due to clinical trials conducted by large national and international study groups such as the COG, BFM, AEIOP, and I-BFM-SG. However, even these large groups may not be able to effectively conduct clinical trials on their own for certain patient subgroups. Larger scale international cooperative Phase III trials may be needed for at least two reasons. First, advances in understanding the prognostic factors and molecular basis of childhood ALL are increasingly leading to the subdivision of patients into risk groups with different survival profiles. This has led to the identification of relatively rare subpopulations that account for less than 5% of ALL patients for whom specific therapeutic questions are warranted, such as infants with *MLL* translocations and patients with Ph+ ALL. The second reason is that, even in more common subpopulations (like ALL patients at intermediate or low-risk of failure), the optimal sample size for a randomized trial can easily reach thousands of patients if it is powered to detect a "modest" improvement (i.e., 6–8% absolute increase in EFS) or to test non-inferiority (i.e., ruling out an unacceptable 3–4% decrease in EFS). While Phase III trials for such populations may be less "interesting" because they do not test novel drugs or treatment strategies, but rather seek to optimize existing treatments, they are very important to clinical practice as they help to define the best treatment for the large majority of newly diagnosed ALL patients. Expansion of recruitment from national to international communities can be successful, although it may sometimes need an innovative approach to study design and conduct. For example, a study design that prospectively used the principles of meta-analysis was adopted in the international trial on the addition of vincristine/dexamethasone Maintenance pulses discussed earlier (Valsecchi and Masera 1996; Conter et al. 2007). Characterization of subgroups which differ in their risk of failure and therapeutic needs continues to grow in importance. This means that statistical design of clinical studies in ALL will be increasingly influenced by the discovery of biomarkers that are predictive of outcome and by the need to develop appropriate prognostic stratification systems (Hoering et al. 2008; DeLore nzoe ta l. 2009).

4.7.2 Endpoints for Clinical Trials

In drug development in oncology, Phase II studies are used to assess whether a novel drug (or combination regimen) has sufficient *activity* to justify the conduct of a Phase III trial on *efficacy*. When the goal is to assess the biologic activity, objective response, measured relatively early in time after the start of treatment, is traditionally the endpoint. When the goal is to assess efficacy, an outcome measure that unequivocally reflects tangible benefits to patients is of interest. The most convincing and direct evidence of such a "definitive" benefit for a cancer patient is survival. Treatments that affect survival are very likely to have a fundamental biological action. Regulatory authorities from Canada, Europe and the USA have provided guidance on the definition of endpoints, and survival is regarded as the gold standard for Phase III trials on anti-cancer drugs (Administration 2007; Canada 2007; Agency 2008). However, in recent years, other outcomes have become important for new drug approval, particularly progression free survival (PFS). This development has generated a debate in the scientific community on whether PFS is a surrogate for overall survival (Fleming et al. 2009). Recent developments in Phase II trial design are also starting to use endpoints other than objective clinical responses. The advent of biologically targeted cytostatic anti-cancer agents has led the way to the design of randomized Phase II studies, with PFS as the primary endpoint rather than the traditional objective response (Dhani et al. 2009). Phase III trials that are designed to guide clinical practice, rather than satisfy requirements for drug development, deserve a specific discussion of best outcome measures, as will be done in the following section, after defining surrogate endpoints from a methodological point of view.

4.7.3 Surrogate Endpoints: Principles

The choice of the endpoint depends strongly on whether the researcher identifies an endpoint of activity as a surrogate for efficacy. In ALL, the advent of reliable methods to measure MRD has created new perspectives in trial design. The potential gain in shortening duration of clinical trials is evident, as MRD can be measured early to detect response, while EFS needs long follow-up, especially if the event rate is initially low. The gain in efficiency may come from the fact that a novel drug given early during treatment may potentially affect MRD levels quite markedly even in a population that is expected to have a relatively good long-term outcome. However, deciding that efficacy of treatment can be assessed in terms of MRD response requires that this response measure is properly validated as a surrogate endpoint. This is a difficult task; examples of definitive validation of putative surrogate endpoints are rare in oncology, and usually require a meta-analysis of several trials (Burzykowski et al. 2008). Validation of a surrogate requires that: (1) the candidate endpoint is a prognostic factor for an established clinical endpoint (EFS or survival); and that (2) it captures fully the treatment effect on the clinical endpoint. While the first condition is easily met since, in practice, candidate surrogates are often selected because of their strong correlation with clinical outcome; the second condition is much more difficult to prove. Indeed it means not only that treatment must affect both the potential surrogate biomarker and the clinical outcome, but also requires that all mechanisms of action of treatment are reflected in the effect on the surrogate biomarker (De Gruttola et al. 2001). The behavior of a response parameter that is a perfect surrogate is illustrated in Fig. 4.5. The scenario is that of an experimental treatment that shows a marked effect on response, with an absolute increase of 20% on the 60% baseline level in the control arm. Here responders (and non-responders) have exactly the same failure rate whether they were treated with the experimental or standard therapy. This is because, by definition of surrogate, response is able to fully capture the effect of treatment on clinical outcome. So, with a 20% long-term failure rate in responders and 50% in non-responders (or a corresponding 80% or 50% 4-year EFS in responders and non-responders, respectively), the effect on clinical outcome is that failure rate changes from 32% in the standard arm to 26% in the experimental arm, with an absolute gain of 6%. Even if simplified, this is not an unrealistic scenario and shows that a high activity on a valid surrogate biomarker may translate into a modest effect on clinical outcome. In other words, even if early response is a

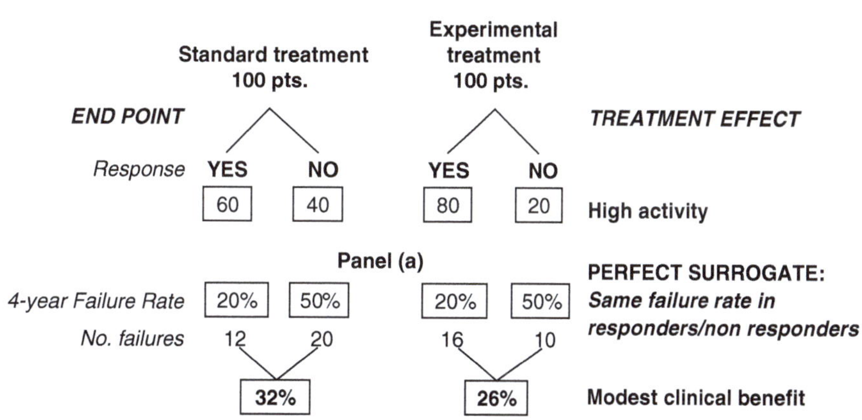

Fig. 4.5 Effect of the experimental relative to the standard treatment in a scenario in which early response is a perfect surrogate of clinical benefit

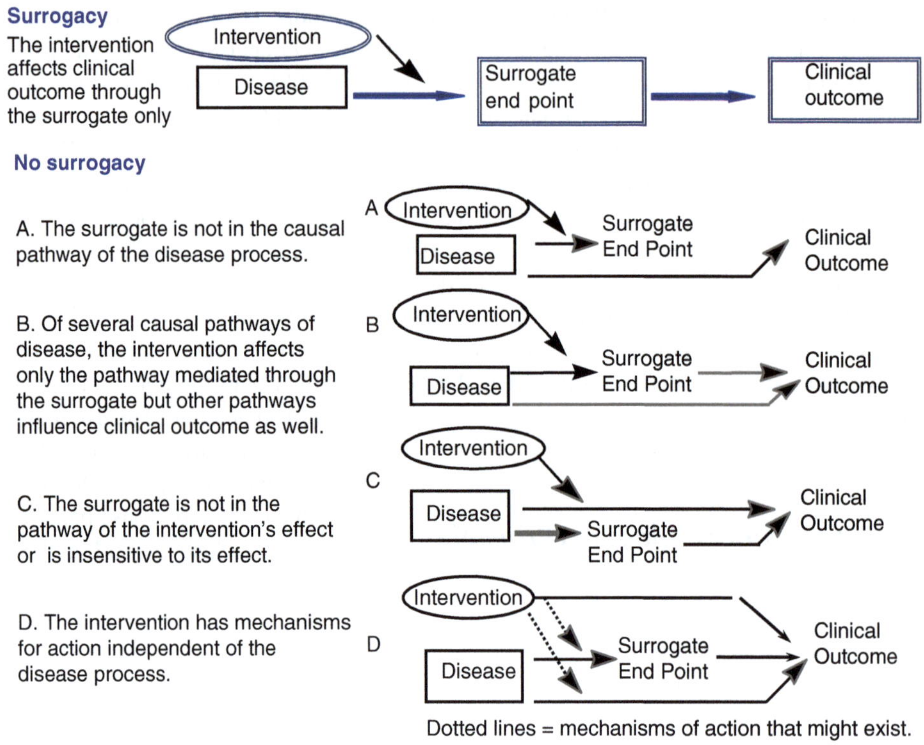

Fig. 4.6 Thec oncept of surrogacy

perfect surrogate, a fairly large increase in early response rate is required to translate into detectable EFS or survival gain. There are many reasons why a biomarker that is candidate to be a surrogate endpoint may not be a valid surrogate of the clinical endpoint, as illustrated in Fig. 4.6 (Fleming and DeMets 1996).

Table 4.4 Methodologicalc onsiderationsone ndpoints

Characteristics	Meaning
Relevant	Clinically important/useful
Quantifiable	Measured or scored on an appropriate scale
Valid	Measures the intended effect
Objective	Interpreted the same by all observers
Reliable	Same effect yields consistent measurements
Sensitive	Responds to small changes in the effect
Specific	Unaffected by extraneous influences

4.7.4 Primary Endpoint in ALL Trials: EFS or Survival?

The choice of the primary endpoint in a Phase III trial is of paramount importance as it defines the outcome on which the main results will be reported, serves as the basis for sample size calculation, and determines the length of follow-up. The primary endpoint needs to be well defined biologically and important to the study question. Also, when possible, a "hard" end point is preferred, which is not prone to observer bias or subjective evaluation. The methodological principles that should be kept in mind when selecting a study endpointa res ummarizedinT able 4.4(Pia ntadosi 2005).

In childhood ALL, Phase III trials not aimed at drug development are largely planned with EFS time rather than survival time as the primary endpoint. Event-free survival is a composite endpoint that includes all types of events that clinically represent important treatment failures. The EFS time is typically the time from the date of study entry until the time of first event, which is classically defined as relapse, death, disease resistance such as Induction failure (not counted if the study includes only patients that have already entered remission) or second malignant neoplasm (especially important in long-term evaluation). In the following, relapse and death will mostly be referred to as competing events as, by far, these are quantitatively and qualitatively the most important types of treatment failures that occur in childhood ALL. With this, EFS in childhood ALL corresponds to what is more generally termed PFS in oncology clinical trials. In childhood ALL, EFS is generally used as the primary outcome in frontline clinical trials as it is more specific than survival, while also satisfying the other characteristics listed in Table 4.4. Children treated for newly diagnosed ALL who relapse are treated with relapse regimens which, depending on type and time of relapse, can be relatively successful. Thus, long-term survival is also modified by the effect of second line treatment and confounded by that, in some cases. The definition of progression may be ambiguous in some cancers. In ALL, relapse and resistance are usually precisely defined in the protocol according to criteria that are standardized and universally accepted, with little room for interpretation on the biologic event and possibly only some arbitrariness in timing of ascertainment. However, if this timing is the same in different treatment arms, with the same time schedule for follow-up, conditions for internal validity of the study comparison are fulfilled.

It is known from many years of research that longer remission is strongly associated with longer survival in ALL, and that the relapse rate diminishes toward zero the longer the patient is in remission. Generally, in modern childhood ALL trials, long-term results show a 10-year OS that is approximately 10% higher in absolute value than the 10-year EFS of approximately 75% (Conter et al. 2010; Gaynon et al. 2010; Kamps et al. 2010; Mitchell et al. 2010; Moricke et al. 2010; Pui et al. 2010; Salzer et al. 2010; Silverman et al. 2010). It is also interesting to see how different eras of protocols that have improved EFS have also improved survival, which is a relevant result from the perspective of the ultimate clinical benefit to the patient and stimulated research to elaborate on a definition of "cure" (Shah et al. 2008).

It is a good principle that a new drug should be marketed and used only if it is superior (or, in some cases not-inferior) to the standard counterpart in terms of mortality outcomes. Nonetheless, in ALL trials that focus on optimizing frontline therapy, it may be worthwhile to adopt a new schedule that induces a relevant improvement in EFS but has only a minor effect on OS. As an extreme example, suppose that a new schedule for Maintenance therapy is tested compared to a standard treatment and its effect is only that of reducing long-term relapses. If it is then supposed that all these patients that relapse can be cured with salvage therapy, then EFS would be improved but long-term OS would be the same as in the standard Maintenance. If EFS is considered as a surrogate for OS, this is an extreme example of what was demonstrated in Fig. 4.5, with a marked effect on EFS having little impact on OS. However, the new Maintenance treatment would be worthwhile to adopt, even though it only affects EFS, because it would prevent relapses, which are very serious conditions that generally lead to intensive retrieval therapies. This assumes that the new Maintenance treatment does not cause major morbidities, as those might also impair survival or subject all patients to toxicity rather than only those that relapse and require retrieval therapy.

This raises another issue in the debate between EFS, which is a composite endpoint, and survival (which may also be seen as a composite endpoint if cancer-related deaths are distinguished from other causes of death; however survival for any cause is regarded here as the best way to analyze survival in childhood ALL trials). As for any composite endpoint, it is of interest to evaluate also the effect of treatment on single types of events, to better understand how treatment affects the rate of relapse/death from cancer, and at what cost in terms of deaths from toxicity. A difficult situation arises, for instance, when a treatment intervention leads to better disease control (fewer relapses), but is associated with increased toxicity and more deaths. This can be the case in some trials that compare HSCT to chemotherapy. It is important to note that even with an increase in toxic deaths; there can still be an advantage for the experimental arm in both EFS and survival, if the mortality increase is very low. In contrast, if the experimental intervention improves disease control but leads to an excess number of deaths, survival can be inferior. Because of these considerations, the description and comparison of different "components" of the EFS is very important for the interpretation of trial results and selection of optimal therapy. The separate analysis of relapse by the so called "relapse free interval" (RFI) (more generally termed time to progression (TTP) in many oncology trials) is done by censoring death as first event (i.e., death not following relapse). RFI is indeed estimating the time to relapse in the hypothetical setting where patients are not at risk of death from any cause other than progression. Instead, methods that account for competing risks can appropriately describe the effect of treatment separately on relapse and death that is not due to progression (Putter et al. 2007). Properly analyzed, EFS as primary endpoint will allow one to dissect the relative issues of toxicity vs. disease control.

Thus, EFS is generally the best primary measure of ALL treatment outcomes, as opposed to what may be the case in studies focused on new drug development. Overall survival should always be reported as the main secondary outcome, and increasingly more attention is being focused on health-related quality of life following treatment for childhood cancer.

4.8 Summarya ndFut ureDi rections

ALL is the most common malignancy that occurs during childhood and the treatment of this disease is a paradigm for how cancer can be treated successfully. Subgroups of children with ALL can now be identified that have expected cure rates in excess of 95%; for these children, future investigations will focus on maintaining excellent cure rates and minimizing toxicity. However, there are other subgroups of childhood ALL for which current treatments are unsatisfactory and for which intensification of myelosuppressive chemotherapy is unlikely to substantially improve outcomes. Biological investigations of ALL are evolving rapidly and high throughput genomic technologies and whole genome nucleotide sequence analyses are identifying new potential therapeutic targets in ALL. Future treatments for ALL, particularly for high-risk subsets, will likely focus on integration of molecularly targeted therapies with combination chemotherapy in order to improve cure rates. Better understanding of the genomic predictors of toxicity will also likely lead to new strategies to prevent or ameliorate the most debilitatinglong-te rme ffectsofA LLthe rapy.

References

Abshire TC, Buchanan GR et al (1992) Morphologic, immunologic and cytogenetic studies in children with acute lymphoblastic leukemia at diagnosis and relapse: a Pediatric Oncology Group study. Leukemia 6(5):357–362

ACUTE LEUKEMIA GROUP B, Freireich EJ et al (1963) The effect of 6-mercaptopurine on the duration of steroid-induced remissions in acute leukemia: a model for evaluation of other potentially useful therapy. Blood 21(6):699–716

Administration, U. S. F. a. D. (2007) Guidance for industry: clinical trial endpoints for the approval of cancer drugs and biologics. Silver Spring, MD

Agency EM (2008) Methodological considerations for using progression free survival (PFS) as primary endpoint in confirmatory trials for registration. www.emea.europa.eu/pdfs/human/ewp/2799408en.pdf

Angiolillo AL, Yu AL et al (2009) A phase II study of Campath-1H in children with relapsed or refractory acute lymphoblastic leukemia: a Children's Oncology Group report. Pediatr Blood Cancer 53(6):978–983

Arico M, Valsecchi MG et al (2000) Outcome of treatment in children with Philadelphia chromosome-positive acute lymphoblastic leukemia. N Engl J Med 342(14):998–1006

Arico M, Schrappe M et al (2008) Clinical outcome of 640 children with newly diagnosed Philadelphia chromosome-positive acute lymphoblastic leukemia treated between 1995 and 2005. Blood (ASH Annu Meet Abstr) 112(11): 568

Atkinson K, Thomas PR et al (1976) Radiosensitivity of the acute leukaemic infiltrate. Eur J Cancer 12(7):535–540

Attarbaschi A, Mann G et al (2008) Minimal residual disease values discriminate between low and high relapse risk in children with B-cell precursor acute lymphoblastic leukemia and an intrachromosomal amplification of chromosome 21: the Austrian and German acute lymphoblastic leukemia Berlin-Frankfurt-Munster (ALL-BFM) trials. J Clin Oncol 26(18):3046–3050

Aur RJ, Simone JV et al (1972) A comparative study of central nervous system irradiation and intensive chemotherapy early in remission of childhood acute lymphocytic leukemia. Cancer29(2):381–391

Aversa F, Reisner Y et al (2008) The haploidentical option for high-risk haematological malignancies. Blood Cells Mol Dis40(1):8–12

Bader P, Kreyenberg H et al (2009) Prognostic value of minimal residual disease quantification before allogeneic stem-cell transplantation in relapsed childhood acute lymphoblastic leukemia: the ALL-REZ BFM Study Group. J Clin Oncol 27(3):377–384

Balduzzi A, Valsecchi MG et al (2005) Chemotherapy versus allogeneic transplantation for very-high-risk childhood acute lymphoblastic leukaemia in first complete remission: comparison by genetic randomisation in an international prospective study. Lancet 366(9486):635–642

Barredo JC, Devidas M et al (2006) Isolated CNS relapse of acute lymphoblastic leukemia treated with intensive systemic chemotherapy and delayed CNS radiation: a pediatric oncology group study. J Clin Oncol 24(19):3142–3149

Barrett AJ, Horowitz MM et al (1994) Bone marrow transplants from HLA-identical siblings as compared with chemotherapy for children with acute lymphoblastic leukemia in a second remission. N Engl J Med 331(19):1253–1258

Behm FG, Raimondi SC et al (1996) Rearrangement of the MLL gene confers a poor prognosis in childhood acute lymphoblastic leukemia, regardless of presenting age. Blood 87(7): 2870–2877

Bercovich D, Ganmore I et al (2008) Mutations of JAK2 in acute lymphoblastic leukaemias associated with Down's syndrome. Lancet 372(9648):1484–1492

Berg SL, Blaney SM et al (2005) Phase II study of nelarabine (compound 506U78) in children and young adults with refractory T-cell malignancies: a report from the Children's Oncology Group. J Clin Oncol 23(15):3376–3382

Beyermann B, Adams HP et al (1997) Philadelphia chromosome in relapsed childhood acute lymphoblastic leukemia: a matched-pair analysis. Berlin-Frankfurt-Munster Study Group. J Clin Oncol 15(6):2231–2237

Biondi A, Valsecchi MG et al (2000) Molecular detection of minimal residual disease is a strong predictive factor of relapse in childhood B-lineage acute lymphoblastic leukemia with medium risk features. A case control study of the International BFM study group. Leukemia 14(11): 1939–1943

Biondi A, Baruchel A et al (2009) The Eleventh International Childhood Acute Lymphoblastic Leukemia Workshop Report: Ponte di Legno, Italy, 6–7 May 2009. Leukemia

Blaney SM, Bernstein M et al (2004) Phase I study of the proteasome inhibitor bortezomib in pediatric patients with refractory solid tumors: a Children's Oncology Group study (ADVL0015). J Clin Oncol 22(23):4804–4809

Bleyer WA, Sather HN et al (1991) Monthly pulses of vincristine and prednisone prevent bone marrow and testicular relapse in low-risk childhood acute lymphoblastic leukemia: a report of the CCG-161 study by the Childrens Cancer Study Group. J Clin Oncol 9(6):1012–1021

Boissel N, Auclerc MF et al (2003) Should adolescents with acute lymphoblastic leukemia be treated as old children or young adults? Comparison of the French FRALLE-93 and LALA-94 trials. J Clin Oncol 21(5):774–780

Borgmann A, Baumgarten E et al (1997) Allogeneic bone marrow transplantation for a subset of children with acute lymphoblastic leukemia in third remission: a conceivable alternative? Bone Marrow Transplant 20(11):939–944

Borgmann A, von Stackelberg A et al (2003) Unrelated donor stem cell transplantation compared with chemotherapy for children with acute lymphoblastic leukemia in a second remission: a matched-pair analysis. Blood 101(10):3835–3839

Borkhardt A, Cazzaniga G et al (1997) Incidence and clinical relevance of TEL/AML1 fusion genes in children with acute lymphoblastic leukemia enrolled in the German and Italian multicenter therapy trials. Associazione Italiana Ematologia Oncologia Pediatrica and the Berlin-Frankfurt-Munster Study Group. Blood 90(2):571–577

Borowitz MJ, Devidas M et al (2008) Clinical significance of minimal residual disease in childhood acute lymphoblastic leukemia and its relationship to other prognostic factors: a Children's Oncology Group study. Blood 111(12):5477–5485

Bostrom BC, Sensel MR et al (2003) Dexamethasone versus prednisone and daily oral versus weekly intravenous mercaptopurine for patients with standard-risk acute lymphoblastic leukemia: a report from the Children's Cancer Group. Blood101(10):380 9–3817

Brecher ML, Weinberg V et al (1986) Intermediate dose methotrexate in childhood acute lymphoblastic leukemia resulting in decreased incidence of testicular relapse. Cancer 58(5): 1024–1028

Brochstein JA, Kernan NA et al (1987) Allogeneic bone marrow transplantation after hyperfractionated total-body irradiation and cyclophosphamide in children with acute leukemia. N Engl J Med 317(26):1618–1624

Brown P, Levis M et al (2006) Combinations of the FLT3 inhibitor CEP-701 and chemotherapy synergistically kill infant and childhood MLL-rearranged ALL cells in a sequence-dependent manner. Leukemia 20(8):1368–1376

Buchanan GR, Boyett JM et al (1991) Improved treatment results in boys with overt testicular relapse during or shortly after initial therapy for acute lymphoblastic leukemia. A Pediatric Oncology group study. Cancer 68(1):48–55

Buchanan GR, Rivera GK et al (2000) Alternating drug pairs with or without periodic reinduction in children with acute lymphoblastic leukemia in second bone marrow remission: a Pediatric Oncology Group Study. Cancer 88(5): 1166–1174

Buhrer C, Hartmann R et al (1993) Superior prognosis in combined compared to isolated bone marrow relapses in salvage therapy of childhood acute lymphoblastic leukemia. Med Pediatr Oncol 21(7):470–476

Buhrer C, Hartmann R et al (1994) Importance of effective central nervous system therapy in isolated bone marrow relapse of childhood acute lymphoblastic leukemia. BFM (Berlin-Frankfurt-Munster) Relapse Study Group. Blood 83(12):3468–3472

Burzykowski T, Buyse M et al (2008) Evaluation of tumor response, disease control, progression-free survival, and time to progression as potential surrogate end points in metastatic breast cancer. J Clin Oncol 26(12):1987–1992

Carnahan J, Stein R et al (2007) Epratuzumab, a CD22-targeting recombinant humanized antibody with a different mode of action from rituximab. Mol Immunol 44(6): 1331–1341

Castillo LA, Craft AW et al (1990) Gonadal function after 12-Gy testicular irradiation in childhood acute lymphoblastic leukaemia. Med Pediatr Oncol 18(3):185–189

Cave H, van der Werff ten Bosch J et al (1998) Clinical significance of minimal residual disease in childhood acute lymphoblastic leukemia. European Organization for Research and Treatment of Cancer – Childhood Leukemia Cooperative Group. N Engl J Med 339(9):591–598

Chessells JM (1998) Relapsed lymphoblastic leukaemia in children: a continuing challenge. Br J Haematol 102(2):423–438

Chessells JM, Leiper AD et al (1994) A second course of treatment for childhood acute lymphoblastic leukaemia: long term follow-up is needed to assess results. Br J Haematol 86(1):48–54

Chessells JM, Hall E et al (1998) The impact of age on outcome in lymphoblastic leukaemia; MRC UKALL X and XA compared: a report from the MRC Paediatric and Adult Working Parties. Leukemia 12(4):463–473

Chessells JM, Harrison CJ et al (2002) Treatment of infants with lymphoblastic leukaemia: results of the UK Infant Protocols 1987–1999. Br J Haematol 117(2):306–314

Chessels JM, Swansbury GJ et al (1997) Cytogenetics and prognosis in childhood lymphoblastic leukaemia: results of MRC UKALL X. Medical Research Council Working Party in Childhood Leukaemia. Br J Haematol 99(1):93–100

Conter V, Valsecchi MG et al (2007) Pulses of vincristine and dexamethasone in addition to intensive chemotherapy for children with intermediate-risk acute lymphoblastic leukaemia: a multicentre randomised trial. Lancet 369(9556): 123–131

Conter V, Arico M et al (2010) Long-term results of the Italian Association of Pediatric Hematology and Oncology (AIEOP) Studies 82, 87, 88, 91 and 95 for childhood acute lymphoblastic leukemia. Leukemia 24(2):255–264

Coustan-Smith E, Sancho J et al (2000) Clinical importance of minimal residual disease in childhood acute lymphoblastic leukemia. Blood 96(8):2691–2696

Coustan-Smith E, Mullighan CG et al (2009) Early T-cell precursor leukaemia: a subtype of very high-risk acute lymphoblastic leukaemia. Lancet Oncol 10(2):147–156

Crist W, Boyett J et al (1986) Clinical and biologic features predict poor prognosis in acute lymphoid leukemias in children and adolescents: a Pediatric Oncology Group review. Med Pediatr Oncol 14(3):135–139

Culbert SJ, Shuster JJ et al (1991) Remission induction and continuation therapy in children with their first relapse of acute lymphoid leukemia. A Pediatric Oncology Group study. Cancer67(1):37–42

Dahlke J, Kroger N et al (2006) Comparable results in patients with acute lymphoblastic leukemia after related and unrelated stem cell transplantation. Bone Marrow Transplant 37(2):155–163

Daser A, Rabbitts TH (2005) The versatile mixed lineage leukaemia gene MLL and its many associations in leukaemogenesis. Semin Cancer Biol 15(3):175–188

de Bont JM, Holt B et al (2004) Significant difference in outcome for adolescents with acute lymphoblastic leukemia treated on pediatric vs adult protocols in the Netherlands. Leukemia 18(12):2032–2035

De Gruttola VG, Clax P et al (2001) Considerations in the evaluation of surrogate endpoints in clinical trials. summary of a National Institutes of Health workshop. Control Clin Trials 22(5):485–502

De Lorenzo P, Antolini L et al (2009) Evaluation of alternative prognostic stratifications by prediction accuracy measures on individual survival with application to childhood leukaemia. Eur J Cancer 45(8):1432–1437

DeAngelo DJ, Dahlberg S et al (2007) A multicenter phase II study using a dose intensified pediatric regimen in adults with untreated acute lymphoblastic leukemia. Blood 110:587

Dhani N, Tu D et al (2009) Alternate endpoints for screening phase II studies. Clin Cancer Res 15(6):1873–1882

Domenech C, Mercier M et al (2008) First isolated extramedullary relapse in children with B-cell precursor acute lymphoblastic leukaemia: results of the Cooprall-97 study. Eur J Cancer44(16):2461–2469

Dopfer R, Henze G et al (1991) Allogeneic bone marrow transplantation for childhood acute lymphoblastic leukemia in second remission after intensive primary and relapse therapy according to the BFM- and CoALL-protocols: results of the German Cooperative Study. Blood 78(10): 2780–2784

Dreyer ZE, Dinndorf P et al (2007a) Unexpected toxicity with intensified induction in infant acute lymphoid leukemia. Blood (ASH Annu Meet Abstr) 110(11):852

Dreyer ZE, Dinndorf P et al (2007b) Hematopoietic stem cell transplant (HSCT) versus intensive chemotherapy in infant acute lymphoblastic leukemia (ALL). J Clin Oncol 25(18s):9514

Druker BJ (2009) Perspectives on the development of imatinib and the future of cancer research. Nat Med 15(10):1149–1152

Dunsmore KP, Devidas M et al (2008) Nelarabine in combination with intensive modified BFM AALL00P2: a pilot study for the treatment of high-risk T-ALL a report from the Children's Oncology Group. J Clin Oncol (ASCO Annu Meet Proc 26:539s

Eapen M, Raetz E et al (2006a) Outcomes after HLA-matched sibling transplantation or chemotherapy in children with B-precursor acute lymphoblastic leukemia in a second remission: a collaborative study of the Children's Oncology Group and the Center for International Blood and Marrow Transplant Research. Blood 107(12):4961–4967

Eapen M, Rubinstein P et al (2006b) Comparable long-term survival after unrelated and HLA-matched sibling donor hematopoietic stem cell transplantations for acute leukemia in children younger than 18 months. J Clin Oncol 24(1): 145–151

Eapen M, Zhang MJ et al (2008) Outcomes after HLA-matched sibling transplantation or chemotherapy in children with acute lymphoblastic leukemia in a second remission after an isolated central nervous system relapse: a collaborative study of the Children's Oncology Group and the Center for International Blood and Marrow Transplant Research. Leukemia22(2):281–286

Eckert C, Biondi A et al (2001) Prognostic value of minimal residual disease in relapsed childhood acute lymphoblastic leukaemia. Lancet 358(9289):1239–1241

Einsiedel HG, von Stackelberg A et al (2005) Long-term outcome in children with relapsed ALL by risk-stratified salvage therapy: results of trial acute lymphoblastic leukemia-relapse study of the Berlin-Frankfurt-Munster Group 87. J Clin Oncol 23(31):7942–7950

Evans PA, Short MA et al (1998) Residual disease detection using fluorescent polymerase chain reaction at 20 weeks of therapy predicts clinical outcome in childhood acute lymphoblastic leukemia. J Clin Oncol 16(11):3616–3627

Farber S, Diamond LK (1948) Temporary remissions in acute leukemia in children produced by folic acid antagonist, 4-aminopteroyl-glutamic acid. N Engl J Med 238(23):787–793

Fleming TR, DeMets DL (1996) Surrogate end points in clinical trials: are we being misled? Ann Intern Med 125(7):605–613

Fleming TR, Rothmann MD et al (2009) Issues in using progression-free survival when evaluating oncology products. J Clin Oncol27(17):2874–2880

Fletcher JA, Lynch EA et al (1991) Translocation (9;22) is associated with extremely poor prognosis in intensively treated children with acute lymphoblastic leukemia. Blood 77(3): 435–439

Flohr T, Schrauder A et al (2008) Minimal residual disease-directed risk stratification using real-time quantitative PCR analysis of immunoglobulin and T-cell receptor gene rearrangements in the international multicenter trial AIEOP-BFM ALL 2000 for childhood acute lymphoblastic leukemia. Leukemia22(4):771–782

Forestier E, Izraeli S et al (2008) Cytogenetic features of acute lymphoblastic and myeloid leukemias in pediatric patients with Down syndrome: an iBFM-SG study. Blood 111(3):1575–1583

Freeman AI, Weinberg V et al (1983) Comparison of intermediate-dose methotrexate with cranial irradiation for the post-induction treatment of acute lymphocytic leukemia in children. N Engl J Med 308(9):477–484

Gajjar A, Ribeiro R et al (1995) Persistence of circulating blasts after 1 week of multiagent chemotherapy confers a poor prognosis in childhood acute lymphoblastic leukemia. Blood 86(4):1292–1295

Galimberti S, Sasieni P et al (2002) A weighted Kaplan-Meier estimator for matched data with application to the comparison of chemotherapy and bone-marrow transplant in leukaemia. Stat Med 21(24):3847–3864

Gassas A, Sung L et al (2006) Comparative outcome of hematopoietic stem cell transplantation for pediatric acute lymphoblastic leukemia following cyclophosphamide and total body irradiation or VP16 and total body irradiation conditioning regimens. Bone Marrow Transplant 38(11): 739–743

Gassas A, Sung L et al (2007) Graft-versus-leukemia effect in hematopoietic stem cell transplantation for pediatric acute lymphoblastic leukemia: significantly lower relapse rate in unrelated transplantations. Bone Marrow Transplant 40(10): 951–955

Gaynon PS, Bleyer WA et al (1990) Day 7 marrow response and outcome for children with acute lymphoblastic leukemia and unfavorable presenting features. Med Pediatr Oncol 18(4): 273–279

Gaynon PS, Steinherz PG et al (1993) Improved therapy for children with acute lymphoblastic leukemia and unfavorable presenting features: a follow-up report of the Childrens Cancer Group Study CCG-106. J Clin Oncol 11(11): 2234–2242

Gaynon PS, Desai AA et al (1997) Early response to therapy and outcome in childhood acute lymphoblastic leukemia: a review. Cancer 80(9):1717–1726

Gaynon PS, Qu RP et al (1998) Survival after relapse in childhood acute lymphoblastic leukemia: impact of site and time to first relapse – the Children's Cancer Group experience. Cancer82(7):1387– 1395

Gaynon PS, Trigg ME et al (2000) Children's Cancer Group trials in childhood acute lymphoblastic leukemia: 1983–1995. Leukemia 14(12):2223–2233

Gaynon PS, Angiolillo AL et al (2010) Long-term results of the Children's Cancer Group studies for childhood acute lymphoblastic leukemia 1983–2002: a Children's Oncology Group report. Leukemia 24(2):285–297

Gluckman E, Rocha V (2008) Indications and results of cord blood transplant in children with leukemia. Bone Marrow Transplant 41(Suppl 2):S80–82

Goldberg JM, Silverman LB et al (2003) Childhood T-cell acute lymphoblastic leukemia: the Dana-Farber Cancer Institute acute lymphoblastic leukemia consortium experience. J Clin Oncol21(19):3616 –3622

Goldstone AH, Richards SM et al (2008) In adults with standard risk acute lymphoblastic leukemia, the greatest benefit is achieved from a matched sibling allogeneic transplantation in first complete remission, and an autologous transplantation is less effective than conventional consolidation/maintenance chemotherapy in all patients: final results of the International ALL Trial (MRC UKALL XII/ECOG E2993). Blood111(4):1827 –1833

Goulden NJ, Knechtli CJ et al (1998) Minimal residual disease analysis for the prediction of relapse in children with standard-risk acute lymphoblastic leukaemia. Br J Haematol 100(1):235–244

Greaves MF, Wiemels J (2003) Origins of chromosome translocations in childhood leukaemia. Nat Rev Cancer 3(9): 639–649

Grundy RG, Leiper AD et al (1997) Survival and endocrine outcome after testicular relapse in acute lymphoblastic leukaemia. Arch Dis Child 76(3):190–196

Hagedorn N, Acquaviva C et al (2007) Submicroscopic bone marrow involvement in isolated extramedullary relapses in childhood acute lymphoblastic leukemia: a more precise definition of "isolated" and its possible clinical implications, a collaborative study of the Resistant Disease Committee of the International BFM study group. Blood 110(12): 4022–4029

Handgretinger R, Chen X et al (2007) Feasibility and outcome of reduced-intensity conditioning in haploidentical transplantation. Ann NY Acad Sci 1106:279–289

Harker-Murray PD, Thomas AJ et al (2008) Allogeneic hematopoietic cell transplantation in children with relapsed acute lymphoblastic leukemia isolated to the central nervous system. Biol Blood Marrow Transplant 14(6): 685–692

Harris MB, Shuster JJ et al (1992) Trisomy of leukemic cell chromosomes 4 and 10 identifies children with B-progenitor cell acute lymphoblastic leukemia with a very low risk of treatment failure: a Pediatric Oncology Group study. Blood 79(12):3316–3324

Harrison CJ (2009) Cytogenetics of paediatric and adolescent acute lymphoblastic leukaemia. Br J Haematol 144(2): 147–156

Hastings C, Sather HN et al (2006) Outcomes in children and adolescents with a markedly elevated white blood cell count (>200, 000) at diagnosis of high risk acute lymphoblastic leukemia (ALL): a report from the Children's Oncology Group. Blood (ASH Annu Meet Abstr) 108(11):1870

Heerema NA, Nachman JB et al (1999) Hypodiploidy with less than 45 chromosomes confers adverse risk in childhood acute lymphoblastic leukemia: a report from the children's cancer group. Blood 94(12):4036–4045

Heerema NA, Sather HN et al (2000) Prognostic impact of trisomies of chromosomes 10, 17, and 5 among children with acute lymphoblastic leukemia and high hyperdiploidy (>50 chromosomes). J Clin Oncol 18(9):1876–1887

Henze G (1997) Childhood acute lymphoblastic leukaemia. Eur J Cancer 33(1):8–9

Henze G, Langermann HJ et al (1981a) The BFM 76/79 acute lymphoblastic leukemia therapy study (author's transl). Klin Pädiatr193(3):145–154

Henze G, Langermann HJ et al (1981b) Thymic involvement and initial white blood count in childhood acute lymphoblastic leukemia. Am J Pediatr Hematol Oncol 3(4):369–376

Henze G, Fengler R et al (1989) Chemotherapy for bone marrow relapse of childhood acute lymphoblastic leukemia. Cancer Chemother Pharmacol 24(Suppl 1):S16–19

Henze G, Fengler R et al (1991) Six-year experience with a comprehensive approach to the treatment of recurrent childhood acute lymphoblastic leukemia (ALL-REZ BFM 85). A relapse study of the BFM group. Blood 78(5):1166–1172

Herold R, von Stackelberg A et al (2004) Acute lymphoblastic leukemia-relapse study of the Berlin-Frankfurt-Munster Group (ALL-REZ BFM) experience: early treatment intensity makes the difference. J Clin Oncol 22(3):569–570, author reply 570–561

Hijiya N, Gaynon P et al (2009) A multi-center phase I study of clofarabine, etoposide and cyclophosphamide in combination in pediatric patients with refractory or relapsed acute leukemia. Leukemia 23(12):2259–2264

Hoering A, Leblanc M et al (2008) Randomized phase III clinical trial designs for targeted agents. Clin Cancer Res 14(14):4358–4367

Horton TM, Gannavarapu A et al (2006) Bortezomib interactions with chemotherapy agents in acute leukemia *in vitro*. Cancer Chemother Pharmacol 58(1):13–23

Horton TM, Pati D et al (2007) A phase 1 study of the proteasome inhibitor bortezomib in pediatric patients with refractory leukemia: a Children's Oncology Group study. Clin Cancer Res 13(5):1516–1522

Huget F, Pigneux A et al (2008) Outcome of a pediatric-inspired therapy in adults with Philadelphia chromosome-neagative acute lymphoblastic leukemia (ALL): final results for the GRAALL-2003 study. J Clin Oncol (ASCO Annu Meet Proc)26:373s

Hunger SP (1996) Chromosomal translocations involving the E2A gene in acute lymphoblastic leukemia: clinical features and molecular pathogenesis. Blood 87(4):1211–1224

Hunger SP, Tkachuk DC et al (1993) HRX involvement in *de novo* and secondary leukemias with diverse chromosome 11q23 abnormalities. Blood 81(12):3197–3203

Hunger SP, Devaraj PE et al (1994) Two types of genomic rearrangements create alternative E2A-HLF fusion proteins in t(17;19)-ALL. Blood 83(10):2970–2977

Hunger SP, Winick NJ et al (2005) Therapy of low-risk subsets of childhood acute lymphoblastic leukemia: when do we say enough? Pediatr Blood Cancer 45(7):876–880

Hunger SP, Sung L et al (2009) Treatment strategies and regimens of graduated intensity for childhood acute lymphoblastic leukemia in low-income countries: a proposal. Pediatr Blood Cancer 52(5):559–565

Jahnukainen K, Salmi TT et al (1998) The clinical indications for identical pathogenesis of isolated and non-isolated testicular relapses in acute lymphoblastic leukaemia. Acta Paediatr87(6):638–643

Jeha S, Gandhi V et al (2004) Clofarabine, a novel nucleoside analog, is active in pediatric patients with advanced leukemia. Blood 103(3):784–789

Jeha S, Pei D et al (2009) Increased risk for CNS relapse in pre-B cell leukemia with the t(1;19)/TCF3-PBX1. Leukemia 23(8):1406–1409

Kager L, Cheok M et al (2005) Folate pathway gene expression differs in subtypes of acute lymphoblastic leukemia and influences methotrexate pharmacodynamics. J Clin Invest 115(1):110–117

Kamps WA, van der Pal-de Bruin KM et al (2010) Long-term results of Dutch Childhood Oncology Group studies for children with acute lymphoblastic leukemia from 1984 to 2004. Leukemia 24(2):309–319

Kang H, Chen IM et al (2010) Gene expression classifiers for relapse-free survival and minimal residual disease improve risk classification and outcome prediction in pediatric B-precursor acute lymphoblastic leukemia. Blood 115(7): 1394–1405

Kaspers GJ, Pieters R et al (1994) Glucocorticoid resistance in childhood leukemia. Leuk Lymphoma 13(3–4): 187–201

Kawamura M, Kikuchi A et al (1995) Mutations of the p53 and ras genes in childhood t(1;19)-acute lymphoblastic leukemia. Blood 85(9):2546–2552

Klumper E, Pieters R et al (1995) *In vitro* cellular drug resistance in children with relapsed/refractory acute lymphoblastic leukemia. Blood 86(10):3861–3868

Konrad M, Metzler M et al (2003) Late relapses evolve from slow-responding subclones in t(12;21)-positive acute lymphoblastic leukemia: evidence for the persistence of a preleukemic clone. Blood 101(9):3635–3640

Kreyenberg H, Eckert C et al (2009) Immunoglobulin and T-cell receptor gene rearrangements as PCR-based targets are stable markers for monitoring minimal residual disease in acute lymphoblastic leukemia after stem cell transplantation. Leukemia23(7):1355–1358

Lal A, Kwan E et al (1998) Molecular detection of acute lymphoblastic leukaemia in boys with testicular relapse. Mol Pathol51(5):277–281

Land VJ, Thomas PR et al (1985) Comparison of maintenance treatment regimens for first central nervous system relapse in children with acute lymphocytic leukemia. A Pediatric Oncology Group study. Cancer 56(1):81–87

Lang P, Handgretinger R (2008) Haploidentical SCT in children: an update and future perspectives. Bone Marrow Transplant 42(Suppl2) :S54–59

Lange BJ, Bostrom BC et al (2002) Double-delayed intensification improves event-free survival for children with intermediate-risk acute lymphoblastic leukemia: a report from the Children's Cancer Group. Blood 99(3):825–833

Langlands K, Craig JI et al (1993) Clonal selection in acute lymphoblastic leukaemia demonstrated by polymerase chain reaction analysis of immunoglobulin heavy chain and T-cell receptor delta chain rearrangements. Leukemia 7(7):1066–1070

Lanino E, Sacchi N et al (2008) Strategies of the donor search for children with second CR ALL lacking a matched sibling donor. Bone Marrow Transplant 41(Suppl 2):S75–79

Lawson SE, Harrison G et al (2000) The UK experience in treating relapsed childhood acute lymphoblastic leukaemia: a report on the medical research council UKALLR1 study. Br J Haematol 108(3):531–543

Leiper AD, Grant DB et al (1986) Gonadal function after testicular radiation for acute lymphoblastic leukaemia. Arch Dis Child 61(1):53–56

Liang DC, Yang CP et al (2010) Long-term results of Taiwan Pediatric Oncology Group studies 1997 and 2002 for childhood acute lymphoblastic leukemia. Leukemia 24(2): 397–405

Lipshultz SE, Rifai N et al (2004) The effect of dexrazoxane on myocardial injury in doxorubicin-treated children with acute lymphoblastic leukemia. N Engl J Med 351(2):145–153

Lo Nigro L, Cazzaniga G et al (1999) Clonal stability in children with acute lymphoblastic leukemia (ALL) who relapsed five or more years after diagnosis. Leukemia 13(2):190–195

Locatelli F, Testi AM et al (2009) Clofarabine, cyclophosphamide and etoposide as single-course re-induction therapy for children with refractory/multiple relapsed acute lymphoblastic leukaemia. Br J Haematol 147(3):371–378

Loh ML, Rubnitz JE (2002) TEL/AML1-positive pediatric leukemia: prognostic significance and therapeutic approaches. Curr Opin Hematol 9(4):345–352

Loh ML, Silverman LB et al (1998) Incidence of TEL/AML1 fusion in children with relapsed acute lymphoblastic leukemia. Blood 92(12):4792–4797

Loh ML, Goldwasser MA et al (2006) Prospective analysis of TEL/AML1-positive patients treated on Dana-Farber Cancer Institute Consortium Protocol 95-01. Blood 107(11):4508–4513

Lori AP, Arcese W et al (2007) Unrelated cord blood transplant in children with high-risk acute lymphoblastic leukemia: a long-term follow-up. Haematologica 92(8):1051–1058

MacMillan ML, Davies SM et al (2008) Twenty years of unrelated donor bone marrow transplantation for pediatric acute leukemia facilitated by the National Marrow Donor Program. Biol Blood Marrow Transplant 14(9 Suppl):16–22

Mahmoud HH, Rivera GK et al (1993) Low leukocyte counts with blast cells in cerebrospinal fluid of children with newly diagnosed acute lymphoblastic leukemia. N Engl J Med 329(5):314–319

Maloney KW, Shuster JJ et al (2000) Long-term results of treatment studies for childhood acute lymphoblastic leukemia: Pediatric Oncology Group studies from 1986–1994. Leukemia 14(12):2276–2285
Maloney KW, Carroll WL et al (2010) Down syndrome childhood acute lymphoblastic leukemia has a unique spectrum of sentinel cytogenetic lesions that influences treatment outcome: a report from the Children's Oncology Group. Blood 2010 May 4 ePub
Marubini E, Valsecchi MG (1995) Analysing survival data from clinical trials and observational studies. Wiley, Chichester
Matloub Y, Angiolillo A et al (2006) Double delayed intensification (DDI) is equivalent to single DI (SDI) in children with National Cancer Institute (NCI) standard-risk acute lymphoblastic leukemia (SR-ALL) Treated on Children's Cancer Group (CCG) clinical trial 1991 (CCG-1991). Blood (ASH Annu Meet Abstr) 108(11):146
Matloub Y, Bostrom BC et al (2008) Escalating dose intravenous methotrexate without leucovorin rescue during interim maintenance is superior to oral methotrexate for children with standard risk acute lymphoblastic leukemia (SR-ALL): Children's Oncology Group Study 1991. Blood (ASH Annu Meet Abstr) 112(11):9
Mehta PA, Davies SM (2008) Allogeneic transplantation for childhood ALL. Bone Marrow Transplant 41(2):133–139
Messinger Y (2010) Phase I study of bortezomib combined with chemotherapy in children with relapsed childhood acute lymphoblastic leukemia (ALL). a report from the therapeutic advances in Childhood Leukemia (TACL) consortium. Pediatr Blood Cancer 55: 254–9
Miniero R, Saracco P et al (1995) Relapse after first cessation of therapy in childhood acute lymphoblastic leukemia: a 10-year follow-up study. Italian Association of Pediatric Hematology-Oncology (AIEOP). Med Pediatr Oncol 24(2): 71–76
Mitchell CD, Richards SM et al (2005) Benefit of dexamethasone compared with prednisolone for childhood acute lymphoblastic leukaemia: results of the UK Medical Research Council ALL97 randomized trial. Br J Haematol 129(6): 734–745
Mitchell C, Richards S et al (2010) Long term follow-up of the United Kingdom medical research council protocols for childhood acute lymphoblastic leukaemia, 1980–2001. Leukemia 24(2):406–418
Moorman AV, Richards SM et al (2007) Prognosis of children with acute lymphoblastic leukemia (ALL) and intrachromosomal amplification of chromosome 21 (iAMP21). Blood 109(6):2327–2330
Moricke A, Reiter A et al (2008) Risk-adjusted therapy of acute lymphoblastic leukemia can decrease treatment burden and improve survival: treatment results of 2169 unselected pediatric and adolescent patients enrolled in the trial ALL-BFM 95. Blood 111(9):4477–4489
Moricke A, Zimmermann M et al (2010) Long-term results of five consecutive trials in childhood acute lymphoblastic leukemia performed by the ALL-BFM study group from 1981 to 2000. Leukemia 24(2):265–284
Morland BJ, Shaw PJ (1996) Induction toxicity of a modified Memorial Sloan-Kettering-New York II Protocol in children with relapsed acute lymphoblastic leukemia: a single institution study. Med Pediatr Oncol 27(3):139–144
Moussalem M, Esperou Bourdeau H et al (1995) Allogeneic bone marrow transplantation for childhood acute lymphoblastic leukemia in second remission: factors predictive of survival, relapse and graft-versus-host disease. Bone Marrow Transplant15(6):943–947
Mullighan CG, Goorha S et al (2007) Genome-wide analysis of genetic alterations in acute lymphoblastic leukaemia. Nature 446(7137):758–764
Mullighan CG, Su X et al (2009a) Deletion of IKZF1 and prognosis in acute lymphoblastic leukemia. N Engl J Med 360(5): 470–480
Mullighan CG, Zhang J et al (2009b) JAK mutations in high-risk childhood acute lymphoblastic leukemia. Proc Natl Acad Sci USA 160:9414–9418
Mullighan CG, Collins-Underwood JR et al (2009c) Rearrangement of CRLF2 in B-progenitor- and Down syndrome-associated acute lymphoblastic leukemia. Nat Genet 41(11): 1243–1246
Nachman J, Palmer NF et al (1990) Open-wedge testicular biopsy in childhood acute lymphoblastic leukemia after two years of maintenance therapy: diagnostic accuracy and influence on outcome–a report from Children's Cancer Study Group. Blood 75(5):1051–1055
Nachman JB, Sather HN et al (1998) Augmented post-induction therapy for children with high-risk acute lymphoblastic leukemia and a slow response to initial therapy. N Engl J Med 338(23):1663–1671
Nachman JB, Heerema NA et al (2007) Outcome of treatment in children with hypodiploid acute lymphoblastic leukemia. Blood110(4):1112–1115
Nachman JB, La MK et al (2009) Young adults with acute lymphoblastic leukemia have an excellent outcome with chemotherapy alone and benefit from intensive postinduction treatment: a report from the children's oncology group. J Clin Oncol 27(31):5189–5194
Neale GA, Pui CH et al (1994) Molecular evidence for minimal residual bone marrow disease in children with "isolated" extra-medullary relapse of T-cell acute lymphoblastic leukemia. Leukemia 8(5):768–775
Nguyen K, Devidas M et al (2008) Factors influencing survival after relapse from acute lymphoblastic leukemia: a Children's Oncology Group study. Leukemia 22(12): 2142–2150
Ortega JA, Nesbit ME Jr et al (1977) L-Asparaginase, vincristine, and prednisone for induction of first remission in acute lymphocytic leukemia. Cancer Res 37(2):535–540
Oudot C, Auclerc MF et al (2008) Prognostic factors for leukemic induction failure in children with acute lymphoblastic leukemia and outcome after salvage therapy: the FRALLE 93 study. J Clin Oncol 26(9):1496–1503
Panzer-Grumayer ER, Schneider M et al (2000) Rapid molecular response during early induction chemotherapy predicts a good outcome in childhood acute lymphoblastic leukemia. Blood95(3):790–794
Piantadosi S (2005) Clinical trials: a metholologic perspective. Wiley, New York
Pieters R, Schrappe M et al (2007) A treatment protocol for infants younger than 1 year with acute lymphoblastic leukaemia (Interfant-99): an observational study and a multicentre randomised trial. Lancet 370(9583):240–250
Pinkel D (1971) Five-year follow-up of "total therapy" of childhood lymphocytic leukemia. JAMA 216:648–652

Pritchard-Jones K, Dixon-Woods M et al (2008) Improving recruitment to clinical trials for cancer in childhood. Lancet Oncol9(4):392–399

Pui CH, Howard SC (2008) Current management and challenges of malignant disease in the CNS in paediatric leukaemia. Lancet Oncol 9(3):257–268

Pui CH, Bowman WP et al (1988) Cyclic combination chemotherapy for acute lymphoblastic leukemia recurring after elective cessation of therapy. Med Pediatr Oncol 16(1):21–26

Pui CH, Behm FG et al (1990) Heterogeneity of presenting features and their relation to treatment outcome in 120 children with T-cell acute lymphoblastic leukemia. Blood 75(1): 174–179

Pui CH, Boyett JM et al (1999) Sex differences in prognosis for children with acute lymphoblastic leukemia. J Clin Oncol 17(3):818–824

Pui CH, Boyett JM et al (2000) Long-term results of TOTAL THERAPY STUDIES 11, 12 and 13A for childhood acute lymphoblastic leukemia at St Jude Children's Research Hospital. Leukemia 14(12):2286–2294

Pui CH, Gaynon PS et al (2002) Outcome of treatment in childhood acute lymphoblastic leukaemia with rearrangements of the 11q23 chromosomal region. Lancet 359(9321): 1909–1915

Pui CH, Chessells JM et al (2003) Clinical heterogeneity in childhood acute lymphoblastic leukemia with 11q23 rearrangements. Leukemia 17(4):700–706

Pui CH, Robison LL et al (2008) Acute lymphoblastic leukaemia. Lancet 371(9617):1030–1043

Pui CH, Campana D et al (2009) Treating childhood acute lymphoblastic leukemia without cranial irradiation. N Engl J Med360(26):2730–2741

Pui CH, Pei D et al (2010) Long-term results of St Jude Total Therapy Studies 11, 12, 13A, 13B, and 14 for childhood acute lymphoblastic leukemia. Leukemia 24(2):371–382

Pulte D, Gondos A et al (2008) Trends in 5- and 10-year survival after diagnosis with childhood hematologic malignancies in the United States, 1990–2004. J Natl Cancer Inst 100(18): 1301–1309

Pulte D, Gondos A et al (2009) Improvement in survival in younger patients with acute lymphoblastic leukemia from the 1980s to the early 21st century. Blood 113(7):1408–1411

Putter H, Fiocco M et al (2007) Tutorial in biostatistics: competing risks and multi-state models. Stat Med 26(11): 2389–2430

Putti MC, Rondelli R et al (1998) Expression of myeloid markers lacks prognostic impact in children treated for acute lymphoblastic leukemia: Italian experience in AIEOP-ALL 88-91 studies. Blood 92(3):795–801

Raetz EA, Borowitz MJ et al (2008a) Reinduction platform for children with first marrow relapse of acute lymphoblastic Leukemia: A Children's Oncology Group Study[corrected]. J Clin Oncol 26(24):3971–3978

Raetz EA, Cairo MS et al (2008b) Chemoimmunotherapy reinduction with epratuzumab in children with acute lymphoblastic leukemia in marrow relapse: a Children's Oncology Group Pilot Study. J Clin Oncol 26(22): 3756–3762

Ramakers-van Woerden NL, Pieters R et al (2000) TEL/AML1 gene fusion is related to *in vitro* drug sensitivity for L-asparaginase in childhood acute lymphoblastic leukemia. Blood96(3):1094–1099

Reiter A, Schrappe M et al (1994) Chemotherapy in 998 unselected childhood acute lymphoblastic leukemia patients. Results and conclusions of the multicenter trial ALL-BFM 86. Blood 84(9):3122–3133

Ribeiro RC, Rivera GK et al (1995) An intensive re-treatment protocol for children with an isolated CNS relapse of acute lymphoblastic leukemia. J Clin Oncol 13(2):333–338

Ribera JM, Ortega JJ et al (2007) Comparison of intensive chemotherapy, allogeneic, or autologous stem-cell transplantation as postremission treatment for children with very high risk acute lymphoblastic leukemia: PETHEMA ALL-93 Trial. J Clin Oncol 25(1):16–24

Ribera JM, Oriol A et al (2008) Comparison of the results of the treatment of adolescents and young adults with standard-risk acute lymphoblastic leukemia with the Programa Espanol de Tratamiento en Hematologia pediatric-based protocol ALL-96. J Clin Oncol 26(11):1843–1849

Richards S, Gray R et al (1996) Duration and intensity of maintenance chemotherapy in acute lymphoblastic leukemia: Overview of 42 trials involving 12000 randomized children. Childhood ALL Collaborative Group. Lancet 347: 1783–1788

Riehm H, Gadner H et al (1977) The west-berlin therapy study of acute lymphoblastic leukemia in childhood–report after 6 years (author's transl). Klin Pädiatr 189(8):89–102

Riehm H, Gadner H et al (1980) The Berlin childhood acute lymphoblastic leukemia therapy study, 1970–1976. Am J Pediatr Hematol/Oncol 2:299–306

Riehm H, Gadner H et al (1990) Results and significance of six randomized trials in four consecutive ALL-BFM studies. Haematol Blood Transfus 33:439–450

Ries LA, Smith MA et al (1999). Cancer incidence and survival among children and adolescents: United States SEER Program 1975–1995. NCIS Program. Bethesda, MD. NIH Pub. No 99–4649

Ritchey AK, Pollock BH et al (1999) Improved survival of children with isolated CNS relapse of acute lymphoblastic leukemia: a pediatric oncology group study. J Clin Oncol 17(12):3745–3752

Rivera GK, Pinkel D et al (1993) Treatment of acute lymphoblastic leukemia. 30 years' experience at St. Jude Children's Research Hospital. N Engl J Med 329(18):1289–1295

Rivera GK, Zhou Y et al (2005) Bone marrow recurrence after initial intensive treatment for childhood acute lymphoblastic leukemia. Cancer 103(2):368–376

Roberts WM, Estrov Z et al (1997) Measurement of residual leukemia during remission in childhood acute lymphoblastic leukemia. N Engl J Med 336(5):317–323

Ross ME, Zhou X et al (2003) Classification of pediatric acute lymphoblastic leukemia by gene expression profiling. Blood 102(8):2951–2959

Roy A, Bradburn M et al (2005a) Early response to induction is predictive of survival in childhood Philadelphia chromosome positive acute lymphoblastic leukaemia: results of the Medical Research Council ALL 97 trial. Br J Haematol 129(1):35–44

Roy A, Cargill A et al (2005b) Outcome after first relapse in childhood acute lymphoblastic leukaemia – lessons from the United Kingdom R2 trial. Br J Haematol 130(1):67–75

Rubnitz JE, Link MP et al (1994) Frequency and prognostic significance of HRX rearrangements in infant acute lymphoblastic leukemia: a Pediatric Oncology Group study. Blood 84(2):570–573

Rubnitz JE, Shuster JJ et al (1997) Case-control study suggests a favorable impact of TEL rearrangement in patients with B-lineage acute lymphoblastic leukemia treated with antimetabolite-based therapy: a Pediatric Oncology Group study. Blood 89(4):1143–1146

Rubnitz JE, Behm FG et al (1999) Low frequency of TEL-AML1 in relapsed acute lymphoblastic leukemia supports a favorable prognosis for this genetic subgroup. Leukemia 13(1):19–21

Rubnitz JE, Wichlan D et al (2008) Prospective analysis of TEL gene rearrangements in childhood acute lymphoblastic leukemia: a Children's Oncology Group study. J Clin Oncol 26(13):2186–2191

Russell LJ, Capasso M et al (2009) Deregulated expression of cytokine receptor gene, CRLF2, is involved in lymphoid transformation in B-cell precursor acute lymphoblastic leukemia. Blood 114(13):2688–2698

Sadowitz PD, Smith SD et al (1993) Treatment of late bone marrow relapse in children with acute lymphoblastic leukemia: a Pediatric Oncology Group study. Blood 81(3): 602–609

Sallan SE, Cammita BM et al (1978) Intermittent combination chemotherapy with adriamycin for childhood acute lymphoblastic leukemia: clinical results. Blood 51(3):425–433

Sallan SE, Hitchcock-Bryan S et al (1983) Influence of intensive asparaginase in the treatment of childhood non-T-cell acute lymphoblastic leukemia. Cancer Res 43(11):5601–5607

Salzer WL, Devidas M et al (2010) Long-term results of the pediatric oncology group studies for childhood acute lymphoblastic leukemia 1984–2001: a report from the children's oncology group. Leukemia 24(2):355–370

Sather HN (1986) Age at diagnosis in childhood acute lymphoblastic leukemia. Med Pediatr Oncol 14(3):166–172

Schmiegelow K, Nyvold C et al (2001) Post-induction residual leukemia in childhood acute lymphoblastic leukemia quantified by PCR correlates with *in vitro* prednisolone resistance. Leukemia 15(7):1066–1071

Schoenfeld DA, Hui Z et al (2009) Bayesian design using adult data to augment pediatric trials. Clin Trials 6(4):297–304

Schrappe M (2004) Evolution of BFM trials for childhood ALL. Ann Hematol 83(Suppl 1):S121–123

Schrappe M, Camitta B et al (2000a) Long-term results of large prospective trials in childhood acute lymphoblastic leukemia. Leukemia 14(12):2193–2194

Schrappe M, Reiter A et al (2000b) Improved outcome in childhood acute lymphoblastic leukemia despite reduced use of anthracyclines and cranial radiotherapy: results of trial ALL-BFM 90. German-Austrian-Swiss ALL-BFM Study Group. Blood95(11):3310 –3322

Schrappe M, Zimmermann M et al (2008) Dexamethasone in induction can eliminate one third of all relapses in childhood acute lymphoblastic leukemia (ALL): results of an international randomized trial in 3655 patients (Trial AEIOP-BFM ALL 2000). Blood (ASH Annu Meet Abstr) 112:7

Schrauder A, von Stackelberg A et al (2008) Allogeneic hematopoietic SCT in children with ALL: current concepts of ongoing prospective SCT trials. Bone Marrow Transplant 41(Suppl2):S71–74

Schroeder H, Garwicz S et al (1995) Outcome after first relapse in children with acute lymphoblastic leukemia: a population-based study of 315 patients from the Nordic Society of Pediatric Hematology and Oncology (NOPHO). Med Pediatr Oncol25(5):372–378

Schultz KR, Pullen DJ et al (2007) Risk- and response-based classification of childhood B-precursor acute lymphoblastic leukemia: a combined analysis of prognostic markers from the Pediatric Oncology Group (POG) and Children's Cancer Group (CCG). Blood 109(3):926–935

Schultz KR, Bowman WP et al (2009) Improved early event-free survival with imatinib in Philadelphia chromosome-positive acute lymphoblastic leukemia: a children's oncology group study. J Clin Oncol 27(31):5175–5181

Seeger K, Adams HP et al (1998) TEL-AML1 fusion transcript in relapsed childhood acute lymphoblastic leukemia. The Berlin-Frankfurt-Munster Study Group. Blood 91(5): 1716–1722

Seibel NL, Steinherz PG et al (2008) Early postinduction intensification therapy improves survival for children and adolescents with high-risk acute lymphoblastic leukemia: a report from the Children's Oncology Group. Blood 111(5): 2548–2555

Shah A, Stiller CA et al (2008) Childhood leukaemia: long-term excess mortality and the proportion "cured". Br J Cancer 99(1):219–223

Shuster JJ, Wacker P et al (1998) Prognostic significance of sex in childhood B-precursor acute lymphoblastic leukemia: a Pediatric Oncology Group Study. J Clin Oncol 16(8): 2854–2863

Silverman LB, Gelber RD et al (1999) Induction failure in acute lymphoblastic leukemia of childhood. Cancer 85(6): 1395–1404

Silverman LB, Declerck L et al (2000) Results of Dana-Farber Cancer Institute Consortium protocols for children with newly diagnosed acute lymphoblastic leukemia (1981–1995). Leukemia 14(12):2247–2256

Silverman LB, Gelber RD et al (2001) Improved outcome for children with acute lymphoblastic leukemia: results of Dana-Farber Consortium Protocol 91-01. Blood 97(5):1211–1218

Silverman LB, Stevenson KE et al (2010) Long-term results of Dana-Farber Cancer Institute ALL Consortium protocols for children with newly diagnosed acute lymphoblastic leukemia (1985–2000). Leukemia 24(2):320–334

Smith M, Arthur D et al (1996) Uniform approach to risk classification and treatment assignment for children with acute lymphoblastic leukemia. J Clin Oncol 14(1):18–24

Sramkova L, Muzikova K et al (2007) Detectable minimal residual disease before allogeneic hematopoietic stem cell transplantation predicts extremely poor prognosis in children with acute lymphoblastic leukemia. Pediatr Blood Cancer 48(1):93–100

Steinherz PG, Gaynon PS et al (1996) Cytoreduction and prognosis in acute lymphoblastic leukemia – the importance of early marrow response: report from the Childrens Cancer Group. J Clin Oncol 14(2):389–398

Steward CG, Goulden NJ et al (1994) A polymerase chain reaction study of the stability of Ig heavy-chain and T-cell receptor delta gene rearrangements between presentation and relapse of childhood B-lineage acute lymphoblastic leukemia. Blood 83(5):1355–1362

Stock W, La M et al (2008) What determines the outcomes for adolescents and young adults with acute lymphoblastic leukemia treated on cooperative group protocols? A comparison of Children's Cancer Group and Cancer and Leukemia Group B studies. Blood 112(5):1646–1654

Strefford JC, van Delft FW et al (2006) Complex genomic alterations and gene expression in acute lymphoblastic leukemia with intrachromosomal amplification of chromosome 21. Proc Natl Acad Sci USA 103(21):8167–8172

Sutcliffe MJ, Shuster JJ et al (2005) High concordance from independent studies by the Children's Cancer Group (CCG) and Pediatric Oncology Group (POG) associating favorable prognosis with combined trisomies 4, 10, and 17 in children with NCI standard-risk B-precursor acute lymphoblastic leukemia: a Children's Oncology Group (COG) initiative. Leukemia 19(5):734–740

Szczepanski T (2007) Why and how to quantify minimal residual disease in acute lymphoblastic leukemia? Leukemia 21(4): 622–626

Takahashi Y, Horibe K et al (1998) Prognostic significance of TEL/AML1 fusion transcript in childhood B-precursor acute lymphoblastic leukemia. J Pediatr Hematol Oncol 20(3): 190–195

Thall PF (2008) A review of phase 2–3 clinical trial designs. Lifetime Data Anal 14(1):37–53

Thorley-Lawson DA, Allday MJ (2008) The curious case of the tumour virus: 50 years of Burkitt's lymphoma. Nat Rev Microbiol6(12):91 3–924

Trueworthy R, Shuster J et al (1992) Ploidy of lymphoblasts is the strongest predictor of treatment outcome in B-progenitor cell acute lymphoblastic leukemia of childhood: a Pediatric Oncology Group study. J Clin Oncol 10(4):606–613

Tsurusawa M, Yumura-Yagi K et al (2007) Survival outcome after the first central nervous system relapse in children with acute lymphoblastic leukemia: a retrospective analysis of 79 patients in a joint program involving the experience of three Japanese study groups. Int J Hematol 85(1):36–40

Tubergen DG, Gilchrist GS et al (1993) Improved outcome with delayed intensification for children with acute lymphoblastic leukemia and intermediate presenting features: a Childrens Cancer Group phase III trial. J Clin Oncol 11(3):527–537

Uckun FM, Gaynon PS et al (1997a) Clinical features and treatment outcome of childhood T-lineage acute lymphoblastic leukemia according to the apparent maturational stage of T-lineage leukemic blasts: a Children's Cancer Group study. J Clin Oncol 15(6):2214–2221

Uckun FM, Sather HN et al (1997b) Clinical features and treatment outcome of children with myeloid antigen positive acute lymphoblastic leukemia: a report from the Children's Cancer Group. Blood 90(1):28–35

Uckun FM, Gaynon PS et al (1999) Paucity of leukemic progenitor cells in the bone marrow of pediatric B-lineage acute lymphoblastic leukemia patients with an isolated extramedullary first relapse. Clin Cancer Res 5(9):2415–2420

Uckun FM, Stork L et al (2000) Residual bone marrow leukemic progenitor cell burden after induction chemotherapy in pediatric patients with acute lymphoblastic leukemia. Clin Cancer Res 6(8):3123–3130

Uderzo C, Grazia Zurlo M et al (1990) Treatment of isolated testicular relapse in childhood acute lymphoblastic leukemia: an Italian multicenter study. Associazione Italiana Ematologia ed Oncologia Pediatrica. J Clin Oncol 8(4): 672–677

Uderzo C, Rondelli R et al (1995) High-dose vincristine, fractionated total-body irradiation and cyclophosphamide as conditioning regimen in allogeneic and autologous bone marrow transplantation for childhood acute lymphoblastic leukaemia in second remission: a 7-year Italian multicentre study. Br J Haematol 89(4):790–797

Valsecchi MG, Masera G (1996) A new challenge in clinical research in childhood ALL: the prospective meta-analysis strategy for intergroup collaboration. Ann Oncol 7(10): 1005–1008

van Dongen JJ, Seriu T et al (1998) Prognostic value of minimal residual disease in acute lymphoblastic leukaemia in childhood. Lancet 352(9142):1731–1738

Veerman AJ, Kamps WA et al (2009) Dexamethasone-based therapy for childhood acute lymphoblastic leukaemia: results of the prospective Dutch Childhood Oncology Group (DCOG) protocol ALL-9 (1997–2004). Lancet Oncol 10(10):957–966

von Stackelberg A, Hartmann R et al (2008) High-dose compared with intermediate-dose methotrexate in children with a first relapse of acute lymphoblastic leukemia. Blood 111(5):2573–2580

Vora A, Frost L et al (1998) Late relapsing childhood lymphoblastic leukemia. Blood 92(7):2334–2337

Weyman C, Graham-Pole J et al (1993) Use of cytosine arabinoside and total body irradiation as conditioning for allogeneic marrow transplantation in patients with acute lymphoblastic leukemia: a multicenter survey. Bone Marrow Transplant 11(1):43–50

Wheeler K, Richards S et al (1998) Comparison of bone marrow transplant and chemotherapy for relapsed childhood acute lymphoblastic leukaemia: the MRC UKALL X experience. Medical Research Council Working Party on Childhood Leukaemia. Br J Haematol 101(1):94–103

Whitehead VM, Vuchich MJ et al (1992) Accumulation of high levels of methotrexate polyglutamates in lymphoblasts from children with hyperdiploid (greater than 50 chromosomes) B-lineage acute lymphoblastic leukemia: a Pediatric Oncology Group study. Blood 80(5): 1316–1323

Whitlock JA (2006) Down syndrome and acute lymphoblastic leukaemia. Br J Haematol 135(5):595–602

Wiersma SR, Ortega J et al (1991) Clinical importance of myeloid-antigen expression in acute lymphoblastic leukemia of childhood. N Engl J Med 324(12):800–808

Winick NJ, Smith SD et al (1993) Treatment of CNS relapse in children with acute lymphoblastic leukemia: a Pediatric Oncology Group study. J Clin Oncol 11(2):271–278

Wofford MM, Smith SD et al (1992) Treatment of occult or late overt testicular relapse in children with acute lymphoblastic leukemia: a Pediatric Oncology Group study. J Clin Oncol 10(4):624–630

Yeoh EJ, Ross ME et al (2002) Classification, subtype discovery, and prediction of outcome in pediatric acute lymphoblastic leukemia by gene expression profiling. Cancer Cell 1(2):133–143

Treatmento fA cuteMyel oidL eukemia

5

Brenda Gibson, John Perentesis, Todd A. Alonzo, and Gertjan J.L. Kaspers

Contents

B.G ibson
Consultant Paediatric Haematologist, Royal Hospital forSic kC hildren, Glasgow, Scotland UnitedK ingdom
e-mail:brenda.gibson@ggc.scot.nhs.uk

J.Pe rentesis (✉)
Cincinnati Children's Hospital Medical Center, OncologyProgra m,
CHRF-2372, Mail Location 7015; 3333 Burnet Avenue, Cincinnati,O H45229, USA
e-mail:john.pe rentesis@cchmc.org

G.J.L.K aspers
Head, Pediatric Oncology/Hematology, VU University Medical CenterA msterdam, DeB oelelaan1117, NL-1081H V Amsterdam, TheN etherlands
e-mail:gjl.ka spers@vumc.nl

T.A.A lonzo
University of Southern California, Department of Preventive Medicine Children's Oncology Group, 440 E. Huntington Dr, Suite400 Arcadia,C A91006,U SA
email:ta lonzo@childrensoncologygroup.org

5.1 AcuteMyel oidL eukemia in Children: Overview

The acute myeloid leukemias (AML) represent a heterogeneous group of malignancies derived from the pluripotent hematopoietic stem cell. These leukemias

G.H. Reaman and F.O. Smith (eds.), *Childhood Leukemia*,
DOI: 10.1007/978-3-642-13781-5_5,

are generally characterized by genetic lesions that result in a combination of defects causing unregulated proliferation of cells and defects in cellular maturation (Gilliland and Griffin 2002). AML accounts for approximately 15–20% of acute leukemia in children. In contrast to acute lymphoblastic leukemia (ALL) in childhood, for which an age-related peak incidence in children is associated with unique genetics, biology, and response to therapy, AML in children is very heterogeneous with large subsets representing disease that is generally similar to that in adults. Pediatric AML does not exhibit a dramatic peak in childhood other than for infants with disease involving translocation of the mixed lineage leukemia (MLL) gene. In both children and adults, AML is a relatively drug-resistant disease. Progress in improving outcome over the past 40 years has been associated with the use of pulses of high-dose, high systemic exposure intensive chemotherapy approaches. Refinements in chemotherapy regimens and major improvements in supportive care practices have resulted in the ability to achieve complete remission (CR) in 80–90% of pediatric patients and long-term event free survival (EFS) in 40–60% of patients. While high-dose chemotherapy Consolidation with hematopoietic stem cell transplantation (HSCT) once represented the predominant treatment approach, recent studies have revealed that large subgroups of patients characterized by specific cytogenetic and molecular features do not require transplantation as initial therapy. Conversely, other molecular analyses have identified very high risk subgroups at the time of initial diagnosis that possess highly resistant stem cell disease and are likely to benefit from stem cell transplantation.

The key recent advances in treatment of AML have reflected the recent identification of molecular and cytogenetic risk groups and the development of new risk-adapted therapy approaches. In accordance with these findings, clinical and morphological classifications for AML in children and adults have now been largely replaced by cytogenetic and molecular risk classification schemes, such as that outlined by the World Health Organization (WHO) in collaboration with the Society for Hematopathology and the European Association of Haematopathology (Vardiman et al. 2009). These new classification approaches have not only effectively identified patients who benefit from different chemotherapy approaches, but they also hold promise to help identify subsets of patients who may potentially benefit from targeted molecular therapies.

5.2 AcuteMyel oidL eukemia: Diagnosis and Classification

5.2.1 Diagnosis: Clinical Manifestations

The clinical presentation of AML most commonly reflects the consequences of diffuse leukemic infiltration of the bone marrow. The suppression of normal hematopoiesis results in laboratory findings of anemia and thrombocytopenia with leukopenia or leukocytosis and variable numbers of blasts in the peripheral blood. Associated symptoms include anemia, fevers, and bleeding, with relatively frequent findings of organ infiltration including hepatosplenomegaly, skin involvement, and thromboses. Common clinical features are summarized in Table 5.1. Hepatosplenomegaly

Table 5.1 Clinical features of Down syndrome and non-Down syndrome AML. Patients enrolled onto CCG 2891(1989–1999) (FromG amise ta l. 2003)

	Down syndrome	Non-Down syndrome	*p*-value
Patients enrolled (No.)	161	947	
Mediana ge (years)	1.8	7.5	<0.001
Enlarged liver (%)	50.6	40.2	0.015
Enlarged spleen (%)	49.4	41.2	0.057
Enlarged nodes (%)	25.6	45.2	<0.001
CNSdi sease (+CSF)	4.5	20.1	<0.001
WBC			
Median/mm^3	6,800	19,900	<0.001
<20,000(%)	80	50.1	<0.001
20–100,000(%)	19.4	33.8	
>100,000(%)	0.6	16.2	
BM blast (%)			
0–5	2.6	3.5	<0.001
5–30	31.6	13.2	
>30	65.8	83.2	
Median platelets/mm^3	26,000	53,000	<0.001

is noted in approximately 15–30% of AML patients (Hurwitz et al. 1993; Lange et al. 2008). Approximately 5–10% of patients present with disease involving the central nervous system (CNS) (Hurwitz et al. 1993; Lie et al. 1996; Hann et al. 1997; Woods et al. 2001; Lie et al. 2003). Monocytic leukemias are characterized by skin involvement as well as gingival swelling. Leukemias with the t(8;21) translocation and FAB-M2 morphology can present with extramedullary mass disease in the orbits, skull and other bones, skin, lymph nodes, gastrointestinal and genitourinary tracts, and brain (Tallman et al. 1993; Krishnan et al. 1994; Pui et al. 1994).

5.2.2 Overview of Laboratory Diagnostic Studies

The development of risk-adapted therapies has provided extraordinary improvements in the outcome for children and adults with AML. The accurate diagnosis and classification of AML is essential for the selection of appropriate effective therapy regimens and interpretation of results from clinical trials. Including clinical and laboratory experts from the United States and Europe, the European LeukemiaNet recently issued expert opinion-based recommendations for the use and interpretation of laboratory studies in the diagnosis and management of AML (Dohner et al. 2010).

5.2.3 Clinical Diagnosis: Morphologic Classification Schemes

A bone marrow aspirate and biopsy should generally be a central part of the routine diagnostic evaluation of potential AML unless the patient's clinical status precludes the procedure. Marrows with extensive leukemic infiltration or fibrosis often have technically suboptimal aspirate specimens which are either unable to be successfully aspirated or diluted by peripheral blood. Bone marrow biopsies and touch imprints have particular utility in these circumstances and are often critical for establishing a diagnosis. Standard evaluation should be conducted using a May-Grunwald-Giemsa or a Wright-Giemsa stain with evaluation and counting of a minimum of 200 leukocytes on the blood smears and 500 nucleated cells on marrow smears (Dohner et al. 2010). In addition, a lumbar puncture should be conducted for the assessment of CNS involvement and presymptomatic intrathecal therapy. Some patients may have clinical complications (e.g., coagulopathy or hypotension) that necessitate a delay in evaluation of the CNS.

As discussed above, AML is characterized by dysregulated proliferation and arrest of differentiation along pathways normally found in hematopoietic development. The French–American–British (FAB) classification system was developed in 1972 and provided the primary morphologic classification of acute myeloid leukemia (Bennett et al. 1976; Bennett et al. 1985). The FAB classification system is based on cytochemical and morphologic analyses of blasts and includes ten different subtypes (Table 5.2). Use of the

Table 5.2 FAB classification of AML (From Bennett et al. 1985)

FAB	AMLs ubtype	Common cytogenetic alteration
M0	Acute myeloblastic leukemia minimally differentiated	
M1	Acutem yeloblasticl eukemia without maturation	
M2	Acutem yeloblastic leukemia with maturation	t(8;21)(q22;q22), t(6;9)
M3	Hypergranular promyelocytic leukemia Microgranular variant	t(15;17)
M4	Acutem yelomonocytic leukemia	inv(16)(p13q22), del(16q)
M4eo	Acutem yelomonocytic leukemia with bone marrow eosinophilia	inv(16),t (16;16)
	Acutem onoblastic/acute monocytic leukemia	
M5a	Poorlydi fferentiated(M5A)	del (11q), t(9;11), t(11;19)
M5b	Differentiated(M5B)	
M6a M6b	Acute erythroid leukemia (erythroid/myeloid and pure erythroleukemia)	
M7	Acutem egakaryoblastic leukemia	t(1;22)
M8	Acuteba sophilicl eukemia	

FAB classification in conjunction with early therapies helped to identify key therapeutic differences within AML subgroups and particularly between AML and ALL. Immunophenotyping has largely superseded the use of cytochemical staining techniques emphasized in the FAB classification, and the WHO classification (see below) has superseded use of the FAB because it incorporates cytogenetic and other classification features that guide application of contemporary risk-adapted therapies for AML.

5.2.4 Clinical Diagnosis: Immunophenotyping

Expression cell surface and cytoplasmic markers aid in the classification of acute myeloid leukemia by definition of precursor stage, as well as markers of granulocytic, monocytic, megakaryocytic, and erythroid pathway maturation. Lineage-specific AML cell surface antigens include CD33, CD13, CD14, CDw41 (platelet IIB/IIIA), CD15, CD11b, CD36, and glycophorin A (Dinndorf et al. 1986; Kuerbitz et al. 1992; Smith et al. 1992). B-lymphocytic antigens, CD10, and T-lymphocyte antigens are present on a proportion of AML, but have not clearly had prognostic significance. However, specific antigen expression can be associated with certain AML subgroups. The expression of glycoprotein IB, glycoprotein IIB/IIIA, and factor VIII antigen is associated with megakaryocytic leukemias (Creutzig et al. 1990). In addition, the expression of CD34 and CD15 with heterogeneous expression of CD13, along with rare expression of HLA-DR, is highly characteristic of the presence of *PML-RAR alpha* gene rearrangements (Orfao et al. 1999). Though there is no uniform consensus regarding interpretation of blast expression levels, generally when 20% or more of leukemic cells express a marker, it is considered to be positive, though select markers, including cytoplasmic CD3, myeloperoxidase, TDT, CD34, and CD117, may be considered positive at lower levels. European LeukemiaNet guidelines outline criteria for determining lineage involvement for *de novo* AML (Table 5.3), and also for the approach to diagnostic characterization of mixed phenotype acute leukemias (MPAL). Notably, sophisticated multicolor flow cytometry analyses are able to detect heterogeneity in blast cell populations that may reflect prognostic significance.

Table 5.3 European LeukemiaNet Guidelines for determining lineage involvement in leukemia (From Döhner et al. 2010)

Expression of markers for diagnoses	
Diagnosis of acute myeloid leukemia (AML)[a]	
Precursor stage	CD34, CD38, CD117, CD133, HLA-DR
Granulocytic markers	CD13, CD15, CD16, CD33, CD65, cytoplasmic myeloperoxidase (cMPO)
Monocyticm arkers	Nonspecific esterase (NSE), CD11c, CD14, CD64, lysozyme, CD4, CD11b, CD36, NG2 homologue
Megakaryocytic markers	CD41 (glycoprotein IIb/IIIa), CD61 (glycoprotein IIIa), CD42 (glycoprotein 1b)
Erythroid marker	CD235a (glycophorin A)
Diagnosis of mixed phenotype acute leukemia (MPAL)	
Myeloid lineage	MPO or evidence of monocytic differentiation (at least two of the following: NSE, CD11c, CD14, CD64, lysozyme)
B-lineage	CD19 (strong) with at least one of the following: CD79a, cCD22, CD10, or CD19 (weak) with at least two of the following: CD79a, cCD22, CD10

[a]For the diagnosis of AML, the table provides a list of selected markers rather than a mandatory marker panel

Requirements for assigning more than one lineage to a single blast population adopted from the WHO classification.[3] Note that the requirement for assigning myeloid lineage in MPAL is more stringent than for establishing a diagnosis of AML. Note also that MPAL can be diagnosed if there are separate populations of lymphoid and myeloid blasts

Most cases with 11q23 abnormalities express the NG2 homologue (encoded by *CSPG4*) reacting with the monoclonal antibody 7.1

5.2.5 Clinical Diagnosis: Conventional and Molecular Cytogenetics

Conventional cytogenetics is a requisite investigation for the contemporary classification and therapeutic planning for AML. In parallel, fluorescence in situ hybridization (FISH) is a powerful tool to complement cytogenetics in the detection of key gene rearrangements. The identification of recurrent balanced translocations and inversions and other recurrent genetic abnormalities is the core element for the current WHO Classification system for acute myeloid leukemia. In general, a minimum of 20 metaphase cells is required to exclude abnormal karyotypes. Notably, cytogenetic analyses from peripheral blood specimens may also be helpful when the marrow specimen is inadequate or unable to be obtained. Alternatively, if the patient's clinical condition permits, a repeat bone marrow aspirate for cytogenetic and molecular analyses should be obtained if the initial sample was inadequate.

5.2.6 Clinical Diagnosis: Molecular Genetic Analyses

Molecular genetic analyses of blasts for key leukemogenic mutations are a critical aspect of contemporary AML diagnosis (see below). Screening for somatically acquired mutations in the *FLT3*, *NPM1*, and *CEBPA* genes has potential prognostic and therapeutic implications, and is strongly encouraged by the European LeukemiaNet expert panel in the initial evaluation of patients with AML. In this regard, the recently updated WHO Classification includes AML with mutations in *NPM1* or *CEBPA* as new provisional entities. Current investigations are analyzing the role of somatic mutations in the *MLL, NRAS, WT1, KIT, RUNX1, TET2, TP53* and *IDH1* genes, and gene expression alteration in *ERG, MN1, EVI1*, and *BAALC*.

5.2.7 World Health Organization Classification System

The presence of recurring cytogenetic abnormalities is the most prognostically significant finding in acute myeloid leukemias. The World Health Organization (WHO) Classification of the Myeloid Neoplasms incorporated diagnostic cytogenetic information into an AML classification system in 2002 (Vardiman et al. 2002). Two key differences between the WHO and previous FAB classification included: (1) a lower blast threshold (from 30% to 20% blasts in the blood or marrow) for the diagnosis of AML, and (2) the primary use of recurring clonal cytogenetic abnormalities as a basis for categorizing AML cases with unique clinical and biological subgroups. Notably, the presence of key clonal recurring cytogenetic abnormalities including t(8;21)(q22;q22), inv(16)(p13;q22), or t(16;16)(p13;q22), and t(15;17)(q22;q12) were considered to be AML regardless of blast percentage. In 2008, the WHO classification of myeloid neoplasms in acute leukemia was revised in the light of new genetic and biological information (Table 5.4) (Vardiman et al. 2009). This diagnostic classification system included new provisional entities, including

Table 5.4 The 2008 revision of the World Health Organization (WHO) classification of myeloid neoplasms. (From Vardiman eta l. 2009)

Acute myeloid leukemia and related neoplasms
Acute myeloid leukemia with recurrent genetic abnormalities
AML with t(8;21)(q22;q22); *RUNX1-RUNX1T1*
AML with inv(16)(p13.1q22) or t(16;16)(p13.1;q22); *CBFB-MYH11*
APL with t(15;17)(q22;q12); *PML-RARA*
AML with t(9;11)(p22;q23); *MLLT3-MLL*
AML with t(6;9)(p23;q34); *DEK-NUP214*
AML with inv(3)(q21q26.2) or t(3;3)(q21;q26.2); *RPN1-EVI1*
AML (megakaryoblastic) with t(1;22)(p13;q13); *RBM15-MKL1*
Provisional entity: AML with mutated NPM1
Provisional entity: AML with mutated CEBPA
Acute myeloid leukemia with myelodysplasia-related changes
Therapy-related myeloid neoplasms
Acute myeloid leukemia, not otherwise specified
AML with minimal differentiation
AML without maturation
AML with maturation
Acute myelomonocytic leukemia
Acute monoblastic/monocytic leukemia
Acute erythroid leukemia
Pure erythroid leukemia
Erythroleukemia,e rythroid/myeloid
Acute megakaryoblastic leukemia
Acute basophilic leukemia
Acute panmyelosis with myelofibrosis
Myeloids arcoma
Myeloid proliferations related to Down syndrome
Transient abnormal myelopoiesis
Myeloid leukemia associated with Down syndrome
Blastic plasmacytoid dendritic cell neoplasm
Acute leukemias of ambiguous lineage
Acute undifferentiated leukemia
Mixed phenotype acute leukemia with t(9;22)(q34;q11.2); *BCR-ABL1*
Mixed phenotype acute leukemia with t(v;11q23); *MLLr* earranged
Mixed phenotype acute leukemia, B-myeloid, NOS
Mixed phenotype acute leukemia, T-myeloid, NOS
Provisional entity: natural killer(NK) cell lymphoblastic leukemia/lymphoma

AML with mutated *NPM1* and AML with mutated *CEBPA*. The 2008 revision of the WHO also included a new category incorporating transient abnormal myelopoiesis as well as MDS and AML that is Down syndrome-related. MDS and AML related to Down syndrome are biologically identical and thus are considered together as "Myeloid leukemia associated with Down syndrome" (see Table 5.4). Incorporation of the WHO revised classification into contemporary treatment regimens permits sophisticated correlation and identification of activity of conventional chemotherapy and novel targeted agents in defined biological subgroups.

5.3 Overviewo fR isk-Stratified Approaches

5.3.1 Overview

The main relevance of prognostic factors in AML is to predict the likelihood of achieving remission and/or the risk of relapse, and thereby to identify patients for whom conventional combination chemotherapy may be inadequate and HSCT in first complete remission (CR1) is indicated. It is suggested that allogeneic HSCT may only benefit patients with a relapse risk of greater than 35% (Cornelissen et al. 2007). While this figure must be dependent on the anticipated procedure-related mortality, patients at low risk of relapse are unlikely to benefit. Predictors of relapse can include pre- or post-treatment characteristics, but will always be protocol dependent. The major pre-treatment characteristics are cytogenetics, age, white blood cell (WBC) count, secondary leukemia and *FLT3*/ITD, *NPM1* and *CEBPA* mutations. The major post-treatment prognostic predictor is the speed and depth of response to treatment, which may be assessed morphologically, immunologically or molecularly. While cytogenetics and response to treatment are the main prognostic factors that drive risk stratification in current treatment protocols, risk group stratification is becoming increasingly complicated. There are many potential future predictors of outcome, but most have not undergone sufficient assessment or validation in children, or indeed adults, to be reliably used to stratify treatment at present. Amongst these are *WT1, MLL–PTD, RUNX1, TET2, IDH1* and *TP53* mutations; *BAALC, ERG, EVI1* and *MN1* gene expression levels, microRNA and gene expression profiles and resistance proteins. While new markers identify targets for novel therapies, combinations of markers may interact to further refine risk group stratification.

5.3.2 Age and White Blood Cell Count at Presentation

Age and WBC count at presentation are recognized as prognostically important but are not routinely used to risk-stratify treatment in children. Increasing age in both children and adults is independently associated with a worse outcome, with children greater than 10 years doing less well than younger children (Razzouk et al. 2006). Within the pediatric age range, a higher white cell count at presentation is associated with a lower CR rate, higher relapse risk, and worse overall survival.

5.3.3 FAB Classification

As outlined above, cytogenetics and use of the WHO classification have largely replaced FAB classification. Notably, the previously reported inferior outcome for acute megakaryoblastic leukemia (AMKL) (M7) in non-Down syndrome (non-DS) AML (Athale et al. 2001; Dastugue et al. 2002; Barnard et al. 2007) and the benefit for HSCT (Athale et al. 2001; Garderet et al. 2005) have recently been challenged (Reinhardt et al. 2005). The Berlin-Frankfurt-Münster (BFM) study group reported an improved outcome for non-DS patients with megakaryoblastic leukemia, treated on recent more intensive trials and found no benefit for HSCT (Reinhardt et al. 2005). Non-DS M7 AML may be a heterogenous disease, and a better outcome has recently been reported for non-DS M7 AML in association with t(1;22) compared to non-DS M7 AML without this karyotypic abnormality (Dastugue et al. 2002).

5.3.4 Acute Promyelocytic Leukemia and Down Syndrome AML

Both acute promyelocytic leukemia (APL) and DS AML are recognized as distinct subtypes of AML in the 2008 WHO classification, with unique features and favorable outcomes when treated on appropriate protocols that recognize their individual chemotherapy sensitivities, including anthracyclines and differentiating agents in APL and high-dose cytarabine in DS AML. Each of the entities is discussed in detail below.

5.3.5 Cytogenetic Abnormalities

The leukemia blast karyotype is a key determinant of outcome in AML (Grimwade et al. 1998; Raimondi et al. 1999). However, the usefulness of the diagnostic karyotype is limited by conflicting data on the prognostic significance of some primary cytogenetic aberrations, including t(8,21), various translocations involving the *MLL* locus on 11q23, and the definition of a complex karyotype. The main limiting factor is that approximately 25% of children (Harrison et al. 2010, Raimondi et al. 1999) (and approximately 40% of adults) with AML have a normal karyotype (cytogenetically normal: CN AML), although molecularly heterogenous disease. Based on multivariable analysis of results from the Medical Research Council (MRC) AML 10 trial, a cytogenetically based risk group classification (Grimwade et al. 1998; Wheatley et al. 1999) has been validated and adopted by a number of cooperative groups. Differences in outcome among these groups are probably explained by small numbers or by differences in the treatment delivered. This cytogenetic risk score classifies good-risk patients as those with t(15,17), t(8,21), inv(16)/t(16,16); poor risk as those with those with −5, del(5q), monosomy 7 (−7), abnormalities of 3q and a complex karyotype (5 or >); and all others as intermediate-risk (Grimwade et al. 1998; Wheatley et al. 1999). The successor trial MRC AML 12 adopted this cytogenetic risk score and reported children (455 with a cytogenetic result) aged less than 15 years old and with favorable (excluding APL), normal, and other intermediate and adverse karyotypes to have a 10-year overall survival (OS) of 64%, 60% and 43%, respectively. Based on 5,876 adult cases (age 16–59 years), the original MRC cytogenetic classification has been further refined to include rarer abnormalities not previously considered separately. The only karyotypes associated with a favorable outcome remain t(15,17), t(8,21), and inv(16)/t(16,16), but the adverse cytogenetic risk group has been extended to include abn(3q) (excluding t(3;5)), inv(3)/t(3,3), −5/del(5q)/add(5q), −7/add(7q), t(6,11), t(10,11), t(9,22), −17/abn(17p) with other changes and complex (>3 unrelated abnormalities) (Grimwade et al. 2009a). Analysis of 729 children treated on MRC AML 10 and 12 reported the interesting new findings that 12p abnormalities and t(6;9) (p23;q34) predict a poor outcome. Additionally, abnormalities of 3q and complex karyotypes do not appear to have the same degree of adverse outcome as reported for adults (Harrison et al. 2010). Recently an adverse prognosis has been reported in an adult study for autosomal monosomy in conjunction with at least one other autosomal monosomy or structural abnormality (Breems et al. 2008).

The core binding factor leukemias (CBF), t(8;21) and inv(16), are heterogeneous (Marcucci et al. 2005; Appelbaum et al. 2006) and adult studies suggest that the OS may be significantly inferior for patients with t(8;21) compared to those with inv(16)/t(16,16), predominantly because of a lower salvage rate after relapse (Marcucci et al. 2005). Outcome is treatment dependent and patients with CBF leukemias may do particularly well when they receive high-dose cytarabine (Bloomfield et al. 1998; Byrd et al. 1999; Appelbaum et al. 2006). Gemtuzumab ozogamicin (Mylotarg), a recombinant humanized anti-CD33 monoclonal antibody linked to the potent anti-tumor intercalating agent, calicheamicin, has recently been reported to preferentially benefit CBF leukemias (Burnett et al. 2006).

Rearrangements of the *MLL* gene are the most common abnormalities in children with AML, although the frequency varies among studies (10–20%) (Rubnitz et al. 2002; Harrison 2010). A recent retrospective international study of 756 children with 11q23-rearranged AML demonstrated significant heterogeneity within this abnormality (Balgobind et al. 2009). This study failed to confirm the previously reported favorable prognosis for t(9;11)(p22;q23) (Rubnitz et al. 2002), but multivariate analysis identified t(1;11)(q21;q23) to be an independent predictor of a favorable outcome while t(10;11)(p12;q23), t(10;11)(p11.2;q23) and t(6;11)(q27;q23) independently predicted an inferior outcome (Balgobind et al. 2009). Patients in this study were treated on different chemotherapy protocols, which may in part explain differences in outcome between groups across *MLL*-rearranged subtypes.

An international collaborative study (Hasle et al. 2007) of 258 children with AML and −7 (n = 172) or del(7q) (n = 86), both with or without other cytogenetic changes, demonstrated heterogeneity within chromosome 7 abnormalities. Monosomy 7 was associated with a lower CR rate (61% vs 89%, $p < 0.001$) and inferior 5-year survival (30% vs 51%, $p < 0.01$)

compared to patients with del(7q). Additional cytogenetic abnormalities impacted outcome. Favorable risk cytogenetics were strongly associated with del(7q) and retained their favorable 5-year survival compared to del(7q) without additional favorable cytogenetics (75% vs 46%, $p = 0.03$). By contrast, patients with −7 and adverse cytogenetics (inv(3), −5/del(5q), or +21) had a dismal outcome (5-year OS 5%), which was not improved by HSCT.

5.3.6 Molecular Mutations

Patients with AML and a cytogenetically normal karyotype (CN-AML) are classified within the intermediate-risk group, despite having molecularly heterogenous AML. CN–AML and those within cytogenetically defined subgroups may be further risk group stratified by prognostically significant molecular characteristics. Class I mutations (*RAS, FLT 3, c-KIT*) activate signaling pathways, increasing proliferation and inhibiting apoptosis while class II mutations (*CEBPA, MLL*-PTD and probably *NPM1*) affect transcriptional processes leading to impaired differentiation. In addition to these mutations regulating signaling and transcription pathways, the expression levels of a number of genes (*BAALC, ERG, EVI1*) may have independent prognostic significance in AML. Many patients with AML harbor more than one mutation, and these mutations interact with each other and do not influence outcome in isolation. The complexity of these interactions is illustrated in Fig. 5.1.

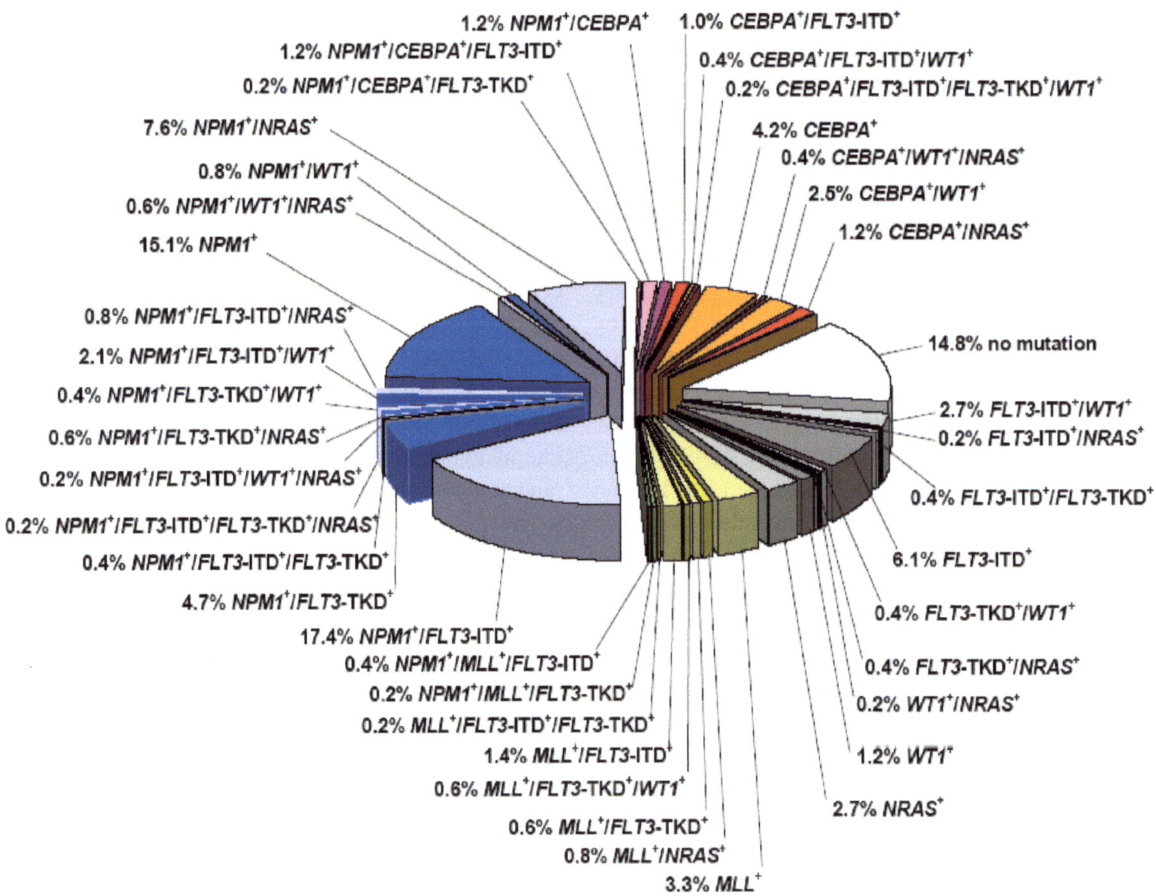

Fig. 5.1 Pie chart illustrating the molecular heterogeneity of cytogenetically normal AML based on mutations in the *NPM1*, *CEBPA*, *MLL*, *FLT3* (internal tandem duplication [ITD] and tyrosine kinase domain [TKD] mutations at codons D835 and I836], *NRAS*, and *WT1* genes. The bluish colors denote *NPM1* mutated subsets, the orange/red colors *CEBPA* mutated subsets, and the yellow/green colors *MLL* mutated subsets; the grey colors depict subsets without hypothetical class II mutations, and the white sector shows the subset without any mutation in the above mentioned genes. Data are derived from mutational analysis of 485 younger adult patients with cytogenetically normal AML from AMLSG (From Dohner et al. 2010. On behalf of the European LeukemiaNet. Blood 2009; Oct 30. Epub)

5.3.6.1 Fms-LikeT yrosine Kinase 3: *FLT3*Mut ations

FLT3 is a tyrosine kinase receptor and therefore of both prognostic and clinical importance because of the potential for targeted therapy with FLT 3 inhibitors. Normal FLT3 signaling is involved in regulation of hematopoietic stem cell development. Internal mutations in the FLT3 receptor have been identified in a large subset of AML. The FLT3 receptor is a tyrosine kinase expressed on the surface of hematopoietic stem cells. Two predominant types of mutations are found in *FLT3* and AML, including internal tandem duplications (ITD) mapping to the juxta-membrane portion of the receptor, and activating mutations in the kinase domain. Mutations in either the ITD or kinase domain both constitutively activate FLT3 signaling. There is an age-associated increase in incidence of AML with *FLT3*/ITD mutations, accounting for 12–17% of AML in children and adolescents, and rising to approximately 34% of adults (Meshinchi et al. 2001; Zwaan et al. 2003a; Meshinchi et al. 2006). Approximately 10% of patients exhibit leukemic blasts with point mutations primarily in the kinase domain at aspartic acid 835 or isoleucine 836. Tandem duplications of *FLT3* (*FLT3*/ITD) are associated with an increased relapse risk and inferior survival in both children and adults (Abu-Duhier et al. 2000; Kottaridis et al. 2001; Meshinchi et al. 2001; Zwaan et al. 2003a; Meshinchi et al. 2006) and in two pediatric studies were the strongest predictor of relapse in multivariate analysis (Meshinchi et al. 2001; Zwaan et al. 2003a). The prognostic impact of *FLT3*/ITD for both adults and children is reported to be dependent on the mutant/wild type allele ratio (Whitman et al. 2001; Thiede et al. 2002; Zwaan et al. 2003; Gale et al. 2008) with high *FLT3*/ITD allelic ratios, indicative of homozygous mutations generated by acquired uniparental disomy, being associated with a particularly poor outcome. The impact of *FLT 3* mutations in the tyrosine kinase domain (*FLT3*–TKD) are variably reported (Mead et al. 2007). Current clinical trials are examining the potential activity of small molecule FLT3 receptor tyrosine kinase inhibitors in conjunction with chemotherapy, and it is yet unclear if these regimens can obviate the role for allogeneic HSCT in these patients.

5.3.6.2 Nucleophosmin: *NPM1* Mutations

The nucleophosmin member 1 (*NPM1*) gene product functions as a likely chaperone molecule between the nucleus and cytoplasm. *NPM1* functions in ribosome biogenesis, maintenance and duplication of centrosomes, and regulation of genomic stability proteins including p53 and ARF. Mutation of the *NPM1* gene is the most common mutation in adult AML (up to 35%) and is present in about 50% of adult CN-AML (Falini et al. 2005; Thiede et al. 2006), but only occurs in about 8% of children (Cazzaniga et al. 2005; Brown et al. 2007) and then mainly in older children. *NPM1* mutation alters the distribution of the protein and causes predominantly a cytoplasmic localization. *NPM1* mutations interact prognostically with *FLT3* ITD and in the absence of *FLT3*/ITD predict a better response to Induction chemotherapy and a favorable overall survival (Dohner et al. 2005; Falini et al. 2005; Thiede et al. 2006; Brown et al. 2007; Mrozek et al. 2007; Schlenk et al. 2008), but this advantage is lost in the presence of *FLT3*/ITD mutation. *NPM1* mutations commonly co-exist with *FLT3*/ITD in CN-AML. Recently it has been suggested that patients with wild type *FLT3*/ ITD, and *NPM1* mutations have a favorable disease, should be classified as good-risk, and should not be candidates for HSCT in CR1 (Schlenk et al. 2008).

5.3.6.3 CCAAT/EnhancerB inding Protein Alpha: *CEBPA* Mutations

CEBPA mutations are found in about 5–15% of adult AML (Schlenk et al. 2008; Wouters et al. 2009) and generally in association with CN-AML. *CEBPA* mutations carry a favorable outcome when biallelic mutations are present (Wouters et al. 2009).

There is growing evidence that *NPM1* and *CEPBA* mutations are class II mutations and primary genetic lesions which impair hematopoietic differentiation.

5.3.6.4 *c-kit*Mut ations

c-kit mutations are detected in 3–11% of pediatric AML cases (Meshinchi et al. 2003; Goemans et al. 2005) and are strongly associated with CBF leukemias. *c-kit* co don 816 mutations negatively impact adult patients with t(8;21) compared to those with wild type *c-kit* (Boissel et al. 2006; Paschka et al. 2006; Schnittger et al. 2006) and may explain the heterogeneity in outcome reported for this cytogenetic group. *c-kit* mutations are likely to have the same negative impact in patients with inv(16), although the evidence is less clear (Boissel et al. 2006; Paschka et al. 2006). The prognostic significance of *c-kit* mutations in children with CBF leukemia is limited by study size. A BFM study found a c-kit mutation in 31% of 16 patients with t(8,21) AML and reported no difference in outcome between patients with and without the mutation (Goemans et al. 2005), while the Japanese Childhood AML Cooperative Study Group reported an inferior outcome for 8 of 46 (17%) patients with t(8;21) and *c-kit* mutation (Shimada et al. 2006). c-kit is a tyrosine kinase receptor and offers the potential for treatment with a tyrosine kinase inhibitor.

5.3.6.5 *MLL-PTD* Mutations

Partial tandem duplication of the mixed lineage leukemia *MLL* (*MLL*-PTD) gene occurs in 5–10% of adult CN-AML and is reported to be associated with an inferior disease free survival (DFS) (Schlenk et al. 2008). *MLL*-PTD mutations usually coexist with *FLT3*/ITD (30–40%) (Schlenk et al. 2008) and the impact of co-existence on outcome is not clear. *MLL*-PTD AML may respond to demethylating agents.

5.3.6.6 BAALC (Brain and Acute Leukemia Cytoplasmic Protein), EVI1 and ERG

High level *BAALC* (brain and acute leukemia cytoplasmic protein), EVI1 and ERG expression independently negatively impact on outcome in CN AML. *BAALC* interacts with *FLT3*/ITD, and the presence of both abnormalities confers a particularly poor prognosis (Balduse ta l. 2006).

5.3.6.7 *RAS* and *WT1* Mutations

RAS mutations are more common in CBF inv(16) leukemias, but their prognostic impact is unclear. They may be targets for farnesyl transferase inhibitors. WT1 gene mutations have been reported to confer an adverse prognosis (Paschka et al. 2008), although not consistently.

Molecular genetic aberrations and their clinical implications have recently been the subject of extensive review (Schlenk and Dohner 2009; Scholl et al. 2009).

5.3.7 Correlation of Prognostic Signature with Clinical Data

The inter-relationship between mutations/cytogenetics/clinical features and outcome is complex. The LeukemiaNet international expert panel has recently recommended a new standardized reporting for the correlation of cytogenetics and molecular genetic data with clinical data in AML (Table 5.5) (Dohner et al. 2010). This re-defines favorable risk disease as CBF leukemias, CN-AML *NPM1* mutated/*FLT3* negative and CN-AML *CEPBA* mutated. These patients are at low risk of relapse and unlikely to benefit from HSCT. CN-AML continues to be classified as intermediate-risk but is subclassified by *NPM1* and *FLT3*/ITD status. A risk classification schema for the management of adult AML patients with normal karyotypes that incorporates the status of *FLT3, NPM1, BAALC, MLL*-PTD and *CEBPA* has been proposed (Mrozek et al. 2007). Others propose the incorporation of additional poor prognostic factors including *WT1, ERG* and *EVI-1* expression (Scholl et al. 2009). However, many of these molecular markers have not been extensively studied in children. Before new prognostic markers can be used to direct treatment in children with AML, their prognostic/predictive value must be validated in children and their benefit tested within the setting of a clinical trial.

5.3.8 Initial Response to Treatment

Current risk group stratification based on cytogenetic and molecular characterization fails to identify all patients at risk of relapse within cytogenetic/molecularly characterized risk groups. Early response to therapy is a powerful predictor of outcome, but morphological assessment is relatively crude. The EFS at 5 years for children treated on BFM 83 and 87 was inferior for those with more than 5% blasts on day 15 compared to those with less than 5% blasts (56% vs 27%, $p = 0.0001$ and 61% vs 40%, $p = 0.001$) (Creutzig et al. 1999). In the MRC trial, patients are

Table 5.5 European LeukemiaNet Guidelines for standardized reporting for correlation of cytogenetic and molecular data in AML with clinical data. Dohner et al, 2010. Standardized reporting for correlation of cytogenetic and molecular genetic data in AML with clinical data[a] (From Dohner et al. 2010. On behalf of the European LeukemiaNet. Blood 2009; Oct 30. Epub)

Geneticgroup	Subsets
Favorable	t(8;21)(q22;q22); *RUNX1-RUNX1T1*
	inv(16)(p13.1q22) or t(16;16)(p13.1; q22); *CBFB-MYH11*
	Mutated *NPM1* without *FLT3*-ITD (normal karyotype)
	Mutated *CEBPA* (normal karyotype)
Intermediate-I	Mutated *NPM1* and *FLT3*-ITD (normal karyotype)
	Wild type *NPM1* and *FLT3*-ITD (normal karyotype)
	Wild type *NPM1* without *FLT3*-ITD (normal karyotype)
Intermediate-II	t(9;11)(p22;q23); *MLLT3-MLL*
	Cytogenetic abnormalities not classified as favorable or adverse
Adverse	inv(3)(q21q26.2)or t (3;3)(q21;q26.2); *RPN1-EVI1*
	t(6;9)(p23;q34); *DEK-NUP214*
	t(v;11)(v;q23); *MLLr* earranged
	−5 or del(5q); −7; abnl(17p); complex karyotype[b]

[a]Frequencies, response rates and outcome measures should be reported by genetic group, and, if sufficient numbers are available, by specific subsets indicated; excluding cases of acute promyelocytic leukemia

[b]Three or more chromosome abnormalities in the absence of one of the WHO designated recurring translocations or inversions, i.e., t(15;17), t(8;21), inv(16) or t(16;16), t(9;11), t(v;11)(v;q23), t(6;9), inv(3)/t(3;3); indicate how many complex karyotype cases have involvement of chromosome arms 5q, 7q, and 17p

assigned to one of three risk groups based on diagnostic cytogenetics and morphological response after course 1 of chemotherapy. Based on 467 patients treated on AML 12, patients in CR (<5% blasts), partial response (PR) (5–15% blasts) and residual disease (RD) (>15% blasts) after course 1 had 10 year survival rates of 76%, 55% and 25% and relapse rates of 31%, 42%, and N/A (because patients with refractory disease were unevaluable for relapse), respectively. When combined with cytogenetics, the OS at 10 years for good, standard and poor-risk patients was 83%, 70% and 39%, respectively with relapse risks of 21%, 36% and 53% respectively. While discriminatory, the MRC risk score unfortunately only identifies about 20% of the patients destined to relapse, and about 60% of relapses come from standard-risk and 20% from good-risk groups.

5.3.9 Minimal Residual Disease Assays and Markers

Minimal residual disease (MRD) assays provide sensitive measurements for detecting low levels of leukemic cells that cannot be detected morphologically (Campana 2003). MRD can be assessed molecularly by real-time quantitative polymerase chain reaction (RT PCR) of leukemic specific targets (gene fusions, e.g., AML-*ETO*; gene mutations, e.g., *NPM1*; and overexpressed genes, e.g., *WT1*) or immunologically by multiparameter flow cytometry identifying an aberrant leukemia-associated immunophenotype (LAIP). The advantage of the latter is that an immunophenotypic AML "signature" can be identified in more than 90% of AML cases, while the molecular heterogeneity of AML is quite extensive and not easily amenable to the development of specific RT PCR assays in most cases. The sensitivity of flow cytometry is at least a log less than RT PCR assays at 10^3–10^4 compared to RT PCR 10^3–10^6, but the sensitivity of flow cytometry may improve with six to eight color laser technology. The usefulness of MRD measurement includes early assessment of response to therapy to improve risk stratification and to guide Consolidation therapy, and subsequent monitoring to detect impending relapse and guide pre-emptive therapy.

The kinetics of AML1-*ETO* and *CBFb-MYH11* fusion transcripts monitored by RT PCR, including the transcript level at diagnosis, extent of reduction after Induction chemotherapy and any increase in transcript level after attainment of CR, are thought to be predictive of outcome. *WT1* transcripts and *NPM1* may be useful for monitoring levels of disease and predicting outcome.

5.3.10 Minimal Residual Disease Studies

There is a paucity of prospective studies of the usefulness of MRD measurement. Pediatric studies on the predictive value of minimal residual disease have reported conflicting results. Sixteen percent of 252 children who achieved morphological remission on the Children's Cancer Group (CCG)-2961 trial had detectable MRD (defined as greater than 0.5% blasts with an aberrant phenotype) after Induction therapy, and on multivariate analysis this was shown to be the most powerful independent prognostic factor associated with poor outcome (Sievers et al. 2003). A study from St. Jude Children's Research Hospital mirrored these findings and reported a 2 year OS of 33% for patients with detectable MRD at the end of Induction therapy compared to 72% for MRD-negative patients ($p = 0.022$) (Coustan-Smith et al. 2003). However, multivariate analysis of 150 children treated on AML BFM 98 study failed to show additional predictive value for MRD measured by flow cytometry compared to other routinely employed risk factors (Langebrake et al. 2006).

5.3.11 Summary

Current approaches to risk group stratification are unrefined and confined to cytogenetics, response to treatment (assessed by different criteria and methods), and limited molecular characterization for some groups. While able to discriminate risk groups, these parameters fail to identify the majority of patients who will relapse. AML is a very heterogenous disease both within CN-AML and within cytogenetically-defined risk groups, and molecular characterization may further refine these risk groups and identify targets for therapy. Systematic evaluation of MRD assessment in conjunction with refined molecular/cytogenetic risk groups will further inform post-remission therapy. While it is important to establish a hierarchy of prognostic factors, their prognostic and predictive value needs to be validated in children with AML and not assumed from adult data, and must be tested within the context of a specific protocol or treatment. At present, refinement of risk stratification helps define the need for HSCT, but increasingly molecular characterization will offer the potential of novel targeted therapy. New prognostic/predictive indicators can only be adopted into clinical practice when properly validated for childhood as well as adult AML.

5.4 Treatmento fPedi atricA ML

5.4.1 Overview

Clinical trials for the therapy of pediatric acute myeloid leukemia have exhibited steady improvement in initial remission induction rates, disease-free survival, event-free survival, and overall survival over the past 5 decades. The key advances in treatment have been as a result of identification and optimization of the dosing and schedule of active drugs (predominantly cytarabine and anthracyclines, as outlined above), the identification of key subgroups of patients benefiting from specialized treatment approaches, and improved supportive care for infections and other complications. Contemporary treatment approaches incorporate four to six courses of intensive chemotherapy, and most groups do not use lower dose "Maintenance" therapy approaches. The use of myeloablative high-dose chemotherapy Consolidation with allogeneic HSCT in CR1 is controversial and under investigation. It is generally not employed in patients with favorable-risk and standard-risk cytogenetics, but it is used in some groups for patients with intermediate-risk disease and a matched related donor. Alternative donor HSCT approaches are generally reserved for patients with high risk cytogenetic or molecular features, or with resistant or residual disease.

Refinements in the treatment of pediatric AML have largely resulted from the development of biologic and risk-stratified approaches to therapy. Early cancer clinical trials in the 1950s and 1960s for children with leukemia included patients with ALL and AML on the same regimen, and identified early major differences in the response of these two diseases to different chemotherapy drugs. Subsequent clinical trials treated patients with AML on separate regimens and identified unique distinguishing biology and response in patients with APL, Down syndrome leukemia, and various cytogenetic subgroups of AML. These observations were paralleled by the development of active risk-adapted regimens for different subgroups, and have in turn provided a foundation for improvements in the overall cure rate of pediatric AML as the overall survival was increased in each subgroup.

5.4.2 Childhood AML Therapy: MRC Experience

Intensive anthracycline- and cytosine-based chemotherapy combined with advances in supportive care have resulted in a dramatic improvement in the survival of children with AML treated on United Kingdom (UK) MRC trials. For the past 2 decades, children (n = 1,053) and adults have been treated on the same or very similar protocols within three trials: MRC AML 10 (1988–1995), MRC AML 12 (1995–2002) and MRC AML 15 (2002–2008).

5.4.2.1 InductionT herapy

Primary areas of investigation in MRC studies have been the comparison of anthracyclines/anthracenediones and testing the benefit of the addition of active agents to the intensive cytarabine and anthracycline core regimen. Successive MRC trials have failed to show any significant superiority in CR rate or OS for any of the four tested intensive Induction regimens. MRC AML 10 tested the comparative benefits of thioguanine with etoposide by comparing DAT (ara-C, daunorubicin, thioguanine) with ADE (ara-C, daunorubicin, etoposide). There was no significant difference in CR rate (DAT 90% vs ADE 93%, p = 0.3, odds ratio (OR) = 1.58 (0.68,3.51)), EFS (DAT 48% vs ADE 45%, p = 0.5, hazard ratio(HR) = 0.89 (0.65,1.23)) or OS (DAT 57% vs ADE 51%, p = 0.3, HR = 0.83 (0.59,1.17)), but there was a non-significant excess of deaths in CR in the ADE arm (8% vs 15% p = 0.09) (Stevens et al. 1998). There was no evidence that children with monocytic involvement (FAB type M4 or M5) in particular benefited from an etoposide-containing regimen (p = 0.9). ADE was brought forward into MRC AML 12 in the belief that the observed lack of advantage for ADE was in part due to the excess of deaths in CR, which could be negated by improved supportive care.

MRC AML 12 found mitoxantrone (MAE) and daunorubicin (ADE) to be of equal efficacy in Induction when combined with similar doses of cytarabine and etoposide. No significant difference was noted in CR rates (ADE 92% vs MAE 90%, p = 0.3, OR = 1.30(0.70, 2.4)) or deaths in CR or EFS. Induction deaths were not significantly higher for MAE (MAE 6% vs ADE 3%, p = 0.2) (Gibson et al. 2005). There was a possibility that MAE was superior for both DFS (p = 0.03, HR = 0.72 (0.54, 0.96)) and relapse risk (RR) (p = 0.05, HR = 0.73 (0.54, 1.00)), but OS was not significantly different (ADE 61% vs MAE 65%, p = 0.2, HR = 0.84 (0.63, 1.12)).

AML 15 compared ADE with FLAG-Ida (fludarabine, cytarabine, granulocyte colony stimulating factor (G-CSF), and idarubicin) with or without the addition of gemtuzumab ozogamicin at 3 mg/m^2 in Induction. The data are unpublished and premature. However, in adult patients there appears to be no difference in the CR rate; an apparent reduction in the relapse risk in the FLAG–Ida arm fails to translate into an improvement in OS because of an increase in deaths in CR for patients receiving FLAG-Ida (Burnett et al. 2009). Gemtuzumab ozogamicin at 3 mg/m^2 combined with Induction chemotherapy appears to benefit predominantly favorable prognosis CBF leukemias.

In summary, no intensive regimen has resulted in a superior CR rate or OS, and any advantage of one regimen over another in terms of a reduction in relapse rate has been balanced by an increase in deaths in Induction or CR.

5.4.2.2 Consolidation/Post-remissionT herapy

MRC AML 12 failed to show an advantage for an additional course of post-remission chemotherapy (four versus five courses of treatment in total) in any risk group of patients already receiving intensive treatment, irrespective of whether HSCT was included, although confidence intervals were wide: deaths in CR, four courses 2% versus five courses 1% (p = 0.6, HR = 0.64 (0.11, 3.7)); relapse risk, four courses 37% versus five courses 37% (p = 1.0, HR = 1.01 (0.67, 1.50)); OS, four courses 74% versus five courses 74% (p = 1.0, HR = 1.01 (0.63,1.62)). This suggests that the benefit from conventional post-remission chemotherapy may reach a plateau and that further improvement may only be achieved by alternative or targeted therapies.

MRC AML trials have traditionally delivered high cumulative doses of anthracycline and anthracenedione therapy (AML 10: 550 mg/m^2; AML 12: 300–610 mg/m^2 calculated on a conversion factor, with mitoxantrone 1 mg/m^2 being equivalent to daunorubicin 5 mg/m^2). AML 15 tested whether the cumulative dose could be safely reduced and high-dose (HD) Ara-C substituted without loss of anti-leukemic efficacy by comparing two blocks of anthracycline-driven MRC Consolidation with two blocks of HD Ara-C

(550 vs 300 mg/m^2). Follow-up is too short to answer this important question, but preliminary data suggest that there may be no detriment to substituting anthracyclines with HD Ara-C in Consolidation (Burnett et al. 2009). Gemtuzumab ozogamicin 3 mg/m^2 has also been tested in combination with chemotherapy in Consolidation. Preliminary results suggest no benefit.

5.4.2.3 Hematopoietic Stem Cell Transplantation

The combined data from MRC AML 10 and AML 12 suggest no survival benefit for allogeneic HSCT in first CR for any risk group in children. While allogeneic HSCT was associated with a significant reduction in RR for good and standard risk patients ($p = 0.02$), but not for poor risk patients, this did not translate into a survival advantage for any risk group ($p = 0.3$) because the reduced relapse risk was counterbalanced by an increase in procedure-related deaths ($p = 0.001$). It may be argued that these data date from 1998 to 2002 and that more recent improvements in transplant-related mortality may allow an advantage for HSCT to emerge. However, the MRC data failed to show a reduction in relapse risk for poor-risk patients, without which a survival advantage cannot be achieved.

In MRC AML 10, autologous HSCT in CR 1 reduced relapse ($p = 0.03$) and improved DFS ($p = 0.02$) but did not significantly improve long-term survival ($p = 0.2$), not because of a counter-balancing effect on procedural mortality, which was low (3%), but because of an inferior survival after relapse (autologous HSCT 7% vs Stop 27%, $p = 0.05$).

MRC studies thus suggest that the role of allogeneic HSCT is limited in first CR and that the ceiling of benefit for chemotherapy may have been reached. Successor studies aim to improve outcome by molecular characterization and the use of targeted therapies in appropriate risk groups or biological subtypes. This will include exploring dosing and scheduling in children. The measurement of MRD by flow cytometry and molecular markers where possible may improve risk stratification and offer the potential for treatment intensification, which may include targeted therapies or stem cell transplantation. Alternatively, MRD may suggest that allogeneic HSCT can appropriately be restricted, reducing the risk of associated procedure-related mortality and morbidity.

5.4.3 Childhood AML Therapy: European and Japanese Experience

Although international collaboration is being expanded, there are still several groups in the mainland of Europe (exclusive of the UK) that conduct independent clinical trials for newly diagnosed pediatric AML. From North to South these groups include the NOPHO (Nordic Society for Pediatric Hematology/Oncology), the BFM group, LAME (the French *Leucémies Aiguës Myéloblastiques de l'Enfant* group), and AIEOP (the Italian *Associazione Italiana Ematologia Oncologia Pediatrica).* Worldwide, other than the Children's Oncology Group (COG) and the St. Jude consortium, Japan also has an active clinical trial for newly diagnosed AML. In other countries, investigators either participate in COG or MRC protocols, or have adapted protocols from the BFM-AML group. The Netherlands and Belgium are currently establishing a pilot study, with collaboration with the NOPHO/Hong Kong consortium in the near future. The main aspects of pediatric AML trials conducted by these groups will be discussed, focusing on Induction therapy, Consolidation therapy, the use of HSCT, and Maintenance therapy. In many cases, the hypotheses tested in the European and Japanese studies are linked to results from investigations by other pediatric and adult groups.

5.4.3.1 Induction Therapy

The backbone of treatment to induce remission is two courses of intensive chemotherapy. The classic combination is 3 days of daunorubicin and 7 days of cytarabine. Usually, a third drug like etoposide or thioguanine is added to this combination. NOPHO applies even four drugs, by adding both etoposide and thioguanine to cytarabine and idarubicin. More than 80% of patients achieve CR with a 3- (or 4-) drug regimen and adequate supportive care (Yates et al. 1973; Weinstein et al. 1980; Yates et al. 1982; Pui 1995; Hann et al. 1997; Lowenberg et al. 1999; Pui et al. 2004; Zwaan and Kaspers 2004; Kaspers and Ravindranath 2005).

Various strategies have been used to increase CR rates and subsequent survival: substitution of daunorubicin with idarubicin or mitoxantrone, increased dosages of cytarabine, and reduced intervals between the initial cycles of chemotherapy (intensive timing) (Ravindranath et al. 1996; Woods et al. 1996; Creutzig et al. 2001b; O'Brien et al. 2002; Perel et al. 2002; Pui et al. 2004). The general conclusion that can be drawn from these studies is that a more intensive remission induction chemotherapy improves the quality of remission, which favorably affects the likelihood of long-term disease-free survival. In particular, a comparison of different schedules in relation to the rate of resistant disease and prognosis suggested that a cumulative anthracycline dose of less than 100 mg/m^2 after one Induction course is associated with a worse outcome (Kaspers and Ravindranath 2005). However, it has to be kept in mind that death due to toxicity during Induction can offset the expected benefits of some of these strategies. In that perspective, it is interesting that rates for CR and overall survival are by and large similar for MRC, COG and NOPHO trials, when MRC does not advocate intensively timed Induction chemo therapy but COG and NOPHO protocols have incorporated this strategy.

The addition of a third drug, thioguanine or etoposide, to intensive anthracycline and cytarabine Induction platforms has been tested by the BFM and the MRC groups, similar to approaches in the North American Pediatric Oncology Group (POG) and CCG groups. Yet, the contribution of a third drug in Induction chemotherapy is not clear (Creutzig et al. 1987; Steuber et al. 1990; Ravindranath et al. 1991; Woods et al. 1996; Stevens et al. 1998; Kaspers and Ravindranath 2005). A direct comparison of etoposide and thioguanine, added to cytarabine and daunorubicin, did not reveal statistically significant differences in remission rates, event-free or overall survival (Stevens et al. 1998). The MRC group has recently tested the efficacy and safety of gemtuzumab ozogamicin as a third drug in Induction therapy in adult AML (Kell et al. 2003; Zwaan and Kaspers 2004). The clinical efficacy of this drug in childhood relapsed and refractory AML does suggest its usefulness, and so do the preliminary results from the MRC trial, which, however, mainly concerned adults (Zwaan et al. 2003a, b). It remains to be proven if long-term outcome will improve with the implementation of this drug in up-front combination chemotherapy in children, but COG is studying that (Zwaan et al. 2003a, b).

Currently, the best approach is not apparent, and neither CR rates nor EFS or OS rates differ significantly among study groups. A goal for current European studies it to enhance drug exposure to potentially result in high quality complete remissions with as low as possible amounts of MRD. Underlying this goal is a strategy to combine drugs with different mechanisms of action, as long as toxicity remains manageable.

Supporting strategies to intensify high-dose cytarabine in pediatric AML Induction therapy are adult studies demonstrating superior post-remission outcome with this approach (Weick et al. 1996; Bishop et al. 1998). The recently complete MRC AML15 study may also provide information on this issue, including information on pediatric AML, since it did include a comparison of standard low-dose and high-dose cytarabine at Induction and enrolled children as well. Unfortunately, other differences in that Induction therapy may confound the results.

5.4.3.2 Consolidation/Post-remissionT herapy

Most groups now use multiple courses of intensive chemotherapy as Consolidation therapy. Higher-risk patients theoretically may benefit from an additional (fifth) course of chemotherapy, but such a risk-group-adapted therapy has not been proven to be better in pediatric AML. Including two courses for Induction, the minimum total number is four as applied by the MRC group, and results of that group are among the best in the world. Study MRC AML 12 did not show a statistically significant benefit for five total courses as compared to four, but that question continued to be studied in AML15, and pediatric results have not yet been reported. The NOPHO is studying the role of two doses of gemtuzumab ozogamicin as post-Consolidation therapy, which one might consider to be an extra course of chemotherapy. The Japanese group reported that they could safely reduce the number of Consolidation courses from eight to six to five for standard-risk patients and to six for higher-risk patients (Tomizawa et al. 2007; Tsukimoto et al. 2009). One may conclude that between four and six courses of chemotherapy in total are usually needed in pediatric AML (i.e., two to four courses of Consolidation therapy). Depending on the content of each course, the number of courses will also influence the cumulative dose of anthracyclines or related drugs. It seems fair to state that the optimal cumulative dose is unknown but that cumulative doses at Induction should not be less than 100 mg/m^2. On the other hand, it is quite clear that cumulative doses of anthracyclines above 300 mg/m^2 are associated with increasing risk of cardiotoxicity (Kremer et al. 2001).

Most studies have included several courses of intermediate- or high-dose cytarabine in their post-remission chemotherapy strategy. The POG 8821 study, for example, used a six-dose schedule, and the CCG and Nordic trials used an eight-dose timed split-dose schedule (Capizzi and Powell 1987; Capizzi et al. 1988; Lie et al. 1996, 2003; Woods et al. 1996; Kaspers and Ravindranath 2005). Some studies combined cytarabine with non-cross-resistant agents. The MRC group, for instance, included the combination of amsacrine, cytarabine, and etoposide (MACE), mitoxantrone/cytarabine, and cytarabine/L-asparaginase (CLASP). The LAME 89/91 and the BFM93 trials combined high-dose cytarabine with mitoxantrone (HAM) (Wells et al. 1994a; Michel et al. 1996; Dahl et al. 2000; Creutzig et al. 2001a, b).

A majority of European groups now assume that high-dose cytarabine should be incorporated into treatment, although there are no recent randomized studies in pediatric AML that have been reported yet to support that policy. An older study by the POG with overall inferior outcome as compared to currently achievable survival rates did not reveal an improvement with higher doses of cytarabine as part of Consolidation therapy (Ravindranath et al. 1991). However, in adult AML it has been shown that high-dose cytarabine at Induction results in better post-remission outcome (Weick et al. 1996; Bishop et al. 1998). High-dose cytarabine as post-remission strategy especially benefited adults with core binding factor or normal karyotype AML (Bloomfield et al. 1998). Knowing that pediatric AML on average includes better risk and thus more chemosensitive patients than adult AML, it seems reasonable to extrapolate these data and to indeed incorporate higher doses of cytarabine in pediatric protocols. Moreover, preclinical studies have shown that AML cells from some patients are more resistant to cytarabine and that in some patients the active transport of cytarabine into the AML cells is limited, a mechanism which is necessary in the case of lower concentrations of cytarabine (Zwaan and Kaspers 2004; Hubeek et al. 2005). Both mechanisms of resistance theoretically can be overcome by higher-dose cytarabine. However, these studies do not identify the optimal moment to use high-dose cytarabine.

5.4.3.3 Hematopoietic Stem Cell Transplantation

All European groups except the BFM-AML group still recommend allogeneic HSCT for certain risk groups. In contrast, all groups except AIEOP do not recommend autologous HSCT (stem cell reinfusion would be more appropriate) anymore, in view of several randomized studies that did not demonstrate a benefit from autologous stem cell reinfusion as compared to chemotherapy (Ravindranath et al. 1996; Woods et al. 2001). Several studies seem in favor of using allogeneic HSCT in AML subgroups. However, with contemporary chemotherapy that results in DFS of more than 50%, the number of studies with appropriate data-analysis (correcting at least for time-to-transplant) that demonstrated significantly improved OS with allogeneic HSCT is actually limited to two studies reported by the LAME (Perel et al. 2005) and the European Organisation for Research and Treatment of Cancer (EORTC) (Entz-Werle et al. 2005) groups. These two studies both have a major confounder, which was the Maintenance therapy given only to patients that were not transplanted. Such Maintenance therapy was proven to have an adverse effect on outcome (Perel et al. 2005; Wells et al. 1994a, b), thus negatively influencing the outcome for chemotherapy-only patients but not for patients that were treated with allogeneic HSCT. The BFM-AML group reported no improved OS with allogeneic HSCT in either studies –87 and –93 analyzed together or in study AML-BFM-98 (Langebrake et al. 2005; Creutzig et al. 2006; Reinhardt et al. 2006). Therefore, since 2006 this group has not advocated the use of allogeneic HSCT in AML patients in CR1, while other groups still recommend allogeneic HSCT for higher-risk patients.

With respect to the risk of relapse, some European studies have suggested that allogeneic HSCT may offer a benefit. The ability to retrieve relapsed AML appears to be lower after allogeneic HSCT in CR1 than that of relapsed AML after chemotherapy only. This observation was reported by the NOPHO group (Lie et al. 2005; Abrahamsson et al. 2007). The relative benefit of allogeneic HSCT in CR1 depends on the effectiveness and type of chemotherapy. For patients in CR1, allogeneic HSCT does not consistently exhibit a significant benefit in overall survival, it is costly, and it is associated with increased late effects. These issues must be carefully balanced against the reported reduced risk of relapse with allogeneic HSCT.

5.4.3.4 Maintenance Therapy

Maintenance chemotherapy has been used in the past by several groups and is still being used by the

BFM-AML group. However, most of the other studies in pediatric AML have not observed improved outcome with Maintenance therapy in the context of contemporary high-dose intensive Induction and Consolidation treatment regimens. Two studies have suggested an adverse impact on OS, apparently because of reduced salvagability after relapse (Wells et al. 1994a, b; Perel et al. 2005). Therefore, the use of Maintenance chemotherapy in pediatric AML cannot be generally recommended. An obvious exception is the treatment of APL, in which Maintenance treatment with all-trans retinoic acid (ATRA) and low-dose chemotherapy including methotrexate and mercaptopurine does provide benefit for patients (Testi et al. 2005). It cannot be excluded that specific subgroups benefit from Maintenance chemotherapy, as well as the possibility that other types of Maintenance therapy are beneficial. For example, the NOPHO is studying the value of two doses of gemtuzumab ozogamicin as post-Consolidation therapy in a randomized study, while LAME is studying the effect of interleukin-2.

5.4.4 Childhood AML Therapy: North American Experience

5.4.4.1 InductionT herapy

Based upon single agent efficacy data in adults and children, early studies demonstrated significant activity for combinations of cytarabine and anthracyclines in pediatric AML remission induction. The CCG 241 study (1975–1979) incorporated cytarabine and daunomycin into multi-agent (5-azacytidine, vincristine and prednisone) therapy for newly diagnosed pediatric AML (Chard et al. 1978). The POG 8101 (1981–1986) study provided pivotal data demonstrating that a "3+7+7 DAT" combination regimen of 3 days of 45 mg/m^2/day daunorubicin, 7 days of continuous infusional low-dose (100 mg/m^2/day) cytarabine and 7 days of 6-thioguanine provided superior outcomes for children with AML when compared to a vincristine, dexamethasone and cytarabine regimen originally designed for ALL (Steuber et al. 1991). In this study, the DAT regimen was established as a standard element in pediatric AML therapy with a complete remission rate of 82% (compared to 61% for the other regimen; $p = 0.02$). Combinations of anthracycline and cytarabine remain at the core of AML Induction regimens, and the CCG 213 study (1986–1989) did not demonstrate benefit with the addition of etoposide, thioguanine and dexamethasone (Wells et al. 1994a, b). Similarly, the CCG-2961 study (1996–1999) was not able to identify a benefit for the addition of idarubicin and fludarabine into an intensive timing remission Induction/Consolidation regimen (Lange et al. 2008).

Building upon observations suggesting benefit with enhanced cytarabine exposure, the POG 8498 study (1984–1988) tested the effect of dose intensification during the second Induction course using additional high-dose 3 g/m^2 q12 h × 6 doses of cytarabine followed by L-asparaginase. POG 8498 showed a trend toward higher EFS (34% vs 29%) and DFS (42% vs 34%) when compared with standard dose DAT platforms (Ravindranath et al. 1991). The POG 9421 study (1995–1999) examined incorporation of high-dose cytarabine as part of the first Induction course and the use of the multidrug resistance modulator cyclosporine. However, intensifying Induction with high-dose DAT and the addition of cyclosporine to Consolidation chemotherapy did not prolong the duration of remission or improve overall survival (Becton et al. 2006). In combination with data from MRC and BFM studies (see below), these observations have helped define effective cytarabine schedules (e.g., 7–10 days of dosing) or high-dose cytarabine exposure in second Induction course, which remains at the core of contemporary Induction regimens.

Although these early improvements in Induction regimens resulted in significant increases in remission induction rates, the impact on EFS and OS was less dramatic. These observations suggested that a small population of residual blasts or leukemia stem cells survives after Induction and later cause relapse. The mechanisms of drug-resistance in AML are complex and multifactorial; however, preclinical data suggest that the leukemic stem cells found in the endosteal region of the marrow are cell cycle quiescent and escape the effects of chemotherapy (Mikkola et al. 2010; Saito et al. 2010). Cytarabine generally requires active cell division to exert full anti-leukemic activity, and in mouse models, it appears that the use of hematopoietic growth factors mobilizes quiescent AML stem cells and stimulates proliferation, rendering them sensitive to the cytotoxic effects of cytarabine (Saito et al. 2010). Exposure to chemotherapy has been hypothesized to exert similar effects on cell cycle quiescent leukemia stem cells (i.e., recruitment into the cell cycle and increased sensitivity to subsequent chemotherapy, particularly S phase active agents such as cytarabine [Vaughan et al. 1984]). In the pivotal CCG 2891 study (1989–1995), Woods and colleagues tested the hypothesis that intensively timed sequential chemotherapy with concurrent G-CSF in Induction would overcome resistance based upon leukemia cell cycle quiescence. CCG 2891 employed a core regimen of a 4-day cycle of dexamethasone, cytarabine, 6-thioguanine, etoposide and daunorubicin (DCTER) and enrolled 589 patients. The randomized study design compared two Induction approaches involving either (1) "intensive timing" in which the second cycle of chemotherapy was administered after a 6-day rest regardless of low or dropping blood counts, or (2) "standard timing" in which the second cycle of chemotherapy was administered at least 14 days or more from the beginning of the first cycle, depending on bone marrow status and recovery of hematopoiesis (Woods et al. 1996). This study demonstrated that intensively timed Induction therapy resulted in a marked improvement in actuarial EFS at 3 years of 42% versus 27% for patients on the standard timing arm ($p = 0.0005$). In addition, patients receiving intensively timed Induction therapy had superior DFS results at 3 years from the end of Induction, 55% versus 37% for standard timing patients ($p = 0.0002$).

5.4.4.2 Consolidation/Post-remission Therapy

In post-Induction therapy, cycles of non-cross resistant drugs or high-dose exposure to limited agents (e.g., high-dose cytarabine) are administered to eradicate minimal residual disease and increase potential for cure. The biological heterogeneity of AML poses difficulties in identifying straightforward conclusions regarding the intensity or number of post-remission cycles required for high cure rates. The CCG 213P study (1983–1985) investigated the utility and timing of cycles of very high-dose cytarabine in therapy intensification in children with AML who had achieved remission after Induction therapy. This study suggested that Maintenance therapy did not appear to benefit patients who had received intensively timed high-dose cytarabine Intensification therapy, though patients receiving non-aggressive Intensification appeared to have improved outcome with Maintenance therapy. Patients who received two intensive courses of high-dose cytarabine and asparaginase administered at 7-day intervals exhibited a significant increase in DFS when compared with patients receiving the same therapy administered at 28-day intervals (OS 58% vs 41% from the end of Induction, $p < 0.04$) (Woods et al. 1990). Using a randomized design, the successor CCG 213 study (1986–1989) also demonstrated no benefit for Maintenance therapy after intensive cytarabine exposure in post-Induction/Consolidation therapy (Wells et al. 1994a, b). The hypothesis that immunologic interventions could initiate an anti-leukemia response in the post-remission setting and eliminate MRD was tested in the CCG-2961 study. However, the use of interleukin-2 in Maintenance did not show a benefit in reduction of relapse (Lange et al. 2008).

5.4.4.3 Hematopoietic Stem Cell Transplantation

The majority of randomized North American studies incorporating analysis by intent to treat have consistently indicated efficacy for myeloablative high-dose chemotherapy Consolidation therapy with stem cell rescue from an HLA-matched family donor (MFD) (Dahl et al. 1990; Feig et al. 1993; Nesbit et al. 1994; Dinndorf and Bunin 1995; Appelbaum 1997; Cassileth et al. 1998). However, improvements in contemporary chemotherapy approaches have suggested that large subsets of children with AML in CR1 have equivalent outcomes without need for stem cell transplantation and its increased risk for immediate and long-term toxicities (Creutzig and Reinhardt 2002). The relatively modest number of children receiving HSCT as part of AML therapy has created difficulties in the clear identification of risk factors and patients who will likely benefit from the procedure.

A recent large multi-cooperative group analysis of factors impacting transplant outcome by Horan and colleagues combined data on 1,373 patients drawn from four cooperative group Phase III trials: POG 8821, CCG 2891, CCG 2961, and MRC 10 (Ravindranath et al. 1996; Stevens et al. 1998; Woods et al. 2001; Horan et al. 2008; Lange et al. 2008). The data set aggregated from the four studies compared 893 patients assigned to chemotherapy alone with 480 assigned to allogeneic HSCT. The majority of the 480 allogeneic HSCT patients included in this intent-to-treat analysis were from the CCG studies ($n = 334$), with additional patients from the POG ($n = 70$) and MRC ($n = 76$) studies.

This analysis confirmed that OS and DFS were superior for the HSCT group. At 8 years, estimates for OS for HSCT and chemotherapy groups were 63% and 57% (HR = 0.77; $p < 0.007$), respectively, and DFS estimates were 56% and 46% (HR = 0.70; $p < 0.001$), respectively. The incidence of relapse was much lower in patients assigned to HSCT compared with those receiving chemotherapy alone (28% vs 47% (HR = 0.51; $p < 0.001$)). However, patients assigned to HSCT had a higher rate of treatment-related mortality compared to those receiving chemotherapy alone (16% vs 7% (HR = 1.97; $p < 0.001$)).

The Horan study also stratified into favorable-, intermediate-, and poor-risk disease groups. Favorable-risk disease included patients with inv(16) and t(8;21). Patients with monosomy 7, monosomy 5, deletions of 5q, or more than 15% blasts after the first course of chemotherapy were considered to have high-risk disease. All other patients were classified as having intermediate-risk disease. In addition, a small number of MRC patients with abnormalities of 3q and patients with five or more cytogenetic abnormalities were classified in the high-risk disease subgroup. The risk-stratified analysis showed a significant benefit in OS for patients who received a transplant in CR1. No significant overall benefit was seen in patients with favorable-risk or poor-risk disease. In the intermediate-risk group, the estimated OS at 8 years was 51% for the patients assigned to chemotherapy alone, compared with 62% for the patients assigned to HSCT (HR = 0.69; $p <0 .006$). As might be expected, the predominant beneficial effect of allogeneic transplant was in reducing the risk of relapse in this subgroup of patients; the relapse incidence was 26% in the HSCT patients compared to 54% in the chemotherapy-only patients (HR = 0.42; $p < 0.001$). In the favorable-risk disease group, a higher incidence of HSCT treatment-related mortality negated the beneficial effects of a modest reduction in the risk for relapse.

5.4.4.4 CurrentA reaso fI nvestigation

A review of five consecutive St. Jude AML studies clearly identified challenges for future directions in pediatric AML therapy. Similar to other studies, incremental progress was achieved by identification of active agents and refinements in dose and schedule of administration. However, these investigations elegantly identified limits in the benefit of increasing the intensity of chemotherapy (AML-87) or prolongation of post-remission therapy by adding sequential myeloablative (AML-80) or nonmyeloablative (AML- 83) chemotherapy cycles. A powerful result of these studies is that risk-adapted and risk-targeted approaches will be necessary to further improve approaches for pediatric AML(R ibeiroe ta l. 2005).

The COG-AAML0531 study for children with *de novo* AML is investigating whether the addition of gemtuzumab ozogamicin to contemporary therapy will improve EFS over treatment with chemotherapy alone. AAML0531 introduces gemtuzumab ozogamicin into the first Induction course and in Intensification/ Consolidation courses of a regimen similar to MRC AML12 therapy with five courses of total treatment. In AAML0531, high-risk patients receive a HSCT if a matched family donor (MFD) or alternative donor is available. Intermediate-risk patients receive a HSCT only if a MFD is available. High and intermediate-risk patients without an appropriate HSCT donor and all low-risk patients receive additional chemotherapy with or without gemtuzumab ozogamicin consistent with the initial randomization.

5.4.4.5 Summary

Recent MRC, European, Japanese and North American studies parallel findings in other groups and observe overall survival rates of 45–65% for most children with AML with contemporary treatment approaches. These studies have highlighted key elements of current approaches for AML therapy, including: (a) the benefit of dose-intensification early in therapy, including timed-sequential therapy approaches, (b) the need for intensive Consolidation therapy, and (c) the key importance of stratification approaches with cytogenetics/molecular genetics and response to therapy as the key predictors of response. In parallel, these approaches to risk stratification have assisted in the development of tailored less intensive but highly effective therapies for patients with Down syndrome, and the use of tailored therapy for patients with acute promyelocytic leukemia (see below). In addition, these investigations are generating improved methods to predict which patients will benefit from allogeneic transplantation in CR1, and a rationale for the use of novel targeted therapy approaches for patients with an extremely poor prognosis, including *FLT3* high allelic ratio internal tandem duplications, and patients with leukemic cells with high-risk cytogenetic features.

5.4.5 Extramedullary and CNS-Directed Therapy

The incidence of AML cells in the cerebrospinal fluid at initial diagnosis differs between studies, but is in the range of 5–30%. Moreover, CNS involvement at relapse is observed in up to 10% of patients, while it was up to 20% in studies in which CNS prophylaxis had not been used (Pui et al. 2004; Kaspers et al. 2008). Therefore, there are good arguments to administer prophylaxis for CNS relapse. Most groups successfully use intrathecal (IT) chemotherapy given four to six times, in that their CNS relapse rates or cumulative incidence of any relapse do not seem to be higher than that reported by the BFM-AML group, which still uses cranial irradiation. The latter policy is based on a single randomized study, and cranial irradiation provided a statistically significant benefit only when randomized and non-randomized patients were pooled. Of interest, the main benefit concerned less bone marrow relapses (Creutzig et al. 1993). Indeed, a St. Jude study showed that even CNS leukemia at initial diagnosis can be successfully treated with chemotherapy only (Abbott et al. 2003). In conclusion, prophylaxis of CNS relapse is indicated using intrathecal chemotherapy, either single-agent cytarabine or cytarabine in combination with prednisolone and methotrexate, while there seems to be no place for prophylactic cranial irradiation in the setting of current intensive chemotherapy. There are no data in favor of either single-agent cytarabine or triple chemotherapy.

Children with CNS disease at diagnosis have traditionally received intrathecal chemotherapy and cranial radiotherapy. The CCG-2891 study showed that children with CNS leukemia at diagnosis can be cured without the use of cranial irradiation (Woods et al. 1996)

5.4.6 Hematopoietic Stem Cell Transplantation

Acute myeloid leukemia can be modulated by the graft versus leukemia effect of allogeneic HSCT, and both allogeneic and autologous HSCT have been reported to result in a reduction in relapse risk in children (Stevens et al. 1998; Burnett et al. 2002). However, the benefit of allogeneic transplantation in CR1 is increasingly challenged by a DFS approximating 60% reported for chemotherapy alone. Importantly, many studies fail to translate a reduction in relapse rate into an improvement in OS (Stevens et al. 1998; Burnett et al. 2002; Reinhardt et al. 2006), and others only demonstrate improved survival for specific risk groups (Horan et al. 2008). Differences in reported benefits for allogeneic transplantation may be explained by differences in the intensity, effectiveness and outcome of chemotherapy (Creutzig et al. 2001a, b; Woods et al. 2001; Entz-Werle et al. 2005; Perel et al. 2005) and the method of data analysis (Wheatley 2002).

The lack of benefit found by the MRC for allogeneic HSCT in CR1 mirrors the experience of the BFM, who also find no improvement in OS, but is contradictory to experience reported by the COG (Woods et al. 2001). Cytogenetics and speed of response to treatment, variably assessed, are powerful indicators of outcome in AML and may be used to target the most intensive therapy to those patents at greatest risk of relapse. However, it is questionable whether allogeneic transplantation benefits even high-risk patients. The MRC report a reduction in the relapse risk for good and standard-risk patients only undergoing allogeneic HSCT (although no benefit in OS), but not for poor-risk disease patients. Without a reduction in relapse rate, allogeneic HSCT cannot benefit patients. Interestingly, the COG reported a significant improvement in DFS and OS for HLA-matched related HSCT in intermediate-risk patients only but not good or poor risk patients (Horan et al. 2008).

Allogeneic HSCT only provides an advantage for patients with AML if the observed reduction in relapse rate is sufficiently great to absorb the procedure-related mortality and the relapse rate post-transplant. Supporters of allogeneic HSCT in CR1 cite the high procedure-related mortality associated with older trials used to assess the benefit of allogeneic HSCT as unfavorably compromising HSCT outcomes, and argue that improvements in current HSCT practice might alter the balance in favor of HSCT. There is some evidence that current low procedure-related mortality, improved transplant procedures and more effective rescue of patients relapsing after transplant have improved HSCT outcomes (Vicente et al. 2007), but it remains to be proven that these will be significantly superior to chemotherapy, which is also improving over time.

While allogeneic HSCT can reduce the relapse risk, at least in some risk groups, benefit in overall survival will require a low procedure-related mortality and innovative modulation of the graft versus leukemia effect. Some studies report both a reduction in relapse rate and an improvement in DFS. The failure to translate this benefit into an improvement in OS is due to improved salvage, particularly in those patients not previously transplanted, and raises the question of whether HSCT might best be reserved for second CR. HSCT may benefit some risk groups more than others, and improved risk group stratification by molecular characterization and MRD may help identify these groups. Most studies have involved the use of matched family or volunteer donors and the benefit of haplo-identical donors and cord stem cells remains untested. The role of any improvement in outcome must also be balanced against the long-term morbidity in children and must be cost effective.

5.5 TreatmentSt rategies in Special Subgroups

5.5.1 Acute Promyelocytic Leukemia

5.5.1.1 Introduction

APL is a rare subtype of AML characterized by distinctive morphology (M3 or M3v), the t(15;17) translocation, a potentially fatal coagulopathy at presentation and unique sensitivity to anthracycline-containing chemotherapy and differentiating agents all-trans retinoic acid (ATRA) and arsenic trioxide (ATO). Children with APL treated with a combination of anthracycline-based chemotherapy and ATRA are reported to have a 5 year OS of 87–90%, DFS of 78–82% and EFS of 71–77% (Mann et al. 2001; de Botton et al. 2004; Ortega et al. 2005; Testi et al. 2005). Unpublished data suggest that outcomes have improved further with the increased use of ATRA, adherence to supportive care guidelines and the use of ATO in salvage therapy. However, these results are achieved with high cumulative anthracycline doses, with their potential for cardiotoxicity in children. ATRA and ATO target the APL-associated PML-RARα oncoprotein and offer a low or non-chemotherapy treatment approach, which is being increasingly tested in adult patients with this subtype of AML. While theoretically an attractive approach in children, there is limited information on the use of ATO in frontline therapy or on its long-term toxicity in this age group.

5.5.1.2 DemographicFeat ures

APL represents approximately 4–8% of pediatric AML (Gregory and Feusner 2003), although a higher incidence has been reported in children of Hispanic and Mediterranean origin, which may suggest a genetic predisposition and/or exposure to environmental factor(s) in the causation. The median age at presentation has been reported between 12 and 15 years (de Botton et al. 2004; Ortega et al. 2005; Testi et al. 2005). It rarely occurs in the first year of life. Therapy-related APL has been described in children previously exposed to epipodophyllotoxins (Detourmignies et al. 1992).

5.5.1.3 Pathogenesis

APL is characterized by rearrangements of the retinoic acid receptor-α (*RARα*) gene on chromosome 17q21. Several partner genes have been identified, but *RARα* is most commonly (>95 %) fused to the *PML* gene (Promyelocytic Leukemia) on chromosome 15q22 as a result of the t(15,17) (q22;q21) translocation. Identification of the underlying molecular lesion is critical to the management of APL because it determines sensitivity to molecularly targeted therapies, ATRA and ATO. *PML- RARα* / t(15,17) (q22;q21) APL is retinoid sensitive as are the rarer APL subtypes seen in children of *NPM1-RARα* / t(5;17) (q35;q21) and *NuMA-RARα* / t(11;17) (q13;q21) translocations. The sensitivity of these rarer subtypes to ATO has not been established. *PLZF-RARα* / t(11;17) (q23;q21) and *STAT5b-RARα* / t(17;17) (q11.2;q21) fusions are retinoid resistant (Grimwade et al. 2000; Mistry et al. 2003). *PRKAR1A – RARα* / t (17;17) (q21;q24) and *FIP1L1-RARα*/ t(4;17) (q12;q21) have also been described. Secondary chromosomal changes can be present at diagnosis.

RARα is a ligand-dependent transcriptional activator that binds to specific DNA sequences found in the promoters of retinoic acid-responsive genes, which are involved in normal myeloid development. In APL, the chimeric oncoprotein (i.e., *PML-RAR α*, *NPM1-RARα*, etc.) is capable of DNA binding but prevents transcription of *RARα* target genes and myeloid cell differentiation. ATRA functions by binding to the *RARα* moiety of *PML-RARα*, causing degradation of the fusion protein and thus allowing terminal differentiation of leukemiapro myelocytes.

5.5.1.4 Diagnosis

APL is classified amongst Acute Myeloid Leukemia with recurrent genetic abnormalities by the WHO classification and as AML M3 or M3v by the FAB classification.

Morphology: The morphology of APL is distinctive, with two subtypes, M3 and M3v (15–30%): classical hypergranular M3 is characterized by hypergranular promyelocytes containing heavy azurophilic granules, bundles of Auer rods (faggots) and bilobed nuclei, while hypogranular/microgranular variant M3v blasts have an apparent paucity of granules.

Immunophenotype: APL has a distinctive, but not diagnostic, phenotype of positivity for CD33, CD13, CD9 and rare expression of HLA-DR, CD34, CD7, CD11b and CD14. Antigen profiles (CD2 and CD56) may correlate with inferior outcome.

Immunohistochemistry: Immunohistochemical staining provides a rapid diagnosis. The characteristic (microspeckled) nuclear PML distribution pattern of APL blasts is readily distinguishable from the wild-type (speckled) PML nuclear staining of normal cells.

Cytogenetics: Conventional cytogenetics or fluorescence hybridization identifies both common and rarer *RARα* translocations. Conventional cytogenetics fail to identify the t(15;17) in approximately 10% of patients with *PML-RARα* transcripts, including those in whom the fusion gene is generated through insertion events in which chromosomes 15 and 17 may appear normal (Grimwade et al. 2000).

Molecular analysis: Molecular diagnosis by reverse transcriptase polymerase chain reaction is important in cases lacking the t(15;17) by conventional cytogenetics and is critical to determine *PML-RARα* isoform type (bcr1,bcr2,bcr3) to allow subsequent, MRD monitoring of fusion gene transcripts by RT PCR assays (Sanze ta l. 2009).

5.5.1.5 PrognosticFac tors

The strongest predictors of outcome are the persistence of MRD, followed by the WBC count (Grimwade and Lo Coco 2002; Grimwade et al. 2009a, b). M3v morphology, *FLT 3* length mutations, *bcr3 PML* breakpoint and higher *PML-RARα* expression ratios have been variably reported to be of independent significance but are interrelated and often found in association with a high WBC count.

MRD: Persistence or recurrence of *PML–RARα* or *RARα-PML* fusion transcripts detected by RT PCR monitoring is the strongest independent predictor of clinical relapse and exceeds WBC count ($p = 0.02$) on multivariatea nalysis(Grimwadee ta l. 2009a, b).

WBC count at diagnosis: The presenting WBC count strongly predicts for the risk of Induction death and relapse (Burnett et al. 1999; Ortega et al. 2005; Testi et al. 2005). The Sanz criteria classify APL into low, intermediate and high-risk based on the WBC count and platelet count (Sanz et al. 2000), but other groups have not found the platelet count to be of predictive value. In the GIMEMA-AIEOP study, the EFS was 83% versus 59% at 10 years ($p = 0.7$) for standard (WBC < 10×10^9/L) versus high-risk (WBC =/> 10×10^9/L) children respectively, and all Induction deaths (4%) were in high-risk patients (Testi et al. 2005). Children more commonly have high-risk disease (35–40%) than adults (de Botton et al. 2004; Ortega et al. 2005;T estie ta l. 2005).

5.5.1.6 Treatment

Children with APL treated on anthracycline- and ATRA-based protocols have a CR rate of around 95% and an EFS of 70–80% (Mann et al. 2001; de Botton et al. 2004; Ortega et al. 2005; Testi et al. 2005). These results have been achieved with heterogeneous regimens. APL is uniquely sensitive to anthracyclines, ATRA and ATO. This presents two challenges for the treatment of children with APL. Firstly, high cumulative anthracycline doses (650 mg/m^2) (Testi et al. 2005) are commonly used, and reducing cardiotoxicity should be a priority in a leukemia with such a favorable outcome. Secondly, there are limited data on the use of ATO in frontline therapy in children both in terms of efficacy and late toxicities.

Induction therapy: The diagnosis of APL is generally considered an oncologic emergency, and therapy with ATRA should be initiated immediately in patients presenting with leukemia and characteristic peripheral blood blast morphology, particularly with evidence of coagulopathy. Patients are at high risk for early fulminant fatal coagulopathy, with deaths predominantly occurring within the first 5–10 days of presentation, and amenable to treatment with ATRA. The simultaneous use of ATRA and anthracycline monotherapy is currently considered optimal Induction chemotherapy (Mandelli et al. 1997; Fenaux et al. 1999; Sanz et al. 2003, 2009). In two separate trials employing simultaneous anthracycline (idarubicin) and ATRA as Induction therapy, the CR and Induction death rates for children were reported at 92% and 96% and 4% and 7.5% respectively (Ortega et al. 2005; Testi et al. 2005). Primary resistance to ATRA and idarubicin is extremely rare. However, children who do not have retinoid sensitive APL should receive standard intensive AML type therapy with anthracyclines and cytarabine.

Consolidation therapy: Comparable results are reported for anthracycline monotherapy (anthracyclines and ATRA) and combination chemotherapy (anthracyclines, ATRA, cytarabine with or without intercalating agents). Any advantage for the addition of any drug to anthracycline monotherapy is protocol dependent and may relate to the anthracycline and to its cumulative dose, cumulative doses of the other drugs and to the risk group. Whilst anthracycline monotherapy in Consolidation has the advantage of reduced morbidity and mortality, there were no remission deaths in four reported pediatric studies (Mann et al. 2001; de Botton et al. 2004; Ortega et al. 2005; Testi et al. 2005) using variable Consolidation courses.

The benefit of cytarabine in Consolidation is uncertain. Combined analysis of the GIMEMA and PETHEMA APL trials, which differed only in the inclusion or exclusion of drugs other than anthracyclines during Consolidation, showed that the omission of non-anthracycline drugs was not associated with an inferior anti-leukemia effect (Sanz et al. 2000). In contrast, the European APL 2000 study reported benefit for cytarabine in combination with daunorubicin (495 mg/m^2) and ATRA in newly diagnosed patients with APL (Ades et al. 2006). Cytarabine was given in both Induction and Consolidation. The benefit of cytarabine may be dependent on the anthracycline and its cumulative dose. A comparison of PETHEMA LPA 99 (high cumulative dose of idarubicin and mitoxantrone, no cytarabine) and APL 2000 (lower cumulative dose of daunorubicin and cytarabine) found benefit for cytarabine in high-risk patients with a WBC count of $>10 \times 10^9$/L($p = 0.026$) (Ades et al. 2006).

Patients with high-risk disease may benefit from more intensive Consolidation. The PETHEMA LPA 99 study employing anthracycline monotherapy in Consolidation reported a reduction in the relapse rate in high and intermediate-risk patients from 20.1% to 8.7% ($p = 0.004$) when ATRA was added to Consolidation and the anthracycline dose intensified (750 mg/m^2 daunorubicin equivalent) (Sanz et al. 2004). High risk patients treated on AIDA 2000 received identical Induction and Consolidation to those treated on AIDA 0493 with the addition of ATRA to each Consolidation block. The relapse rate for high-risk patients in AIDA 2000 was 2% at a median follow-up of 2 years compared to 29% for AIDA 0493 at a median follow-up of 4.5 years ($p = 0.0004$) (Lo Coco et al. 2004).

Maintenance treatment: The benefit of Maintenance therapy with intermittent ATRA (15 days every 3 months) in combination with 6-mercaptopurine and methotrexate has been variably reported (Tallman et al. 1997; Fenaux et al. 1999; Testi et al. 2005). It is unclear if ATRA in Maintenance is of benefit to patients who receive prolonged exposure in earlier phases of treatment or to those who are in molecular remission at the end of Consolidation.

Molecular monitoring in APL: Serial molecular MRD monitoring by RT PCR during and after therapy can detect persistent or recurrent molecular disease and guide pre-emptive therapy. The persistence of *PML-RARA* transcripts at the end of Consolidation (but not Induction) predicts for the risk of hematological relapse as does the recurrence of PCR positivity; both situations may be averted by pre-emptive therapy (Diverio et al. 1998; Burnett et al. 1999). The results from two pediatric studies suggest that less than 5% of children are MRD positive at the end of Consolidation (Ortega et al. 2005; Testi et al. 2005).

Hematopoietic stem cell transplantation: The only role for HSCT in frontline therapy is for the small number of patients with persistent or recurrence of MRD who may benefit from either allogeneic or autologous transplantation dependent on their molecular status after salvage therapy.

All-trans retinoic acid: An ATRA dose of 25 mg/m^2 appears to be effective in children (de Botton et al. 2004; Ortega et al. 2005; Testi et al. 2005), which is considerably lower than that of 45 mg/m^2 routinely employed in adults. Three studies using an ATRA dose of 25 mg/m^2 report EFS of 71–82% and OS of 76–90%, suggesting efficacy.

Hemorrhage: Death from hemorrhage, particularly intracranial hemorrhage (ICH), is the most common cause of failure to achieve CR, and children with a WBC count >10 × 10^9/L and the M3 variant are at particular risk. This classifies APL as a medical emergency. The coagulopathy can be initiated or exacerbated by chemotherapy, and ATRA, which improves the coagulopathy, must be started immediately on morphological suspicion and not delayed until the diagnosis is molecularly confirmed. Patients with a high WBC count should not undergo leukopheresis as this can exacerbate the coagulopathy. The incidence of death from ICH in children is reported at 3–4% despite increased awareness, pre-emptive therapy and the use of ATRA (de Botton et al. 2004; Ortega et al. 2005; Testi et al. 2005). Fibrinogen levels should be maintained above 1.5–2 g/L with fresh frozen plasma (FFP) or cryoprecipitate and the platelet count above 50 × 10^9/L until the coagulopathy resolves (Milligan et al. 2006). There is no proven benefit for the use of heparin, tranexamic acid or anti-fibrinolytic drugs. NovoSeven may be considered in life-threatening hemorrhage unresponsive to platelets, FFP and cryoprecipitate.

APL differentiation syndrome: APL differentiation syndrome is associated with high mortality if not promptly treated (De Botton et al. 1998; de Botton et al. 2003). It is thought to be related to surface adhesion molecule modulation and cytokine release following ATRA- or ATO-induced differentiation of APL cells (Frankel et al. 1992). Dexamethasone should be introduced at the earliest signs of APL differentiation syndrome, and if the condition progresses, ATRA/ATO should be temporarily discontinued. Although there is no proven benefit for prophylactic dexamethasone, it is usually given simultaneously with chemotherapy to patients with high WBC count who are at particular risk (De Botton et al. 1998, 2003). The incidence of APL differentiating syndrome is similar in children and adults (definite 3–5%, indeterminate 5–15%) with a mortality rate of less than 1% (Mann et al. 2001; de Botton et al. 2004; Ortega et al. 2005; Testi et al. 2005).

Pseudotumour cerebri: Children have a higher incidence of ATRA-associated headache and pseudotumour cerebri than adults: 13–30% and 5–9%, respectively for children receiving ATRA at a dose of 25 mg/m^2 (Mann et al. 2001; Ortega et al. 2005; Testi et al. 2005) and 39% and 16%, respectively for those receiving 45 mg/m^2 (de Botton et al. 2004). In addition, these studies suggest that there is no relative benefit in terms of disease control in treating children with doses higher than 25 mg/m^2.

Arsenic trioxide (ATO): Preliminary data from adult studies suggests at least comparability between ATO and single agent ATRA in terms of the achievement of CR (>90%) and that combined ATO and ATRA is superior to ATO or ATRA alone (Niu et al. 1999; Soignet et al. 2001; Shen et al. 2004). A small single center pediatric study using monotherapy with ATO reported a hematological and molecular remission rate of 91% with a relapse-free survival (RFS) and OS of 81% and 91%, respectively at 30 months (George et al. 2004). ATO and ATRA with or without the addition of gemtuzumab ozogamicin have shown favorable results in adults (Estey et al. 2006; Ravandi et al. 2009). The addition of ATO to Consolidation (Consolidation blocks 1 and 2: ATO 0.15 mg/kg/day for 5 days/week for 5 weeks) following remission induction with ATRA and chemotherapy has been reported to significantly improve the EFS and OS in adults with newly diagnosed APL (Powell 2007). ATO is usually well tolerated, although its use in Induction and hematological relapse is associated with hyperleukocytosis and APL differentiation syndrome. Other adverse effects include prolongation of the QT interval, reversible peripheral neuropathy and skin hyperpigmentation. Little is known of late ATO cardiac and neurological toxicity, but hyperpigmentation, palmar keratosis, distal neuropathy and muscular atrophy have been observed with long-term use. There is a need to define toxicity in children and to assess the role and best strategy for the use of ATO in this age group.

5.5.1.7 Refractoryo rR elapsedDi sease

Approximately 3–5% of children have persistent molecular disease at the end of Consolidation and 20–25% have either a molecular or hematological relapse. The outcome following molecular relapse with pre-emptive therapy is superior to that following hematological relapse. Approximately 3–5% of APL patients develop extramedullary (EM) relapse, usually involving the CNS or the skin.

ATO has emerged as the single most active agent in patients with relapsed APL, with CR rates of approximately 80–90% and most patients achieving molecular remission after two cycles (Ghavamzadeh et al. 2006; Lo Coco et al. 2007; Tallman 2007). There appears to be no advantage for combining ATRA with ATO in the relapsed setting.

The best Consolidation strategy after ATO-induced second remission is unknown, but options include additional cycles of ATO, ATRA, gemtuzumab ozogamicin, and standard chemotherapy and HSCT. Gemtuzumab ozogamicin offers the combination of calicheamicin – a cytotoxic agent with similarities to anthracyclines, and an anti-CD33 antibody; CD33 is homogenously expressed in virtually 100% of APL. Data from the European Bone Marrow Transplant (EBMT) Registry report a 5-year cumulative incidence of leukemia-free survival (LFS) of 51% for 195 patients autografted in CR2 and a 5-year LFS of 59% for the 137 patients allografted in CR2 (Sanz et al. 2007). The appropriate procedure is guided by the molecular status, age, availability of an HLA-identical donor and the time from diagnosis to transplant.

Extramedullary relapse has been increasingly reported since the introduction of ATRA in the treatment of APL (Evans and Grimwade 1999; Specchia et al. 2001; Breccia et al. 2003; de Botton et al. 2006). This may be due to longer survival increasing the number of patients at risk, although the role of ATRA in mediating increased expression of adhesion molecules has been questioned. It has also been suggested that APL differentiation syndrome and intracerebral bleeding during Induction might be associated with an increased risk of extramedullary relapse (Evans and Grimwade 1999; Specchia et al. 2001; Breccia et al. 2003; de Botton et al. 2006).

EM relapse usually occurs in the CNS and is typically accompanied by overt or molecular bone marrow relapse. EM relapse in APL should be regarded as a systemic relapse and both CNS directed and systemic therapy given (Sanz et al. 2009). Irrespective of the intensity of treatment, patients with an EM relapse have an OS comparable with those with a hematological relapse. Although ATO crosses the blood–brain barrier, the concentrations in cerebral spinal fluid (CSF) achieved by intravenous infusion are probably insufficient for the treatment of meningeal leukemia (Knipp et al. 2007). This combined with the potential for increased ATO neurological toxicity in individuals receiving concomitant intrathecal chemotherapy and cranial irradiation may limit its usefulness in CNS relapse. This argues in favor of the use of CNS intrathecal prophylaxis in the frontline protocols (starting with Consolidation), at least for patients with unfavorable presenting features associated with a higher risk of CNS relapse, expecting that this might result in a significant proportion of patients being over-treated.

5.5.1.8 New Drugs

FLT-3 inhibitors: FLT-3 inhibitors offer the possibility of using combination therapy that targets both mutations contributing to the pathogenesis of APL: FLT-3 inhibitors for *FLT3*/ITD and ATRA for the *PML/RARα* fusion. However, *FLT3* mutations may only exist in subclones or be lost at relapse, and FLT3 inhibitors and ATRA may not work synergistically *in vivo* (Gale et al. 2005). Histone deacetylase (HDAC) inhibitors (Fazi et al. 2005) may have a potential role in the treatment of APL in the future.

5.5.1.9 Conclusions

The outcome for children with APL is likely to continue to improve as novel approaches such as the addition of ATO and gemtuzumab ozogamicin to conventional frontline therapy and the possibilities of low- or non-chemotherapy approaches are explored. The anti-leukemia effect of reducing the cumulative anthracycline dose, or substituting lipsomal anthracyclines, should be tested within a clinical trial. The benefit, content and duration of Maintenance merit clarification. Risk stratification may be more accurately defined by molecular monitoring than by the WBC count, and targeting treatment to the risk of relapse may reduce unnecessary toxicity to standard-risk patients. The ideal frequency of molecular monitoring, the best pre-emptive therapy, and the role of novel agents should be established. Finally cardiotoxicity and treatment-related myelodysplasia deserve careful monitoring, as do the toxicities of new agents as they are introduced.

5.5.2 Down Syndrome Transient Myeloproliferative Disorder and Myeloid Leukemia

5.5.2.1 Epidemiology and Incidence

Children with Down syndrome are at an increased risk for developing both acute myeloid and acute lymphoblastic leukemia. The increased incidence of acute myeloid leukemia in children with Down syndrome was first described in 1957 by Krivit and Good, and is predominately observed during the first 4 years of life (Krivit and Good 1957). The risk for the development of hematologic abnormalities including leukemia is relatively high in early childhood though it decreases with age. Hasle and co-workers conducted a Danish population-based study of 2,814 individuals with Down syndrome and found that the risk for leukemia decreased dramatically as patients became older, with a standardized incidence ratio (SIR) of 56 for children aged between 0 and 4 years, decreasing to 10 for individuals between 5 and 29 years of age. Significantly, no cases of leukemia were observed after 29 years of age. The cumulative risk of leukemia is 2.7% by age 30 (Hasle et al. 2000). Among Down syndrome leukemia patients, malignancies derived from primitive megakaryocytic and erythroid blood progenitors predominate (FAB-M7 subtype), with a 600-fold increase in relative risk for acute megakaryocytic leukemia (AMLK) as compared to other children (Zipursky et al. 1994). The biological and clinical features of AMKL in children with Down syndrome are distinctly different from other forms of AMKL, and Down syndrome AMKL is now considered a specific sub-type of AML in DS in the World Health Organization (WHO) classification (see above). In addition, the risk for myelodysplastic syndrome (MDS) with marrow fibrosis is also markedly increased in children with Down syndrome, with an estimated relative risk of 175, and in many cases the MDS precedes the development of leukemia (Creutzig et al. 1996; Lange et al. 1998).

Newborns with Down syndrome are also at risk for development of an abnormal myeloproliferative disorder, and approximately 5–10% may exhibit leukocytosis with circulating blast-like cells (Zipursky 2003). This is often accompanied by hepatosplenomegaly, reflecting a proliferation of a hematopoietic progenitor from the liver. Most cases of the myeloproliferation resolve spontaneously, and the main thrust of therapy is to protect the patient from life-threatening complications of hyperleukocytosis, liver injury, or related metabolic complications. This transient myeloproliferative disorder (TMD) almost exclusively presents in infants less than 2–3 months of age, and is associated with an estimated 10–20% risk for the development of subsequent characteristic acute myeloid leukemia of infants with Down syndrome in 3–4 years (Massey et al. 2006; Klusmann et al. 2008; Muramatsu et al. 2008). While all children with Down syndrome share the additional genes from chromosome 21, the reason why only a small subset develops acute leukemia or exhibits neonatal transient myeloproliferative disorder is unknown.

5.5.2.2 Biologyo fT MDandA ML in Children with Down Syndrome

Human chromosome 21 contains over 300 genes and other regulatory transcripts, including the Down syndrome critical region at 21q22, which is associated with the predominance of phenotypic characteristics of Down syndrome. Multiple lines of evidence clearly implicate additional copies of this region of chromosome 21 as at least partially responsible for the initiation of Down syndrome leukemia. Notably, in individuals who are mosaic for Down syndrome, if a leukemia or transient myeloproliferative disorder occurs, it is always found to harbor additional copies of chromosome 21. Chromosome 21, and particularly the 21q22 region, includes a variety of genes implicated in leukemia. These include oncogenes such as *ERG, ETS2, RUNX1,* and *SON*, as well as other genes critical in folate/single carbon metabolism and oxidant stress. Limited detailed examination of oncogenes found on chromosome 21q22 has, as of yet, not identified consistent frequent patterns of mutation leading to pathologically constitutive activation. In addition, various mouse models with trisomy of syntenic regions of chromosome 21 variably exhibit hematologic disorders such as anemia, macrocytosis and platelet abnormalities, but they are not consistently associated with spontaneous leukemia. These observations have led to the search for other associated genetic mutations that may be responsible for or contribute to the evolution of leukemia in patients with Down syndrome.

In the context of AMKL, a key observation has been the identification of somatic mutations in the megakaryocyte-erythroid transcription factor, *GATA1*, located at chromosome Xp11.23 (Wechsler et al. 2002). The blasts in the vast majority of patients with Down syndrome and transient myeloproliferative disorder and AMKL, possess N-terminal truncating mutations in *GATA1* that produce a shortened version of the protein (GATA1s), and result in a block in differentiation and proliferation of megakaryocytic precursors (Wechsler et al. 2002; Groet et al. 2003; Hitzler et al. 2003;

Mundschau et al. 2003; Rainis et al. 2003; Xu et al. 2003; Shimada et al. 2004). The reason for the particular propensity of *GATA1s* mutations to be found in Down syndrome, TMD and AMKL is unknown, and it appears likely that additional cancer-causing mutations, or genetic "hits," are also necessary for the full development of AMKL. In the absence of Down syndrome, an inherited mutation of *GATA1* results in the expression of only the short isoform and causes anemia and neutropenia, but not leukemia (Hollanda et al. 2006). A variety of mutations in other oncogenes (e.g., *JAK3* genes, *FLT3,* and *RAS)* have been described as occurring at variable frequencies in the AMKL of Down syndrome patients, as have alterations of tumor suppressor genes including *TP53* (Malinge et al. 2009). Recently, the chromosome 21 micro-RNA, miR-125b-2, has been identified as increasing proliferation and enhancing self-renewal of megakaryocytic and megakaryocytic/erythroid progenitors, and it appears to interact with the *GATA1s* in preclinical Down syndrome AMKL models. The target genes of miR-125b are down-regulated in DS-AMKL, and miR-125b-2 has been proposed as an onco-miR involved in the pathogenesis of Down syndrome AMKL (Klusmann et al. 2010). These additional mutations and genetic alterations may provide clues to other pathways that specifically cooperate with trisomy 21q22 and GATA1s mutations in the development of TMD and AMKL.

This emerging data suggests a stochastic pathway for the development of AMKL in children with Down syndrome, with additional copies of chromosome region 21q22 representing a "first hit," the subsequent acquisition of *GATA1s* mutations representing a "second hit," and transformation to leukemia also requiring altered expression or mutations in other pathways. The leukemias in children with Down syndrome may share common early "hits" with a variety of subsequent parallel common pathways to leukemia. The acquisition of late leukemogenic mutations may be influenced by other features associated with increased genotoxicity in Down syndrome (e.g., alterations in oxidant and single carbon/folate metabolism, etc.), and various models for leukemogenesis have been proposed (Cabelof et al. 2009; Malinge et al. 2009; Roy et al. 2009).

The unique biology of myeloid leukemia in children with Down syndrome may also offer insight into the superior clinical response of these patients to cytarabine and anthracycline regimens, and parallel *in vitro* studies that demonstrated marked sensitivity of DS leukemia blasts to chemotherapy (Taub et al. 1999; Frost et al. 2000; Zwaan et al. 2002; Taub and Ge 2005). Leukemia cells from patients with Down syndrome also exhibit marked sensitivity to anthracyclines (2–7-fold), mitoxantrone (ninefold), amsacrine (16-fold), etoposide (20-fold), 6-thioguanine (threefold), busulfan (fivefold), vincristine (23-fold), and prednisolone (more than 1.1-fold), when compared to leukemia cells from patients without Down syndrome (Zwaan et al. 2002). Elegant studies from the laboratory of Taub and co-workers also demonstrate that AMKL blasts generate significantly higher levels of the active intracellular cytarabine metabolite, ara-CTP, when compared to blasts from AML patients without Down syndrome. This group has developed the hypothesis that mutated *GATA1s* reduces expression of cytidine deaminase (CDA), the enzyme that deaminates and inactivates cytarabine, rendering cells more sensitive to cytotoxicity. Supporting this notion, they have demonstrated significantly lower CDA expression in megakaryoblasts from patients with Down syndrome when compared to blasts from other AML patients. In addition, transfection of the full-length *GATA1* cDNA resulted in significantly increased CDA expression and reduced cytarabine sensitivity in a DS AMKL cell line (Ge et al. 2005). Related investigations have linked alterations in single carbon metabolism with increased expression of chromosome 21q22.3 genes, including cystathionine-β-synthase (CBS). CBS catalyzes an intermediate step in the synthesis of cysteine, and increased activity in patients with Down syndrome is associated with significantly lower levels of homocysteine, methionine and *S*-adenosylmethionine, and potentially altered folate metabolism. These observations may also explain in part sensitivity to cytarabine as well as methotrexate (Taub et al. 1999; Taub and Ge 2005). Overexpression of chromosome 21-localized genes, including superoxide dismutase, may be linked to increased chemotherapy drug sensitivity.

5.5.2.3 ClinicalFeat uresandManag ement of TMD in Children with Down Syndrome

In TMD, immature megakaryoblasts accumulate in the liver predominantly and to a lesser extent in the bone marrow and peripheral blood; this results in leukocytosis, which can be severe. Transient myeloproliferative disorder is most commonly a disorder of hepatic hematopoiesis and, thus, a prenatal presentation or *in utero* diagnosis is not uncommon. TMD exhibits a variable clinical presentation and course, and it is likely that most patients are asymptomatic and do not come to medical attention. However, a subset of patients may develop life-threatening leukocytosis, hydrops fetalis, liver dysfunction and bleeding diathesis, or pericardial and/or pleural effusions, as well as hepatosplenomegaly, lymphadenopathy or leukemia cutis. Approximately 70–80% of patients with TMD exhibit a spontaneous remission. Causes of death in TMD are largely associated with organ failure secondary to hyperviscosity affecting the heart, lungs or kidneys, bowel ischemia and necrotizing enterocolitis, or liver failure secondary to fibrosis. Liver abnormalities in patients with TMD can often present insidiously and manifest only with a persistently and progressively increasing conjugated bilirubinemia. Immunophenotypic evaluation of TMD blasts reflect largely myeloid and megakaryoblastic differentiation with expression of CD33, CD38, CD117, CD34, CD7, CD56, CD36, CD71, CD42b, and receptors for thrombopoietin and erythropoietin (Yumura-Yagi et al. 1992; Girodon et al. 2000; Karandikar et al. 2001; Langebrake et al. 2005). Leukemia-associated recurring chromosomal abnormalities are uncommon in TMD (Forestier et al. 2008).

TMD generally resolves slowly over several months, and is most commonly managed with supportive treatment including low-dose chemotherapy, exchange transfusion or leukapheresis. Patients with severe leukocytosis or symptomatic disease, including those with hepatic dysfunction and evolving fibrosis, have been successfully managed with low-dose cytarabine. Several low-dose cytarabine regimens have been employed by the cooperative cancer groups and include: (1) POG 9481 cytarabine dosing of 10 mg/m^2 per dose twice a day for 7 days (Massey et al. 2006), (2) COG 2971 dosing of 3.33 mg/kg/24 h as continuous intravenous infusion for 5 days (Gamis 2005), and the (3) AML-BFM 93, 98 and 04 series dosing of 0.5–1.5 mg/kg for 3–12 days (Klusmann et al. 2008). In most circumstances, there is a prompt response to cytarabine with eradication of peripheral blasts in the first 1–2 weeks of therapy. Mortality from symptomatic TMD is approximately 15–20%, and multivariate analysis has revealed severe leukocytosis (WBC > 10^9/L), preterm delivery, ascites, and bleeding diathesis as risk factors for poor outcome (Zipursky 2003; Klusmann et al. 2008; Muramatsu et al. 2008). Approximately 20% of patients with TMD will progress or recur with acute megakaryoblastic leukemia. After successful recovery from an episode of TMD, patients require close monitoring for residual complications, but also for the potential increased risk for the development of leukemia in the next 2–4 years of life. General recommendations include monthly hemogram with white cell differential and platelet count for the first year and, if normal, every 2 months for the subsequent years.

5.5.2.4 ClinicalFeat uresandManag ement of AML in Children with Down Syndrome

AMKL in patients with Down syndrome has significantly different clinical features when compared with AML in other children, and in the CCG 2861/2891 study of 118 patients with Down syndrome and 1,088 patients without Down syndrome, some of the characteristic differences were: a younger median age of presentation (1.8 vs 7.5 years), lower presenting white blood cell counts (7.6 × 10^9/L vs 19.9 × 10^9/L), lower platelet count at diagnosis (29.0 × 10^3/μL vs 52.0 × 10^3/μL), a greater frequency of antecedent MDS (20% vs 8%), and an under-representation of characteristic t(8;21); t(15;17); 16q22 AML chromosomal translocations (Lange et al. 1998). Down syndrome AMKL represents a unique biology and is now recognized as a distinct diagnostic entity in the WHO classification of myeloid leukemias. Central nervous system involvement is also less frequent, and the bone marrow morphology can reveal accompanying varying levels of dysplasia and fibrosis with abnormalities in megakaryocytes (Gamis et al. 2003; Creutzig et al. 2005; Zeller et al. 2005; Rao et al. 2006). Paralleling the biology of AMKL, immunophenotypic characterization of blasts generally reflects the differentiation along pathways in early myeloid differentiation (expression of CD33, CD38, CD117, CD34, and CD7), megakaryocytic lineage markers (expression of CD42b and CD41), and erythroid lineage markers (expression of CD36 and Glycophorin A) (Yumura-Yagi et al. 1992; Girodon et al. 2000; Karandikar et al. 2001; Langebrake et al. 2005). Consistent with the unique biology of this disease, the characteristic translocations t(1;22) and t(1;3) that occur in other forms of AMKL are generally not observed in Down syndrome AMKL (Lange 2000;

Forestier et al. 2008). Compared to other pediatric patients with AML, children with Down syndrome and AMKL exhibit significantly increased frequencies of dup(1q), del(6q), del(7p), dup(7q), +8, +11, del(16q), and +21 (Forestier et al. 2008).

Recent clinical findings indicate that AMKL in younger children with Down syndrome often responds well to multi-agent chemotherapy regimens of modest intensity, with cure rates in excess of those observed in children with acute myeloid leukemia without Down syndrome. Ravindranath was the first to observe superior outcomes for patients with Down syndrome and AML who were treated with high-dose cytarabine on POG 8498 (Ravindranath et al. 1992). This finding paralleled biological investigations of cytarabine and anthracycline sensitivity in AMKL blasts from patients with Down syndrome (see above), and Down syndrome patients consistently exhibited relatively low relapse rates in multiple subsequent small and large-scale clinical studies in pediatric AML (Table 5.6). However, these studies also indicated that children with Down syndrome have an increased risk of side effects with chemotherapy, and high rates of regimen-related mortality may compromise overall outcome. This phenomenon was most clearly identified in the CCG 2891 study, which was a randomized trial for children with AML comparing intensive timing versus standard timing of the same five-drug cytarabine and anthracycline-based Induction chemotherapy regimen. The intensive timing Induction delivered the two Induction chemotherapy courses separated by a 6-day rest interval, regardless of marrow recovery, while in the standard timing Induction, the second course was administered after marrow recovery if the day-14 marrow had less than 5% blasts or on days 14–17 if significant residual leukemia was present. The CCG 2861 and 2891 studies enrolled 1,206 children with AML, including 118 children with Down syndrome and 1,088 children without Down syndrome, and the results revealed a marked excess of regimen-related mortality in the children with Down syndrome treated on the intensive timing arm (32%) when compared to children with Down syndrome treated with standard timing (2%), or compared with other children with AML but without Down syndrome (5% mortality in standard timing; 11% with intensive timing) (Lange et al. 1998). The optimal chemotherapy regimen for children with Down syndrome and AMKL remains under investigation, and most cooperative groups have developed separate strata within larger AML studies or independent clinical studies for patients with Down syndrome and AMKL. As indicated in Table 5.6, contemporary treatment regimens exhibit approximately 74–85% EFS for children with Down syndrome and AMKL. The intensity of therapy has been successfully significantly reduced in clinical regimens for children with Down syndrome and AMKL without compromising relapse rates.

In addition to infectious complications and mortality, children with Down syndrome appear to have increased risk for clinical cardiotoxicity. The POG 9421 study included 57 patients with Down syndrome and AMKL and treated patients with five cycles of chemotherapy, including daunorubicin 135 mg/m^2 and mitoxantrone 80 mg/m^2. Symptomatic cardiomyopathy was seen in ten patients (17.5%) relatively soon after completion of treatment, and three died as a result of congestive heart failure. It is postulated that increased dosage of genes located on chromosome 21, including carbonyl reductase and superoxide dismutase, predisposes to risk of anthracycline-related cardiomyopathy (O'Brien et al. 2008).

AML in the older child and young adult with Down syndrome appears to have a somewhat more resistant biology, paralleling that seen in other children without Down syndrome, and current therapy recommendations include treatment on standard acute myeloid leukemia regimens. This may be reflected in part in recent observations that Down syndrome patients who had TMD and subsequently developed AMKL exhibited superior EFS and fewer relapses when compared with Down syndrome patients with AMKL and no previous history of TMD (91% vs 70%; log-rank $p = 0.039$) (Klusmann et al. 2008). The results of the CCG 2891 study indicated inferior outcomes with increasing age at diagnosis of Down syndrome-AML, particularly for children older than 4 years; this was mirrored in the CCG 2971 study (Gamis et al. 2003). These data continue to support the notions that tailoring therapy to the unique biology of Down syndrome-AML in the younger patient may hold great promise to preserve excellent relapse-free survival with markedly reduced toxicity. Current COG approaches treat older children (>4 years of age) with Down syndrome leukemia on the same pediatric AML regimens with other children without Down syndrome.

Table 5.6 Down syndrome-AML clinical studies: outcomes and chemotherapy drug exposure. (From Ravindranath et al. 1992; Creutzig et al. 1996; Ravindranath et al. 1996; Lange et al. 1998; Craze et al. 1999; Kojima et al. 2000; Creutzig et al. 2005; Abildgaarde ta l. 2006;A l-Ahmarie t al. 2006;O 'Briene ta l. 2008)

Regimen	Number of patients	Cytarabine dose (g/m^2)	Anthracycline dose (mg/m^2)	EFS (%)	Treatment-related mortality (%)	Refractory (%)	Relapse (%)
Japanese Consortium (Kojimae ta l. 2000)	33	4.2	300	80	9	0	9
HSC-Toronto (Al-Ahmarie ta l. 2006)	18	6.7	0	67	NR	–	33
MRC AML 10 (Crazee ta l. 1999)	32	10.6	650	59	34	0	8
MRC AML 10 Modified (Crazee ta l. 1999)	13	ND	ND	46	8	8	38
CCG2861/2891 STDtiming (Langee ta l. 1998)	85	15.2	320	74	2	2	ND
CCG2861/2891 INTtiming (Langee ta l. 1998)	25	15.2	320	52	32	4	ND
POG9421 (O'Briene ta l. 2008)	57	20.7	135/80	77	4	–	14
BFM-98 (Creutzige ta l. 2005)	66	23–29	220–240	89	5	0	6
BFM-87/93 (Creutzige ta l. 1996)	21	23–43	220–400	48	33	0	14
POG8498 (Ravindranathe ta l. 1992)	12	40.7	230	100	0	0	0
POG8821 (Ravindranathe ta l. 1996)	34	48.1	350	68	18	–	17
NOPHO-AML93 (Abildgaarde ta l. 2006)	41	49.6	150/30	85	5	5	7
NOPHO-AML88 (Abildgaarde ta l. 2006)	15	50.1	450	47	33	13	7

Abildgaarde ta l. (2006)A nnH ematol8 5:275–280
Al-Ahmarie ta l. (2006)B rJ H aematol133: 646–648
Crazee ta l. (1999)A rchD isC hild81: 32–37
Creutzige ta l. (2005)Le ukemia19: 1355–1360
Creutzige ta l. (1996)Le ukemia10: 1677–1686
Kojimae ta l. (2000)Le ukemia14: 786–791
Langee ta l. (1998)B lood91: 608–615
O'Briene ta l. (2008)J C linO ncol26: 414–420
Ravindranathe ta l. (1992)B lood80: 2210–2214
Ravindranath et al. (1996) N Engl J Med 334:1428–1434

5.6 RefractoryandR elapsedA ML

About 5% of children with newly diagnosed AML still have ≥5% blasts in their bone marrow after two courses of combination chemotherapy, which is called resistant (or refractory) disease. Moreover, about 20% of patients conventionally defined as achieving CR have minimal residual leukemia (0.1–4% blasts) at the end of two cycles of Induction therapy. The prognosis of these children with resistant, MRD-positive or relapsed AML is relatively poor (Webb et al. 1999; Pui et al. 2004;K aspersa ndR avindranath 2005).

The most frequent event for newly diagnosed patients with AML is a relapse, occurring in about one in three children. Bone marrow usually is involved, and the CNS in up to 10% of cases (including combined relapses). About 50% of patients suffer an early relapse, arbitrarily defined as within 1 year from initial diagnosis, and 50% suffer a late relapse, after 1 year. Outcome from relapse is significantly better in case of a longer duration of CR1 (Stahnke et al. 1998; Webb et al. 1999; Kaspers et al. 2009). However, the international study Relapsed AML 2001/01 showed early treatment response to be an even more important prognostic factor (Kaspers et al. 2009). In that study, early response was determined by morphological examination of the bone marrow obtained at day 28 from start of re-Induction, and defined as good in case of less than 20% AML blasts, and poor in case of 20% or more of such blasts. Day 28 in practice is between days 28 and 42 from the start of re-Induction therapy. In addition to treatment response, favorable cytogenetics t(8;21) and inv(16), as initially identified in studies with newly diagnosed children, also seem to be a favorable prognostic factor at relapsed AML (Webb et al. 1999; Kaspers et al. 2009). Study Relapsed AML 2001/01 and several other recently published studies report a probability of long-term survival from relapsed AML of more than 30%, as summarized by Goemans et al. (2008). Therefore, re-Induction chemotherapy should be offered to all children and adolescents with relapsed AML who can tolerate intensive treatment. However, patients that respond poorly to the first course of re-Induction chemotherapy, patients that do not achieve a second complete remission, and patients that relapse again could be offered more experimental therapy in that setting of a very dismal prognosis. Fortunately, innovative treatment seems achievable within 10–20 years from now.

Whether or not treatment of a patient with relapsed AML with curative intention should be attempted may depend on many factors, such as age, duration of first remission, cytogenetic findings, the treatment modalities the patient received before relapse, and especially the physical and psychological condition of the patient and his/her parents. There are only a few studies on the treatment of relatively unselected groups of children with relapsed AML. High-dose chemotherapy with two or more of the agents cytarabine, mitoxantrone, etoposide, idarubicin, and fludarabine, can induce complete remission in 50–80% of the relapsed AML cases. Patients with AML that express CD33 can be treated with gemtuzumab ozogamicin alone or in combination with other agents, although responses in CD33-negative cases have been reported. Children who achieve subsequent CR should receive HSCT including autografts or allografts from related or unrelated HLA-matched donors. The survival rate from relapsed AML is about 20%, but is significantly higher in late relapses (Lowenberg et al. 1999; Pui et al. 2004; Kaspers and Ravindranath 2005).

In the setting of the so-called "International Pediatric AML Group," and coordinated by the AML committee of the International BFM Study Group, a large intergroup randomized study in pediatric relapsed and refractory AML is ongoing. For the first re-Induction course, the FLAG regimen is being compared with FLAG plus liposomal daunorubicin, followed by another course of FLAG. Stem cell transplantation is intended in all patients, either from a matched sibling donor (preferred) or an unrelated matched donor. Results are encouraging and survival is demonstrated in both early and late relapses. Moreover, the study proves the possibility to run an international study in pediatric AML with more than ten groups participating worldwide.

5.7 New/RecentA pproachest oT herapy

5.7.1 Approaches to MRD

Another group with unfavorable prognosis is the group of patients with minimal residual disease (MRD). These patients have persistent measurable AML blast cells after one to two courses of intensive chemotherapy (Coustan-Smith et al. 2003; Pui et al. 2004). MRD can be detected by polymerase chain reaction (PCR) amplification of antigen receptor genes and/or of fusion transcripts, and by flowcytometric detection of ectopic or aberrant immunophenotypes. Flowcytometry is applicable in the majority of patients with AML. There is a strong correlation between MRD levels detected during clinical remission and treatment outcome (Sievers et al. 2003; Campana and Coustan-Smith 2004). Monitoring of MRD will probably allow the identification of patients at high risk for a subsequent relapse and to adjust further treatment (Campana and Coustan-Smith 2004; Kaspers and Creutzig 2005). However, the prediction of a subgroup with an excellent prognosis based on MRD measurements still is difficult, probably because of the limited sensitivity of flow cytometry in comparison to PCR-based techniques (which unfortunately are useful in only a minority of AML patients).

5.7.2 Targeted Therapy Approaches

Significant improvements have already been achieved with conventional drugs that have been available for the treatment of AML for decades. Therefore, it seems realistic to expect major advances with the development of new drugs and especially novel treatment modalities. Discussion of all of these challenges is beyond the scope of this chapter, but they have been reviewed elsewhere (Kaspers and Zwaan 2007). In brief, innovative treatment will consist of at least four different modalities. First, the development of novel but conventional drugs. A good example might be clofarabine, a relatively novel nucleoside analogue that is being studied in both children and adults with AML. Second, the design of drugs with novel mechanisms of action, often targeted at leukemia-specific abnormalities. Typical examples are monoclonal-antibody mediated treatment such as with gemtuzumab ozogamicin (targeting CD33-positive cells) and with tyrosine kinase inhibitors (targeting *FLT3*- or *kit*-mutated AML cells). Third, improving the graft-versus-leukemia effect of donor cells without an increase in graft-versus-host-disease. And finally, the development of vaccination and other immunotherapy approaches. Innovative treatment will become more and more tailored and personalized, which will necessitate large-scale and thus international collaboration. Such collaborative efforts will be the only way to enroll a sufficient number of patients with a specific subtype of AML in a given study. Despite such an international setting, randomized studies in large cohorts of patients will more and more become impossible because of limited patient numbers eligible for subgroup-directed therapy. Thus, innovative trial designs will also be necessary. Fortunately, international large-scale collaboration has been realized in the past 10–20 years, especially in the setting of the International BFM Study Group, the so-called International Pediatric AML Group, and the International Consortium for Childhood APL. These collaborations together with the efforts of many professionals in pediatric AML will undoubtedly further improve the outcome of this disease in terms of cure, side-effects and late effects.

5.8 Summary: Advances in Therapies for Pediatric Acute Myeloid Leukemia

Advances in cytogenetics and molecular biology have yielded significant insight into the biological heterogeneity of acute myeloid leukemia, and the response of different biological subgroups to specific chemotherapy approaches. These insights have led to the development of targeted therapies (e.g., all-trans-retinoic acid and arsenic trioxide for acute promyelocytic leukemia with the *PML/RAR* translocation), or modified conventional chemotherapy treatment regimens tailored for host and disease biology (e.g., Down syndrome acute megakaryoblastic leukemia and Fanconi anemia with AML). However, for the majority of patients with AML, chemotherapy dose-exposure appears to have reached a maximum level now limited by significant toxicity, and for many patients, treatment outcomes remain unsatisfactory. The core chemotherapeutic regimens were developed over 3 decades ago and are based largely upon anthracyclines and cytarabine. Significant incremental progress in improving outcomes has been based upon refinements in chemotherapy dose and scheduling and parallel advances in supportive care with reduction in the risk of complications. Primary recent advances in pediatric AML therapy include:

1. Molecularly targeted therapy for acute promyelocyticle ukemia
2. Therapies tailored to the unique disease biology and host sensitivity of patients with Down syndrome and AML
3. Improved outcomes with dose exposure and intensity in Induction

4. Better characterization of patients who do and do not derive benefit from allogenic transplantation
5. Importance of cytogenetics and molecular classification to predict response
6. Early insights into the number of post-remission cycles of Intensification needed for curative approaches

References

Abbott BL, Rubnitz JE et al (2003) Clinical significance of central nervous system involvement at diagnosis of pediatric acute myeloid leukemia: a single institution's experience. Leukemia 17(11):2090–2096

Abildgaard L, Ellebaek E et al (2006) Optimal treatment intensity in children with Down syndrome and myeloid leukaemia: data from 56 children treated on NOPHO-AML protocols and a review of the literature. Ann Hematol 85(5):275–280

Abrahamsson J, Clausen N et al (2007) Improved outcome after relapse in children with acute myeloid leukaemia. Br J Haematol136(2):229–236

Abu-Duhier FM, Goodeve AC et al (2000) FLT3 internal tandem duplication mutations in adult acute myeloid leukaemia define a high-risk group. Br J Haematol 111(1):190–195

Ades L, Chevret S et al (2006) Is cytarabine useful in the treatment of acute promyelocytic leukemia? Results of a randomized trial from the European Acute Promyelocytic Leukemia Group. J Clin Oncol 24(36):5703–5710

Al-Ahmari A, Shah N et al (2006) Long-term results of an ultra low-dose cytarabine-based regimen for the treatment of acute megakaryoblastic leukaemia in children with Down syndrome. Br J Haematol 133(6):646–648

Appelbaum FR (1997) Allogeneic hematopoietic stem cell transplantation for acute leukemia. Semin Oncol 24(1):114–123

Appelbaum FR, Kopecky KJ et al (2006) The clinical spectrum of adult acute myeloid leukaemia associated with core binding factor translocations. Br J Haematol 135(2):165–173

Athale UH, Razzouk BI et al (2001) Biology and outcome of childhood acute megakaryoblastic leukemia: a single institution's experience. Blood 97(12):3727–3732

Baldus CD, Thiede C et al (2006) BAALC expression and FLT3 internal tandem duplication mutations in acute myeloid leukemia patients with normal cytogenetics: prognostic implications. J Clin Oncol 24(5):790–797

Balgobind BV, Raimondi SC et al (2009) Novel prognostic subgroups in childhood 11q23/MLL-rearranged acute myeloid leukemia: results of an international retrospective study. Blood114(12):248 9–2496

Barnard DR, Alonzo TA et al (2007) Comparison of childhood myelodysplastic syndrome, AML FAB M6 or M7, CCG 2891: report from the Children's Oncology Group. Pediatr Blood Cancer 49(1):17–22

Becton D, Dahl GV et al (2006) Randomized use of cyclosporin A (CsA) to modulate P-glycoprotein in children with AML in remission: Pediatric Oncology Group Study 9421. Blood 107(4):1315–1324

Bennett JM, Catovsky D et al (1976) Proposals for the classification of the acute leukaemias. French-American-British (FAB) co-operative group. Br J Haematol 33(4): 451–458

Bennett JM, Catovsky D et al (1985) Proposed revised criteria for the classification of acute myeloid leukemia. A report of the French-American-British Cooperative Group. Ann Intern Med103(4):620–625

Bishop JF, Matthews JP et al (1998) Intensified induction chemotherapy with high dose cytarabine and etoposide for acute myeloid leukemia: a review and updated results of the Australian Leukemia Study Group. Leuk Lymph 28(3–4): 315–327

Bloomfield CD, Lawrence D et al (1998) Frequency of prolonged remission duration after high-dose cytarabine intensification in acute myeloid leukemia varies by cytogenetic subtype. Cancer Res 58(18):4173–4179

Boissel N, Leroy H et al (2006) Incidence and prognostic impact of c-Kit, FLT3, and Ras gene mutations in core binding factor acute myeloid leukemia (CBF-AML). Leukemia 20(6):965–970

Breccia M, Carmosino I et al (2003) Early detection of meningeal localization in acute promyelocytic leukaemia patients with high presenting leucocyte count. Br J Haematol 120(2):266–270

Breems DA, Van Putten WL et al (2008) Monosomal karyotype in acute myeloid leukemia: a better indicator of poor prognosis than a complex karyotype. J Clin Oncol 26(29): 4791–4797

Brown P, McIntyre E et al (2007) The incidence and clinical significance of nucleophosmin mutations in childhood AML. Blood110(3):979–985

Burnett AK, Grimwade D et al (1999) Presenting white blood cell count and kinetics of molecular remission predict prognosis in acute promyelocytic leukemia treated with all-trans retinoic acid: result of the randomized MRC trial. Blood 93(12):4131–4143

Burnett AK, Wheatley K et al (2002) The value of allogeneic bone marrow transplant in patients with acute myeloid leukaemia at differing risk of relapse: results of the UK MRC AML 10 trial. Br J Haematol 118(2):385–400

Burnett AK, Kell WJ et al (2006) The addition of Gemtuzumab Ozogamicin to induction chemotherapy for AML improves disease free survival without extra toxicity: preliminary analysis of 1115 patients in the MRC AML15 trial. ASH Annu Meeting Abstracts 108(11):13

Burnett AK, Hills RK et al (2009) Attempts to optimise induction and consolidation chemotherapy in patients with acute myeloid leukaemia: results of the MRC AML15 trial. ASH Annu Meeting Abstracts 114(22):484

Byrd JC, Dodge RK et al (1999) Patients with t(8;21)(q22;q22) and acute myeloid leukemia have superior failure-free and overall survival when repetitive cycles of high-dose cytarabine are administered. J Clin Oncol 17(12):3767–3775

Cabelof DC, Patel HV et al (2009) Mutational spectrum at GATA1 provides insights into mutagenesis and leukemogenesis in Down syndrome. Blood 114(13):2753–2763

Campana D (2003) Determination of minimal residual disease in leukaemia patients. Br J Haematol 121(6):823–838

Campana D, Coustan-Smith E (2004) Minimal residual disease studies by flow cytometry in acute leukemia. Acta Haematol 112(1–2):8–15

Capizzi RL, Powell BL (1987) Sequential high-dose ara-C and asparaginase versus high-dose ara-C alone in the treatment of patients with relapsed and refractory acute leukemias. Semin Oncol 14(2 Suppl 1):40–50

Capizzi RL, Davis R et al (1988) Synergy between high-dose cytarabine and asparaginase in the treatment of adults with refractory and relapsed acute myelogenous leukemia – a Cancer and Leukemia Group B study. J Clin Oncol 6(3):499–508

Cassileth PA, Harrington DP et al (1998) Chemotherapy compared with autologous or allogeneic bone marrow transplantation in the management of acute myeloid leukemia in first remission. N Engl J Med 339(23):1649–1656

Cazzaniga G, Dell'Oro MG et al (2005) Nucleophosmin mutations in childhood acute myelogenous leukemia with normal karyotype. Blood 106(4):1419–1422

Chard RL, Finklestein JZ et al (1978) Increased survival in childhood acute nonlymphocytic leukemia after treatment with prednisone, cytosine arabinoside, 6-thioguanine, cyclophosphamide, and oncovin (PATCO) combination chemotherapy. Med Pediatr Oncol 4(3):263–273

Cornelissen JJ, van Putten WL et al (2007) Results of a HOVON/SAKK donor versus no-donor analysis of myeloablative HLA-identical sibling stem cell transplantation in first remission acute myeloid leukemia in young and middle-aged adults: benefits for whom? Blood 109(9):3658–3666

Coustan-Smith E, Ribeiro RC et al (2003) Clinical significance of residual disease during treatment in childhood acute myeloid leukaemia. Br J Haematol 123(2):243–252

Craze JL, Harrison G et al (1999) Improved outcome of acute myeloid leukaemia in Down's syndrome. Arch Dis Child 81(1):32–37

Creutzig U, Reinhardt D (2002) Current controversies: which patients with acute myeloid leukaemia should receive a bone marrow transplantation? – a European view. Br J Haematol 118(2):365–377

Creutzig U, Ritter J et al (1987) The childhood AML studies BFM-78 and -83: treatment results and risk factor analysis. Haematol Blood Transfus 30:71–75

Creutzig U, Ritter J et al (1990) Identification of two risk groups in childhood acute myelogenous leukemia after therapy intensification in study AML-BFM-83 as compared with study AML-BFM-78. AML-BFM Study Group. Blood 75(10):1932–1940

Creutzig U, Ritter J et al (1993) Does cranial irradiation reduce the risk for bone marrow relapse in acute myelogenous leukemia? Unexpected results of the Childhood Acute Myelogenous Leukemia Study BFM-87. J Clin Oncol 11(2):279–286

Creutzig U, Ritter J et al (1996) Myelodysplasia and acute myelogenous leukemia in Down's syndrome. A report of 40 children of the AML-BFM Study Group. Leukemia 10(11): 1677–1686

Creutzig U, Zimmermann M et al (1999) Definition of a standard-risk group in children with AML. Br J Haematol 104(3):630–639

Creutzig U, Reinhardt D et al (2001a) Intensive chemotherapy versus bone marrow transplantation in pediatric acute myeloid leukemia: a matter of controversies. Blood 97(11): 3671–3672

Creutzig U, Ritter J et al (2001b) Improved treatment results in high-risk pediatric acute myeloid leukemia patients after intensification with high-dose cytarabine and mitoxantrone: results of Study Acute Myeloid Leukemia-Berlin-Frankfurt-Munster 93. J Clin Oncol 19(10):2705–2713

Creutzig U, Reinhardt D et al (2005) AML patients with Down syndrome have a high cure rate with AML-BFM therapy with reduced dose intensity. Leukemia 19(8):1355–1360

Creutzig U, Zimmermann M et al (2006) Less toxicity by optimizing chemotherapy, but not by addition of granulocyte colony-stimulating factor in children and adolescents with acute myeloid leukemia: results of AML-BFM 98. J Clin Oncol24(27):4499–4506

Dahl GV, Kalwinsky DK et al (1990) Allogeneic bone marrow transplantation in a program of intensive sequential chemotherapy for children and young adults with acute nonlymphocytic leukemia in first remission. J Clin Oncol 8(2): 295–303

Dahl GV, Lacayo NJ et al (2000) Mitoxantrone, etoposide, and cyclosporine therapy in pediatric patients with recurrent or refractory acute myeloid leukemia. J Clin Oncol 18(9): 1867–1875

Dastugue N, Lafage-Pochitaloff M et al (2002) Cytogenetic profile of childhood and adult megakaryoblastic leukemia (M7): a study of the Groupe Francais de Cytogenetique Hematologique (GFCH). Blood 100(2):618–626

De Botton S, Dombret H et al (1998) Incidence, clinical features, and outcome of all trans-retinoic acid syndrome in 413 cases of newly diagnosed acute promyelocytic leukemia. The European APL Group. Blood 92(8):2712–2718

de Botton S, Chevret S et al (2003) Early onset of chemotherapy can reduce the incidence of ATRA syndrome in newly diagnosed acute promyelocytic leukemia (APL) with low white blood cell counts: results from APL 93 trial. Leukemia 17(2):339–342

de Botton S, Coiteux V et al (2004) Outcome of childhood acute promyelocytic leukemia with all-trans-retinoic acid and chemotherapy. J Clin Oncol 22(8):1404–1412

de Botton S, Sanz MA et al (2006) Extramedullary relapse in acute promyelocytic leukemia treated with all-trans retinoic acid and chemotherapy. Leukemia 20(1):35–41

Detourmignies L, Castaigne S et al (1992) Therapy-Related Acute Promyelocytic Leukemia – a Report on 16 Cases. J Clin Oncol 10(9):1430–1435

Dinndorf P, Bunin N (1995) Bone marrow transplantation for children with acute myelogenous leukemia. J Pediatr Hematol Oncol 17(3):211–224

Dinndorf PA, Andrews RG et al (1986) Expression of normal myeloid-associated antigens by acute leukemia cells. Blood 67(4):1048–1053

Diverio D, Rossi V et al (1998) Early detection of relapse by prospective reverse transcriptase-polymerase chain reaction analysis of the PML/RARalpha fusion gene in patients with acute promyelocytic leukemia enrolled in the GIMEMA-AIEOP multicenter "AIDA" trial. GIMEMA-AIEOP Multicenter "AIDA" Trial. Blood 92(3):784–789

Dohner K, Schlenk RF et al (2005) Mutant nucleophosmin (NPM1) predicts favorable prognosis in younger adults with acute myeloid leukemia and normal cytogenetics: interaction with other gene mutations. Blood 106(12): 3740–3746

Dohner H, Estey EH et al (2010) Diagnosis and management of acute myeloid leukemia in adults: recommendations from an international expert panel, on behalf of the European LeukemiaNet. Blood 115(3):453–474

Entz-Werle N, Suciu S et al (2005) Results of 58872 and 58921 trials in acute myeloblastic leukemia and relative value of chemotherapy vs allogeneic bone marrow transplantation in first complete remission: the EORTC Children Leukemia Group report. Leukemia 19(12):2072–2081

Estey E, Garcia-Manero G et al (2006) Use of all-trans retinoic acid plus arsenic trioxide as an alternative to chemotherapy in untreated acute promyelocytic leukemia. Blood 107(9): 3469–3473

Evans GD, Grimwade DJ (1999) Extramedullary disease in acute promyelocytic leukemia. Leuk Lymph 33(3–4): 219–229

Falini B, Mecucci C et al (2005) Cytoplasmic nucleophosmin in acute myelogenous leukemia with a normal karyotype. N Engl J Med 352(3):254–266

Fazi F, Travaglini L et al (2005) Retinoic acid targets DNA-methyltransferases and histone deacetylases during APL blast differentiation *in vitro* and *in vivo*. Oncogene 24(11): 1820–1830

Feig SA, Lampkin B et al (1993) Outcome of BMT during first complete remission of AML: a comparison of two sequential studies by the Children's Cancer Group. Bone Marrow Transplant12(1):65–71

Fenaux P, Chastang C et al (1999) A randomized comparison of all transretinoic acid (ATRA) followed by chemotherapy and ATRA plus chemotherapy and the role of maintenance therapy in newly diagnosed acute promyelocytic leukemia. Blood94(4):1192– 1200

Forestier E, Izraeli S et al (2008) Cytogenetic features of acute lymphoblastic and myeloid leukemias in pediatric patients with Down syndrome: an iBFM-SG study. Blood 111(3): 1575–1583

Frankel SR, Eardley A et al (1992) The "retinoic acid syndrome" in acute promyelocytic leukemia. Ann Intern Med 117(4): 292–296

Frost BM, Gustafsson G et al (2000) Cellular cytotoxic drug sensitivity in children with acute leukemia and Down's syndrome: an explanation to differences in clinical outcome? Leukemia 14(5):943–944

Gale RE, Hills R et al (2005) Relationship between FLT3 mutation status, biologic characteristics, and response to targeted therapy in acute promyelocytic leukemia. Blood 106(12): 3768–3776

Gale RE, Green C et al (2008) The impact of FLT3 internal tandem duplication mutant level, number, size, and interaction with NPM1 mutations in a large cohort of young adult patients with acute myeloid leukemia. Blood 111(5): 2776–2784

Gamis AS (2005) Acute myeloid leukemia and Down syndrome evolution of modern therapy – state of the art review. Pediatr Blood Cancer 44(1):13–20

Gamis AS, Woods WG et al (2003) Increased age at diagnosis has a significantly negative effect on outcome in children with Down syndrome and acute myeloid leukemia: a report from the Children's Cancer Group Study 2891. J Clin Oncol 21(18):3415–3422

Garderet L, Labopin M et al (2005) Hematopoietic stem cell transplantation for *de novo* acute megakaryocytic leukemia in first complete remission: a retrospective study of the European Group for Blood and Marrow Transplantation (EBMT). Blood 105(1):405–409

Ge Y, Stout ML et al (2005) GATA1, cytidine deaminase, and the high cure rate of Down syndrome children with acute megakaryocytic leukemia. J Natl Cancer Inst 97(3):226–231

George B, Mathews V et al (2004) Treatment of children with newly diagnosed acute promyelocytic leukemia with arsenic trioxide: a single center experience. Leukemia 18(10): 1587–1590

Ghavamzadeh A, Alimoghaddam K et al (2006) Treatment of acute promyelocytic leukemia with arsenic trioxide without ATRA and/or chemotherapy. Ann Oncol 17(1):131–134

Gibson BE, Wheatley K et al (2005) Treatment strategy and long-term results in paediatric patients treated in consecutive UK AML trials. Leukemia 19(12):2130–2138

Gilliland DG, Griffin JD (2002) The roles of FLT3 in hematopoiesis and leukemia. Blood 100(5):1532–1542

Girodon F, Favre B et al (2000) Immunophenotype of a transient myeloproliferative disorder in a newborn with trisomy 21. Cytometry42(2):118–122

Goemans BF, Zwaan CM et al (2005) Mutations in KIT and RAS are frequent events in pediatric core-binding factor acute myeloid leukemia. Leukemia 19(9): 1536–1542

Goemans BF, Tamminga RY et al (2008) Outcome for children with relapsed acute myeloid leukemia in the Netherlands following initial treatment between 1980 and 1998: survival after chemotherapy only? Haematologica 93(9): 1418–1420

Gregory J, Feusner J (2003) Acute promyelocytic leukaemia in children. Best Pract Res Clin Haematol 16(3):483–494

Grimwade D, Lo Coco F (2002) Acute promyelocytic leukemia: a model for the role of molecular diagnosis and residual disease monitoring in directing treatment approach in acute myeloid leukemia. Leukemia 16(10):1959–1973

Grimwade D, Walker H et al (1998) The importance of diagnostic cytogenetics on outcome in AML: analysis of 1, 612 patients entered into the MRC AML 10 trial. The Medical Research Council Adult and Children's Leukaemia Working Parties. Blood 92(7):2322 2333

Grimwade D, Biondi A et al (2000) Characterization of acute promyelocytic leukemia cases lacking the classic t(15;17): results of the European Working Party. Blood 96(4): 1297 1308

Grimwade D, Jovanovic JV et al (2009a) Prospective minimal residual disease monitoring to predict relapse of acute promyelocytic leukemia and to direct pre-emptive arsenic trioxide therapy. J Clin Oncol 27(22):3650–3658

Grimwade J, Hills R et al (2010) National Cancer Research Institute Adult Leukaemia Working Group. Refinement of cytogenetic classification in acute myeloid leukaemia :determination of prognostic significance of rare recurring chromosomal abnormalities among 5876 younger adult patients treated on United Kingdom Medical research Council trials. Blood116(3):354–365

Groet J, McElwaine S et al (2003) Acquired mutations in GATA1 in neonates with Down's syndrome with transient myeloid disorder. Lancet 361(9369):1617–1620

Hann IM, Stevens RF et al (1997) Randomized comparison of DAT versus ADE as induction chemotherapy in children and younger adults with acute myeloid leukemia. Results of the Medical Research Council's 10th AML trial (MRC AML10). Adult and Childhood Leukaemia Working

Parties of the Medical Research Council. Blood 89(7): 2311–2318
Harrison CJ, Hills RK et al (2010) Cytogenetics of childhood acute myeloid leukemia: United Kingdom Medical Research Council Treatment trials AML 10 and 12. J Clin Oncol. Jun 1;28(16):2674–81. Epub 2010 May 3
Hasle H, Clemmensen IH et al (2000) Risks of leukaemia and solid tumours in individuals with Down's syndrome. Lancet 355(9199):165–169
Hasle H, Alonzo TA et al (2007) Monosomy 7 and deletion 7q in children and adolescents with acute myeloid leukemia: an international retrospective study. Blood 109(11): 4641–4647
Hitzler JK, Cheung J et al (2003) GATA1 mutations in transient leukemia and acute megakaryoblastic leukemia of Down syndrome. Blood 101(11):4301–4304
Hollanda LM, Lima CS et al (2006) An inherited mutation leading to production of only the short isoform of GATA-1 is associated with impaired erythropoiesis. Nat Genet 38(7): 807–812
Horan JT, Alonzo TA et al (2008) Impact of disease risk on efficacy of matched related bone marrow transplantation for pediatric acute myeloid leukemia: the Children's Oncology Group. J Clin Oncol 26(35):5797–5801
Hubeek I, Stam RW et al (2005) The human equilibrative nucleoside transporter 1 mediates *in vitro* cytarabine sensitivity in childhood acute myeloid leukaemia. Br J Cancer 93(12): 1388–1394
Hurwitz CA, Schell MJ et al (1993) Adverse prognostic features in 251 children treated for acute myeloid leukemia. Med Pediatr Oncol 21(1):1–7
Karandikar NJ, Aquino DB et al (2001) Transient myeloproliferative disorder and acute myeloid leukemia in Down syndrome. An immunophenotypic analysis. Am J Clin Pathol 116(2):204–210
Kaspers GJ, Creutzig U (2005) Pediatric acute myeloid leukemia: international progress and future directions. Leukemia 19(12):2025–2029
Kaspers GLJ, Ravindranath Y (2005) Acute myeloid leukemia in children and adolescents. In: Degos L, Griffin JD, Linch DC, Lowenberg B (eds) Textbook of malignant haematology. London, Martin Dunitz, pp 617–632
Kaspers GJ, Zwaan CM (2007) Pediatric acute myeloid leukemia: towards high-quality cure of all patients. Haematologica 92(11):1519–1532
Kaspers GJL, Zimmermann M et al (2008) Prognostic significance of time to relapse in pediatric AML: results from the International Randomised Phase III Study Relapsed AML 2001/01. Blood (ASH Annu Meeting Abstracts) 112(11): 2976
Kaspers G, Gibson B et al (2009) Central nervous system involvement in relapsed acute promyelocytic leukemia. Pediatr Blood Cancer 53(2):235–236, author reply 237
Kell WJ, Burnett AK et al (2003) A feasibility study of simultaneous administration of gemtuzumab ozogamicin with intensive chemotherapy in induction and consolidation in younger patients with acute myeloid leukemia. Blood 102(13):4277–4283
Klusmann J-H, Creutzig U et al (2008) Treatment and prognostic impact of transient leukemia in neonates with Down syndrome. Blood 111(6):2991–2998
Klusmann J-H, Li Z et al (2010) miR-125b-2 is a potential oncomiR on human chromosome 21 in megakaryoblastic leukemia. Gene Dev 24(5):478–490
Knipp S, Gattermann N et al (2007) Arsenic in the cerebrospinal fluid of a patient receiving arsenic trioxide for relapsed acute promyelocytic leukemia with CNS involvement. Leuk Res 31(11):1585–1587
Kojima S, Sako M et al (2000) An effective chemotherapeutic regimen for acute myeloid leukemia and myelodysplastic syndrome in children with Down's syndrome. Leukemia 14(5):786–791
Kottaridis PD, Gale RE et al (2001) The presence of a FLT3 internal tandem duplication in patients with acute myeloid leukemia (AML) adds important prognostic information to cytogenetic risk group and response to the first cycle of chemotherapy: analysis of 854 patients from the United Kingdom Medical Research Council AML 10 and 12 trials. Blood98(6):1752–1759
Kremer LCM, van Dalen EC et al (2001) Anthracycline-induced clinical heart failure in a cohort of 607 children: long-term follow-up study. J Clin Oncol 19(1):191–196
Krishnan K, Ross CW et al (1994) Neural cell-adhesion molecule (CD 56)-positive, t(8;21) acute myeloid leukemia (AML, M-2) and granulocytic sarcoma. Ann Hematol 69(6):321–323
Krivit W, Good RA (1957) Simultaneous occurrence of mongolism and leukemia; report of a nationwide survey. AMA J Dis Child94(3):289–293
Kuerbitz SJ, Civin CI et al (1992) Expression of myeloid-associated and lymphoid-associated cell-surface antigens in acute myeloid leukemia of childhood: a Pediatric Oncology Group study. J Clin Oncol 10(9):1419–1429
Lange B (2000) The management of neoplastic disorders of haematopoiesis in children with Down's syndrome. Br J Haematol110(3):512–524
Lange BJ, Kobrinsky N et al (1998) Distinctive demography, biology, and outcome of acute myeloid leukemia and myelodysplastic syndrome in children with Down syndrome: Children's Cancer Group Studies 2861 and 2891. Blood 91(2):608–615
Lange BJ, Smith FO et al (2008) Outcomes in CCG-2961, a children's oncology group phase 3 trial for untreated pediatric acute myeloid leukemia: a report from the children's oncology group. Blood 111(3):1044–1053
Langebrake C, Creutzig U et al (2005) Immunophenotype of Down syndrome acute myeloid leukemia and transient myeloproliferative disease differs significantly from other diseases with morphologically identical or similar blasts. Klin Padiatr 217(3):126–134
Langebrake C, Creutzig U et al (2006) Residual disease monitoring in childhood acute myeloid leukemia by multiparameter flow cytometry: the MRD-AML-BFM Study Group. J Clin Oncol 24(22):3686–3692
Lie SO, Jonmundsson G et al (1996) A population-based study of 272 children with acute myeloid leukaemia treated on two consecutive protocols with different intensity: best outcome in girls, infants, and children with Down's syndrome. Nordic Society of Paediatric Haematology and Oncology (NOPHO). Br J Haematol 94(1):82–88
Lie SO, Abrahamsson J et al (2003) Treatment stratification based on initial *in vivo* response in acute myeloid leukaemia in children without Down's syndrome: results of NOPHO-AML trials. Br J Haematol 122(2):217–225
Lie SO, Abrahamsson J et al (2005) Long-term results in children with AML: NOPHO-AML Study Group – report of three consecutive trials. Leukemia 19(12): 2090–2100

Lo Coco F, Avvisati G et al (2004) Front-line treatment of acute promyelocytic leukemia with AIDA induction followed by risk-adapted consolidation: results of the AIDA-2000 trial of the Italian GIMEMA Group. ASH Annu Meeting Abstracts 104(11):392

Lo Coco F, Ammatuna E et al (2007) Current treatment of acute promyelocytic leukemia. Haematologica 92(3): 289–291

Lowenberg B, Downing JR et al (1999) Acute myeloid leukemia. N Engl J Med 341(14):1051–1062

Malinge S, Izraeli S et al (2009) Insights into the manifestations, outcomes, and mechanisms of leukemogenesis in Down syndrome. Blood 113(12):2619–2628

Mandelli F, Diverio D et al (1997) Molecular remission in PML/RAR alpha-positive acute promyelocytic leukemia by combined all-trans retinoic acid and Idarubicin (AIDA) therapy. Blood90(3):1014–1021

Mann G, Reinhardt D et al (2001) Treatment with all-trans retinoic acid in acute promyelocytic leukemia reduces early deaths in children. Ann Hematol 80(7):417–422

Marcucci G, Mrozek K et al (2005) Prognostic factors and outcome of core binding factor acute myeloid leukemia patients with t(8;21) differ from those of patients with inv(16): a Cancer and Leukemia Group B study. J Clin Oncol 23(24): 5705–5717

Massey GV, Zipursky A et al (2006) A prospective study of the natural history of transient leukemia (TL) in neonates with Down syndrome (DS): Children's Oncology Group (COG) study POG-9481. Blood 107(12):4606–4613

Mead AJ, Linch DC et al (2007) FLT3 tyrosine kinase domain mutations are biologically distinct from and have a significantly more favorable prognosis than FLT3 internal tandem duplications in patients with acute myeloid leukemia. Blood 110(4):1262–1270

Meshinchi S, Woods WG et al (2001) Prevalence and prognostic significance of Flt3 internal tandem duplication in pediatric acute myeloid leukemia. Blood 97(1):89–94

Meshinchi S, Stirewalt DL et al (2003) Activating mutations of RTK/ras signal transduction pathway in pediatric acute myeloid leukemia. Blood 102(4):1474–1479

Meshinchi S, Alonzo TA et al (2006) Clinical implications of FLT3 mutations in pediatric AML. Blood 108(12): 3654–3661

Michel G, Baruchel A et al (1996) Induction chemotherapy followed by allogeneic bone marrow transplantation or aggressive consolidation chemotherapy in childhood acute myeloblastic leukemia. A prospective study from the French Society of Pediatric Hematology and Immunology (SHIP). Hematol Cell Ther 38(2): 169–176

Mikkola HKA, Radu CG et al (2010) Targeting leukemia stem cells. Nat Biotech 28(3):237–238

Milligan DW, Grimwade D et al (2006) Guidelines on the management of acute myeloid leukaemia in adults. Br J Haematol 135(4):450–474

Mistry AR, Pedersen EW et al (2003) The molecular pathogenesis of acute promyelocytic leukaemia: implications for the clinical management of the disease. Blood Rev 17(2):71–97

Mrozek K, Marcucci G et al (2007) Clinical relevance of mutations and gene-expression changes in adult acute myeloid leukemia with normal cytogenetics: are we ready for a prognostically prioritized molecular classification? Blood 109(2):431–448

Mundschau G, Gurbuxani S et al (2003) Mutagenesis of GATA1 is an initiating event in Down syndrome leukemogenesis. Blood101(11):4298–4300

Muramatsu H, Kato K et al (2008) Risk factors for early death in neonates with Down syndrome and transient leukaemia. Br J Haematol142(4):610–615

Nesbit ME Jr, Buckley JD et al (1994) Chemotherapy for induction of remission of childhood acute myeloid leukemia followed by marrow transplantation or multiagent chemotherapy: a report from the Childrens Cancer Group. J Clin Oncol 12(1):127–135

Niu C, Yan H et al (1999) Studies on treatment of acute promyelocytic leukemia with arsenic trioxide: remission induction, follow-up, and molecular monitoring in 11 newly diagnosed and 47 relapsed acute promyelocytic leukemia patients. Blood94(10):3315–3324

O'Brien TA, Russell SJ et al (2002) Results of consecutive trials for children newly diagnosed with acute myeloid leukemia from the Australian and New Zealand Children's Cancer Study Group. Blood 100(8):2708–2716

O'Brien MM, Taub JW et al (2008) Cardiomyopathy in children with Down syndrome treated for acute myeloid leukemia: a report from the Children's Oncology Group Study POG 9421. J Clin Oncol 26(3):414–420

Orfao A, Chillon M et al (1999) The flow cytometric pattern of CD34, CD15 and CD13 expression in acute myeloblastic leukemia is highly characteristic of the presence of PML-RARalpha gene rearrangements. Haematologica 84(5): 405–412

Ortega JJ, Madero L et al (2005) Treatment with all-trans retinoic acid and anthracycline mono chemotherapy for children with acute promyelocytic leukemia: a multicenter study by the PETHEMA group. J Clin Oncol 23(30):7632–7640

Paschka P, Marcucci G et al (2006) Adverse prognostic significance of KIT mutations in adult acute myeloid leukemia with inv(16) and t(8;21): a Cancer and Leukemia Group B Study. J Clin Oncol 24(24):3904–3911

Paschka P, Marcucci G et al (2008) Wilms' tumor 1 gene mutations independently predict poor outcome in adults with cytogenetically normal acute myeloid leukemia: a cancer and leukemia group B study. J Clin Oncol 26(28): 4595–4602

Perel Y, Auvrignon A et al (2002) Impact of addition of maintenance therapy to intensive induction and consolidation chemotherapy for childhood acute myeloblastic leukemia: results of a prospective randomized trial, LAME 89/91. Leucamie Aique Myeloide Enfant. J Clin Oncol 20(12): 2774–2782

Perel Y, Auvrignon A et al (2005) Treatment of childhood acute myeloblastic leukemia: dose intensification improves outcome and maintenance therapy is of no benefit – multicenter studies of the French LAME (Leucemie Aigue Myeloblastique Enfant) Cooperative Group. Leukemia 19(12):2082–2089

Powell BL (2007) Effect of consolidation with arsenic trioxide (As_2O_3) on event-free survival (EFS) and overall survival (OS) among patients with newly diagnosed acute promyelocytic leukemia (APL): North American Intergroup Protocol C9710. ASCO Meeting Abstracts 25(18 Suppl):2

Pui CH (1995) Childhood leukemias. N Engl J Med 332(24): 1618–1630

Pui MH, Fletcher BD et al (1994) Granulocytic sarcoma in childhood leukemia: imaging features. Radiology 190(3): 698–702

Pui CH, Schrappe M et al (2004) Childhood and adolescent lymphoid and myeloid leukemia. Hematol Am Soc Hematol Educ Program 2004(1):118–145

Raimondi SC, Chang MN et al (1999) Chromosomal abnormalities in 478 children with acute myeloid leukemia: clinical characteristics and treatment outcome in a cooperative pediatric oncology group study-POG 8821. Blood 94(11): 3707–3716

Rainis L, Bercovich D et al (2003) Mutations in exon 2 of GATA1 are early events in megakaryocytic malignancies associated with trisomy 21. Blood 102(3):981–986

Rao A, Hills RK et al (2006) Treatment for myeloid leukaemia of Down syndrome: population-based experience in the UK and results from the Medical Research Council AML 10 and AML 12 trials. Br J Haematol 132(5):576–583

Ravandi F, Estey E et al (2009) Effective treatment of acute promyelocytic leukemia with all-trans-retinoic acid, arsenic trioxide, and gemtuzumab ozogamicin. J Clin Oncol 27(4): 504–510

Ravindranath Y, Steuber CP et al (1991) High-dose cytarabine for intensification of early therapy of childhood acute myeloid leukemia: a Pediatric Oncology Group study. J Clin Oncol9(4):572–580

Ravindranath Y, Abella E et al (1992) Acute myeloid leukemia (AML) in Down's syndrome is highly responsive to chemotherapy: experience on Pediatric Oncology Group AML Study 8498. Blood 80(9):2210–2214

Ravindranath Y, Yeager AM et al (1996) Autologous bone marrow transplantation versus intensive consolidation chemotherapy for acute myeloid leukemia in childhood. Pediatric Oncology Group. N Engl J Med 334(22):1428–1434

Razzouk BI, Estey E et al (2006) Impact of age on outcome of pediatric acute myeloid leukemia: a report from 2 institutions. Cancer 106(11):2495–2502

Reinhardt D, Diekamp S et al (2005) Acute megakaryoblastic leukemia in children and adolescents, excluding Down's syndrome: improved outcome with intensified induction treatment. Leukemia 19(8):1495–1496

Reinhardt D, Kremens B et al (2006) No improvement of overall-survival in children with high-risk acute myeloid leukemia by stem cell transplantation in 1st complete remission. ASH Annu Meeting Abstracts 108(11):320

Ribeiro RC, Razzouk BI et al (2005) Successive clinical trials for childhood acute myeloid leukemia at St Jude Children's Research Hospital, from 1980 to 2000. Leukemia 19(12): 2125–2129

Roy A, Roberts I et al (2009) Acute megakaryoblastic leukaemia (AMKL) and transient myeloproliferative disorder (TMD) in Down syndrome: a multi-step model of myeloid leukaemogenesis. Br J Haematol 147(1):3–12

Rubnitz JE, Raimondi SC et al (2002) Favorable impact of the t(9;11) in childhood acute myeloid leukemia. J Clin Oncol 20(9):2302–2309

Saito Y, Uchida N et al (2010) Induction of cell cycle entry eliminates human leukemia stem cells in a mouse model of AML. Nat Biotech 28(3):275–280

Sanz MA, Lo Coco F et al (2000) Definition of relapse risk and role of nonanthracycline drugs for consolidation in patients with acute promyelocytic leukemia: a joint study of the PETHEMA and GIMEMA cooperative groups. Blood 96(4): 1247–1253

Sanz MA, Martin G et al (2003) Choice of chemotherapy in induction, consolidation and maintenance in acute promyelocytic leukaemia. Best Pract Res Clin Haematol 16(3):433–451

Sanz MA, Martin G et al (2004) Risk-adapted treatment of acute promyelocytic leukemia with all-trans-retinoic acid and anthracycline monochemotherapy: a multicenter study by the PETHEMA group. Blood 103(4):1237–1243

Sanz MA, Labopin M et al (2007) Hematopoietic stem cell transplantation for adults with acute promyelocytic leukemia in the ATRA era: a survey of the European Cooperative Group for Blood and Marrow Transplantation. Bone Marrow Transplant39(8):461–469

Sanz MA, Grimwade D et al (2009) Management of acute promyelocytic leukemia: recommendations from an expert panel on behalf of the European LeukemiaNet. Blood 113(9):1875–1891

Schlenk RF, Dohner K (2009) Impact of new prognostic markers in treatment decisions in acute myeloid leukemia. Curr Opin Hematol16(2):98–104

Schlenk RF, Dohner K et al (2008) Mutations and treatment outcome in cytogenetically normal acute myeloid leukemia. N Engl J Med 358(18):1909–1918

Schnittger S, Kohl TM et al (2006) KIT-D816 mutations in AML1-ETO-positive AML are associated with impaired event-free and overall survival. Blood 107(5):1791–1799

Scholl S, Fricke HJ et al (2009) Clinical implications of molecular genetic aberrations in acute myeloid leukemia. J Cancer Res Clin Oncol 135(4):491–505

Shen ZX, Shi ZZ et al (2004) All-trans retinoic acid/As2O3 combination yields a high quality remission and survival in newly diagnosed acute promyelocytic leukemia. Proc Natl Acad Sci USA 101(15):5328–5335

Shimada A, Xu G et al (2004) Fetal origin of the GATA1 mutation in identical twins with transient myeloproliferative disorder and acute megakaryoblastic leukemia accompanying Down syndrome. Blood 103(1):366

Shimada A, Taki T et al (2006) KIT mutations, and not FLT3 internal tandem duplication, are strongly associated with a poor prognosis in pediatric acute myeloid leukemia with t(8;21): a study of the Japanese Childhood AML Cooperative Study Group. Blood 107(5):1806–1809

Sievers EL, Lange BJ et al (2003) Immunophenotypic evidence of leukemia after induction therapy predicts relapse: results from a prospective Children's Cancer Group study of 252 patients with acute myeloid leukemia. Blood 101(9): 3398–3406

Smith FO, Lampkin BC et al (1992) Expression of lymphoid-associated cell surface antigens by childhood acute myeloid leukemia cells lacks prognostic significance. Blood 79(9): 2415–2422

Soignet SL, Frankel SR et al (2001) United States multicenter study of arsenic trioxide in relapsed acute promyelocytic leukemia. J Clin Oncol 19(18):3852–3860

Specchia G, Lo Coco F et al (2001) Extramedullary involvement at relapse in acute promyelocytic leukemia patients treated or not with all-trans retinoic acid: a report by the Gruppo Italiano Malattie Ematologiche dell'Adulto. J Clin Oncol 19(20):4023–4028

Stahnke K, Boos J et al (1998) Duration of first remission predicts remission rates and long-term survival in children with relapsed acute myelogenous leukemia. Leukemia 12(10): 1534–1538

Steuber CP, Culbert SJ et al (1990) Therapy of childhood acute nonlymphocytic leukemia: the Pediatric Oncology Group experience (1977–1988). Haematol Blood Transfus 33: 198–209

Steuber CP, Civin C et al (1991) A comparison of induction and maintenance therapy for acute nonlymphocytic leukemia in childhood: results of a Pediatric Oncology Group study. J Clin Oncol 9(2):247–258

Stevens RF, Hann IM et al (1998) Marked improvements in outcome with chemotherapy alone in paediatric acute myeloid leukemia: results of the United Kingdom Medical Research Council's 10th AML trial. MRC Childhood Leukaemia Working Party. Br J Haematol 101(1):130–140

Tallman MS (2007) Treatment of relapsed or refractory acute promyelocytic leukemia. Best Pract Res Clin Haematol 20(1):57–65

Tallman MS, Hakimian D et al (1993) Granulocytic sarcoma is associated with the 8;21 translocation in acute myeloid leukemia. J Clin Oncol 11(4):690–697

Tallman MS, Andersen JW et al (1997) All-trans-retinoic acid in acute promyelocytic leukemia. N Engl J Med 337(15): 1021–1028

Taub JW, Ge Y (2005) Down syndrome, drug metabolism and chromosome 21. Pediatr Blood Cancer 44(1):33–39

Taub JW, Huang X et al (1999) Expression of chromosome 21-localized genes in acute myeloid leukemia: differences between Down syndrome and non-Down syndrome blast cells and relationship to *in vitro* sensitivity to cytosine arabinoside and daunorubicin. Blood 94(4):1393–1400

Testi AM, Biondi A et al (2005) GIMEMA-AIEOP AIDA protocol for the treatment of newly diagnosed acute promyelocytic leukemia (APL) in children. Blood 106(2):447–453

Thiede C, Steudel C et al (2002) Analysis of FLT3-activating mutations in 979 patients with acute myelogenous leukemia: association with FAB subtypes and identification of subgroups with poor prognosis. Blood 99(12):4326–4335

Thiede C, Koch S et al (2006) Prevalence and prognostic impact of NPM1 mutations in 1485 adult patients with acute myeloid leukemia (AML). Blood 107(10):4011–4020

Tomizawa D, Tabuchi K et al (2007) Repetitive cycles of high-dose cytarabine are effective for childhood acute myeloid leukemia: long-term outcome of the children with AML treated on two consecutive trials of Tokyo Children's Cancer Study Group. Pediatr Blood Cancer 49(2):127–132

Tsukimoto I, Tawa A et al (2009) Risk-stratified therapy and the intensive use of cytarabine improves the outcome in childhood acute myeloid leukemia: the AML99 trial from the Japanese Childhood AML Cooperative Study Group. J Clin Oncol27(24):4007–4013

Vardiman JW, Harris NL et al (2002) The World Health Organization (WHO) classification of the myeloid neoplasms. Blood 100(7):2292–2302

Vardiman JW, Thiele J et al (2009) The 2008 revision of the World Health Organization (WHO) classification of myeloid neoplasms and acute leukemia: rationale and important changes. Blood 114(5):937–951

Vaughan W, Karp J et al (1984) Two-cycle timed-sequential chemotherapy for adult acute nonlymphocytic leukemia. Blood 64(5):975–980

Vicente D, Lamparelli T et al (2007) Improved outcome in young adults with *de novo* acute myeloid leukemia in first remission, undergoing an allogeneic bone marrow transplant. Bone Marrow Transplant 40(4):349–354

Webb DK, Wheatley K et al (1999) Outcome for children with relapsed acute myeloid leukaemia following initial therapy in the Medical Research Council (MRC) AML 10 trial. MRC Childhood Leukaemia Working Party. Leukemia 13(1):25–31

Wechsler J, Greene M et al (2002) Acquired mutations in GATA1 in the megakaryoblastic leukemia of Down syndrome. Nat Genet32(1):148–152

Weick JK, Kopecky KJ et al (1996) A randomized investigation of high-dose versus standard-dose cytosine arabinoside with daunorubicin in patients with previously untreated acute myeloid leukemia: a Southwest Oncology Group study. Blood88(8):2841–2851

Weinstein HJ, Mayer RJ et al (1980) Treatment of acute myelogenous leukemia in children and adults. N Engl J Med 303(9):473–478

Wells R, Woods W et al (1994a) Treatment of newly diagnosed children and adolescents with acute myeloid leukemia: a Childrens Cancer Group study. J Clin Oncol 12(11): 2367–2377

Wells RJ, Odom LF et al (1994b) Cytosine arabinoside and mitoxantrone treatment of relapsed or refractory childhood leukemia: initial response and relationship to multidrug resistance gene 1. Med Pediatr Oncol 22(4):244–249

Wheatley K (2002) Current controversies: which patients with acute myeloid leukaemia should receive a bone marrow transplantation? A statistician's view. Br J Haematol 118(2):351–356

Wheatley K, Burnett AK et al (1999) A simple, robust, validated and highly predictive index for the determination of risk-directed therapy in acute myeloid leukaemia derived from the MRC AML 10 trial. United Kingdom Medical Research Council's Adult and Childhood Leukaemia Working Parties. Br J Haematol 107(1):69–79

Whitman SP, Archer KJ et al (2001) Absence of the wild-type allele predicts poor prognosis in adult *de novo* acute myeloid leukemia with normal cytogenetics and the internal tandem duplication of FLT3: a cancer and leukemia group B study. Cancer Res 61(19):7233–7239

Woods WG, Ruymann FB et al (1990) The role of timing of high-dose cytosine arabinoside intensification and of maintenance therapy in the treatment of children with acute nonlymphocytic leukemia. Cancer 66(6):1106–1113

Woods WG, Kobrinsky N et al (1996) Timed-sequential induction therapy improves postremission outcome in acute myeloid leukemia: a report from the Children's Cancer Group. Blood87(12):4979–4989

Woods WG, Neudorf S et al (2001) A comparison of allogeneic bone marrow transplantation, autologous bone marrow transplantation, and aggressive chemotherapy in children with acute myeloid leukemia in remission: a report from the Children's Cancer Group. Blood 97(1):56–62

Wouters BJ, Lowenberg B et al (2009) Double CEBPA mutations, but not single CEBPA mutations, define a subgroup of acute myeloid leukemia with a distinctive gene expression

profile that is uniquely associated with a favorable outcome. Blood113(13):3088–3091
Xu G, Nagano M et al (2003) Frequent mutations in the GATA-1 gene in the transient myeloproliferative disorder of Down syndrome. Blood 102(8):2960–2968
Yates JW, Wallace HJ Jr et al (1973) Cytosine arabinoside (NSC-63878) and daunorubicin (NSC-83142) therapy in acute non-lymphocytic leukemia. Cancer Chemother Rep 57(4):485–488
Yates J, Glidewell O et al (1982) Cytosine arabinoside with daunorubicin or adriamycin for therapy of acute myelocytic leukemia: a CALGB study. Blood 60(2):454–462
Yumura-Yagi K, Hara J et al (1992) Mixed phenotype of blasts in acute megakaryocytic leukaemia and transient abnormal myelopoiesis in Down's syndrome. Br J Haematol 81(4): 520–525
Zeller B, Gustafsson G et al (2005) Acute leukaemia in children with Down syndrome: a population-based Nordic study. Br J Haematol128(6):797–804
Zipursky A (2003) Transient leukaemia – a benign form of leukaemia in newborn infants with trisomy 21. Br J Haematol 120(6):930–938
Zipursky A, Thorner P et al (1994) Myelodysplasia and acute megakaryoblastic leukemia in Down's syndrome. Leuk Res 18(3):163–171
Zwaan CM, Kaspers GJL (2004) Possibilities for tailored and targeted therapy in paediatric acute myeloid leukaemia. Br J Haematol127(3):264–279
Zwaan CM, Kaspers GJ et al (2002) Different drug sensitivity profiles of acute myeloid and lymphoblastic leukemia and normal peripheral blood mononuclear cells in children with and without Down syndrome. Blood 99(1):245–251
Zwaan CM, Meshinchi S et al (2003a) FLT3 internal tandem duplication in 234 children with acute myeloid leukemia: prognostic significance and relation to cellular drug resistance. Blood 102(7):2387–2394
Zwaan CM, Reinhardt D et al (2003b) Gemtuzumab ozogamicin: first clinical experiences in children with relapsed/ refractory acute myeloid leukemia treated on compassionate-useba sis.B lood101(10):3868–3871

Part IV

The Impact of Pharmacogenetics and Pharmacogenomics on Childhood Leukemia

Pharmacogenetic and Pharmacogenomic Considerations in the Biology and Treatmento fC hildhoodL eukemia

6

Jun J. Yang, Parinda A. Mehta, Mary V. Relling, and Stella M. Davies

Contents

J.J. Yang
St. Jude Children's Research Hospital
262 DannyThoma sPl ace
Memphis, TN38105
e-mail:j un.yang@stjude.org

P.A.M etha
Division of Bone Marrow Transplantation and Immune Deficiency, Cancer and Blood Diseases Institute, Cincinnati Children'sH ospitalM edicalC enter, 3333B urnetA venue
Cincinnati Ohio45229- 3039
e-mail:pa rinda.mehta@cchmc.org

M.V.R elling (✉)
St. Jude Children's Research Hospital
Pharmaceutical Sciences, 262 Danny Thomas Place, MS313 , Memphis, TN38105- 3678, USA
e-mail:ma ry.relling@stjude.org

S.M.D avies
Division of Bone Marrow Transplantation and Immune Deficiency, Cancer and Blood Diseases Institute, Cincinnati Children's Hospital Medical Center, 3333 Burnet Avenue, CHRF-2323, Cincinnati,O H45229 , USA
e-mail:s tella.davies@cchmc.org

6.1 Concepto fPhar macogenetics and Pharmacogenomics

Pharmacogenetics and pharmacogenomics refer to the study of the genetic basis for variation in drug response. Pharmacogenomics agnostically surveys the entire genome for genetic factors affecting response to medication, while pharmacogenetics primarily focuses on a handful of genomic loci based on prior knowledge. Still rapidly evolving, pharmacogenetics and pharmacogenomics have already significantly changed many fields of medicine. Thus, genetic variation has been implicated in drug efficacy (e.g., *CYP2D6* and tamoxifen in breast cancer [Hoskins et al. 2009], *CYP2C19* and clopidogrel in platelet aggregation [Shuldiner et al. 2009; Simon et al. 2009]), and toxicity (e.g., *TPMT* and 6-mercaptopurine-related myelosuppression (Relling et al. 1999b), *CYP2C9* and warfarin-induced bleeding (International Warfarin Pharmacogenetics et al. 2009), *HLA-B*5701* and flucloxacillin-induced liver damage (Daly et al. 2009).

6.1.1 Types of Genetic Variations

Genetic variations can be either inherited (germline polymorphisms) or acquired (somatic mutations). Common forms of inherited genetic variations include sequence

G.H. Reaman and F.O. Smith (eds.), *Childhood Leukemia*,
DOI: 10.1007/978-3-642-13781-5_6, © Springer-Verlag Berlin Heidelberg 2011

variations such as single-nucleotide polymorphisms (SNPs; a single base difference in DNA sequence among individuals), genomic insertions and deletions (gain or loss of short segments of sequence in the genome of an individual, usually less than 100 base pairs), and structural variations such as copy number variants (gain or loss of large segments of sequence in the genome of an individual, inversions, or translocations). Genetic changes in tumors are more frequent and more commonly include functionally deleterious sequence and structural variations, and may also include aneuploidy and uniparental disomy (deletion of one copy of a chromosomal segment followed by duplication of the remaining copy).

The most common type of germline sequence variations are SNPs. There are 17.8 million SNPs deposited in dbSNP (http://www.ncbi.nlm.nih.gov/projects/SNP/), the central SNP repository maintained by the National Institutes of Health, through submission by individual investigators as well as large-scale genetic variation discovery consortia (e.g., International HapMap project; www.hapmap.org). Recent advances in high-throughput parallel sequencing technology (next generation sequencing) have inaugurated an era of genomics in which complete sequencing of individual human genomes can be accomplished with fewer resources (2 months with $3 million) compared to when the Human Genome Project was conducted (10 years and $3 billion). Complete sequences of a handful of human genomes determined by next generation sequencing confirm that the total number of SNPs in any individual genome is approximately three to four million, 30% of which are unique to the individual of interest (private SNPs) (Ley et al. 2008; Wang et al. 2008; Wheeler et al. 2008). On average, only 0.2% of SNPs are considered deleterious (resulting in change in amino acid sequence nonsynonymous). It should be noted that SNPs can also affect gene function by regulating transcription activity (*UGT1A1*28* promoter SNPs) (Fisher et al. 2000), mRNA stability and microRNA binding (*DHFR 3′UTR* SNP) (Mishra et al. 2007), translation efficiency and protein folding (*ABCB1 C3435T*) (Kimchi-Sarfaty et al. 2007).

Another common form of inherited polymorphism is copy number variation (CNV), which has received increasing attention in recent years. It is estimated that up to 12% of human genome is subject to CNV, and the resultant alterations in gene dosage and expression have been implicated in disease predisposition and progression (Ouahchi et al. 2006; Wain et al. 2009). Copy number changes can also occur in drug target and drug metabolizing genes, and are therefore important subjects of pharmacogenetic and pharmacogenomic studies. For instance, the epidermal growth factor receptor (*EGFR*) gene copy number is predictive of clinical response to EGFR antibodies (cetuximab) or small molecule inhibitors (gefitinib) (Hirsch et al. 2009). Copy number variation in the glutathione transferase genes is also well documented, with 50% and 20% of the Caucasian population affected by the *GSTM1* and *GSTT1* deletions, respectively (Moyer et al. 2007, 2008). *CYP2D6* deletion (*CYP2D6*5*) and duplication (*CYP2D6×2*) are observed in 5.1% and 7.2% of the Caucasian population, respectively (Ledesma and Agundez 2005).

6.1.2 Phenotype–Genotype Relationships and Goals of Pharmacogenetics and Pharmacogenomics

Drug response phenotypes can be largely classified as drug efficacy and drug toxicity. Efficacy phenotypes can be clinical response such as minimal residual disease (MRD), risk of relapse, or primary tumor cell *in vitro* sensitivity to antileukemic agents. Identification of patients who are likely or unlikely to benefit from a particular therapy will allow clinicians to design more effective and individualized treatment. Another important type of phenotypic trait is drug-related toxicity. In pediatric leukemia therapy, patients are treated for an extended period of time with intense chemotherapeutic drugs, many of which are associated with serious adverse effects. Because of the developmental stage of this patient population, some toxicities of leukemia therapy have prolonged negative impacts. For instance, a fraction of children who receive etoposide as acute lymphoblastic leukemia (ALL) therapy also go on to develop secondary cancer (therapy-induced acute myeloid leukemia [AML]) (Pui 1991), to which most patients succumb. Therefore, a single chemotherapeutic agent can manifest side effects in multiple forms and the underlying mechanisms as well as genetic basis can be distinct. Another type of phenotype of interest in pharmacogenetics and pharmacogenomics is the pharmacologic properties of the drug, such as variability in plasma clearance (e.g., pharmacokinetics of methotrexate (MTX)) and metabolism/activation of a drug (e.g., leukemia intracellular accumulation of MTX polyglutamates). Such pharmacologic variability can contribute to the variability in clinical response or toxicity. While systemic drug disposition and drug

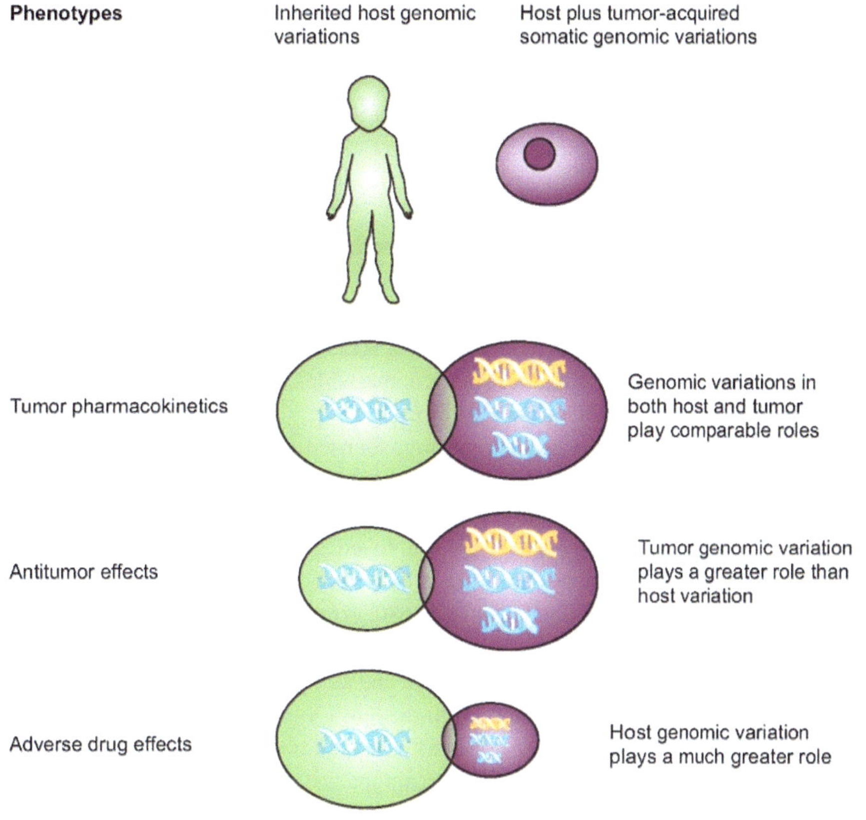

Fig. 6.1 Bothinhe ritedhos t (constitutional) genomic variations (green circles) and somatically acquired genomic variation specific to the leukemic cells (purple circles) can affect phenotypes of interest in children with leukemia

toxicities are more likely associated with germline genetic variations, tumor response is determined by genetic factors of both host and tumor (Fig. 6.1).

There are multiple goals of pharmacogenetics and pharmacogenomics. Genetic variations associated with clinically relevant phenotypes with sufficient intergenotype differences (large odds ratios between risk allele carriers and noncarriers) can be utilized to direct dosing, and/or choice of specific medications. Although much interpatient variability in pharmacokinetics and dynamics is due to inherited variation, if each genetic polymorphism associated with drug response has only a small effect size, these variants will be unlikely to be amenable for clinical application. Even for drugs for which response variability is highly inheritable, the possibility exists that multiple genetic variations contribute to efficacy/toxicity, each with a relatively moderate effect. Such pharmacogenetic and pharmacogenomic results are still valuable in better understanding the biology and pharmacology of the drug, although they may not be useful for patient care decisions.

6.2 AcuteL ymphoblasticL eukemia

ALL is the most common type of cancer in children with 3,500 new cases every year in the US (Pui and Evans 2006). The use of combination chemotherapy to cure ALL in children has emerged as a paradigm for treating disseminated cancers (Simone 1979, 2003). Similarly, elucidation of the pharmacogenomics of ALL and its translation to clinic practice has clearly exemplified the value of pharmacogenomics in optimizing pharmacotherapy of human cancers and non-malignant conditions in general (Cheok and Evans 2006).

6.2.1 Genetic Variations Related to Drug Efficacy

Although the overall cure rate of childhood ALL is approaching 90%, significant variability exists in response to ALL therapy, with some subtypes at a higher risk of relapse (Pui and Evans 2006). Clinical response to chemotherapy is most certainly multifactorial and is dictated by genetic factors of both host and tumor.

6.2.1.1 GeneticA berrationsi nT umorA ffecting Anti-leukemic Drugs

A remarkable feature of pharmacogenomics of ALL is the early and extensive utilization of genome-wide screening technology. While initial studies using DNA microarray-based gene expression profiling, focused on molecular classification of leukemia (AML vs ALL, T-cell vs B-cell ALL, genetic subtypes of ALL) (Yeoh et al. 2002), this technology was soon employed to identify genetic changes in the leukemia cells responsible for chemosensitivity. Interrogating 9,670 genes across the genome, Cheok et al. compared expression patterns in primary ALL cells sampled before and after exposure to four upfront treatments (high-dose MTX plus 6-mercaptopurine, low-dose MTX plus 6-mercaptopurine, high-dose MTX alone, and 6-mercaptopurine alone) (Cheok et al. 2003). Distinct gene expression signatures (up- or down-regulated following chemotherapy) were identified for each treatment regimen, suggesting highly specific cellular responses to each agent. Of note, only 14% of genes whose expression changed when these drugs were given as single agents also changed when they were given in combination; thus the effects of combination therapy are not simply the sum of effects of each single agent. Similar analyses of asparaginase-treated ALL patient samples revealed increased expression in tRNA synthetases, solute transporters and CCAAT/enhancer binding protein family members, reminiscent of effects of amino acid starvation(Fine e ta l. 2005).

Global gene expression patterns were also associated with *in vitro* sensitivity of primary ALL cells to antileukemic agents. Holleman et al. studied primary leukemia cells from 173 children with ALL for both gene expression profile and *in vitro* sensitivity to prednisolone, vincristine, asparaginase, and daunorubicin (Holleman et al. 2004). Distinct sets of genes were identified for association with sensitivity to each agent (Fig. 6.2), suggesting independent mechanisms of drug resistance. In a subsequent study, Lugthart et al. sought to characterize genetic determinants of *de novo* multiple drug cross-resistance of leukemia cells (Lugthart et al. 2005). *In vitro* sensitivity profiles were significantly correlated among chemotherapeutic agents (i.e., cases resistant to asparaginase were also resistant to prednisolone), and cross-resistance was less common in patients older than 10 years at diagnosis and in certain genetic subtypes of ALL (*TEL-AML1* or *E2A-PBX1*). Forty-five genes were identified as associated with cross-resistance to four mechanistically distinct antileukemic agents and this gene expression signature was also predictive of risk of relapse in two independent cohorts of patients with ALL. Of the 108 genes discriminating single drug resistance in the study by Holleman et al., only 15% were also among the genes discriminating cross-resistance, reflecting distinction between single drug and multiple drug resistance.

Efforts continue using gene expression profiling to identify genetic predictors of response to specific agents used in ALL. Sorich et al. studied the genome-wide gene expression pattern of 161 children with ALL and their *in vivo* response to an upfront MTX window therapy (Sorich et al. 2008). They described a 50-gene signature whose expression was significantly correlated with change in circulating leukemic blasts before and after MTX treatment; the signature included genes in the nucleotide biosynthesis pathway (thymidylate synthetase [*TYMS*], dihydrofolate reductase [*DHFR*], and CTP synthetase [*CTPS*]), which exhibited the strongest associations with MTX response. To characterize genetic determinants of tumor cell activation of MTX (i.e., polyglutamation), a recent genome-wide study comprehensively interrogated leukemia cell gene expression, somatic copy number alterations, and inherited SNPs genotypes (French et al. 2009); increased chromosome 18 copy number was predictive of MTX polyglutamate accumulation even after adjusting for hyperdiploidy.

There are genomic variations associated with resistance to glucocorticoids. A recent study by Real et al. demonstrated that expression of genes in the *NOTCH* pathway are important determinants of glucocorticoid sensitivity in T-cell ALL (Real et al. 2009). They elegantly showed that chemical blockade of the *NOTCH* pathway using a γ-secretase inhibitor effectively sensitized leukemia cells to dexamethasone by autoregulation of glucocorticoid receptor. In B-lineage ALL, Cheok et al. showed that components of the SWI/SNF chromatin-remodeling complex, important in

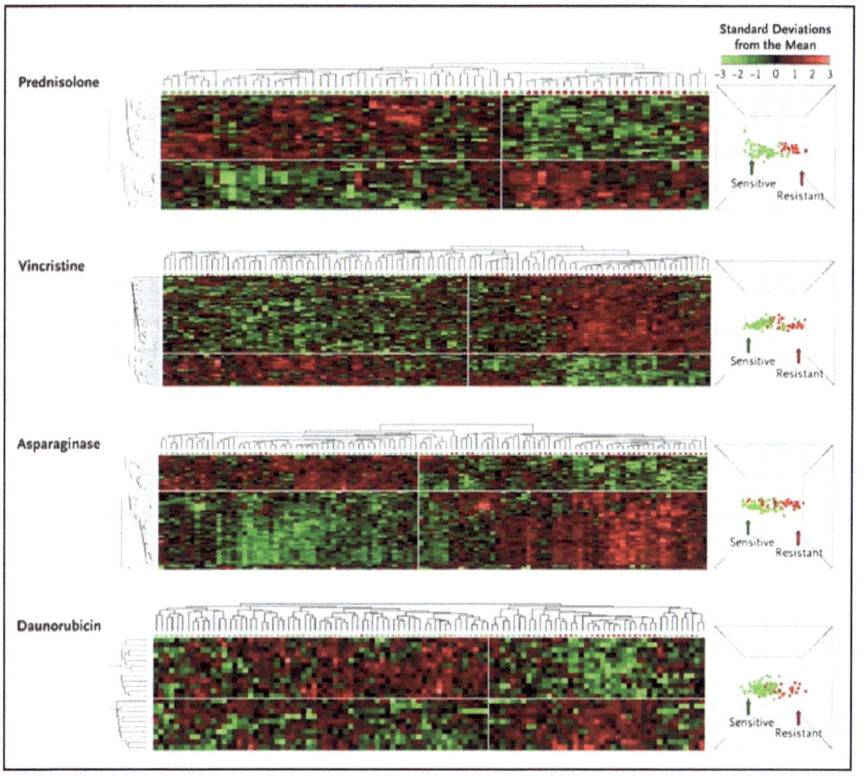

Fig. 6.2 Results of supervised hierarchical-clustering and principal-component analyses of genes whose expression discriminates between drug-resistant and drug-sensitive B-lineage acute lymphoblastic leukemia (ALL) with respect to prednisolone, vincristine, asparaginase, and daunorubicin. Each column represents an ALL sample, labeled according to whether it was sensitive (green) or resistant (red) to a given drug, and each row represents a probe set. The "heat" maps (*left*) indicate a high (red) or a low (green) level of expression. The three-dimensional plots on the right show three principal components based on the significant discriminating genes for each drug. Each circle represents an individual ALL sample; red circles indicate those with drug-resistant ALL, and green circles those with drug-sensitive ALL (© 2004 Massachusetts Medical Society; Holleman et al. 2004)

steroid-induced transcription activation, were significantly associated with dexamethasone sensitivity in 177 children with ALL (Pottier et al. 2008). Experimentally, gene silencing of *SMARCA4* and *SMARCB2* both resulted in glucocorticoid resistance. Of interest, prednisolone resistance in precursor B-ALL is also associated with elevated expression of genes involved in glucose metabolism, and the rate of glycolysis in human ALL cell lines is positively correlated with glucocorticoid resistance. Inhibition of glycolysis (small molecular inhibitors or short hairpin RNA), reversed resistance to prednisolone in both cultured cell lines as well as primary ALL samples (Hulleman et al. 2009). Gene expression signature of glucocorticoid resistance was also used to guide high-throughput screening of small molecules modulating glucocorticoid sensitivity (Wei et al. 2006). The *mTOR* inhibitor rapamycin sensitized ALL cells to glucocorticoid-induced apoptosis by down-regulating antiapoptotic *MCL1*.

Another approach to discover drug resistance genes is to compare genetic aberrations between matched diagnosis and relapse ALL samples, on the premise that relapse disease arises at least partly as a result of drug resistance to chemotherapy (Klumper et al. 1995). Studying 35 matched diagnosis/relapse pairs, Bhojwani et al. (Bhojwani et al. 2006) observed significant differences between diagnosis and relapse in the expression of genes involved in cell-cycle regulation, DNA repair, and apoptosis in patients who relapsed early (within 36 months of first remission). In contrast, no common pattern of changes was noted among late-relapse pairs. Also, early relapse samples were more similar to their respective diagnostic samples, while late-relapse samples exhibited greater divergence in gene expression compared to their diagnostic samples. *Survivin* (*BIRC5*) was significantly up-regulated at relapse in two independent cohorts of relapsed ALL patients and has been shown to effectively modulate sensitivity to chemotherapeutic agents used in ALL. A subsequent study by this group surveyed somatic copy number alterations in 20 diagnosis/relapse ALL pairs (Yang et al. 2008). Most copy number changes were preserved from diagnosis to relapse, while a fraction of genomic lesions (17%) was novel at relapse. A recurrent relapse-specific focal deletion of *MSH6* resulted in reduction of gene expression in respective pairs; reduced expression of *MSH6* was associated with resistance to mercaptopurine and prednisolone. Together, these results provided a plausible mechanism by which acquired genetic aberrations contribute to drug resistance at ALL relapse.

6.2.1.2 GeneticV ariationsi nt heHo stA ffecting Anti-leukemic Drugs

Polymorphisms in genes involved in drug metabolism and transport have been reported to modulate efficacy of antileukemic agents and clinical outcome of ALL (summarized in Table 6.1). The cytochrome P450 enzymes (particularly the CYP3A subfamily) are involved in the Phase I metabolism of many antileukemic agents (e.g., cyclophosphamide, etoposide, doxorubicin, and vinca alkaloids), and polymorphisms in *CYP3A4/3A5* might contribute to variation of ALL therapy outcome (Aplenc et al. 2003; Fleury et al. 2004; Rocha et al. 2005). Importantly, glucocorticoids are potent inducers of CYP3A enzymes, which influence the clearance of glucocorticoids themselves as well agents metabolized by CYP3As (e.g., etoposide; Kishie ta l. 2004).

A number of Phase II metabolism enzymes are involved in inactivation of antileukemic agents. Thiopurine methyltransferase (*TPMT*) inactivates 6-mercaptopurine and genetic variations in this gene profoundly decrease *TPMT* enzymatic activity. In fact, the relationship between *TPMT* polymorphisms and response to the thiopurines in children with ALL (efficacy and toxicity) is among the best established examples of clinical application of pharmacogenetics (Relling et al. 1999; Stanulla et al. 2005a; Schmiegelow et al. 2009a, b); in some protocols, low or intermediate *TPMT* activity phenotypes are associated with lower relapse rates. Through glutathione conjugation, glutathione S-transferases (GSTs) generally inactivate glucocorticoids, vincristine, anthracyclines, methotrexate, cyclophosphamide, and epipodophyllotoxins, and polymorphisms in various *GST* genes (*GSTT1, GSTM1, GSTP1*) have been extensively studied in prognosis of childhood ALL (Chen et al. 1997; Anderer et al. 2000; Stanulla et al. 2000, 2005a, b; Davies et al. 2002; Krajinovic et al. 2002a, b; Rocha et al. 2005;). Genetic variations in the NADPH dehydrogenase, quinine 1 (*NQO1*), have also been linked to treatment outcome of ALL (Krajinovic et al. 2002a, b; da Silva Silveira eta l. 2009).

Both ABC transporters and solute carriers are important in intracellular uptake and efflux of antileukemic agents (Jamroziak et al. 2004; de Jonge et al. 2005; Stanulla et al. 2005a, b; Ansari et al. 2009). Molecular targets of certain antileukemic drugs (e.g., *NR3C1* and the folate pathway) are also polymorphic and therefore plausible sources for response variability (Krajinovic et al. 2002a, b, 2004, 2005; Lauten et al. 2003; Fleury et al. 2004; Aplenc et al. 2005; de Jonge et al. 2005;; Chiusolo et al. 2007; Dulucq et al. 2008; Ansari et al. 2009; da Silva Silveira et al. 2009; Ongaro et al. 2009; Pietrzyk et al. 2009). Recently, Davies et al. studied 16 genetic variations in 529 children with newly diagnosed ALL and found that a promoter polymorphism of *CCR5* was most highly associated with response to remission induction treatment (measured as MRD) (Davies et al. 2008). The authors hypothesized that chemokine receptors retain leukemia cells in the bone marrow stroma, which in turn confers protection against chemotherapeutic agents (Iwamoto et al. 2007).

With the exception of *TPMT*, the prognostic value of genetic variations in most drug metabolizing enzymes and transporters studied thus far has been controversial primarily due to the lack of reproducibility (Table 6.1). While some discrepancy can be attributed to sample size and statistical design, prognostic genotypes are highly treatment-dependent. Because ALL treatment regimens vary from study to study (e.g., antimetabolites-focused vs. not), the importance of certain drug metabolizing enzymes and transporters also differ significantly dependent upon the use of antileukemic agents they target. Therefore, caution should be used in attempting to generalize these results (Table 6.1).

Table 6.1 Candidate genetic polymorphisms investigated for association with childhood acute lymphoblastic leukemia (ALL) outcome

Mechanism of action	Polymorphism	Drugst argeted	dbSNP ID	Clinical phenotype	Conclusion	Ref(samples ize)
Phase I metabolism enzymes	*CYP3A4 *1B*	Glucocorticoid, vincristine, cyclophosphamide, etoposide	rs2740574	Relapse	Not significant	(Fleury et al. 2004) (*N* = 222) (Aplenc et al. 2003) (*N* = 1204) (Rocha et al. 2005) (*N* = 246)
	*CYP3A5*3*	Glucocorticoid, vincristine, cyclophosphamide, etoposide	rs776746	Relapse	Nots ignificant	(Aplence ta l. 2003) (*N* = 1204) (Rocha eta l. 2005) (*N* = 246)
	*CYP3A5*6*	Glucocorticoid, vincristine, cyclophosphamide, etoposide	rs10264272	Relapse	Nots ignificant	(Aplence ta l. 2003) (*N* = 1204)
Phase II metabolism enzymes	*GSTM1*0 (deletion)*	Glucocorticoid, vincristine, doxorubicin, etoposide, methotrexate	Not applicable	Relapse	Significant (deletion is associated with fewer relapse)	(Rochae ta l. 2005) (*N* = 246); (Stanulla eta l. 2000)(*N*= 128); (Chen et al. 1997)(*N* = 416)
				Relapse	Nots ignificant	(Daviese ta l. 2002) (*N* = 710); (Krajinovice ta l. 2002a, b)(*N* = 320)
				In vivo response to prednisolone	Nots ignificant	(Anderere t al. 2000) (*N* = 135)
	GSTT1 deletion	Glucocorticoid, vincristine, doxorubicin, etoposide, methotrexate	Not applicable	Relapse	Significant (deletion is associated with fewer relapse)	(Stanullae ta l. 2000) (*N* = 128)
				In vivo response to prednisolone	Significant	(Anderere ta l. 2000) (*N* = 135)
				Relapse	Nots ignificant	(Rochae ta l. 2005) (*N* = 246) (Davies eta l. 2002)(*N*= 710) (Chen et al. 1997)(*N* = 416)
	*GSTP1*B*	Glucocorticoid, vincristine, doxorubicin, etoposide, methotrexate	rs1695	Relapse (central nervous system)	Significant (variant is associated with fewer relapse)	(Stanulla et al. 2005) (*N* = 68)
				Relapse	Nots ignificant	(Krajinovic et al. 2002) (*N* = 320); (Stanullae ta l. 2000) (*N* = 128); (Rocha eta l. 2005) (*N* = 246)

(continued)

Table 6.1 (continued)

Mechanism of action	Polymorphism	Drugst argeted	dbSNP ID	Clinical phenotype	Conclusion	Ref(samples ize)
	*TPMT*2/*3A*	6-Mercaptopurine, 6-thioguanine	rs1800462/ rs28933403	Minimal residual disease after mercaptopu-rine treatment	Significant (variant is associated with better response)	(Stanulla et al. 2005) (*N* = 814)
				Relapse	Significant (variant is associated with better response)	(Relling et al. 1999) (*N* = 180); (Schmiegelow et al. 2009) (*N* = 599)
	*NQO1*2*	Doxorubicin	rs1800566	Relapse	Significant (variant is associated with more relapse)	(Krajinovic et al. 2002) (*N* = 320); (da Silva Silveira eta l. 2009)(*N* = 95)
Transporters	*ABCB1 C3435T*	Vincristine, doxorubicin, etoposide	rs1045642	Relapse	Significant (variant is associated with fewer relapse)	(Stanulla et al. 2005) (*N* = 68); (Jamroziak eta l. 2004) (*N* = 113)
				Relapse	Nots ignificant	(Rochae ta l. 2005) (*N* = 246);
	ABCB1 G2677T/A		rs2032582	Relapse	Nots ignificant	(Rochae ta l. 2005) (*N* = 246);
	ABCC4 T1393C			Relapse (variant is associated with fewer relapse)	Significant	(Ansarie ta l. 2009) (*N* = 275)
	ABCC4 A934C		rs2274407	Relapse (variant is associated with more relapse)	Significant	(Ansarie ta l. 2009) (*N* = 275)
	SLC19A1 G80A		rs1051266	Relapse	Nots ignificant	(Rochae ta l. 2005) (*N* = 246)
				Methotrexate sensitivity	Nots ignificant	(de Jonge et al. 2005)(*N* = 157)
Drug target	*NR3C1 G198A*	Glucocorticoid	rs6189	Relapse	Nots ignificant	(Fleurye ta l. 2004) (*N* = 222)
	NR3C1 G200A		rs6190	Relapse	Nots ignificant	(Fleurye ta l. 2004) (*N* = 222)
	NR3C1 A1220G		rs6195	Relapse	Nots ignificant	(Rochae ta l. 2005) (*N* = 246); (Fleury eta l. 2004) (*N* = 222)
	NR3C1 A-3807G		rs10052957	Relapse	Significant	(Ansarie ta l. 2009) (*N* = 310)
	NR3C1 C646G		rs41423247	Relapse	Significant	(Ansarie ta l. 2009) (*N* = 310)

Table 6.1 (continued)

Mechanism of action	Polymorphism	Drugst argeted	dbSNP ID	Clinical phenotype	Conclusion	Ref(samples ize)
	NR3C1 9b T/C		rs6198	Relapse	Significant	(Ansarie ta l. 2009) (*N* = 310)
	TYMS enhancer repeat	Methotrexate	rs34743033	Relapse	Significant (variant is associated with higher TYMS activity and more relapse)	(Rochae ta l. 2005) (*N* = 246); (Krajinovic et al. 2002) (*N* = 205); (Krajinovic et al. 2005)(*N* = 259); (da Silva Silveira eta l. 2009)(*N* = 95); (Dulucqe ta l. 2008) (*N* = 277)
				Relapse	Nots ignificant	(Ongaroe ta l. 2009) (*N* = 122); (Lauten eta l. 2003)(*N* = 80)
				Methotrexate sensitivity	Nots ignificant	(de Jonge et al. 2005)(*N* = 157)
	DHFR A-1612G/T	Methotrexate	rs1650694	Relapse	Significant (variant is associated with higher DHFR activity and more relapse)	(Dulucqe ta l. 2008) (*N* = 277)
	DHFR A-317G	Methotrexate	rs408626		Significant	(Dulucqe ta l. 2008) (*N* = 277)
	MTHFR C677T	Methotrexate	rs1801133	Relapse	Significant (variant is associated with more relapse)	(Aplence ta l. 2005) (*N* = 520); (Krajinovic et al. 2004)(*N* = 201); (Pietrzyke ta l. 2009) (*N* = 403); (Ongaro eta l. 2009) (*N* = 122)
				Relapse	Nots ignificant	(Rochae ta l. 2005) (*N* = 246); (Chiusolo eta l. 2007)(*N* = 82)
	MTHFR A1298C	Methotrexate	rs1801131	Methotrexate sensitivity	Significant (variant is associated with lower sensitivity)	(de Jonge et al. 2005)(*N* = 157)
				Relapse	Nots ignificant	(Rochae ta l. 2005) (*N* = 246); (Aplenc et al. 2005) (*N*= 520); (Chiusolo et al. 2007)(*N* = 82); (Krajinovic et al. 2004)(*N* = 201)
	MTHFD1 G1958A	Methotrexate		Relapse	Significant (variant is associated with more relapse)	(Krajinovic et al. 2004)(*N* = 201)

With the advancement in high-throughput genotyping technology, it is now feasible to agnostically screen the entire genome with reasonable resolution for genetic variations associated with response to antileukemic agents. For instance, Yang et al. recently performed a genome-wide association study to identify germline SNPs related to MRD status after remission induction therapy (Yang et al. 2009). Interrogating 476,796 genetic variations in 487 children with ALL, the authors identified 102 SNPs associated with MRD in two independent patient cohorts. Particularly, genotypes at several SNPs in *IL15* exhibited one of the strongest association signals ($p = 8.8 \times 10^{-7}$). *IL15* expression in diagnostic blasts was also correlated with leukemia burden after Induction treatment in both cohorts. A proliferation-stimulatory cytokine, *IL15* can protect hematologic tumors from glucocorticoid-induced apoptosis *in vitro* (Tinhofer et al. 2000), and *IL15* expression in ALL blasts has also been linked to risk of relapse of central nervous system leukemia (Cario et al. 2007). Most notably, of 102 SNPs associated with MRD, 21 were associated with antileukemic drug disposition, generally linking leukemia eradication with greater drug exposure. The fact that this agnostic approach discovered and validated genetic variations with previously unrecognized association with treatment response in childhood ALL, argues for the value of genome-wide screening of inherited polymorphisms in future pharmacogenomic studies of ALL.

6.2.2 Genetic Variations Related to Drug Toxicity

The thiopurines, mercaptopurine (which is a metabolite of the medication azathioprine) and thioguanine, are widely used to treat ALL and AML and their methylation is catalyzed by a highly polymorphic enzyme, thiopurine methyltransferase (*TPMT*) (Remy 1963;Weinshilboum and Sladek 1980; Woodson and Weinshilboum 1983; Lennard et al. 1989; Krynetski and Evans 1998; McBride et al. 2000; Evans and McLeod 2003). Activity is inherited as an autosomal codominant trait, with ~91% of most populations displaying high enzyme activity, 9% having intermediate activity, and 0.3% having undetectable activity (Weinshilboum and Sladek 1980). Polymorphic *TPMT* activity is due to inherited polymorphisms in the *TPMT* gene, most of which involve nonsynonymous SNPs (Table 6.2). Three of these SNPs account for over 85% of all variant alleles, making genotyping for *TPMT* polymorphisms tenable, but at least 28 variant alleles have been identified, most of which have been associated with decreased activity *in vitro* (Lennard et al. 1995; Schaeffeler et al. 2004; von Ahsen et al. 2004; Hamdan-Khalil et al. 2005; Stanulla et al. 2005a, b; Garat et al. 2008; Ujiie et al. 2008). Most of these involve nonsynonymous SNPs (Salavaggione et al. 2005; Ujiie et al. 2008) that result in highly unstable and/or rapidly degraded *TPMT* protein, without affecting *TPMT* gene expression (Krynetski et al. 1995; Tai et al. 1997).

Table6.2 Thiopurinege notypesa ndphe notypes

*TPMT*a lleles	*TPMT* genotype	Phenotype	Population frequency	Recommendeds tarting thiopurine dosages
TPMT *1/*1	Homozygous wild-type	High activity	~91% of most populations	No basis for focusing on thiopurines rather than other agents
*TPMT**1/*X Where X = *2, *3A, *3B, *3C, *9, *16, *17, or *18	Heterozygous	Intermediate activity	~9% of most populations	Focus on dosage decrease of thiopurine rather than other agents; start at 30–50% of normal doses; consider cap on thiopurine dose
*TPMT**X /*Y Where X and Y = *2, *3A, *3B, *3C, *9, *16, *17, or *18	Homozygous variant or homozygous deficient	Low activity	~0.3% of most populations	Focus on dosage decrease of thiopurine rather than other agents; start at 5–10% of normal doses; consider 3 days/week rather than daily dosing

TPMT directly inactivates the parent base drug molecules, shunting drug away from activation, and thus *TPMT* activity is inversely related to the concentrations of the cytotoxic thioguanine nucleotide (TGN) metabolites that are at least partly responsible for both the desired antileukemic and undesired adverse effects of thiopurines. A secondary metabolite of mercaptopurine, but not thioguanine, is metabolized to methylthioinosine monophosphate, which itself inhibits *de novo* purine synthesis and contributes to both antitumor effects and host toxicity (Allan and Bennett 1971; Dervieux et al. 2001; Krynetski and Evans 2003). Thus, high *TPMT* activity (wild-type genotype) has been associated with lower host toxicity and, variably, to a higher risk of leukemic relapse (Lennard et al. 1987, 1990). Conversely, patients with low *TPMT* activity are at higher risk of myelosuppression following thiopurine therapy (Lennard et al. 1989; Evans et al. 1991), but have lower levels of MRD (Stanulla et al. 2005a, b) and may be at lower risk of relapse (Lennard et al. 1990). *TPMT* heterozygotes display a phenotype intermediate between the two homozygous states (Evans et al. 2001). Low *TPMT* activity (or high TGN levels) has been associated with the development of secondary tumors in patients who have received chronic thiopurine therapy (Relling et al. 1998, 1999; Thompsen et al. 1999; Schmiegelow et al. 2009a, b). Thus, many advocate prospective testing for *TPMT* status by genotypic or phenotypic tests to allow preemptive dosage reductions to minimize acute and long-term toxicities. Using an approach to adjust dosages of ALL maintenance therapy based on thiopurine testing and target levels of myelosuppression, *TPMT* heterozygotes received lower mercaptopurine doses than the majority of patients with wild-type *TPMT*, but their relapse risk was not greater (Relling et al. 2006). As of 2009, the product labeling for all three thiopurines highlighted the higher risk of toxicity with low *TPMT*, the availability of testing, and precautions regarding dosing.

Dosing of thiopurines is facilitated not only by genotyping tests, but also by phenotyping tests. Erythrocyte concentrations of TGN reach steady-state levels after 2–4 weeks of constant dosing after all three thiopurines, and are inversely related to *TPMT* activity (Lennard et al. 1995; Lennard and Lilleyman 1996). The complete absence of detectable thioguanine metabolites is an excellent indicator of noncompliance with therapy (Lennard et al. 1995), which can be a significant problem with these orally administered agents. Following azathioprine or mercaptopurine (but not thioguanine), the tertiary metabolite methylmercaptopurine monophosphate is present in red cells, with levels in homozygous wild-type individuals being 10–50 times greater than those for thioguanine nucleotides, 3–15 times greater in *TPMT* heterozygotes, and the methyl metabolites are undetectable in the rare homozygous deficient individuals (Relling et al. 1999). Thus, absolute levels as well as ratios of the nucleotide metabolites can be useful adjuncts to genotyping and phenotyping tests for *TPMT*.

Pharmacogenetic studies of MTX toxicity in childhood ALL have primarily focused on genetic variations in the folate pathway (Fig. 6.3). While in adult patients receiving MTX for prevention of graft-versus-host disease following hematopoietic cell transplant, the variant T allele at *MTHFR C677T* polymorphism predicted higher risk of oral mucositis and slower recovery of platelet counts (Ulrich et al. 2001; Robien et al. 2004), this association was not consistently confirmed in children with ALL (Aplenc et al. 2005; Kishi et al. 2007). In a comprehensive study of chemotherapy-related toxicities in 247 children with ALL, the contribution of genetic variations differed significantly among phase of ALL therapy. During the Induction phase, when drugs subject to the steroid/cytochrome P450 pathway predominated, genotypes in *VDR* intro 8 and *CYP3A5 *3* were related to gastrointestinal toxicity and infection. During the Consolidation and Continuation phases, when antifolates predominated, the *RFC* polymorphism (*A80G*) predicted gastrointestinal toxicity. In a more recent genome-wide screening, genetic variations at the *SLCO1B1* locus exhibited strong, albeit unexpected, association with MTX plasma clearance ($p = 1.5 \times 10^{-10}$) (Trevino et al. 2009). Of interest, genotypes at this *SLCO1B1* SNP were also predictive of grade 3–4 gastrointestinal toxicity of MTX during Consolidation therapy.

Children with ALL receive intensive treatment with glucocorticoid (orally two to three times per day during 4–6 weeks of remission induction and for 5–7 days/month as pulse therapy during Maintenance therapy). Potential adverse effects include osteonecrosis, altered fat distribution, obesity, diabetes, myopathy, hypertension, immune suppression with a resultant increase in infections, and altered mental status. To identify the pharmacogenetic basis for glucocorticoid-induced hypertension, Kamdem et al. determined the

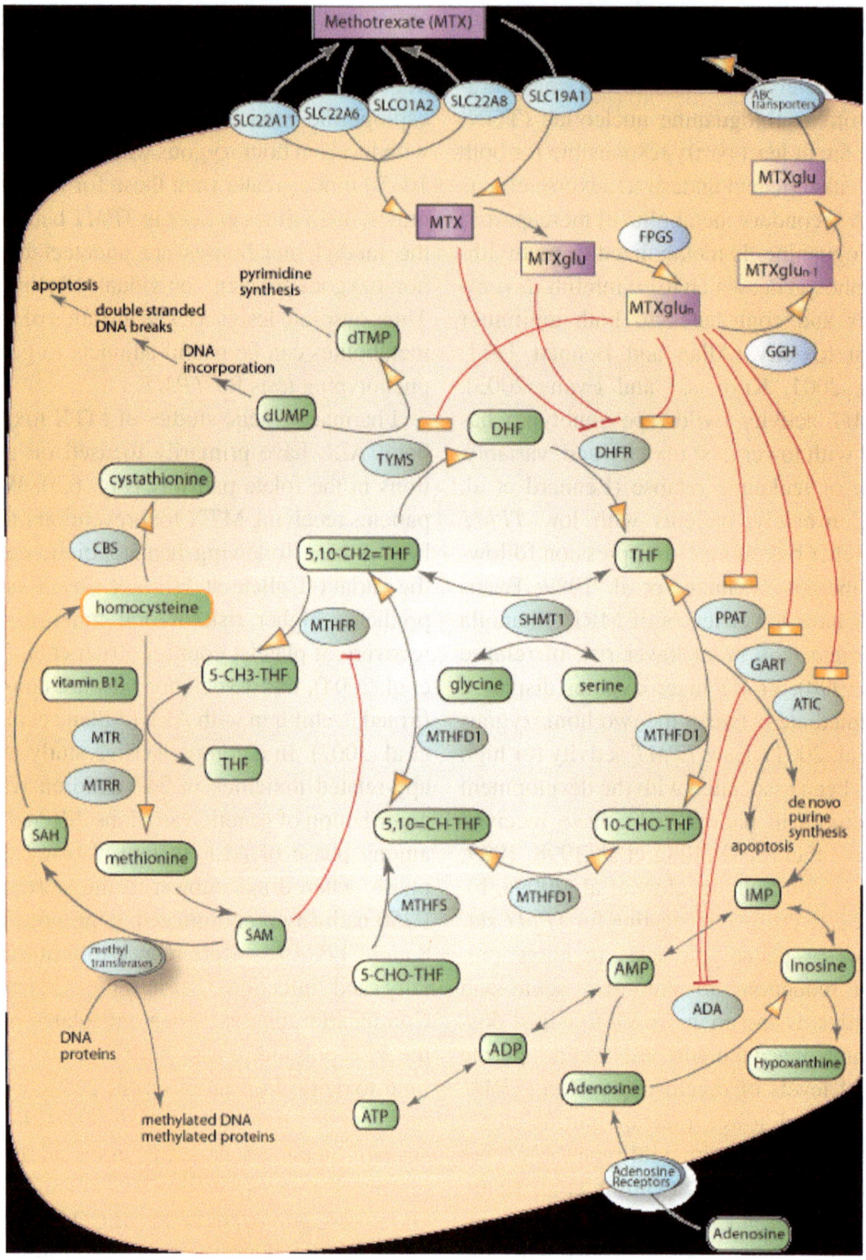

Fig. 6.3 Cellular pathway of methotrexate and major targets. Methotrexate, an analogue of reduced folate, targets endogenous cellular folate metabolism. At pharmacologic concentrations of 0.1–10 uM, cellular entry of methotrexate is by the reduced folate carrier (SLC19A1). Its main intracellular target is dihydrofolate reductase (DHFR), inhibition of which results in accumulation of dihydrofolate (DHF) and a depletion of cellular folates. Cytoplasmic folylpolyglutamyl synthase (FPGS) adds glutamate residues to methotrexate, improving its intracellular retention and the affinity for target enzymes (TYMS, PPAT, GART and ATIC) (© 2009 PharmGKB; Klein et al. 2001)

genotypes for 203 candidate polymorphisms in genes either related to hypertension or likely to affect the pharmacokinetics or pharmacodynamics of antileukemic agents in 698 children with ALL (Kamdem et al. 2008). SNPs in the *ALPL, APOB, BGLAP, CNTNAP2, CRHR, LEPR, NTAN1*, and *SLC12A3* genes exhibited significant associations with drug-related hypertension ($p < 0.05$). A corticotropin-releasing hormone receptor-1 (*CRHR1*) polymorphism, *rs1876828*, is predictive of bone mineral density among patients who have completed glucocorticoid-containing therapy for ALL (Jones et al. 2008), consistent with its correlation with glucocorticoid-induced changes in lung function in patients with asthma (Tantisira et al. 2004). Osteonecrosis (avascular necrosis) occurs in 10–15% of children receiving ALL therapy and is directly linked to the use of corticosteroids (dexamethasone or prednisone) (Mattano et al. 2000; Ribeiro et al. 2001). In a case–control study of ALL patients treated at St. Jude Children's Research Hospital, genetic variants predicted to be high-affinity for *VDR* and low activity for *TYMS* were associated with higher risk for osteonecrosis, suggesting roles for glucocorticoid and antimetabolite (MTX and mercaptopurine) pharmacodynamics in the osteonecrosis risk (Relling et al. 2004). However, a subsequent study of children treated on CCG1882 protocol did not observe any associations of *VDR* and *TYMS* polymorphisms with risk of osteonecrosis, possibly due to differences in ALL therapy (St. Jude patients receive more MTX-intensive treatment) (French et al. 2008). Instead, a *PAI-1* SNP was found to contribute to risk of osteonecrosis after adjusting age, sex, and treatment arm. Further studies are warranted to determine the exact contribution of genetic variation in risk of glucocorticoid-induced osteonecrosis and to investigate specific genetic variations in the context of particular treatment regimens.

In vincristine-containing ALL chemotherapy protocols, impaired motor performance due to peripheral neuropathy is well documented (Hartman et al. 2006). Vinca-alkaloid drugs are metabolized by CYP3A4/3A5 and transported by ABCB1. Both *CYP3A4*1B* and *CYP3A5*3* were associated with neuropathy in children treated on the CCG-1891 protocol (Aplenc et al. 2003), although motor performance was not related to genotypes at *CYP3A5 *3/*3, CYP3A5 *1*3, ABCB1 C3435T, G2677A/T*, or *MAPT* haplotypes in a smaller BFM cohort of 34 children with ALL (Hartman et al. 2009). Variability in plasma clearance of vincristine was not explained by *ABCB1 C3435T, G2677A/T* polymorphisms (Plasschaert et al. 2004). A significantly lower incidence of neuropathy was observed in black children with ALL compared to white patients receiving identical vincristine regimens, implying plausible roles of ancestry-related genetic variations (Renbargere ta l. 2008).

Adverse effects specific to asparaginase include thrombosis, pancreatitis, and allergy. However, thus far, there is little evidence for a genetic basis for these complications among patients with acute leukemia. There are conflicting data as to whether thromboses among children with ALL are related to the frequency of prothrombotic genetic polymorphisms such as those in factor V Leiden, *MTHFR*, and in prothrombin (Nowak-Gottl et al. 1999; Wermes et al. 1999a, b; Mitchell et al. 2003; Chung et al. 2008), although the majority of evidence indicates genetic variants are not strongly predictive of thrombosis risk in patients with leukemia.

6.3 AcuteMyel oidL eukemia

AML constitutes approximately 15–20% of childhood leukemias (Smith et al. 1999). The prognosis of children who have AML has improved greatly during the past 3 decades. Complete remission (CR) rates as high as 80–90% and overall survival (OS) rates of 60% are now reported (Creutzig et al. 2005; Entz-Werle et al. 2005; Gibson et al. 2005; Kaspers et al. 2005; Perel et al. 2005; Pession et al. 2005; Ravindranath et al. 2005; Ribeiro et al. 2005; Smith et al. 2005). This success reflects the use of increasingly intensive Induction chemotherapy followed by post-remission treatment with additional anthracyclines and high-dose cytarabine, as well as myeloablative regimens followed by hematopoietic stem cell transplantation (HSCT) for those with sibling donors, to maintain a durable long-term remission. Thirty to 40% of patients with AML relapse despite improvements in risk-assignment and dose-intensive risk adapted treatment. In addition, the intensive therapy needed for cure is associated with significant morbidity and mortality. The occurrence of a substantial number of deaths in remission caused by toxicity of therapy is an important limitation to success of treatment for AML (Creutzig et al. 2004; Rubnitz et al. 2004; Slats et al. 2005).

Genetically determined variations in response to damage induced by chemotherapy are being intensively investigated as causes of differential susceptibility to leukemogenesis and differential response to therapy (Naoe et al. 2000; Wiemels et al. 2001; Krajinovic et al. 2002a, b). Key drugs currently used in therapy of AML include cytarabine (ara-C), anthracyclines and other anti-metabolites. As in ALL, polymorphisms in genes that encode drug-metabolizing enzymes, transporters, or targets can profoundly influence the efficacy and toxicity of AML therapy, thereby affecting the outcome of therapy.

6.3.1 Genetic Variations in the Host Affecting Antileukemic Drugs

6.3.1.1 RaceandEt hnicity

Recent studies have analyzed the influence of host factors on outcome in pediatric AML. In a Children's Cancer Group study, Aplenc et al. analyzed 791 children treated in the CCG 2891 trial and showed that Hispanic and black children have a poorer outcome (OS) than white children (37% vs 48% ($p = 0.016$) and 34% vs 48% ($p = 0.007$), respectively) (Aplenc et al. 2006). The authors confirmed the reduced survival in black children identified in that trial in the successor trial CCG 2961. There were no significant differences in the characteristics of the leukemias in the different ethnic groups, and all therapy was documented as having been administered according to schedule, suggesting pharmacogenetic differences in drug metabolism as the most likely cause for the differences in outcome.

6.3.1.2 PharmacogeneticV ariation in Metabolism of Cytarabine

Cytosine arabinoside (cytarabine; 1-B-D-arabinofuranosylcytosine), an arabinose-containing analogue of the pyrimidine nucleoside deoxycytidine, is an active chemotherapeutic agent for hematological malignancies, particularly AML (Ellison et al. 1968; Beard et al. 1974; Keating et al. 1982). Cytarabine forms the backbone of both Induction and Consolidation therapy for AML, given at standard or high doses (Bodey et al. 1969). The cytotoxic effect of cytarabine requires transport into the cells followed by metabolic activation. Intracellular transport of cytarabine, when administered in standard doses, is mediated by the human equilibrative transporter hENT1 (Wiley et al. 1983; Galmarini et al. 2002). At high doses, cytarabine diffuses into the cell at a rate that exceeds that of pump-mediated transport (Kessel et al. 1969). Inside the cell, cytarabine is phosphorylated to its active triphosphate form (ara-CTP) through the sequential action of deoxycytidine kinase (dCK), deoxycytidylate kinase and nucleoside diphosphate kinase (Schrecker et al. 1968; Chou et al. 1977; Galmarini et al. 2002). Phosphorylation by dCK is the rate-limiting step in this process. Ara-CTP is incorporated into DNA and inhibits DNA synthesis in a competitive fashion (Furth et al. 1968; Graham et al. 1970). Cytidine deaminase (CDD) is a pyrimidine salvage pathway enzyme that catalyzes the hydrolytic deamination of cytidine and deoxycytidine to their corresponding uracil nucleosides. CDD deaminates cytarabine, resulting in the formation of its inactive metabolite 1-B-D-arabinofuranosyluracil (Chabner et al. 1974; Cacciamani et al. 1991; Betts et al. 1994). Several studies have suggested that increased levels of CDD may play an important role in the development of resistance to cytarabine (Steuart et al. 1971; Yusa eta l. 1992).

A common polymorphism, *A79C*, in the *CDD* gene changes a lysine residue to glutamine, resulting in decreased enzyme activity. Bhatla et al. investigated *CDD A79C* genotypes for 457 children with AML treated on protocols CCG 2941 and 2961 and analyzed the impact of *CDD* genotype on therapy outcomes (Bhatla et al. 2009). Treatment-related mortality following Induction chemotherapy was significantly elevated in children with the CC genotype compared with AA and AC (Fig. 6.4). However, this difference was only significant in children randomized to receive IDA-FLAG (cytarabine=7,590 mg/m^2) as Consolidation therapy, and was not significant in those receiving IDA-DCTER (cytarabine 800 mg/m^2). These data indicate that while host genotype may influence response to therapy, the importance of genotype may vary depending on the dose of drug being used, and also on the dosing schedule; therefore, generating a pharmacogenetic profile to predict response to therapy may be challenging and requires careful consideration of the package of therapy being given.

Polymorphisms or altered expression of proteins involved in cytarabine metabolism, such as deoxycytidine kinase, DNA polymerase, and as nucleoside transporter, play a role in leukemic blast cell sensitivity to this agent. Factors that reduce the intracellular concentration of ara-CTP may induce chemoresistance in AML patients. These factors include reduced influx of cytarabine by the hENT1 transporter, reduced phosphorylation by dCK, and increased degradation by high Km cytoplasmic 5′-nucleotidase (5NT) and/or

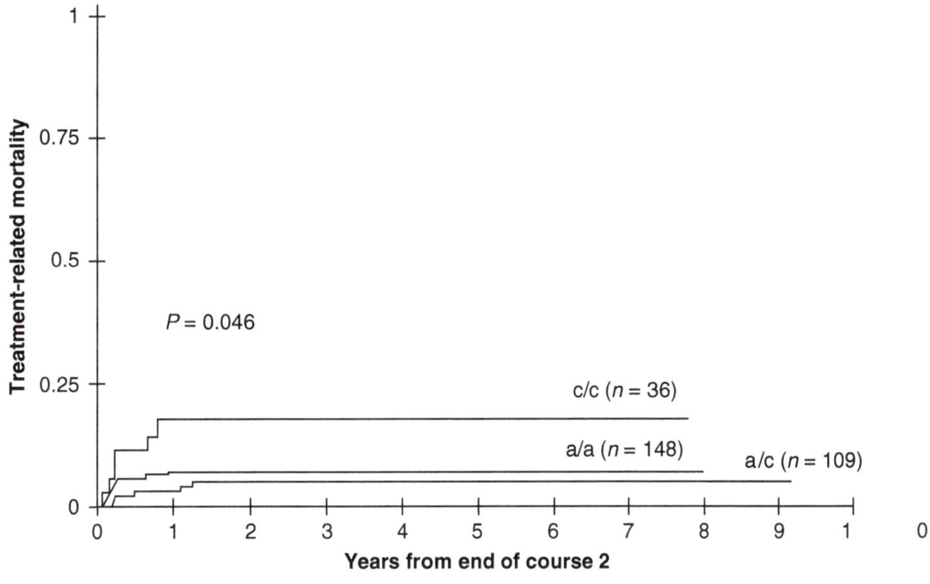

Fig. 6.4 Post-Induction treatment related mortality by cytidine deaminase genotype (Bhatla et al. 2009)

CDD. Increased levels of DNA polymerase alpha (DNA POL) and reduced levels of topoisomerase I (TOPO I) and topoisomerase II (TOPO II) have also been detected in cytarabine-resistant cell lines. Galmarini et al. (2002) analyzed the expression of these parameters at diagnosis, using reverse transcription polymerase chain reaction, in the blast cells of 123 adult AML patients treated with cytarabine to determine whether these factors are important in clinical cytarabine resistance. In univariate analysis, patients with expression of *5NT* or *DNA POL* at diagnosis had significantly shorter disease-free survival (DFS). In multivariate analysis, *DNA POL* positivity and *hENT1* deficiency were related to a shorter DFS. In univariate analysis, patients with *5NT*-positive blasts had significantly shorter OS. In multivariate analysis, shorter OS was related to *DNA POL* positivity. These results suggest that expression of *DNA POL, 5NT* and *hENT1* at diagnosis may correlate with resistance to cytarabine in AML patients.

The same group also analyzed dCK and high-Km 5′-nucleotidase (cytosolic Nucleotidase II – cN-II) mRNA expression by the quantitative real-time polymerase chain reaction in leukemic blasts at diagnosis from 115 AML patients treated with cytarabine (Galmarini et al. 2003). In a multivariate analysis taking into account other clinical and laboratory variables, high cN-II expression and a high cN-II/dCK ratio were found to be independent prognostic factors for DFS and also predicted shorter OS. Overall, these authors concluded that dCK and cN-II mRNA expression in leukemic blasts at diagnosis is correlated with clinical outcome and may play a functional role in the resistance to cytarabine in patients with AML.

6.3.2 X-Ray Repair Cross-complementing - 3 (XRCC3)

DNA is at constant risk of damage from both endogenous and exogenous sources. Cells have highly complex pathways to accomplish repair of DNA damage and maintain genomic integrity (Ishikawa et al. 2006; Kennedy et al. 2006). DNA double strand breaks (DSBs) can form in response to a variety of exogenous agents like ionizing radiation and certain chemotherapeutic drugs. Variations in individual DNA repair capacity may also influence chemotherapy response and associated toxicity; genetic polymorphisms have been described in multiple genes associated with DNA repair. During the homologous recombination process of DSBs repair, the XRCC3 protein interacts directly with and stabilizes the RAD51 protein (Bishop et al. 1998; Masson et al. 2001; Yamada et al. 2004). Epidemiological studies have noted positive associations between *XRCC3* polymorphism *C241T*, and development of melanomas, bladder cancer, breast cancer, lung cancer and gliomas (Winsey et al. 2000; Matullo et al. 2001; Kuschel et al. 2002; Popanda et al. 2004; Wang et al. 2004). Similarly, a recent report associated this polymorphism with susceptibility to AML in adults. The authors reported increased susceptibility to both *de novo* and therapy-related AML when both variant alleles were present (Seedhouse et al. 2004).

A recent pediatric study followed up on this observation and evaluated the role of *XRCC3 C241T* polymorphism in childhood AML. The authors reported that *XRCC3* polymorphism did not play a role in susceptibility to childhood AML, but showed that patients heterozygous for the *XRCC3 C241T* allele had improved post-Induction DFS compared to children homozygous for the major or minor allele, each of whom had similar outcomes. Improved survival was due to reduced relapse in the heterozygous children, and this effect was most marked in children randomized to therapy likely to generate DNA double-strand breaks (etoposide, daunomycin) as opposed to anti-metabolite based therapy (fludarabine, cytarabine) (Bhatla et al. 2008).

These data further demonstrate that pharmacogenetic associations may be specific to the therapy protocol in which the observations were made, and that identifying pharmacogenetic profiles that are generalizable to more than one complex therapeutic protocol will likely be challenging. This is a particular challenge in oncology when multiple drugs are almost invariably used, and the whole treatment protocol needs to be considered.

6.3.3 Glutathione S-Transferase Polymorphisms

Polymorphism in *GST*s have been studied in both childhood ALL and AML patients. GSTs are a family of enzymes that add sulfur molecules (as glutathione) to a wide range of acceptor molecules (Salinas et al. 1999). The reaction is generally a detoxification, and the conjugate is degraded by the enzymes of the gamma-glutamyl cycle (Board 1981; Seidegard et al. 1988; Pemble et al. 1994). *GST theta (GSTT1)* and *mu* (*GSTM1*) genes are absent in approximately 15% and 50% of the population, respectively (Rebbeck 1997). *GST* expression has been shown to play an important role in determining the cytotoxicity of some chemotherapeutic drugs, including alkylating agents such as chlorambucil, cyclophosphamide, melphalan, nitrogen mustard, and thiotepa, intercalating agents such as doxorubicin, and mitomycin C and carmustine (Tsuchida et al. 1992). In studies of laboratory cell lines, increased expression of *GST* has been shown to be associated with development of resistance to a range of cytotoxic drugs, including alkylating agents (Hoban et al. 1992), anthracyclines (Chao et al. 1992), and nitrosourea (Smith et al. 1989).

Alkylating agents and anthracyclines are important drugs in the treatment of AML and are subject to detoxification by GST. Three hundred and six children with AML receiving chemotherapy on Children's Cancer Group therapeutic studies were genotyped for *GSTT1* and *GSTM1* to test the hypothesis that toxicity would be greater in children without the genes (Davies et al. 2001). Patients with a *GSTT1*-negative genotype had reduced survival compared with those with at least one *GSTT1* allele (*GSTT1* positive) (52% vs 40% at 5 years; log-rank $p = 0.05$) (Fig. 6.5). A multivariate model of survival adjusted for age group, sex, white blood cell (WBC) count, chloroma, central nervous system involvement, and French–American–British group confirmed the increased risk of death in the *GSTT1*-negative cases (relative risk, AQ 1.6; $p = 0.02$). The frequency of death in remission was increased in *GSTT1*-negative cases compared with *GSTT1*-positive cases (24% vs 12%, log-rank

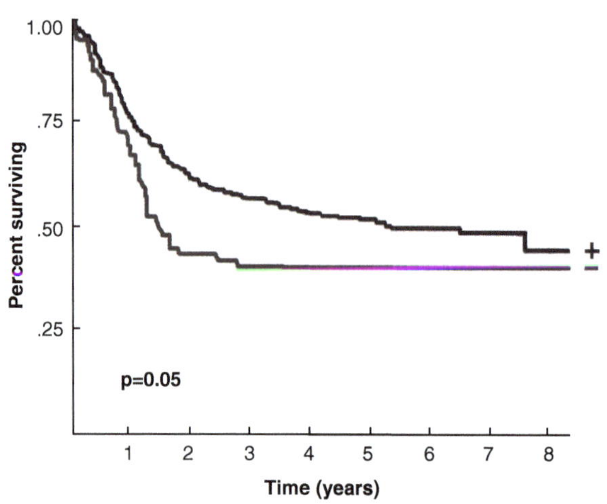

Fig. 6.5 Survival in *GSTT1*-positive (+; $n = 240$) and -null (–; $n = 65$) children with AML (52% vs 40%; $p = 0.05$) (Reprinted with permission. ©2008 American Society of Clinical Oncology. Allr ightsr eserved;D aviese ta l. 2001)

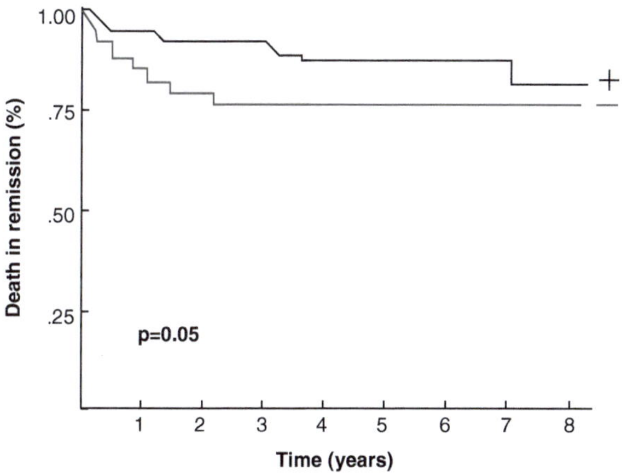

Fig. 6.6 Death in remission in *GSTT1*-positive (+; $n = 172$) and -null (–; $n = 47$) children with AML (24% vs 12%; $p = 0.05$) (Reprinted with permission. ©2008 American Society of ClinicalO ncology.A llr ightsr eserved;D aviese ta l. 2001)

$p = 0.05$) (Fig. 6.6). The frequency of relapse from end of Induction was similar in *GSTT1*-negative and *GSTT1*-positive cases (38% vs 35%, log rank $p = 0.5$).

Data linking *GST* polymorphisms to outcomes in AML were replicated in some, but not all, studies of adult patients with AML (Naoe et al. 2002; Mossallam et al. 2006; Weiss et al. 2006; Barragan et al. 2007; Voso et al. 2008; Lee et al. 2009). These discrepancies between studies may reflect the retrospective nature of the studies, differences in patient populations in terms of age or other prognostic factors, and variable treatment regimens. Taken together, these data indicate that *GST* genotypes affect the outcome of AML therapy, but the effect needs to be measured in context with the patient population and therapy received.

6.3.4 CD33: Coding Region Polymorphisms

Gemtuzumab ozogamicin (GO) (Mylotarg CMA-676;Wyeth Pharmaceuticals, Philadelphia, PA) is a humanized monoclonal antibody directed against the CD33 surface antigen that is conjugated to a derivative of the cytotoxic antibiotic calicheamicin (Hamann et al. 2002), and is associated with a 25% response rate in adult patients with CD33-positive AML in first relapse (Bross et al. 2001; Sievers et al. 2001; Larson et al. 2002). Approximately 90% of patients with AML have myeloid blast cells that express significant levels of CD33 (Dinndorf et al. 1986; Legrand et al. 2000). On binding, the antibody-antigen complex is internalized into target cells, and the calicheamicin molecule is released through hydrolysis. Calicheamicin binds to the minor groove of cellular DNA and causes double-strand breaks that lead to apoptosis (Ikemoto et al. 1995). Based on positive experience in treatment of relapsed/refractory and *de novo* adult patients with AML (Bross et al. 2001; Sievers et al. 2001; Larson et al. 2002), as well as promising early pediatric data (Arceci et al. 2005; Aplenc et al. 2008), an ongoing Phase III trial within the Children's Oncology Group is evaluating the effect of GO when added to standard AML therapy.

In a recent study, Lamba et al. (2009) undertook a comprehensive analysis of CD33 expression, including polymorphisms in the *CD33* gene, and correlated the results to GO response as measured by changes in MRD levels. The authors sequenced the complete coding region of the *CD33* gene from the genomic DNA of 22 pediatric AML patients enrolled on the St Jude AML02 protocol. Eight polymorphisms were identified; however, only *Val14Ala*, *Arg69Gly*, *Arg304Gly*, *Ser305Pro* and a *3′-UTR* SNP occurred with a minimum allele frequency of greater than 10%. None of the SNPs were significantly associated with CD33 expression levels ($p > 0.34$ for each polymorphism). The number of T-alleles of *rs12459419* had a significant positive association with the MRD-change variable ($p = 0.024$), with increasing number of T-alleles associated with a poorer response to GO-containing regimens (either alone or in combination with cytosine arabinoside, daunorubicin, and etoposide (ADE)). All three patients with poor MRD response to GO (MRD level >0.01) were homozygous TT (*Val14Val*) for the *rs12459419* variant (allele frequency 100%), whereas only 2 of 19 patients (11%) with response to GO (MRD levels, <0.01) were homozygous TT.

6.3.5 XPD

Recent data from elderly AML patients treated on MRC11 trial showed reduced event-free survival (EFS) and OS, along with increased risk of developing treatment-related leukemia, in *XPD751* glutamine homozygotes (CC), suggesting that the glutamine variant confers greater protection against chemotherapy-induced leukemic blast cell death, leading to earlier disease relapse and ultimately shorter OS (Allan et al. 2004). However, in contrast to the adult data, *XPD751* did not influence outcome of therapy in 465 children with AML (Mehta et al. 2006).

These different findings in adult and pediatric populations underscore the different biology of AML in children and adults. For example, AML in older adults is more likely to have adverse cytogenetic features compared to children (Dastugue et al. 1995; Leith et al. 1997). Also, over time adult patients have more opportunity to accumulate additional genetic insults (secondary hits), with perhaps increased susceptibility to develop cancers that are more resistant to therapy. Outcomes for treatment of adult AML are commonly inferior to those reported in pediatric series (Rees et al. 1986; Hiddemann et al. 1999; Goldstone et al. 2001; Stone 2002). Moreover, compared to children, older adults have poorer tolerance of combination chemotherapy regimens, leading to the use of less-intensive treatment protocols. Progress in AML therapy in children has largely been made by aggressive intensification of chemotherapy. It is also possible that intensification of chemotherapy in children can overcome a marginal modulating effect of particular genetic variant.

6.3.6 P-Glycoprotein Polymorphism and Outcome of AML

One of the major etiologies for treatment failure in patients with AML is clinical resistance to chemotherapy, which is associated with the expression of multidrug resistance (MDR) proteins (Sonneveld et al. 2001). Among those, members of the family of adenosine triphosphate-binding cassette (ABC) transporter proteins play a role as drug efflux pumps in the plasma membrane (Klein et al. 1999; Sonneveld and List 2001). The classical MDR phenotype results from expression of the *MDR1* gene and its 170-kd protein product, P-glycoprotein (P-gp), also designated as ABC protein transporter, subfamily B, member 1 (ABCB1) (Juliano et al. 1976). The *ABCB1* gene is localized on chromosome 7q21.17 and consists of 28 exons (Ambudkar et al. 2003). P-gp acts as an energy-dependent drug efflux pump for chemotherapeutic drugs such as the anthracyclines and epipodophyllotoxins, commonly used in AML therapy (Ambudkar eta l. 1999).

In patients with AML, increased P-gp expression and enhanced drug efflux have been reported with increasing age. Approximately 35% of AML patients under 60 years of age and 71% of elderly AML patients express detectable Pgp levels in blast cells before treatment (Leith et al. 1999). Pgp activity and expression have been established to represent independent risk factors for treatment failure in AML (Tsimberidou et al. 2002; Mahadevan and List 2004) and increased Pgp expression is also detected in relapsed patients (Guercie ta l. 1995).

Mickley et al. reported the first evidence of the presence of polymorphisms in the human *MDR1* gene (Mickley et al. 1998). Since then, attention has been focused on SNPs located in the *MDR1* coding region and their association with Pgp expression/function (Kantharidis et al. 2000; Marzolini et al. 2004; Wang et al. 2006). Hoffmeyer et al. identified 15 polymorphisms of the *MDR1* gene with various frequencies. The authors described a noncoding sequence change *C3435T* in exon 26 of the *MDR1* gene at a wobble position as being significantly correlated with altered enterocyte P-gp expression and function (Hoffmeyer et al. 2000). Population frequencies of these genetic variants vary according to racial background. As determined by Cascorbi et al., the three most frequent SNPs in the Caucasian population are located in exons 12, 21, and 26 (positions 1236, 2677, and 3435) (Cascorbi eta l. 2001).

In a cohort of 150 AML patients aged 60 years or older, van der Holt et al. investigated whether *C1236T*, *G2677T*, and *C3435T* variants of the *ABCB1* gene in AML correlate with P-gp function and expression in leukemic blasts and with *ABCB1* transcript levels (van der Holt et al. 2006). All patients were treated in a multicenter, randomized, Phase III trial comparing standard Induction treatment with or without the P-gp inhibitor PSC-833 (van der Holt et al. 2005). None of these allelic variations predicted a difference in complete remission rate and survival endpoints, a finding that was later replicated (Hur et al. 2008).

These results are in contrast to a previous report from Illmer et al. involving 410 Caucasian patients with AML, which showed significantly lower OS and an increased risk of relapse in patients with the wild-type variant of *G2677T* (despite lower *MDR1* mRNA expression in bone marrow blasts) and in patients with the wild-type genotype of all three most common SNPs in exons 12, 21, and 26 (Illmer et al. 2002). Authors concluded that these observations indicate that allelic variants of the *MDR1* gene may influence therapy outcome by additional mechanisms, different from P-gp expression on AML blasts, possibly involving pharmacokinetic effects of P-gp.

Another study by Kim et al. analyzed 110 Korean patients with AML, and found that C/C genotype at *−3435* ($p = 0.05$) and G/G at *−2677* ($p = 0.04$) were strongly associated with a higher probability of CR and EFS, but were not found to be associated with improved OS (Kim et al. 2006). In addition, a C/C genotype at exon 26 was significantly associated with a lower expression of P-gp, suggesting that improvement in the CR and EFS were linked to increasing the intracellular accumulation of chemotherapeutic agents related to the lowered Pgp expression. In terms of the lack of effect of *MDR1* genotype on long-term outcome (OS), findings from this study correlated with other similar observations (Leith et al. 1999; Illmer et al. 2002), suggesting the possibility that *MDR1* gene SNPs may affect pharmacokinetics and pharmacodynamics of various drugs, altering the drug clearance, and in turn may influence the treatment outcomes independent of Pgp activity and expression.

To further understanding of the factors that influence Pgp expression in AML blasts, Seedhouse et al. compared the effect of leukemia-specific factors (cytogenetics, WBC count, type of AML, and bcl-2 overexpression), genetic factors (*ABCB1* polymorphisms – *G1199A, G2677T*, and *C3435T*), and age on blast Pgp protein expression and function in a large cohort of AML patients. Presentation bone marrow or peripheral blood samples from 817 patients entered into the United Kingdom AML14 ($n = 323$) and AML15 ($n = 494$) trials were studied prospectively over a 7-year period (1999–2006). AML14 was a trial for patients >60 years of age with AML or high-risk myelodysplastic syndrome (>10% blasts), and AML15 predominantly included patients <60 years of age. Age, low WBC count, high bcl-2, secondary AML and myelodysplastic syndrome, and adverse cytogenetics all correlated strongly with high Pgp protein expression. However, *ABCB1 3435TT* homozygosity was negatively correlated with Pgp. The genetic polymorphism *3435TT* (which results in unstable mRNA) has a significant effect on Pgp expression, but this is only seen in 40% of cases in which mRNA and protein are detectable, indicating that only if Pgp is turned on by leukemia-specific factors do genetic factors secondarily affect expression levels (Seedhouse et al. 2007).

The proximal promoter region controls expression of most *MDR1* transcripts, and several associations of SNPs variants and Pgp expression have been reported, although several of these findings are contradictory (Ueda et al. 1987; Kioka et al. 1992; Cornwell and Smith 1993; Tanabe et al. 2001; Calado et al. 2002; Taniguchi et al. 2003; Takane et al. 2004; Wang et al. 2006; Lourenco et al. 2008). Genotypes determined in tumor and somatic tissues may differ due to cytogenetic and molecular changes associated with malignant transformation and progression. Discordance between germ line and tumor genotypes may be particularly relevant in leukemia because cytogenetic abnormalities are frequent.

6.4 PharmacogeneticsandL eukemia Survivors

Improved survival from leukemia means there are more individuals at risk for late side effects of exposure to chemotherapy. It is crucial to recognize the importance of follow-up of these patients to monitor for and address potential therapy-related long-term complications. There has been increasing interest in using pharmacogenetic markers to predict such complications and potentially modify therapy to avoid these consequences.

Anthracycline-related congestive heart failure (CHF) is an important long-term complication among childhood cancer survivors. Preclinical abnormalities of cardiac structure and function have been reported in 60% of patients who received anthracyclines (Wouters et al. 2005), and the risk of overt, clinically symptomatic CHF has been estimated at 4–5% (Green et al. 2001). Potential risk factors for anthracycline-related CHF include total cumulative dose, female sex, radiation therapy, and younger age at diagnosis (Lipshultz et al. 2005). The pathogenesis of anthracycline-related chronic cardiotoxicity appears to be mediated by a combination of oxidative damage and perturbations in cardiac iron homeostasis induced by anthracycline C-13 alcohol metabolites (Minotti et al. 2004).

The potential role of genetic variability in the pathogenesis of chronic cardiotoxicity remains to be elucidated. Blanco et al. investigated the impact of two functional candidate genetic polymorphisms on the risk of anthracycline-related CHF among childhood cancer survivors (Blanco et al. 2008). Thirty patients with CHF and 115 matched controls were genotyped for polymorphisms in *NQO1 (NQO1*2*) (nicotinamide adenine dinucleotide phosphate: quinone oxidoreductase 1 gene) and *CBR3* (carbonyl reductase 3 gene), the *CBR3* valine [V] to methionine [M] substitution at position 244 [*V244M*]. Enzyme activity assays with recombinant *CBR3* isoforms (*CBR3 V244* and *CBR3 M244*) and the anthracycline substrate doxorubicin were used to investigate the functional impact of the *CBR3 V244M* polymorphism. There was a trend toward an association between the *CBR3 V244M* polymorphism and the risk of CHF (OR, 8.16; $p = 0.056$ for G/G vs A/A; OR, 5.44; $p = 0.092$ for G/A vs A/A). In line, recombinant *CBR3 V244* (G allele) synthesized 2.6-fold more cardiotoxic doxorubicinol per unit of time than *CBR3 M244* (A allele). These preliminary results are limited by a relatively small sample size; therefore, confirmatory larger studies and similar other studies would be useful to help optimize long-term outcomes of these patients.

6.5 Conclusion

Further knowledge of and insight into the role of host genetic polymorphisms will ultimately lead to integration of pharmacodynamic and pharmacogenomic studies in individualizing therapy for children with AML to enhance efficacya ndre ducetox icity.

References

Allan PW, Bennett LL Jr (1971) 6-Methylthioguanylic acid, a metabolite of 6-thioguanine. Biochem Pharmacol 20(4): 847–852

Allan JM, Smith AG et al (2004) Genetic variation in XPD predicts treatment outcome and risk of acute myeloid leukemia following chemotherapy. Blood 104(13):3872–3877

Ambudkar SV, Dey S et al (1999) Biochemical, cellular, and pharmacological aspects of the multidrug transporter. Annu Rev Pharmacol Toxicol 39:361–398

Ambudkar SV, Kimchi-Sarfaty C et al (2003) P-glycoprotein: from genomics to mechanism. Oncogene 22(47): 7468–7485

Anderer G, Schrappe M et al (2000) Polymorphisms within glutathione S-transferase genes and initial response to glucocorticoids in childhood acute lymphoblastic leukaemia. Pharmacogenetics10(8):715–726

Ansari M, Sauty G et al (2009) Polymorphisms in multidrug resistance-associated protein gene 4 is associated with outcome in childhood acute lymphoblastic leukemia. Blood 114(7):1383–1386

Aplenc R, Glatfelter W et al (2003) CYP3A genotypes and treatment response in paediatric acute lymphoblastic leukaemia. Br J Haematol 122(2):240–244

Aplenc R, Thompson J et al (2005) Methylenetetrahydrofolate reductase polymorphisms and therapy response in pediatric acute lymphoblastic leukemia. Cancer Res 65(6): 2482–2487

Aplenc R et al (2006) Ethnicity and survival in childhood acute myeloid leukemia: a report from the Children's Oncology Group. Blood 108(1):74–80

Aplenc R, Alonzo TA et al (2008) Safety and efficacy of gemtuzumab ozogamicin in combination with chemotherapy for pediatric acute myeloid leukemia: a report from the Children's Oncology Group. J Clin Oncol 26(14): 2390–3295

Arceci RJ, Sande J et al (2005) Safety and efficacy of gemtuzumab ozogamicin in pediatric patients with advanced CD33+ acute myeloid leukemia. Blood 106(4):1183–1188

Barragan E, Collado M et al (2007) The GST deletions and NQO1*2 polymorphism confers interindividual variability of response to treatment in patients with acute myeloid leukemia. Leuk Res 31(7):947–953

Beard ME, Fairley GH (1974) Acute leukemia in adults. Semin Hematol11(1):5–24

Betts L, Xiang S et al (1994) Cytidine deaminase. The 2.3 A crystal structure of an enzyme: transition-state analog complex. J Mol Biol 235(2):635–656

Bhatla D, Gerbing RB et al (2008) DNA repair polymorphisms and outcome of chemotherapy for acute myelogenous leukemia: a report from the Children's Oncology Group. Leukemia 22(2):265–272

Bhatla D, Gerbing RB et al (2009) Cytidine deaminase genotype and toxicity of cytosine arabinoside therapy in children with acute myeloid leukemia. Br J Haematol 144(3): 388–394

Bhojwani D, Kang H et al (2006) Biologic pathways associated with relapse in childhood acute lymphoblastic leukemia: a Children's Oncology Group study. Blood 108(2): 711–717

Bishop DK, Ear U et al (1998) Xrcc3 is required for assembly of Rad51 complexes *in vivo*. J Biol Chem 273(34): 21482–21488

Blanco JG, Leisenring WM et al (2008) Genetic polymorphisms in the carbonyl reductase 3 gene CBR3 and the NAD(P) H:quinone oxidoreductase 1 gene NQO1 in patients who developed anthracycline-related congestive heart failure after childhood cancer. Cancer 112(12):2789–2795

Board PG (1981) Biochemical genetics of glutathione-S-transferase in man. Am J Hum Genet 33(1):36–43

Bodey GP, Freireich EJ et al (1969) Cytosine arabinoside (NSC-63878) therapy for acute leukemia in adults. Cancer Chemother Rep 53(1):59–66

Bross PF, Beitz J et al (2001) Approval summary: gemtuzumab ozogamicin in relapsed acute myeloid leukemia. Clin Cancer Res7(6):1490–149 6

Cacciamani T, Vita A et al (1991) Purification of human cytidine deaminase: molecular and enzymatic characterization and inhibition by synthetic pyrimidine analogs. Arch Biochem Biophys2 90(2):285–292

Calado RT, Falcao RP et al (2002) Influence of functional MDR1 gene polymorphisms on P-glycoprotein activity in CD34+ hematopoietic stem cells. Haematologica 87(6): 564–568

Cario G, Izraeli S et al (2007) High interleukin-15 expression characterizes childhood acute lymphoblastic leukemia with involvement of the CNS. J Clin Oncol 25(30):4813–4820

Cascorbi I, Gerloff T et al (2001) Frequency of single nucleotide polymorphisms in the P-glycoprotein drug transporter MDR1 gene in white subjects. Clin Pharmacol Ther 69(3): 169–174

Chabner BA, Johns DG et al (1974) Purification and properties of cytidine deaminase from normal and leukemic granulocytes. J Clin Invest 53(3):922–931

Chao CC, Huang YT et al (1992) Overexpression of glutathione S-transferase and elevation of thiol pools in a multidrug-resistant human colon cancer cell line. Mol Pharmacol 41(1): 69–75

Chen CL, Liu Q et al (1997) Higher frequency of glutathione S-transferase deletions in black children with acute lymphoblastic leukemia. Blood 89(5):1701–1707

Cheok MH, Evans WE (2006) Acute lymphoblastic leukaemia: a model for the pharmacogenomics of cancer therapy. Nat Rev Cancer 6(2):117–129

Cheok MH, Yang W et al (2003) Treatment-specific changes in gene expression discriminate *in vivo* drug response in human leukemia cells. Nat Genet 34(1):85–90

Chiusolo P, Reddiconto G et al (2007) MTHFR polymorphisms' influence on outcome and toxicity in acute lymphoblastic leukemia patients. Leuk Res 31(12):1669–1674

Chou TC, Arlin Z et al (1977) Metabolism of 1-beta-D-arabinofuranosylcytosine in human leukemic cells. Cancer Res 37(10):3561–3570

Chung BH, Ma ES et al (2008) Inherited thrombophilic factors do not increase central venous catheter blockage in children with malignancy. Pediatr Blood Cancer 51(4):509–512

Cornwell MM, Smith DE (1993) SP1 activates the MDR1 promoter through one of two distinct G-rich regions that modulate promoter activity. J Biol Chem 268(26): 19505–19511

Creutzig U, Zimmermann M et al (2004) Early deaths and treatment-related mortality in children undergoing therapy for acute myeloid leukemia: analysis of the multicenter clinical trials AML-BFM 93 and AML-BFM 98. J Clin Oncol 22(21): 4384–4393

Creutzig U, Zimmermann M et al (2005) Treatment strategies and long-term results in paediatric patients treated in four consecutive AML-BFM trials. Leukemia 19(12): 2030–2042

da Silva Silveira V, Canalle R et al (2009) Polymorphisms of xenobiotic metabolizing enzymes and DNA repair genes and outcome in childhood acute lymphoblastic leukemia. Leuk Res33(7):898–901

Daly AK, Donaldson PT et al (2009) HLA-B*5701 genotype is a major determinant of drug-induced liver injury due to flucloxacillin. Nat Genet 41(7):816–819

Dastugue N, Payen C et al (1995) Prognostic significance of karyotype in *de novo* adult acute myeloid leukemia. The BGMT group. Leukemia 9(9):1491–1498

Davies SM, Robison LL et al (2001) Glutathione S-transferase polymorphisms and outcome of chemotherapy in childhood acute myeloid leukemia. J Clin Oncol 19(5): 1279–1287

Davies SM, Bhatia S et al (2002) Glutathione S-transferase genotypes, genetic susceptibility, and outcome of therapy in childhood acute lymphoblastic leukemia. Blood 100(1): 67–71

Davies SM, Borowitz MJ et al (2008) Pharmacogenetics of minimal residual disease response in children with B-precursor acute lymphoblastic leukemia: a report from the Children's Oncology Group. Blood 111(6):2984–2990

de Jonge R, Hooijberg JH et al (2005) Effect of polymorphisms in folate-related genes on *in vitro* methotrexate sensitivity in pediatric acute lymphoblastic leukemia. Blood 106(2): 717–720

Dervieux T, Medard Y et al (2001) Possible implication of thiopurine S-methyltransferase in occurrence of infectious episodes during maintenance therapy for childhood lymphoblastic leukemia with mercaptopurine. Leukemia 15(11): 1706–1712

Dinndorf PA, Andrews RG et al (1986) Expression of normal myeloid-associated antigens by acute leukemia cells. Blood 67(4):1048–1053

Dulucq S, St-Onge G et al (2008) DNA variants in the dihydrofolate reductase gene and outcome in childhood ALL. Blood 111(7):3692–3700

Ellison RR, Holland JF et al (1968) Arabinosyl cytosine: a useful agent in the treatment of acute leukemia in adults. Blood 32(4):507–523

Entz-Werle N, Suciu S et al (2005) Results of 58872 and 58921 trials in acute myeloblastic leukemia and relative value of chemotherapy vs allogeneic bone marrow transplantation in first complete remission: the EORTC Children Leukemia Group report. Leukemia 19(12):2072–2081

Evans WE, McLeod HL (2003) Pharmacogenomics–drug disposition, drug targets, and side effects. N Engl J Med 348(6): 538–549

Evans WE, Horner M et al (1991) Altered mercaptopurine metabolism, toxic effects, and dosage requirement in a thiopurine methyltransferase-deficient child with acute lymphocytic leukemia. J Pediatr 119:985–989

Evans WE, Hon YY et al (2001) Preponderance of thiopurine S-methyltransferase deficiency and heterozygosity among patients intolerant to mercaptopurine or azathioprine. J Clin Oncol19(8):2293–2301

Fine BM, Kaspers GJ et al (2005) A genome-wide view of the *in vitro* response to l-asparaginase in acute lymphoblastic leukemia. Cancer Res 65(1):291–299

Fisher MB, Vandenbranden M et al (2000) Tissue distribution and interindividual variation in human UDP-glucuronosyltransferase activity: relationship between UGT1A1 promoter genotype and variability in a liver bank. Pharmacogenetics 10(8):727–739

Fleury I, Primeau M et al (2004) Polymorphisms in genes involved in the corticosteroid response and the outcome of childhood acute lymphoblastic leukemia. Am J Pharmacogenomics4(5):33 1–341

French D, Hamilton LH et al (2008) A PAI-1 (SERPINE1) polymorphism predicts osteonecrosis in children with acute lymphoblastic leukemia: a report from the Children's Oncology Group. Blood 111(9):4496–4499

French D, Yang W et al (2009) Acquired variation outweighs inherited variation in whole genome analysis of methotrexate polyglutamate accumulation in leukemia. Blood 113(19):4512–4520

Furth JJ, Cohen SS (1968) Inhibition of mammalian DNA polymerase by the 5'-triphosphate of 1-á-D-arabinofuranosyladenine. Can Res 28:2061–2067

Galmarini CM, Thomas X et al (2002) *In vivo* mechanisms of resistance to cytarabine in acute myeloid leukaemia. Br J Haematol117(4):8 60–868

Galmarini CM, Thomas X et al (2003) Deoxycytidine kinase and cN-II nucleotidase expression in blast cells predict survival in acute myeloid leukaemia patients treated with cytarabine. Br J Haematol 122(1):53–60

Garat A, Cauffiez C et al (2008) Characterisation of novel defective thiopurine S-methyltransferase allelic variants. Biochem Pharmacol76(3):404–415

Gibson BE, Wheatley K et al (2005) Treatment strategy and long-term results in paediatric patients treated in consecutive UK AML trials. Leukemia 19(12):2130–2138

Goldstone AH, Burnett AK et al (2001) Attempts to improve treatment outcomes in acute myeloid leukemia (AML) in older patients: the results of the United Kingdom Medical Research Council AML11 trial. Blood 98(5): 1302–1311

Graham FL, Whitmore GF (1970) Studies in mouse L-cells on the incorporation of 1-beta-D-arabinofuranosylcytosine into DNA and on inhibition of DNA polymerase by 1-beta-D-arabinofuranosylcytosine 5'-triphosphate. Cancer Res 30(11):2636–2644

Green DM, Grigoriev YA et al (2001) Congestive heart failure after treatment for Wilms' tumor: a report from the National Wilms' Tumor Study group. J Clin Oncol 19(7): 1926–1934

Guerci A, Merlin JL et al (1995) Predictive value for treatment outcome in acute myeloid leukemia of cellular daunorubicin accumulation and P-glycoprotein expression simultaneously determined by flow cytometry. Blood 85(8):2147–2153

Hamann PR, Hinman LM et al (2002) Gemtuzumab ozogamicin, a potent and selective anti-CD33 antibody-calicheamicin conjugate for treatment of acute myeloid leukemia. Bioconjug Chem 13(1):47–58

Hamdan-Khalil R, Gala JL et al (2005) Identification and functional analysis of two rare allelic variants of the thiopurine S-methyltransferase gene, *TPMT**16 and *TPMT**19. Biochem Pharmacol 69(3):525–529

Hartman A, van den Bos C et al (2006) Decrease in motor performance in children with cancer is independent of the cumulative dose of vincristine. Cancer 106(6):1395–1401

Hartman A, van Schaik RH et al (2009) Polymorphisms in genes involved in vincristine pharmacokinetics or pharmacodynamics are not related to impaired motor performance in children with leukemia. Leuk Res 34:154–159

Hiddemann W, Kern W et al (1999) Management of acute myeloid leukemia in elderly patients. J Clin Oncol 17(11): 3569–3576

Hirsch FR, Varella-Garcia M et al (2009) Predictive value of EGFR and HER2 overexpression in advanced non-small-cell lung cancer. Oncogene 28(Suppl 1):S32–37

Hoban PR, Robson CN et al (1992) Reduced topoisomerase II and elevated alpha class glutathione S-transferase expression in a multidrug resistant CHO cell line highly cross-resistant to mitomycin C. Biochem Pharmacol 43(4): 685–693

Hoffmeyer S, Burk O et al (2000) Functional polymorphisms of the human multidrug-resistance gene: multiple sequence variations and correlation of one allele with P-glycoprotein expression and activity *in vivo*. Proc Natl Acad Sci USA 97(7):3473–3478

Holleman A, Cheok MH et al (2004) Gene-expression patterns in drug-resistant acute lymphoblastic leukemia cells and response to treatment. N Engl J Med 351(6):533–542

Hoskins JM, Carey LA et al (2009) CYP2D6 and tamoxifen: DNA matters in breast cancer. Nat Rev Cancer 9(8):576–586

Hulleman E, Kazemier KM et al (2009) Inhibition of glycolysis modulates prednisolone resistance in acute lymphoblastic leukemia cells. Blood 113(9):2014–2021

Hur EH, Lee JH et al (2008) C3435T polymorphism of the MDR1 gene is not associated with P-glycoprotein function of leukemic blasts and clinical outcome in patients with acute myeloid leukemia. Leuk Res 32(10):1601–1604

Ikemoto N, Kumar RA et al (1995) Calicheamicin-DNA complexes: warhead alignment and saccharide recognition of the minor groove. Proc Natl Acad Sci USA 92(23): 10506–10510

Illmer T, Schuler US et al (2002) MDR1 gene polymorphisms affect therapy outcome in acute myeloid leukemia patients. Cancer Res 62(17):4955–4962

International Warfarin Pharmacogenetics Consortium, Klein TE et al (2009) Estimation of the warfarin dose with clinical and pharmacogenetic data. N Engl J Med 360(8):753–764

Ishikawa K, Ishii H et al (2006) DNA damage-dependent cell cycle checkpoints and genomic stability. DNA Cell Biol 25(7):406–411

Iwamoto S, Mihara K et al (2007) Mesenchymal cells regulate the response of acute lymphoblastic leukemia cells to asparaginase. J Clin Invest 117(4):1049–1057

Jamroziak K, Mlynarski W et al (2004) Functional C3435T polymorphism of MDR1 gene: an impact on genetic susceptibility and clinical outcome of childhood acute lymphoblastic leukemia. Eur J Haematol 72(5):314–321

Jones TS, Kaste SC et al (2008) CRHR1 polymorphisms predict bone density in survivors of acute lymphoblastic leukemia. J Clin Oncol 26(18):3031–3037

Juliano RL, Ling V (1976) A surface glycoprotein modulating drug permeability in Chinese hamster ovary cell mutants. Biochim Biophys Acta 455(1):152–162

Kamdem LK, Hamilton L et al (2008) Genetic predictors of glucocorticoid-induced hypertension in children with acute lymphoblastic leukemia. Pharmacogenet Genom 18(6): 507–514

Kantharidis P, El-Osta S et al (2000) Regulation of MDR1 gene expression: emerging concepts. Drug Resist Updat 3(2): 99–108

Kaspers GJ, Creutzig U (2005) Pediatric acute myeloid leukemia: international progress and future directions. Leukemia 19(12):2025–2029

Keating MJ, McCredie KB et al (1982) Improved prospects for long-term survival in adults with acute myelogenous leukemia. JAMA 248(19):2481–2486

Kennedy RD, D'Andrea AD (2006) DNA repair pathways in clinical practice: lessons from pediatric cancer susceptibility syndromes. J Clin Oncol 24(23):3799–3808

Kessel D, Hall TC et al (1969) Uptake and phosphorylation of cytosine arabinoside by normal and leukemic human blood cells *in vitro*. Cancer Res 29(2):459–463

Kim DH, Park JY et al (2006) Multidrug resistance-1 gene polymorphisms associated with treatment outcomes in *de novo* acute myeloid leukemia. Int J Cancer 118(9): 2195–2201

Kimchi-Sarfaty C, Oh JM et al (2007) A "silent" polymorphism in the MDR1 gene changes substrate specificity1. Science 315(5811):525–528

Kioka N, Yamano Y et al (1992) Heat-shock responsive elements in the induction of the multidrug resistance gene (MDR1). FEBS Lett 301(1):37–40

Kishi S, Yang W et al (2004) Effects of prednisone and genetic polymorphisms on etoposide disposition in children with acute lymphoblastic leukemia. Blood 103(1):67–72

Kishi S, Cheng C et al (2007) Ancestry and pharmacogenetics of antileukemic drug toxicity. Blood 109(10):4151–4157

Klein I, Sarkadi B et al (1999) An inventory of the human ABC proteins. Biochim Biophys Acta 1461(2):237–262

Klein TE, Chang JT et al (2001) Integrating genotype and phenotype information: an overview of the PharmGKB Project. Pharmacogenomics J 1:167–170

Klumper E, Pieters R et al (1995) *In vitro* cellular drug resistance in children with relapsed/refractory acute lymphoblastic leukemia. Blood 86:3861–3868

Krajinovic M, Costea I et al (2002a) Polymorphism of the thymidylate synthase gene and outcome of acute lymphoblastic leukaemia. Lancet 359(9311):1033–1034

Krajinovic M, Labuda D et al (2002b) Polymorphisms in genes encoding drugs and xenobiotic metabolizing enzymes, DNA repair enzymes, and response to treatment of childhood acute lymphoblastic leukemia. Clin Cancer Res 8(3): 802–810

Krajinovic M, Lemieux-Blanchard E et al (2004) Role of polymorphisms in MTHFR and MTHFD1 genes in the outcome of childhood acute lymphoblastic leukemia. Pharmacogenomics J 4(1):66–72

Krajinovic M, Costea I et al (2005) Combining several polymorphisms of thymidylate synthase gene for pharmacogenetic analysis. Pharmacogenomics J 5(6):374–380

Krynetski EY, Evans WE (1998) Pharmacogenetics of cancer therapy: getting personal. Am J Hum Genet 63:11–16

Krynetski E, Evans WE (2003) Drug methylation in cancer therapy: lessons from the *TPMT* polymorphism. Oncogene 22(47):7403–7413

Krynetski EY, Schuetz JD et al (1995) A single point mutation leading to loss of catalytic activity in human thiopurine S-methyltransferase. Proc Natl Acad Sci USA 92: 949–953

Kuschel B, Auranen A et al (2002) Variants in DNA double-strand break repair genes and breast cancer susceptibility. Hum Mol Genet 11(12):1399–1407

Lamba JK, Pounds S et al (2009) Coding polymorphisms in CD33 and response to gemtuzumab ozogamicin in pediatric patients with AML: a pilot study. Leukemia 23(2): 402–404

Larson RA, Boogaerts M et al (2002) Antibody-targeted chemotherapy of older patients with acute myeloid leukemia in first relapse using Mylotarg (gemtuzumab ozogamicin). Leukemia16(9):1627–1636

Lauten M, Asgedom G et al (2003) Thymidylate synthase gene polymorphism and its association with relapse in childhood B-cell precursor acute lymphoblastic leukemia. Haematol ogica88(3):353–354

Ledesma MC, Agundez JA (2005) Identification of subtypes of CYP2D gene rearrangements among carriers of CYP2D6 gene deletion and duplication. Clin Chem 51(6):939–943

Lee HS, Lee JH et al (2009) Clinical significance of GSTM1 and GSTT1 polymorphisms in younger patients with acute myeloid leukemia of intermediate-risk cytogenetics. Leuk Res33(3):426–433

Legrand O, Perrot JY et al (2000) The immunophenotype of 177 adults with acute myeloid leukemia: proposal of a prognostic score. Blood 96(3):870–877

Leith CP, Kopecky KJ et al (1997) Acute myeloid leukemia in the elderly: assessment of multidrug resistance (MDR1) and cytogenetics distinguishes biologic subgroups with remarkably distinct responses to standard chemotherapy. A Southwest Oncology Group study. Blood 89(9): 3323–3329

Leith CP, Kopecky KJ et al (1999) Frequency and clinical significance of the expression of the multidrug resistance proteins MDR1/P-glycoprotein, MRP1, and LRP in acute myeloid leukemia: a Southwest Oncology Group Study. Blood94(3):1086–1099

Lennard L, Lilleyman JS (1996) Individualizing therapy with 6-mercaptopurine and 6-thioguanine related to the thiopurine methyltransferase genetic polymorphism. Ther Drug Monit18: 328–334

Lennard L, Van Loon JA et al (1987) Thiopurine pharmacogenetics in leukemia: correlation of erythrocyte thiopurine methyltransferase activity and 6- thioguanine nucleotide concentrations. Clin Pharmacol Ther 41:18–25

Lennard L, Van Loon JA et al (1989) Pharmacogenetics of acute azathioprine toxicity: relationship to thiopurine methyltransferase genetic polymorphism. Clin Pharmacol Ther 46: 149–154

Lennard L, Lilleyman JS et al (1990) Genetic variation in response to 6-mercaptopurine for childhood acute lymphoblastic leukaemia. Lancet 336:225–229

Lennard L, Welch J et al (1995) Intracellular metabolites of mercaptopurine in children with lymphoblastic leukaemia: a possible indicator of non-compliance? Br J Cancer 72: 1004–1006

Ley TJ, Mardis ER et al (2008) DNA sequencing of a cytogenetically normal acute myeloid leukaemia genome. Nature 456(7218):66–72

Lipshultz SE, Lipsitz SR et al (2005) Chronic progressive cardiac dysfunction years after doxorubicin therapy for childhood acute lymphoblastic leukemia. J Clin Oncol 23(12):2629–2636

Lourenco JJ, Maia RC et al (2008) Genomic variation at the MDR1 promoter and P-glycoprotein expression and activity in AML patients. Leuk Res 32(6):976–979

Lugthart S, Cheok MH et al (2005) Identification of genes associated with chemotherapy crossresistance and treatment response in childhood acute lymphoblastic leukemia. Cancer Cell7(4):375–386

Mahadevan D, List AF (2004) Targeting the multidrug resistance-1 transporter in AML: molecular regulation and therapeutic strategies. Blood 104(7):1940–1951

Marzolini C, Paus E et al (2004) Polymorphisms in human MDR1 (P-glycoprotein): recent advances and clinical relevance. Clin Pharmacol Ther 75(1):13–33

Masson JY, Stasiak AZ et al (2001) Complex formation by the human RAD51C and XRCC3 recombination repair proteins. Proc Natl Acad Sci USA 98(15):8440–8446

Mattano LA Jr, Sather HN et al (2000) Osteonecrosis as a complication of treating acute lymphoblastic leukemia in children: a report from the Children's Cancer Group. J Clin Oncol18(18):3262–3272

Matullo G, Guarrera S et al (2001) DNA repair gene polymorphisms, bulky DNA adducts in white blood cells and bladder cancer in a case-control study. Int J Cancer 92(4): 562–567

McBride KL, Gilchrist GS et al (2000) Severe 6-thioguanine-induced marrow aplasia in a child with acute lymphoblastic leukemia and inhibited thiopurine methyltransferase deficiency. J Pediatr Hematol Oncol 22(5):441–445

Mehta PA, Alonzo TA et al (2006) XPD Lys751Gln polymorphism in the etiology and outcome of childhood acute myeloid leukemia: a Children's Oncology Group report. Blood 107(1):39–45

Mickley LA, Lee JS et al (1998) Genetic polymorphism in MDR-1: a tool for examining allelic expression in normal cells, unselected and drug-selected cell lines, and human tumors. Blood 91(5):1749–1756

Minotti G, Recalcati S et al (2004) Doxorubicin cardiotoxicity and the control of iron metabolism: quinone-dependent and independent mechanisms. Methods Enzymol 378: 340–361

Mishra PJ, Humeniuk R et al (2007) A miR-24 microRNA binding-site polymorphism in dihydrofolate reductase gene leads to methotrexate resistance. Proc Natl Acad Sci USA 104(33): 13513–13518

Mitchell LG, Andrew M et al (2003) A prospective cohort study determining the prevalence of thrombotic events in children with acute lymphoblastic leukemia and a central venous line who are treated with L-asparaginase: results of the Prophylactic Antithrombin Replacement in Kids with Acute Lymphoblastic Leukemia Treated with Asparaginase (PARKAA) Study. Cancer 97(2):508–516

Mossallam GI, Abdel Hamid TM et al (2006) Glutathione S-transferase GSTM1 and GSTT1 polymorphisms in adult acute myeloid leukemia; its impact on toxicity and response to chemotherapy. J Egypt Natl Cancer Inst 18(3): 264–273

Moyer AM, Salavaggione OE et al (2007) Glutathione S-transferase T1 and M1: gene sequence variation and functional genomics. Clin Cancer Res 13(23):7207–7216

Moyer AM, Salavaggione OE et al (2008) Glutathione s-transferase p1: gene sequence variation and functional genomic studies. Cancer Res 68(12):4791–4801

Naoe T, Takeyama K et al (2000) Analysis of genetic polymorphism in NQO1, GST-M1, GST-T1, and CYP3A4 in 469 Japanese patients with therapy-related leukemia/ myelodysplastic syndrome and *de novo* acute myeloid leukemia. Clin Cancer Res 6(10):4091–4095

Naoe T, Tagawa Y et al (2002) Prognostic significance of the null genotype of glutathione S- transferase-T1 in patients with acute myeloid leukemia: increased early death after chemotherapy. Leukemia 16(2):203–208

Nowak-Gottl U, Wermes C et al (1999) Prospective evaluation of the thrombotic risk in children with acute lymphoblastic leukemia carrying the MTHFR TT 677 genotype, the prothrombin G20210A variant, and further prothrombotic risk factors. Blood 93(5):1595–1599

Ongaro A, De Mattei M et al (2009) Gene polymorphisms in folate metabolizing enzymes in adult acute lymphoblastic leukemia: effects on methotrexate-related toxicity and survival. Haematologica 94(10):1391–1398

Ouahchi K, Lindeman N et al (2006) Copy number variants and pharmacogenomics. Pharmacogenomics 7(1):25–29

Pemble S, Schroeder KR et al (1994) Human glutathione S-transferase Theta (GSTT1): cDNA cloning and the characterization of a genetic polymorphism. Biochem J 300: 271–276

Perel Y, Auvrignon A et al (2005) Treatment of childhood acute myeloblastic leukemia: dose intensification improves outcome and maintenance therapy is of no benefit–multicenter studies of the French LAME (Leucemie Aigue Myeloblastique Enfant) Cooperative Group. Leukemia 19(12): 2082–2089

Pession A, Rondelli R et al (2005) Treatment and long-term results in children with acute myeloid leukaemia treated according to the AIEOP AML protocols. Leukemia 19(12): 2043–2053

Pietrzyk JJ, Bik-Multanowski M et al (2009) Additional genetic risk factor for death in children with acute lymphoblastic leukemia: a common polymorphism of the MTHFR gene. Pediatr Blood Cancer 52(3):364–368

Plasschaert SL, Groninger E et al (2004) Influence of functional polymorphisms of the MDR1 gene on vincristine pharmacokinetics in childhood acute lymphoblastic leukemia. Clin Pharmacol Ther 76(3):220–229

Popanda O, Schattenberg T et al (2004) Specific combinations of DNA repair gene variants and increased risk for non-small cell lung cancer. Carcinogenesis 25(12):2433–2441

Pottier N, Yang W et al (2008) The SWI/SNF chromatin-remodeling complex and glucocorticoid resistance in acute lymphoblastic leukemia. J Natl Cancer Inst 100(24): 1792–1803

Pui CH (1991) Epipodophyllotoxin-related acute myeloid leukaemia. Lancet 338(8780):1468

Pui CH, Evans WE (2006) Treatment of acute lymphoblastic leukemia. N Engl J Med 354(2):166–178

Ravindranath Y, Chang M et al (2005) Pediatric Oncology Group (POG) studies of acute myeloid leukemia (AML): a review of four consecutive childhood AML trials conducted between 1981 and 2000. Leukemia 19(12): 2101–2116

Real PJ, Tosello V et al (2009) Gamma-secretase inhibitors reverse glucocorticoid resistance in T cell acute lymphoblastic leukemia. Nat Med 15(1):50–58

Rebbeck TR (1997) Molecular epidemiology of the human glutathione S-transferase genotypes GSTM1 and GSTT1 in cancer susceptibility. Cancer Epidemiol Biomarkers Prev 6(9):733–743

Rees JK, Gray RG et al (1986) Principal results of the Medical Research Council's 8th acute myeloid leukaemia trial. Lancet2(8518):123 6–1241

Relling MV, Yanishevski Y et al (1998) Etoposide and antimetabolite pharmacology in patients who develop secondary acute myeloid leukemia. Leukemia 12:346–352

Relling MV, Hancock ML et al (1999a) Prognostic importance of 6-mercaptopurine dose intensity in acute lymphoblastic leukemia. Blood 93(9):2817–2823

Relling MV, Hancock ML et al (1999b) Mercaptopurine therapy intolerance and heterozygosity at the thiopurine S-methyltransferase gene locus. J Natl Cancer Inst 91: 2001–2008

Relling MV, Rubnitz JE et al (1999c) High incidence of secondary brain tumours after radiotherapy and antimetabolites. Lancet354(9172):3 4–39

Relling MV, Yang W et al (2004) Pharmacogenetic risk factors for osteonecrosis of the hip among children with leukemia. J Clin Oncol 22(19):3930–3936

Relling MV, Pui CH et al (2006) Thiopurine methyltransferase in acute lymphoblastic leukemia1. Blood 107(2):843–844

Remy CN (1963) Metabolism of thiopyrimidines and thiopurines. J Biol Chem 238:1078–1084

Renbarger JL, McCammack KC et al (2008) Effect of race on vincristine-associated neurotoxicity in pediatric acute lymphoblastic leukemia patients. Pediatr Blood Cancer 50(4): 769–771

Ribeiro RC, Fletcher BD et al (2001) Magnetic resonance imaging detection of avascular necrosis of the bone in children receiving intensive prednisone therapy for acute lymphoblastic leukemia or non-Hodgkin lymphoma. Leukemia 15(6):891–897

Ribeiro RC, Razzouk BI et al (2005) Successive clinical trials for childhood acute myeloid leukemia at St Jude Children's Research Hospital, from 1980 to 2000. Leukemia 19(12): 2125–2129

Robien K, Schubert MM et al (2004) Predictors of oral mucositis in patients receiving hematopoietic cell transplants for chronic myelogenous leukemia. J Clin Oncol 22(7): 1268–1275

Rocha JC, Cheng C et al (2005) Pharmacogenetics of outcome in children with acute lymphoblastic leukemia. Blood 105(12):4752–4758

Rubnitz JE, Lensing S et al (2004) Death during induction therapy and first remission of acute leukemia in childhood: the St Jude experience. Cancer 101(7):1677–1684

Salavaggione OE, Wang L et al (2005) Thiopurine S-methyltransferase pharmacogenetics: variant allele functional and comparative genomics. Pharmacogenet Genom 15(11): 801–815

Salinas AE, Wong MG (1999) Glutathione S-transferases – a review. Curr Med Chem 6(4):279–309

Schaeffeler E, Fischer C et al (2004) Comprehensive analysis of thiopurine S-methyltransferase phenotype-genotype correlation in a large population of German-Caucasians and identification of novel *TPMT* variants. Pharmacogenetics 14(7):407–417

Schmiegelow K, Al-Modhwahi I et al (2009a) Methotrexate/6-mercaptopurine maintenance therapy influences the risk of a second malignant neoplasm after childhood acute lymphoblastic leukemia: results from the NOPHO ALL-92 study. Blood113(24):6077–6084

Schmiegelow K, Forestier E et al (2009b) Thiopurine methyltransferase activity is related to the risk of relapse of childhood acute lymphoblastic leukemia: results from the NOPHO ALL-92 study. Leukemia 23(3):557–564

Schrecker AW, Goldin A (1968) Antitumor effect and mode of action of 1-beta-D-arabinofuranosylcytosine 5'-phosphate in leukemia L1210. Cancer Res 28(4):802–803

Seedhouse C, Faulkner R et al (2004) Polymorphisms in genes involved in homologous recombination repair interact to increase the risk of developing acute myeloid leukemia. Clin Cancer Res 10(8):2675–2680

Seedhouse CH, Grundy M et al (2007) Sequential influences of leukemia-specific and genetic factors on p-glycoprotein expression in blasts from 817 patients entered into the National Cancer Research Network acute myeloid leukemia 14 and 15 trials. Clin Cancer Res 13(23):7059–7066

Seidegard J, Vorachek WR et al (1988) Hereditary differences in the expression of the human glutathione transferase active on trans-stilbene oxide are due to a gene deletion. Proc Natl Acad Sci USA 85:7293–7297

Shuldiner AR, O'Connell JR et al (2009) Association of cytochrome P450 2C19 genotype with the antiplatelet effect and clinical efficacy of clopidogrel therapy. JAMA 302(8): 849–857

Sievers EL, Larson RA et al (2001) Efficacy and safety of gemtuzumab ozogamicin in patients with CD33-positive acute myeloid leukemia in first relapse. J Clin Oncol 19(13): 3244–3254

Simon T, Verstuyft C et al (2009) Genetic determinants of response to clopidogrel and cardiovascular events. N Engl J Med 360(4):363–375

Simone JV (1979) Childhood leukemia as a model for cancer research: the Richard and Hinda Rosenthal Foundation Award Lecture. Cancer Res 39(11):4301–4307

Simone JV (2003) Childhood leukemia – successes and challenges for survivors. N Engl J Med 349(7):627–628

Slats AM, Egeler RM et al (2005) Causes of death – other than progressive leukemia – in childhood acute lymphoblastic (ALL) and myeloid leukemia (AML): the Dutch Childhood Oncology Group experience. Leukemia 19(4): 537–544

Smith MT, Evans CG et al (1989) Denitrosation of 1, 3-bis(2-chloroethyl)-1-nitrosourea by class mu glutathione transferases and its role in cellular resistance in rat brain tumor cells. Cancer Res 49(10):2621–2625

Smith MA, Ries LAG et al (1999) In: Ries LAG, Smith MA, Gurney JG, Linet M, Tamra T, Young L et al (eds) Cancer incidence and survival among children and adolescents: United States SEER Program 1975–1995. NIH Pub. No. 99-4649. National Cancer Institute, SEER Program, Bethesda, MD, pp 17–34

Smith FO, Alonzo TA et al (2005) Long-term results of children with acute myeloid leukemia: a report of three consecutive Phase III trials by the Children's Cancer Group:

CCG 251, CCG 213 and CCG 2891. Leukemia 19(12): 2054–2062
Sonneveld P, List AF (2001) Chemotherapy resistance in acute myeloid leukaemia. Best Pract Res Clin Haematol 14(1): 211–233
Sorich MJ, Pottier N et al (2008) *In vivo* response to methotrexate forecasts outcome of acute lymphoblastic leukemia and has a distinct gene expression profile. PLoS Med 5(4):e83
Stanulla M, Schrappe M et al (2000) Polymorphisms within glutathione S-transferase genes (GSTM1, GSTT1, GSTP1) and risk of relapse in childhood B-cell precursor acute lymphoblastic leukemia: a case-control study. Blood 95(4): 1222–1228
Stanulla M, Schaeffeler E et al (2005a) Thiopurine methyltransferase (*TPMT*) genotype and early treatment response to mercaptopurine in childhood acute lymphoblastic leukemia. JAMA293(12):1485–1489
Stanulla M, Schaffeler E et al (2005b) GSTP1 and MDR1 genotypes and central nervous system relapse in childhood acute lymphoblastic leukemia. Int J Hematol 81(1):39–44
Steuart CD, Burke PJ (1971) Cytidine deaminase and the development of resistance to arabinosyl cytosine. Nat New Biol 233(38):109–110
Stone RM (2002) The difficult problem of acute myeloid leukemia in the older adult. CA Cancer J Clin 52(6):363–371
Tai HL, Krynetski EY et al (1997) Enhanced proteolysis of thiopurine S-methyltransferase (*TPMT*) encoded by mutant alleles in humans (*TPMT**3A, *TPMT**2): mechanisms for the genetic polymorphism of *TPMT* activity. Proc Natl Acad Sci USA 94:6444–6449
Takane H, Kobayashi D et al (2004) Haplotype-oriented genetic analysis and functional assessment of promoter variants in the MDR1 (ABCB1) gene. J Pharmacol Exp Ther 311(3): 1179–1187
Tanabe M, Ieiri I et al (2001) Expression of P-glycoprotein in human placenta: relation to genetic polymorphism of the multidrug resistance (MDR)-1 gene. J Pharmacol Exp Ther 297(3):1137–1143
Taniguchi S, Mochida Y et al (2003) Genetic polymorphism at the 5' regulatory region of multidrug resistance 1 (MDR1) and its association with interindividual variation of expression level in the colon. Mol Cancer Ther 2(12): 1351–1359
Tantisira KG, Lake S et al (2004) Corticosteroid pharmacogenetics: association of sequence variants in CRHR1 with improved lung function in asthmatics treated with inhaled corticosteroids. Hum Mol Genet 13(13):1353–1359
Thompsen J, Schroder H et al (1999) Possible carcinogenic effect of 6-mercaptopurine on bone marrow stem cells: relation to thiopurine metabolism. Cancer 86(6):1080–1086
Tinhofer I, Marschitz I et al (2000) Expression of functional interleukin-15 receptor and autocrine production of interleukin-15 as mechanisms of tumor propagation in multiple myeloma. Blood 95(2):610–618
Trevino LR, Shimasaki N et al (2009) Germline genetic variation in an organic anion transporter polypeptide associated with methotrexate pharmacokinetics and clinical effects. J Clin Oncol 27(35):5972–5978
Tsimberidou AM, Paterakis G et al (2002) Evaluation of the clinical relevance of the expression and function of P-glycoprotein, multidrug resistance protein and lung resistance protein in patients with primary acute myelogenous leukemia. Leuk Res 26(2):143–154
Tsuchida S, Sato K (1992) Glutathione transferases and cancer. Crit Rev Biochem Mol Biol 27:337–384
Ueda K, Clark DP et al (1987) The human multidrug resistance (mdr1) gene. cDNA cloning and transcription initiation. J Biol Chem 262(2):505–508
Ujiie S, Sasaki T et al (2008) Functional characterization of 23 allelic variants of thiopurine S-methyltransferase gene (*TPMT**2 - *24). Pharmacogenet Genomics 18(10): 887–893
Ulrich CM, Yasui Y et al (2001) Pharmacogenetics of methotrexate: toxicity among marrow transplantation patients varies with the methylenetetrahydrofolate reductase C677T polymorphism. Blood 98(1):231–234
van der Holt B, Lowenberg B et al (2005) The value of the MDR1 reversal agent PSC-833 in addition to daunorubicin and cytarabine in the treatment of elderly patients with previously untreated acute myeloid leukemia (AML), in relation to MDR1 status at diagnosis. Blood 106(8): 2646–2654
van der Holt B, Van den Heuvel-Eibrink MM et al (2006) ABCB1 gene polymorphisms are not associated with treatment outcome in elderly acute myeloid leukemia patients. Clin Pharmacol Ther 80(5):427–439
von Ahsen N, Armstrong VW et al (2004) Rapid, long-range molecular haplotyping of thiopurine S-methyltransferase (*TPMT*) *3A, *3B, and *3C. Clin Chem 50(9):1528–1534
Voso MT, Hohaus S et al (2008) Prognostic role of glutathione S-transferase polymorphisms in acute myeloid leukemia. Leukemia22(9):1685–1691
Wain LV, Armour JA et al (2009) Genomic copy number variation, human health, and disease. Lancet 374(9686):340–350
Wang LE, Bondy ML et al (2004) Polymorphisms of DNA repair genes and risk of glioma. Cancer Res 64(16): 5560–5563
Wang B, Ngoi S et al (2006) The promoter region of the MDR1 gene is largely invariant, but different single nucleotide polymorphism haplotypes affect MDR1 promoter activity differently in different cell lines. Mol Pharmacol 70(1): 267–276
Wang J, Wang W et al (2008) The diploid genome sequence of an Asian individual. Nature 456(7218):60–65
Wei G, Twomey D et al (2006) Gene expression-based chemical genomics identifies rapamycin as a modulator of MCL1 and glucocorticoid resistance. Cancer Cell 10(4):331–342
Weinshilboum RM, Sladek SL (1980) Mercaptopurine pharmacogenetics: monogenic inheritance of erythrocyte thiopurine methyltransferase activity. Am J Hum Genet 32:651–662
Weiss JR, Kopecky KJ et al (2006) Glutathione S-transferase (GSTM1, GSTT1 and GSTA1) polymorphisms and outcomes after treatment for acute myeloid leukemia: pharmacogenetics in Southwest Oncology Group (SWOG) clinical trials. Leukemia 20(12):2169–2171
Wermes C, Fleischhack G et al (1999a) Cerebral venous sinus thrombosis in children with acute lymphoblastic leukemia carrying the MTHFR TT677 genotype and further prothrombotic risk factors. Klinische Padiatrie 211(4):211–214
Wermes C, von Depka Prondzinski M et al (1999b) Clinical relevance of genetic risk factors for thrombosis in paediatric oncology patients with central venous catheters. Eur J Pediatr 158(Suppl 3):S143–146

Wheeler DA, Srinivasan M et al (2008) The complete genome of an individual by massively parallel DNA sequencing. Nature 452(7189):872–876

Wiemels JL, Smith RN et al (2001) Methylenetetrahydrofolate reductase (MTHFR) polymorphisms and risk of molecularly defined subtypes of childhood acute leukemia. Proc Natl Acad Sci USA 98(7):4004–4009

Wiley JS, Jones SP et al (1983) Cytosine arabinoside transport by human leukaemic cells. Eur J Cancer Clin Oncol 19(8): 1067–1074

Winsey SL, Haldar NA et al (2000) A variant within the DNA repair gene XRCC3 is associated with the development of melanoma skin cancer. Cancer Res 60(20):5612–5616

Woodson LC, Weinshilboum RM (1983) Human kidney thiopurine methyltransferase. Purification and biochemical properties. Biochem Pharmacol 32:819–826

Wouters KA, Kremer LC et al (2005) Protecting against anthracycline-induced myocardial damage: a review of the most promising strategies. Br J Haematol 131(5):561–578

Yamada NA, Hinz JM et al (2004) XRCC3 ATPase activity is required for normal XRCC3-Rad51C complex dynamics and homologous recombination. J Biol Chem 279(22): 23250–23254

Yang JJ, Bhojwani D et al (2008) Genome-wide copy number profiling reveals molecular evolution from diagnosis to relapse in childhood acute lymphoblastic leukemia. Blood 112(10):4178–4183

Yang JJ, Cheng C et al (2009) Genome-wide interrogation of germline genetic variation associated with treatment response in childhood acute lymphoblastic leukemia. JAMA 301(4):393–403

Yeoh EJ, Ross ME et al (2002) Classification, subtype discovery, and prediction of outcome in pediatric acute lymphoblastic leukemia by gene expression profiling. Cancer Cell 1(2):133–143

Yusa K, Oh-hara T et al (1992) Human immunodeficiency virus type 1 induces 1-beta-D-arabinofuranosylcytosine resistance in human H9 cell line. J Biol Chem 267(24): 16848–16850

Part V

The Potential Role of Biologically Targeted Therapy for Childhood Leukemia

Promising Targeted Agents

7

Patrick Brown, Gregory H. Reaman, Nita L. Seibel, and Pamela Kearns

Contents

P. Brown (✉)
Departments of Oncology and Pediatrics, Sidney Kimmel Comprehensive Cancer Center and Johns Hopkins University School of Medicine, Baltimore, MD, USA
e-mail: pbrown2@jhmi.edu

G.H. Reaman
George Washington University School of Medicine & Health Sciences, The Children's National Medical Center, III Michigan Ave. D.C. 20010, NW, Washington
e-mail: greaman@childrensoncologygroup.org

N.L. Seibel
Cancer Therapy Evaluation Program, National Cancer Institute, Bethesda, MD, USA

P. Kearns
School of Cancer Sciences, University of Birmingham, Birmingham, UK

7.1 Introduction

7.1.1 Overview

The past several decades have yielded remarkable improvements in long-term survival of children with acute leukemia, primarily resulting from sequential, controlled, multicenter clinical trials evaluating intensification of chemotherapy in a risk-adjusted paradigm based upon clinical and biologic features (Pui et al. 2004). These improvements have been particularly striking for acute lymphoblastic leukemia (ALL), the most common malignancy in children. In ALL, prolonged event-free survival (EFS) rates now approach 80%. This progress unequivocally represents one of the greatest success stories in modern medicine (Pui and Evans 2006; Moricke et al. 2008). Despite this success, however, many patients with ALL still relapse. Unfortunately, the outlook for children with relapsed ALL is grim, especially if the relapse occurs within 3 years of diagnosis (Nguyen et al. 2008). Also disconcerting are the significant, and not

G.H. Reaman and F.O. Smith (eds.), *Childhood Leukemia*,
DOI: 10.1007/978-3-642-13781-5_7, © Springer-Verlag Berlin Heidelberg 2011

uncommonly debilitating, acute and late complications associated with curative therapeutic approaches for ALL (Pui et al. 2003; Mody et al. 2008).

Therapeutic success has proven more difficult for children with acute myeloid leukemia (AML), although prolonged EFS rates for childhood AML now approximate 50% (Rubnitz 2008). In both AML and the higher risk subsets of ALL, a limit in the effectiveness of chemotherapy intensification to improve outcome has been reached due to offsetting increases in unacceptable toxicities. Furthermore, intensification of therapy with allogeneic hematopoietic stem cell transplantation (HSCT) only modestly improves the outcome of these patients, while introducing even higher risks of acute and late complications (Oliansky et al. 2007; Mulrooney et al. 2008).

Further improvements in outcome for childhood acute leukemia will likely depend on the development of new therapeutic strategies. To accomplish this, several interdependent and complementary areas of research are needed. These include (1) refinement in the definitions of specific subclasses of these diseases, which warrant varying intensities of therapy due to the relative risk of treatment failure (Pui and Evans 2006; Meshinchi and Arceci 2007); (2) an improved understanding of the biology of the leukemic stem cell (LSC), since eradication of the LSC (as opposed to mere reduction in the numbers of bulk leukemia cells) is emerging as a relevant goal of leukemia therapy (Bonnet and Dick 1997); and (3) the discovery and characterization of genetic and epigenetic alterations that are important in the pathogenesis of these diseases, either overall or for specific molecularly defined subsets, and that can be potentially targeted by novel therapeutic approaches. This review will focus on these novel molecularly targeted drug therapies for childhood ALL and AML (Table 7.1, Fig. 7.1). In this context, "targeted" refers to agents that selectively disrupt a tumor-specific biological pathway or a subset of cells within the bulk population that is essential for leukemia maintenance.

7.1.2 *Molecular Pathogenesis of Leukemia: The Basis of Targeted Therapy*

Recurrent translocations provided the most important initial clues to the molecular pathogenesis of leukemia (and cancer in general), and, in some notable cases, have facilitated development of successful molecularly targeted therapies. Perhaps the best example is found in chronic myelogenous leukemia (CML), for which the

Table7.1 Summary of molecularly targeted agents in clinical development for childhood acute leukemia

Class	Moleculart arget	Agent(s)	Disease	Subset	Phase
Monoclonals	CD33	Gemtuzumab ozogamicin	AML	CD33+	III
	CD22	Epratuzumab,C AT-8015	ALL	CD22+	II
	CD19	Blinatumomab	ALL	CD10+	I
TKI	BCR-ABL	Imatinib,D asatinib	ALL	Ph+	II
	FLT3	Lestaurtinib,S orafenib, Midostaurin	AML	FLT3m utated	II
			ALL	MLLr earranged	II
Proteasome inhibitors	NF-kB	Bortezomib	AML,A LL		I
mTORinhibitors	mTOR	Sirolimus,T emsirolimus	AML,A LL		I
Epigenetic modulators	HDAC	Vorinostat,Ent inostat	AML,A LL		I
	DNA methyltransferase	Azacitidine,D ecitabine	AML,A LL		I
Notchinhibitors	Gammas ecretase	MK0752,L Y450139	ALL	T-cell, Notch-mutant	I
Apoptosis modulators	BCL2f amily	Oblimersen,O blatoclax	ALL,A ML		I
	XIAP	AEG35156	AML		I

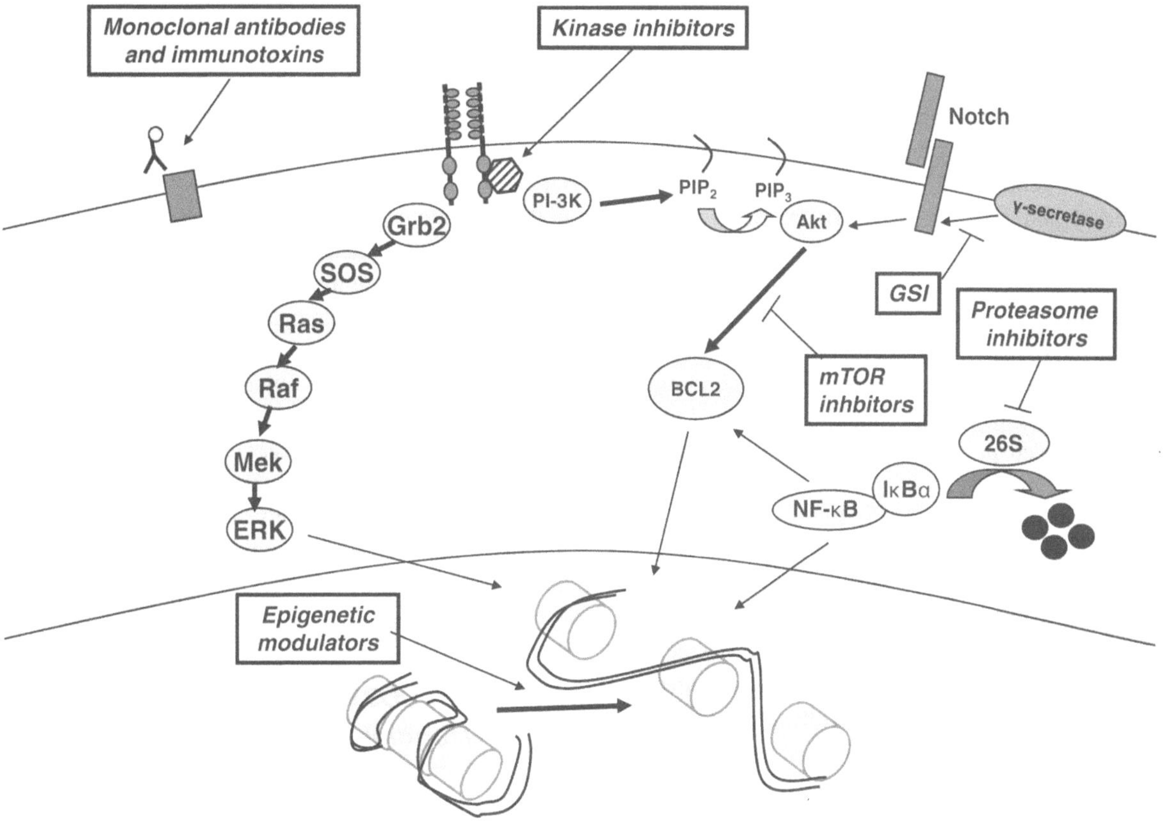

Fig. 7.1 Molecularly targeted agents in childhood leukemia. *GSI* gamma secretase inhibitors, *mTOR* mammalian target of rapamycin

discovery of the reciprocal translocation t(9;22)(q34;q11) (the Philadelphia chromosome, or Ph) led sequentially to identification of the BCR-ABL fusion protein, an understanding that resultant activation of the ABL kinase was central to the pathogenesis of CML, and, finally, the development of novel agents (imatinib and others) that could eradicate CML cells by inhibiting ABL kinase activity. This example is also helpful in understanding the importance of the LSC concept in the development of novel, molecularly targeted therapies. While a high proportion of patients with CML can achieve remission with imatinib therapy alone, it is unknown whether imatinib therapy successfully eradicates the CML stem cell, since it is not yet clear that long-term remissions after cessation of imatinib therapy will be widely achievable (Graham et al. 2002; Michor et al. 2005). Longer follow-up of patients treated in this manner will answer this important question.

Another example is acute promyelocytic leukemia (APL), which is characterized by the reciprocal translocation t(15;17)(q22;q21). The differentiation block induced by the resultant PML-RARα fusion protein has been successfully targeted with all-trans retinoic acid (ATRA), which, in combination with chemotherapy, has transformed a disease with a relatively high risk of relapse into one in which most cases are cured. In this case, the APL stem cell appears to be effectively eradicated by this approach. Interestingly, the APL stem cell seems to have distinct characteristics compared to the stem cell for other subtypes of AML, in that it has the more differentiated phenotype of a committed myeloid precursor (as opposed to the primitive phenotype reminiscent of the normal hematopoietic stem cell, which is characteristic of the other subtypes of AML) (Grimwade and Enver 2004). This may in part explain the relative ease with which APL can be successfully treated in children and adults with the combined use of chemotherapy and differentiating agents.

Other recurrent cytogenetic abnormalities are characteristic of unique biological subsets of childhood acute leukemias. For example, in B-precursor ALL, the t(12;21) translocation that results in the *ETV6-RUNX1* fusion gene is correlated with a good outcome, as are cases with "high" hyperdiploidy (>50 chromosomes). In contrast, cases showing rearrangements of the *MLL* gene (11q23), hypodiploidy (<44 chromosomes), and the t(9;22) (Ph+ ALL) fare poorly. Leukemic stem cells are less well characterized for childhood ALL when compared with AML, but evidence suggests that their phenotype varies depending on the biological subtype (Cox et al. 2004; Castor et al. 2005; le Viseur et al. 2008). While these abnormalities have led to a better understanding of leukemogenesis and improved prognostication, they have not as yet (except in the case of Ph+ ALL, which will be discussed in this chapter) led to the development of targeted therapies analogous to imatinib or ATRA.

The ability to move beyond standard cytogenetic approaches for the discovery and characterization of molecular alterations in ALL and AML has begun to pave the way for development of additional novel, targeted therapies that will hopefully improve the outcome for children with these diseases. The recent development of high throughput technologies to assess global genetic and epigenetic alterations in leukemia is greatly accelerating the identification of potential "targetable" abnormalities. The translation of the identification of molecular targets into effective therapies, however, is proving to be more difficult, resulting in a bottleneck that is unlikely to be relieved without a paradigm shift in how clinical research is conducted in the era of molecular therapeutics.

7.2 MonoclonalA ntibodies and Immunoconjugates

7.2.1 Differentiation Antigens as a Potential Target for Immunotherapy Approaches

The antigen expression profiles of leukemic blasts parallel those of normal stages of B- and T-cell differentiation in ALL and the normal stages of myeloid differentiation in AML. The phenotypic characterization of acute leukemia is an essential component of the diagnostic work-up of both diseases and is increasingly utilized, in concert with other parameters of cell biology in risk-adjusted treatment decisions (Bonnet and Dick 1997; Pui and Evans 2006; Meshinchi and Arceci 2007). In addition, these relatively lineage-specific antigens have been demonstrated to offer potential options for targeted immunotherapy approaches. Targeted immunotherapy includes monoclonal antibodies directed against specific cell surface antigens that destroy leukemia cells through immune mechanisms such as antibody-dependent cellular cytotoxicity (ADCC) and/or complement mediated cytotoxicity. In addition, monoclonal antibodies can be conjugated to additional moieties (e.g., cytotoxins or radioactive isotopes) in an attempt to enhance anticancer activity. Ideally, the differentiation antigens to target are those that are expressed on the overwhelming majority of leukemia cells, but which are not expressed on normal hematopoietic stem cells or on other normal tissues.

7.2.2 Anti-CD33 (Gemtuzumab Ozogamicin)

CD33 is a cell surface sialoglycoprotein that is increasingly expressed on normal myeloid cells as they differentiate; it is expressed on the surface of leukemia cells in 90% of cases of AML in adults and children (Brashem-Stein et al. 1993; Freeman et al. 1995). Gemtuzumab ozogamicin (Mylotarg®, Wyeth) is a humanized, monoclonal anti-CD33 antibody conjugated to the potent cytotoxin, calicheamicin (Sievers et al. 2001; Zwaan et al. 2003; Arceci et al. 2005; Larson et al. 2005). As a single agent in relapsed or refractory primary AML, gemtuzumab ozogamicin demonstrated response rates of 30–35% in both adult and pediatric patients. In a pediatric Phase I/II trial the response rate in children with primary refractory disease was the same as that for patients with relapsed disease, suggesting that the agent might circumvent recognized causes of drug resistance (Linenberger et al. 2001). Major toxicities seen in children at the maximum tolerated dose of 2–3 mg/m^2 (depending on high-dose cytarabine regimen) include myelosuppression and sinusoidal obstruction syndrome (SOS), also known as veno-occlusive disease of the liver, in patients undergoing subsequent allogeneic stem cell transplantation (Aplenc et al. 2008). This was noted to occur in patients who underwent transplantation within 3½ months of exposure to gemtuzumab. A pilot study performed by the Children's Oncology Group (COG) determined the maximum tolerated dose of gemtuzumab when given with high-dose cytarabine and in combination with mitoxantrone. Subsequent pilot studies have established the safety of the agent in combination with multi-drug regimens including the intensive Medical Research Council (MRC)-based chemotherapy in children with newly diagnosed AML. Feasible coadministration of the immunotoxin with both cytarabine, daunomycin and etoposide as well as mitoxantrone and cytarabine have been demonstrated (Franklin et al. 2008). A randomized Phase III study in *de novo* pediatric AML is testing the hypothesis that the immunotoxin improves survival by decreasing the likelihood of primary Induction failure as well as relapse.

Clinical response to gemtuzumab has been inversely correlated with mdr-1, P-glycoprotein expression, presumably related to increased cellular efflux of calicheamicin (Linenberger et al. 2001). The combinations of gemtuzumab with inhibitors of drug efflux are under investigation. A potential limitation of the use of gemtuzumab is the relative and inconsistent expression of CD33 by leukemia stem cells and the hypothesis that the eradication of such is required for long-term disease-free survival and cure. Longer follow-up of current clinical trials will definitively demonstrate the agent's ability to induce initial cytoreduction as well as improve long-term outcome.

7.2.3 Anti-CD22 (Epratuzumab)

Epratuzumab (Immunomedics) is a humanized monoclonal antibody (IgG1) directed against CD22, which is a B-cell-restricted 135 kD glycoprotein, initially present in the cytoplasm of early B-cell precursors and later expressed on the cell surface during B-cell differentiation. The antigen is widely expressed in B-cell lymphomas and B-precursor ALL (Carnahan et al. 2003). The mechanism of cytotoxicity of epratuzumab is thought to include both ADCC as well as complement mediated cytotoxicity and direct induction of apoptosis. In addition to direct cytotoxicity and decrease in CD22-bearing cells, the antibody induces other B-cell modulatory activity. Single-agent studies have demonstrated its tolerability in children and pilot studies in combination with re-Induction chemotherapy in children have demonstrated feasibility and tolerability as well as efficacy when used in combination with vincristine, prednisone, L-asparaginase, and doxorubicin at a dose of 360 mg/m^2 (Raetz et al. 2008). Efficacy evaluation of epratuzumab in combination with conventional chemotherapy in newly diagnosed high-risk B-precursor ALL patients is planned by the COG.

Anti-CD22 immunotoxins are also in development, including BL22, which conjugates a pseudomonas exotoxin-A to anti-CD22 and is undergoing adult clinical trials in chronic lymphocytic and hairy cell leukemia. An additional immunotoxin that combines anti-CD22 and anti-CD19 monoclonal antibodies conjugated to deglycosylated ricin A (Combotox®) has demonstrated preclinical activity in childhood ALL and is undergoing clinical evaluation in adults with relapsed B lineage ALL (Herrera et al. 2000; Herrera et al. 2003).

The second-generation investigational anti-CD22 immunotoxin, CAT-8015(HA22), has demonstrated clinical activity early in a pediatric Phase I trial. However, dose-limiting toxicities of the agent occur and appear to be due to vascular leak syndrome (Wayne et al. 2009).

7.2.4 Anti-CD19

The CD19 antigen is more ubiquitously expressed by normal B-lymphocyte progenitors and more universally expressed by B-precursor ALL cells and provides a better theoretical target for targeted immunotherapeutic approaches. A novel class of bispecific T-cell associated antibodies (BiTE) that redirects T-cells through anti-CD3 for lysis of target cells is under clinical investigation. Blinatumomab (MT103) targets the CD19 antigen on B-cells, the expression of which is ubiquitous in B-cell precursor ALL. In a single-agent Phase II trial of this agent in patients with B-precursor ALL who had evidence of minimal residual disease (MRD) at end Induction, MRD status was reversed in 13 of 16 patients. Thirteen of 16 evaluable patients experiencing molecular complete remission after a single cycle of blinatumomab had extended clinical and molecular and complete remission and two of the patients who failed had isolated extra-medullary relapse (Zugmaier et al. 2009). Based on this compelling clinical activity, plans for pediatric investigation in relapsed ALL (in both the pre- and post-transplant settings) are under consideration. The strong investigational interest in the agent is somewhat tempered by isolated observations of central neurotoxicity, the etiology of which is not clear.

In summary, the early experience of some of these investigational agents provides a sound rationale for their expanded clinical study in relapsed ALL and in patient subgroups at high risk for treatment failure.

7.3 TyrosineK inasel nhibitors(T KI)

7.3.1 BCR-ABL: Imatinib, Dasatinib

Historically, children with Ph+ ALL have had a dismal prognosis, with EFS of only approximately 20% when treated with chemotherapy alone (Arico et al. 2000). As mentioned, efforts to develop small molecular inhibitors of the BCR-ABL protein led to the development of imatinib, which binds to and inhibits its tyrosine kinase activity. Imatinib has potent clinical activity in CML and has revolutionized treatment of this disorder (Druker et al. 2001a, b). However, both *de novo* and acquired imatinib resistance are observed in CML and represent the major cause of treatment failure (Gorre and Sawyers 2002). In Ph+ ALL, 60–70% of previously treated patients respond to single-agent imatinib therapy, but responses are short-lived with median time to progression of 2–3 months (Druker et al. 2001a, b; Ottmann et al. 2002). Clinical trials in adults have shown that addition of imatinib to hyper-CVAD (cyclophosphamide, vincristine, Adriamycin, dexamethasone) is safe and is associated with at least a short-term improvement in survival in Ph+ ALL (Thomas et al. 2004). The combination of imatinib plus Induction chemotherapy has been shown to be superior to Induction chemotherapy alone in quickly lowering disease burden, assessed by Day 14 marrow status, and showed a trend toward improved Induction rate (Lee et al. 2005a, b).

The recently completed COG AALL0031 trial established the safety and tested the efficacy of an intensive chemotherapy backbone plus imatinib in treating children with Ph+ ALL (Schultz et al. 2009). The addition of imatinib was safe and associated with relatively minor additional toxicity (mild asymptomatic transaminitis requiring intermittent rather than continuous dosing during Maintenance therapy). While the long-term impact of imatinib on EFS of pediatric Ph+ ALL patients remains to be determined, recent results in adult and pediatric patients indicate a favorable response in the context of multi-agent chemotherapy as assessed by early endpoints, such as complete response (CR) rate (for patients receiving imatinib in Induction), levels of MRD, and proportion of patients proceeding to transplant (Lee et al. 2005a, b). In addition, the early outcome data from AALL0031 are promising (Schultz et al. 2009). The 3-year EFS of patients receiving continuous imatinib (n = 44) is 80.5 ± 11.2%, including those assigned to a sibling HSCT (n = 13) and those receiving off-protocol alternative donor HSCT (n = 6), and excluding those failing to achieve remission after 4 weeks of standard Induction chemotherapy (n = 6). This is significantly higher than historical controls, both from previous Pediatric Oncology Group studies (n = 120; 3-year EFS 35.0 ± 4.4%) and from other published data (n = 267, 2-year EFS 40.9 ± 5.4%) (64). While these results are encouraging, longer follow-up is needed to determine if these impressive early results will hold up over time. It is hypothesized that further gains in outcome for patients with Ph+ ALL are most likely to derive from integration of more potent targeted agents or incorporation of agents that act synergistically with imatinib into intensive combination chemotherapy regimens.

A variety of newer agents may improve upon the activity of imatinib and thereby increase the efficacy of the current treatment program for Ph+ ALL. The new class of ABL/Src kinase inhibitors, and specifically dasatinib, are the most promising of these agents. Signaling through the Src family kinases HCK, LYN, and FGR is required for leukemic transformation in Ph+ ALL (but not Ph+ CML) (Hu et al. 2004). In June 2006, dasatinib was granted accelerated approval by the Food and Drug Administration (FDA) for treatment of adults with chronic phase, accelerated phase, or myeloid or lymphoid blast phase CML, and regular approval for adults with Ph+ ALL with resistance or intolerance to prior therapy. *In vitro*, dasatinib is 325 times more potent than imatinib at blocking the ABL kinase activity (O'Hare et al. 2005). Furthermore, dasatinib is active *in vitro* against most known imatinib-resistant BCR-ABL mutants (Shah et al. 2004; Carter et al. 2005a, b). Dasatinib has displayed a high level of efficacy for patients with imatinib-resistant CML with minimal side effects, including mild myelosuppression and nausea (Talpaz et al. 2006). Dasatinib is a particularly attractive agent for treatment of Ph+ ALL due to its dual targeting of ABL and the Src kinases, more powerful suppression of BCR/ABL signaling, and efficacy in imatinib-resistant leukemia.

Consequently, an ongoing COG study is testing intensification of tyrosine kinase inhibitor therapy by combining dasatinib with the AALL0031 backbone of intensive chemotherapy beginning in the latter 2 weeks of Induction and continuing with all post-Induction courses. As dasatinib is highly effective as a single agent at targeting imatinib-resistant Ph+ leukemic clones, it is possible that substitution of dasatinib for imatinib will prove effective in preventing resistance and increasing EFS in children with Ph+ ALL.

7.3.2 FLT3: Lestaurtinib, Sorafenib, AC220, Midostaurin

Another aberrantly activated kinase against which targeted therapies are being developed is FLT3 (Brown et al. 2004; Levis et al. 2005a, b). FLT3 is a receptor tyrosine kinase that is expressed in over 90% of cases of AML (Carow et al. 1996). Mutations in *FLT3* that lead to constitutive (ligand-independent) phosphorylation occur in approximately 30–35% of adults and 20–25% of children with AML (Kiyoi et al. 1998; Meshinchi et al. 2001; Yamamoto et al. 2001). About two thirds of these *FLT3* mutations are internal tandem duplications (ITD) in the juxtamembrane region of the receptor, and one third are point mutations (PM) in the kinase domain. Several studies have shown that the presence of FLT3/ITD confers an increased risk of relapse and decreased survival in childhood AML (Iwai et al. 1999; Kondo et al. 1999; Meshinchi et al. 2001, 2006). In a retrospective study of children with *de novo* AML enrolled on the Children's Cancer Group (CCG) CCG-2891 Phase III clinical trial, for example, patients with FLT3/ITD had an 8-year overall survival and EFS of 13% and 7%, respectively, versus 50% and 44% for patients without FLT3/ITD (Meshinchi et al. 2001). Further studies in both adult and pediatric AML have demonstrated that in FLT3/ITD positive samples, the ratio of mutant to wild-type alleles has additional prognostic significance, such that patients with high ITD allelic ratios have a worse prognosis (Whitman et al. 2001; Thiede et al. 2002; Meshinchi et al. 2006).

The demonstrated importance of FLT3 signaling in AML has led to the development of small molecules with selective FLT3 inhibitory activity. Lestaurtinib (CEP-701) is an orally bioavailable indolocarbazole derivative with an inhibitory concentration (IC) 50 of 3 nM for inhibition of phosphorylation of ITD, PM, and wild-type (WT) FLT3 (Levis et al. 2002). Preclinical studies have shown that lestaurtinib selectively kills primary adult and pediatric AML blasts with *FLT3* mutations (Levis et al. 2002; Brown et al. 2004). In the study of pediatric AML samples, for example, those with FLT3/ITD were particularly likely to demonstrate *in vitro* sensitivity to lestaurtinib, with 14 of 15 samples (93%) noted to be responders. While samples with FLT3/PM (4 of 15, or 27%) and those with FLT3/WT (4 of 14, or 29%) were significantly less likely to respond, over one quarter of these samples did demonstrate pronounced sensitivity, and the sensitive samples were shown to express high levels of activated FLT3.

There is growing clinical experience with lestaurtinib. In a Phase II single-agent study in adults with relapsed/refractory *FLT3*-mutant AML, lestaurtinib was well-tolerated at doses up to 80 mg orally twice daily, with common toxicities of mild nausea and fatigue (Smith et al. 2004). Successful inhibition of FLT3 phosphorylation to less than 10% of baseline levels was demonstrated at this dose. Clinical responses (reduction in peripheral blood or bone marrow blast percentage) were seen in 5 of 14 patients, all of whom had been shown to be refractory to chemotherapy. Another Phase II study tested lestaurtinib as frontline monotherapy (80 mg orally twice daily for 8 weeks) for older adults with AML that were not considered eligible for chemotherapy (Knapper et al. 2006). Clinical responses were seen in three of five (60%) patients with *FLT3* mutations, and in 5 of 22 (23%) patients with wild-type *FLT3*. An ongoing study randomizes adults with relapsed/refractory *FLT3*-mutant AML to receive chemotherapy alone (mitoxantrone, etoposide, and cytarabine; or high-dose cytarabine) or chemotherapy in sequential combination with lestaurtinib (80 mg orally twice daily) (Levis et al. 2005a, b). Lestaurtinib has been well-tolerated in this trial, with mild to moderate gastrointestinal symptoms and fatigue attributed to the drug. Ten of 17 (59%) patients on the lestaurtinib arm have achieved a CR or partial response (PR), compared to 4 of 17 (24%) patients randomized to chemotherapy only. Cytotoxicity analysis showed that 80% of pretreatment samples were sensitive to lestaurtinib *in vitro*. Thirteen of 17 (76%) patients on the lestaurtinib arm achieved high enough levels of drug in plasma to fully inhibit FLT3 phosphorylation. Remarkably, the ten patients who met both criteria predictive of a good response (i.e., had pretreatment leukemia cells that were sensitive *in vitro* to lestaurtinib, and achieved sufficient plasma levels of lestaurtinib) were the clinical responders. Conversely, the seven patients with insensitive cells or insufficient drug plasma levels did not respond.

Lestaurtinib is now being tested in the COG for children with relapsed/refractory *FLT3*-mutant AML. Lestaurtinib is given in sequential combination with re-Induction chemotherapy (high-dose cytarabine (HiDAC) and idarubicin). The sequence of exposure in this trial (chemotherapy followed by FLT3 inhibitor) is based upon preclinical studies demonstrating that maximal synergy between FLT3 inhibition and chemotherapy is achieved with this approach, compared to simultaneous exposure (which is additive rather than synergistic) or FLT3 inhibitor followed by chemotherapy (which is antagonistic) (Levis et al. 2004; Brown et al. 2006). The antagonism seen with the sequence of FLT3 inhibition followed by chemotherapy is due to the cell-cycle-arresting properties of FLT3 inhibitors, which protect the arrested cells from the cytotoxic effects of chemotherapy agents (which are most toxic to actively cycling cells).

In addition to lestaurtinib, there are several other small molecule FLT3 inhibitors in clinical development for AML, including sorafenib (Ravandi et al. 2010), AC220 (Zarrinkar et al. 2009) and midostaurin (Stone et al. 2005). Plans to incorporate FLT3 inhibitors into COG Phase III clinical trials for *de novo* pediatric FLT3/ITD positive patients are under consideration.

Similar concerns to those described for CD33-targeted therapy have been raised about the relevance of FLT3-targeted therapy to the goal of eradicating the LSC. The discovery that about 10–20% of patients whose leukemia is FLT3/ITD+ at diagnosis will lack the mutation at relapse (Kottaridis et al. 2002) suggests that in a subset of patients, FLT3 mutations may be a secondary event that arises in a subclone of the leukemic population. However, the presence of FLT3/ITD mutations in the cells responsible for long-term engraftment of AML patient samples in nonobese diabetic/severe combined immunodeficient (NOD/SCID) mice (which is the strongest functional evidence of LSC activity) provides direct evidence that in the majority of cases, FLT3/ITD mutations are present in the LSC (Levis et al. 2005a, b). Further evidence comes from a study showing a correlation between the presence of the FLT3/ITD mutation in CD34+/CD33– myeloid progenitors and a significantly poorer outcome (compared to cases in which FLT3/ITD was present only in more differentiated CD34+/CD33+ progenitors)(Polla rde ta l. 2006).

FLT3 has been implicated in the pathogenesis of some cases of ALL in infants and children. Gene expression studies have shown that the highest levels of FLT3 mRNA expression occur in cases of infant and childhood ALL with rearrangements of the *MLL* gene (which account for 80% of infant and 5% of childhood ALL cases) and in cases of ALL with hyperdiploidy with more than 50 chromosomes (which account for 25% of childhood ALL cases) (Armstrong et al. 2002; Armstrong et al. 2004). The correlation of high FLT3 expression and these cytogenetic abnormalities is very strong. Moreover, several laboratories have demonstrated that leukemic blasts from cases of *MLL*-rearranged and hyperdiploid ALL also express high levels of FLT3 at the protein level, and that FLT3 is constitutively phosphorylated in these cases even in the absence of *FLT3*-activating mutations, suggesting autocrine activation via coexpression of FLT3 ligand (FL) (Armstrong et al. 2003; Zheng et al. 2004; Brown et al. 2005; Stam et al. 2005). In addition, activating mutations of *FLT3* (specifically, point mutations in the activation loop of the kinase domain) occur in approximately 15% of infants and children with ALL with *MLL* gene rearrangements or hyperdiploidy (Armstrong et al. 2003, 2004; Taketani et al. 2004). Small insertion/deletion mutations in the juxtamembrane domain have also been reported in an additional 12% of high-hyperdiploid ALL cases, for a total *FLT3* mutation rate of about 30% in hyperdiploid ALL cases.

Given the importance of FLT3 in the pathogenesis of ALL, FLT3 inhibitors are being evaluated for ALL as well. *In vitro*, lestaurtinib selectively kills those primary infant and childhood ALL cells with high-level expression of constitutively activated FLT3. For those with *MLL* rearrangements, marked lestaurtinib sensitivity was seen in 82% (9 of 11) of *MLL*-rearranged samples versus 8% (1 of 13) of samples that lacked *MLL* rearrangement and expressed low levels of FLT3 (Brown et al. 2005). Since monotherapy with any single molecularly targeted agent is unlikely to be curative in acute leukemia, targeted agents are more likely to be effective as components of combination chemotherapy regimens. Lestaurtinib has been shown to result in synergistic killing of *MLL*-rearranged ALL cells when combined with multiple chemotherapy agents (Brown et al. 2006). The degree of synergy is markedly dependent upon sequence of exposure to the agents. Exposure to chemotherapy followed by lestaurtinib results in consistent and strong synergistic cell killing, while simultaneous exposure, is in most cases, additive. Exposure to lestaurtinib followed by chemotherapy is, in many cases, antagonistic. This sequence dependence is due to the effects of FLT3 inhibition on cell-cycle progression.

Based on these data, lestaurtinib is being tested in the COG for infants with newly diagnosed *MLL*-rearranged ALL. Lestaurtinib is being added in a randomized fashion to the multicourse chemotherapy regimen used in a previous clinical trial for infant ALL. The design of this study takes into account the preclinical data regarding combinations of lestaurtinib and chemotherapy, as lestaurtinib will be given immediately following exposure to standard cytotoxic chemotherapy in an effort to maximize potential synergy, and will not be given for at least 24 h prior to chemotherapy to avoid potential antagonism.

Unlike rearrangements of the *MLL* gene, hyperdiploidy is a favorable prognostic feature in childhood ALL (Pui et al. 2004). Nonetheless, 10–20% of these patients will suffer relapse of their disease. Data indicate that FLT3 delivers crucial survival signals in high-hyperdiploid cells, as indicated by their exquisite sensitivity to FLT3 inhibition in cytotoxicity and apoptosis assays (Brown et al. 2005). FLT3 inhibitors, therefore, may have a role in the treatment of high-hyperdiploid ALL, either in the setting of relapsed disease, or as part of upfront therapy to enable the decreased use of cytotoxic agents (with their significant short and long-term toxicities) while maintaining high cure rates.

7.4 Proteasomel nhibitors

The proteasome is responsible for intracellular protein degradation. Polyubiquitination marks intracellular proteins destined to undergo degradation at the proteasome. Careful control of the degradation of proteins through the ubiquitin-proteasome pathway is essential for multiple processes in the cell, which include orderly progression through cell cycle, p53-mediated responses to cellular stresses, and nuclear factor (NF)-κB activation (Adams 2004; Orlowski and Kuhn 2008).

Proteasome inhibitors were first synthesized to block the proteolytic processes, with the dipeptidyl boronic acid compound bortezomib (PS-341) being the first to proceed into clinical development. Bortezomib induced apoptosis in preclinical studies in leukemic cell lines that were chemotherapy-resistant and radiation-resistant. Based on the multiple signaling pathways affected by proteasome inhibition, there is probably not a single effect of bortezomib that is responsible for all its anti-cancer activity. One effect of bortezomib is to repress NF-κB signaling by stabilizing the inhibitor protein IκB, and allowing IκB to maintain it inhibitory influence over NF-κB. Bortezomib can also stabilize p53, allowing it to function as an apoptotic transcription factor in cells exposed to bortezomib. Proteasome inhibition can induce aggresome formation, endoplasmic reticulum stress, and the unfolded protein response which has special relevance for multiple myeloma cells given their high rates of protein synthesis (Orlowski and Kuhn 2008). Bortezomib is FDA-approved for patients with multiple myeloma and progressive mantle cell lymphoma. The most common moderate-to-serious adverse events observed in adults receiving bortezomib have been asthenia, peripheral neuropathy, thrombocytopenia, and neutropenia (Adams 2004).

Proteasome inhibition is of interest in AML. Although unstimulated CD+34 stem cells do not express activated NF-κB, NF-κB is constitutively activated in primary AML specimens, and specifically in the CD34+/CD38- LSC population (Guzman et al. 2001). The combination of a proteasome inhibitor and idarubicin demonstrates rapid and extensive apoptosis of AML blasts and the LSC population *in vitro* and *in vivo*, while preserving normal hematopoietic stem cells (Guzman et al. 2002). These data have formed the basis for the hypothesis that by selectively targeting the LSC population in AML, more durable responses will be achieved than with standard therapies alone. A Phase I study of bortezomib in adults with refractory or relapsed acute leukemias established tolerability with twice weekly dosing of 1.25 mg/m^2 for 4 weeks of a 6-week cycle (Cortes et al. 2004). The combination of bortezomib and pegylated liposomal doxorubicin in adults with advanced hematologic malignancies showed activity in two of five patients with AML (Orlowski et al. 2005a, b). A Phase I study adding bortezomib to a standard re-Induction regimen using idarubicin and cytarabine demonstrated a good safety profile for the regimen and promising anti-leukemia activity(A ttare ta l. 2008).

Bortezomib is being investigated in pediatric and adolescent leukemias. The Phase I study of bortezomib in pediatric leukemia identified 1.3 mg/m^2 (given twice weekly for 2 out of 3 weeks) as the recommended Phase II dose (Horton et al. 2007). Dose-limiting toxicities seen at the 1.7 mg/m^2 dose were altered mental state and grade 4 hypotension, followed by grade 5 hypoxia in a patient with fever and neutropenia. The COG is conducting a Phase II study in patients with relapsed/secondary AML in which bortezomib is combined with an Induction regimen of either idarubicin/cytarabine or etoposide/cytarabine. COG AAML1031 is a Phase III randomized study in children and adolescents with *de novo* AML who will be randomized at diagnosis to receive standard chemotherapy with or without bortezomib.

Several reports have documented *in vitro* activity against ALL cell lines, although this is a nonspecific observation, since many cancer cell lines are sensitive to bortezomib. In the Pediatric Preclinical Testing Program (PPTP), bortezomib showed some activity against the ALL xenografts, with both of the T-cell ALL xenografts evaluated responding to bortezomib (Houghton et al. 2008a, b). In the Phase I study of bortezomib for children with recurrent leukemias, there were no responses in nine children with B-cell ALL, all heavily pretreated (Horton et al. 2007). Against ALL cell lines, bortezomib was synergistic with dexamethasone and additive with vincristine, asparaginase, cytarabine, and doxorubicin (Horton et al. 2006). Bortezomib can be safely administered with standard re-Induction therapy in the recurrent ALL setting, and eight of ten patients treated as such showed a complete response in the bone marrow (Messenger et al. 2008). This approach is being piloted by the COG in COG AALL07P1, which is a Phase II pilot trial of bortezomib in combination with intensive re-Induction therapy for children with relapsed ALL and lymphoblastic lymphoma.

Since the proteasome has become a valid target for cancer therapy, development of newer inhibitors continues, which may offer additional benefits. Two second-generation proteasome inhibitors have entered Phase I trials in adults: NPI-0052 (salinosporamide A) and carfilzomib (formerly PR-171). In preclinical studies, both of these at least partially overcame bortezomib resistance *in vitro* and may have a broader spectrum of activity and less neurotoxicity than bortezomib (Chauhan et al. 2005; Alsina et al. 2007; Kuhn et al. 2007; Orlowski et al. 2007). Another potential interesting target is the immunoproteasome, whose expression may be more tissue restricted than the constitutive proteasome. Currently, all the proteasome inhibitors target both the immunoproteasome and constitutive proteasome. Since the immunoproteaseome is expressed predominantly in hematopoietic tissues and other tissues express much lower levels of immunoproteasome subunits, less toxicity, such as neurologic and gastrointestinal symptoms, may be observed (Rivett and Hearn 2004; Orlowski et al. 2005a, b; Ho et al. 2007).

7.5 mTORI nhibitorsSi rolimus, Temsirolimus

The mammalian target of rapamycin (mTOR) is a serine/threonine kinase that functions as a key regulator of cell growth, protein synthesis, and cell-cycle progression through interactions with a number of signaling pathways, including PI3K/AKT, ras, TCL1, and BCR/ABL (Meric-Bernstam and Gonzalez-Angulo 2009). Rapamycin (sirolimus), a macrocyclic lactone first noted to have significant anti-cancer activity in preclinical models more than two decades ago, was the first mTOR inhibitor to be used in the clinical setting (Douros and Suffness 1981; Eng et al. 1984). Rapamycin is FDA-approved as an immunosuppressive agent in solid organ transplantation, but the drug has clear anti-neoplastic activity and is in Phase II–III trials against a variety of cancers (Baldo et al. 2008). Rapamycin has poor aqueous solubility and variable bioavailability, requiring therapeutic drug monitoring. A number of second-generation mTOR inhibitors including temsirolimus (CCI-779), everolimus (RAD001), and deferolimus (AP23573) have been developed to circumvent those problems. Temsirolimus was the first mTOR inhibitor to gain FDA approval for any malignancy, when it was approved in 2007 for first-line treatment of poor prognosis patients with advanced renal cell carcinoma. Everolimus is FDA approved as second-line therapy for renal cell carcinoma following progression on a VEGF-targeted therapy (Motzer et al. 2008). When used as monotherapy, mTOR inhibitors are relatively well-tolerated, with the primary toxicities for cancer patients consisting of asthenia, mucositis, thrombocytopenia, hypercholesterolemia, and pneumonitis (Baldo et al. 2008; Meric-Bernstama ndG onzalez-Angulo 2009).

Many hematological malignancies have aberrant activation of mTOR and related signaling pathways. An evaluation of rapamycin by the PPTP showed broad *in vivo* tumor growth inhibition across most of the histologies evaluated, with objective responses (tumor regressions) observed for several diagnoses including ALL (Houghton et al. 2008a, b). The activity observed for rapamycin against the ALL PPTP panel is consistent with other reports showing *in vivo* activity for rapamycin and rapamycin analogs (rapalogs) against ALL xenografts (Teachey et al. 2006, 2008). The mTOR inhibitors appear to be active against both B- and T-cell ALL; however, they may be more active in T-cell disease (Houghton et al. 2008a, b). Pediatric Phase I trials of the rapalogs have been completed with temsirolimus and everolimus (Fouladi et al. 2007). In a Phase I trial of sirolimus in children with relapsed/refractory ALL, all patients tolerated sirolimus (Rheingolde ta l. 2007).

Because mTOR inhibitors are less likely to be effective in the clinical setting when used as single agents against leukemia, combination treatment is being explored. The mTOR inhibitors have been shown to be effective and potentially synergistic in combination with a number of chemotherapeutic agents *in vitro*, such as methotrexate, dexamethasone, etoposide, asparaginases, and doxorubicin (Saydam et al. 2005; Teachey et al. 2008). The PPTP demonstrated that the combinations of rapamycin with cyclophosphamide or vincristine were well tolerated, with the combinations commonly showing significantly greater antitumor activity than the single-agent treatments (Houghton et al. 2008a, b). Combining corticosteroids with mTOR inhibitors was found to hold promise when Wei et al. screened a database of drug-associated gene expression signatures of glucocorticoid sensitivity as compared to resistance. They found the profile generated by sirolimus matched the signature of glucocorticoid sensitivity and demonstrated that sirolimus could restore steroid sensitivity to steroid-resistant ALL (Wei et al. 2006). Other investigators have shown that mTOR inhibitors may reverse glucocorticoid resistance in ALL cells (Gu et al. 2008; Haarman et al. 2008). Additionally, since BCR-ABL is upstream of the PI3K/AKT/mTOR signaling pathway, mTOR inhibitors may be effective in Ph+ALL, including BCR-ABL tyrosine kinase inhibitor resistant disease (Kharas et al. 2004). The COG is planning a pilot study of temsirolimus with re-Induction chemotherapy for patients with recurrent ALL.

As a result of the potential activity of mTOR inhibitors against ALL, and considering that HSCT is used as a major salvage for patients with refractory or relapsed ALL and sirolimus has been used as graft-versus-host disease (GVHD) prophylaxis in a number of transplant trials, the use of sirolimus in the post-HSCT setting is being tested by the COG. COG's Phase III randomized trial, ASCT 0431, is evaluating the addition of sirolimus to GVHD prophylaxis during HSCT for relapsed ALL. The primary hypothesis of this trial is that the addition of sirolimus to GVHD will increase leukemia-free survival compared to a regimen of standard agents, through the novel benefit of using a drug that has the potential to both control GVHD and directly suppress leukemic blasts.

Recent interest has focused on targeting the PI3K/AKT/mTOR pathway in AML, as a majority of patients' blasts have constitutive activation of AKT with subsequent phorphorylation of downstream targets of mTOR (Xu et al. 2003). Promising results have been demonstrated using monotherapy with mTOR inhibitors in preclinical models of AML; however, these have not translated into substantial clinical benefit in early phase trials (Yee et al. 2006; Rizzieri et al. 2008). Despite these findings, there is interest that targeting the mTOR pathway may enhance the cytotoxity of existing chemotherapeutic agents and other targeted agents. Sirolimus has been shown to enhance the sensitivity of AML blasts to etoposide *in vitro* and the combination could prevent engraftment of AML cells in NOD/SCID mice better than either single agent alone, if cells were treated *in vitro* prior to injection (Xu et al. 2005). Blocking the mTOR pathway increases the sensitivity of AML cells to HDAC (histone deacetylase) inhibitors (Nishioka et al. 2008). Since combination therapy with mTOR inhibitors and either cytotoxics or biologicals may be beneficial in patients with AML, clinical trials testing mTOR inhibitors in AML are being conducted in adults. As other inhibitors of the PI3K/AKT/mTOR pathway are developed and tested in clinical trials, these agents may prove to be superior to mTOR inhibitors alone. The dual inhibitor PI103, which targets both mTOR and PI3K, has shown promise in preclinical studies (Park et al. 2008).

7.6 NOTCHPat hwayl nhibitors

The NOTCH signaling pathway helps regulate cell proliferation and apoptosis and is required for normal embryonic development. NOTCH1 is a member of a family of highly conserved receptors that normally signal through a series of ligand-induced proteolytic cleavage events. As a result of these events, the intracellular portion of NOTCH1 (ICN1) gains access to the nucleus where it forms a short-lived transcriptional activation complex, resulting in eventual transcription of target genes (Kopan and Ilagan 2009). The final step of cleavage by γ-secretase liberates ICN1. Activating mutations in the *NOTCH1* gene leading to increased levels of ICN1 are present in over 50% of human T-ALL cases as well as many murine T-ALL models (Aster et al. 2008). Further studies have shown that ICN1 drives the growth of T-ALL cells by up-regulation of *MYC* expression and enhanced signaling of PI3-kinase/AKT/mTOR pathway. The NOTCH pathway has been shown to be a key regulator of human T-cell acute leukemia initiating cell activity (Armstrong et al. 2009). Increases in ICN1 levels caused by *NOTCH1* mutations are counteracted by drugs that inhibit γ-secretase. Since γ-secretase is linked to Alzheimer's disease, a large number of drugs are in preclinical development. Gamma secretase inhibitors (GSI) can induce G_0/G_1 arrest, decrease cell viability, and cause apoptosis of T-ALL cell lines carrying *NOTCH*-activating mutations.

The first attempt to treat patients with refractory/relapsed T-ALL with an oral GSI resulted in treatment failures and significant gastrointestinal toxicity (DeAngelo 2006). The toxicity was probably a result of goblet cell metaplasia, as in the absence of NOTCH signaling the differentiation of epithelial cells lining the small bowel and colon is characterized by a marked increase in goblet cell differentiation and arrested cell proliferation in the intestinal crypts (Milano et al. 2004). The poor results could be due to inadequate inhibition of NOTCH signaling since dosing was limited by gastrointestinal toxicity, or to the limited levels of apoptosis induced in *NOTCH1*-mutant cell lines by GSI (Weng et al. 2004; Lewis et al. 2007). Recently, combination therapy with glucocorticoids and GSIs has been shown to improve the antileukemic effects of GSIs and the glucocorticoids have been shown to abrogate the development of goblet cell metaplasia in mice treated with GSIs. These results suggest that glucocorticoids plus GSIs may have a role in the treatment of glucocorticoid-resistant T-ALL. Additionally, glucocorticoids might ameliorate the clinical toxicity associated with systemic inhibition of NOTCH signaling with GSIs (Real and Ferrando 2009; Real et al. 2009). Altering the schedule of administration of GSIs in mice by using an intermittent, 3-day on/4-day off GSI dosing schedule avoids gut toxicity while maintaining the anti-T-ALL effects (Cullion et al. 2009). Rapamycin has been shown to enhance the efficacy of GSIs in mice, raising the possibility that combination therapy with GSIs, glucocorticoids, and mTOR inhibitors may have a role in the treatment of T-ALL (Cullion et al. 2009).

NOTCH1 mutations are not found in B-ALL and are seen only rarely in AML. The rare human AMLs with *NOTCH1* mutations tend to show minimal myeloid differentiation, frequently express T-cell antigens, and fall into a distinct subgroup by expression profiling (Weng et al. 2004; Palomero et al. 2006; Aster et al. 2008). The relationship between the role of the NOTCH pathway and AML-derived stem cells is suggested by overexpression of Jagged-2, one of the Notch ligands, in leukemic stem cells from AML. Incubation of the leukemic stem cells with a GSI inhibited leukemic stem cell growth in colony formation assays (Gal eta l. 2006).

7.7 EpigeneticMo dulators

7.7.1 Overview

Epigenetic control of gene expression is now recognized as an important mechanism in the initiation and prognosis of human malignancies including leukemias (Esteller 2003, 2008). Both the process of methylation of cytosines in CpG island regions situated within gene promoter regions and changes in chromatin conformation mediated by histone acetylation lead to transcriptional silencing. An increasing number of epigenetically silenced genes are being recognized in cancer and cancer-type-specific patterns of hypermethylation are emerging. In addition, genes predicted as relevant to tumorigenesis have been identified as being under epigenetic control, including tumor suppressor genes, cell cycle regulators, and DNA repair genes. Single gene analyses in acute leukemias have identified promoter hypermethylation in an increasing number of genes, including *E-cadherin* (Melki et al. 2000), *calcitonin* (Leegwater et al. 1997), *estrogen receptor* (Yao et al. 2009), *hypermethylation in cancer-1 (HIC-1)* (Melki et al. 1999a, b) and *p15INK4b* (Quesnel and Fenaux 1999; Tsellou et al. 2005), and methylation studies of multiple gene sets revealed that increased methylation is an independent factor of poor prognosis (Melki et al.

1999a, b; Melki and Clark 2002; Hess et al. 2008). Genome-wide methylation studies have identified disease-specific methylation profiles in acute leukemias (Scholz et al. 2005) and have been successfully used to identify novel methylation target genes in ALL (Taylor eta l. 2007;K uange ta l. 2008).

Unlike genetic alterations, such as gene deletions and mutations, epigenetic events do not alter the primary DNA sequence. Epigenetic processes are biochemical changes that affect DNA and the associated proteins. These processes determine the configuration of chromatin and modify gene expression (Baylin 2005). Importantly, they are reversible and therefore can be therapeutically targeted. Currently, there are two types of clinically applicable epigenetic modulators that are able to up-regulate epigenetically silenced genes: the DNA methyltransferase inhibitors (DNMTi) and the histone deacetylase inhibitors (HDACi). Clinical trials are beginning to demonstrate how they can be best applied in the treatment of hematological malignancies.

7.7.2 DNA Methyltransferase Inhibitors

There are two DNMTi in clinical use: 5-azacytidine and 5-aza-2′-deoxycytidine (decitabine). Both are nucleoside analogues that were originally investigated as cytotoxic agents for leukemias over three decades ago, when they were administered at high doses (5-azacytidine 600–1,500 mg/m^2 and decitabine 1,500–2,500 mg/m^2). Clinical studies in leukemia escalating to the maximum tolerated doses demonstrated promising responses, but the dose-limiting toxicity was prolonged myelosuppression. Dose-dependent antileukemia activity was reported in Phase I trials for pediatric relapsed and refractory leukemia (0.75–80 mg/kg), but the associated significant prolonged myelosuppression limited further development (Rivard et al. 1981; Momparler et al. 1985).

Both 5-azacytidine and decitabine are activated by phosphorylation to their triphosphate forms. 5-Azacytidine is predominantly incorporated into RNA, resulting in disassembly of polyribosomes, altered RNA methylation, and a defective receptor function of transfer RNA. Decitabine triphosphate is incorporated into DNA, depleting DNA methyltransferases, which results in DNA hypomethylation. At the higher doses, decitabine forms DNA adducts that inhibit DNA synthesis and induce cell death, whereas at lower doses, the DNA hypomethylation causes changes in gene expression profiles that induce differentiation, reduce proliferation, and increase apoptosis (Momparler 2005).

The therapeutic potential of the now recognized hypomethylation activity of both 5-azacytidine and decitabine at low doses (5-azacytidine 50–75 mg/m^2 decitabine 100–150 mg/m^2) is under evaluation in several types of leukemia, notably myelodysplastic syndromes (MDS) and myeloid leukemias. The Cancer and Leukemia Group B (CALGB) performed a series of clinical trials investigating low-dose 5-azacytidine in MDS. The outcome of the Phase II trials (CALGB 8421 [Silverman et al. 2006] and CALGB 8921 [Silverman et al. 2006]) and the pivotal randomized Phase III trial (CALGB 9221 [Silverman et al. 2002, 2006]) that compared low-dose 5-azacytidine to best supportive care confirmed the role for low-dose 5-azacytidine in the management of MDS. CALGB 9221 demonstrated 10% CR, 1% PR, and 36% hematological improvement (HI) in the 5-azacytidine arm compared to no CR or PR in the supportive care arm. The crossover design of CALGB 9221 allowing supportive care arm patients to move to the 5-azacytidine arm precluded conclusions on overall survival; however, a subsequent randomized trial reported by Fenaux et al. (2009) confirmed that low-dose 5-azacytidine (20 mg/m^2/day × 14 days every 28 days) conferred a survival advantage in high-risk MDS compared to conventional treatment regimes (51% vs 26% at 2 years) (Fenaux et al. 2009).

Decitabine, a more potent hypomethylating agent inducing a different profile of gene reexpression compared to 5-azacytidine (Flotho et al. 2009), is also being explored at low-dose schedules in the treatment of MDS and AML. As with 5-azacytidine, the early phase clinical trials of decitabine demonstrated that low-dose schedules were associated with promising response rates in MDS. This led to a Phase III trial randomizing decitabine against best supportive care (Kantarjian et al. 2006). Decitabine was administered at 15 mg/m^2 per dose, every 8 h × 3 days every 6 weeks, and produced 9% CR, 8% PR, and 13% HI compared to no responses in the supportive care arm. Although the responses were durable (median 41 weeks), they did not translate to a statistically significant overall survival advantage (time to AML or death 12.1 months vs 7.8 months, $p = 0.16$) (Kantarjian et al. 2006). On the basis of the results of these Phase III trials, the FDA has approved both 5-azacytidine and decitabine for the treatment of MDS. Studies investigating the therapeutic value of DNMTi in pediatric MDS are planned, but will be challenging due to the low patient numbers in the younger age group.

Both the dose and the duration of exposure to hypomethylating agents can influence their ability to inhibit DNA methylation, reduce clonogenicity, and reactivate tumor suppressor genes (Khan et al. 2006; Lemaire et al. 2008). The successful clinical application of DNMTi in MDS and other hematological malignancies will require further optimization of the dose and schedule both as single agents and in combination with other epigenetic modifiers and conventional cytotoxic drugs. An important challenge is the identification of biomarkers that can either predict response or monitor efficacy of hypomethylating agents. Reduction in global methylation is measurable shortly after commencement of treatment and peaks at 10–15 days with recovery at 4–6 weeks; however, attempts to identify reexpression of single genes as biomarkers have produced contradictory results. Some clinical studies have suggested a correlation between response and induced hypomethylation affecting specific genes, but this is not a consistent finding in all studies and indeed an inverse relationship has been reported in CML (Oki et al. 2007). The optimum response biomarker for hypomethylating agents, therefore, remains unclear and is complicated by the multiplicity of the downstream effects of hypomethylation. Epigenetic regulation of genes includes not only the reexpression of methylation-silenced genes in multiple pathways such as pro-apoptosis, proliferation, differentiation, and immune regulation, but also down-regulation of oncogenes via reactivation of epigenetically regulated micro-RNAs.

Beyond MDS, the clinical investigation of DNMTi has been predominantly in AML. Central morphology review of diagnostic samples from the participants in the Kantarjian trial re-classified 12 MDS patients to AML; nine were randomized to receive decitabine treatment and 5/9 (56%) achieved an objective response (Kantarjian et al. 2006). Subsequently, several low-dose, long-exposure schedules of decitabine have been explored in AML, predominantly in the elderly population in whom intensive cytotoxic chemotherapy is not well tolerated. Moderate responses have been reported. Lubbert et al. (Lubbert and Minden 2005) investigated decitabine in patients with AML (median age 72 years) using an Induction regimen of 135 mg/m^2 continuous intravenous (IV) infusion over 72 h every 6 weeks for four courses. Patients in complete remission could receive Maintenance therapy with 20 mg/m^2 IV for 3 days every 8 weeks. Interestingly, the median time to response was 13 weeks and objective responses were observed in 31% (14% CR and 17% PR) (Lubbert and Minden 2005). Similarly, a study of elderly AML patients (median age 69 years) treated with an alternative schedule of decitabine (20 mg/m^2 IV for 5 days every 4 weeks) produced an objective response rate (in patients in CR and those in CR but with incomplete platelet response [CRi]) of 26% (Cashen et al. 2009). Further studies investigating low-dose schedules of both 5-azacytidine and decitabine in AML, including high-risk subgroups, in Induction regimens as well as in Maintenance therapy are ongoing. The results of studies in pediatric AML are awaited.

Although preclinical evidence supports the importance of epigenetic processes in ALL, including in the pediatric age group, to date the clinical exploration of epigenetic modifiers in ALL has been limited and clinical studies using the low-dose schedules in ALL are still awaited. There is evidence to suggest that epigenetic modifiers may have specific application in certain subgroups of pediatric acute leukemias. Several recurrent chromosomal translocations characterize subgroups of childhood acute leukemia. The translocations fuse the DNA-binding domain of a transcriptional activator to a transcriptional repressor, leading to decreased expression of target genes that regulate myeloid differentiation, and causing the block in myeloid differentiation that characterizes acute leukemia (Tenen et al. 1997; Friedman 1999). The processes of histone acetylation and promoter methylation have been shown to contribute to transcriptional repression activity of fusion proteins, including AML1-ETO (Klisovic et al. 2003), PML-RARA (Grignani et al. 1998; Lin et al. 1998), and TEL-AML1 (Heibert et al. 2001). In addition, the constitutive up-regulation of *HOX* genes essential to leukemogenesis associated with abnormalities in the *MLL* gene at 11q23 has been shown to involve DNA methyltransferase and histone acetylase activity (Whitman et al. 2005; Dorrance et al. 2006). Recently, infant ALL with the *MLL* rearrangement was reported to exhibit global hypermethylation. Interestingly, this was associated with increased sensitivity to decitabine (Schafer et al. 2009). Leukemias carrying these fusion proteins may prove to be particularly sensitive to epigenetic modulators and would be an important target group for the development of these agents.

7.7.3 Histone Deacetylase Inhibitors

HDACi are another class of epigenetic modifiers undergoing clinical evaluation in hematological malignancies. Acetylation of the NH2-terminal tails of histones is catalyzed by histone acetylation transferases (HAT) and results in an open chromatin configuration that promotes gene transcription. Conversely, deacetylation is mediated by histone deacetylases (HDAC) and leads to gene repression; HDAC inhibition, therefore, promotes gene reexpression through chromatin relaxation (Marks et al. 2004). Several HDACi have been evaluated clinically in early-phase clinical trials but disappointingly, the results of their use in the treatment of leukemias do not strongly support their efficacy as single agents (Giles et al. 2006; Gojo et al. 2007; Garcia-Manero et al. 2008). Nevertheless, there is clear evidence of synergy *in vitro* between of DNMT inhibitors and HDAC inhibitors, both in reactivation of gene expression (Cameron et al. 1999) and in anti-leukemic activity (Tong et al. 2009). Trials combining decitabine or 5-azacytidine with valproic acid, SAHA, depsipeptide, and other newer HDACi are producing promising results. A randomized Phase II study of decitabine versus decitabine plus valproic acid in MDS, chronic myelomonocytic leukemia (CMML) and AML was recently reported and it did not show a significant difference in overall responses between the two arms. Comparison of molecular responses showed no difference in global hypomethylation (as measured by LINE1) between the two arms and no correlation with responses; however, sustained hypomethylation and reexpression of specific genes, *P15*, *ATM* and *miR124*, did appear to correlate with response (Castoro et al. 2009).

Pediatric studies investigating the use of epigenetic modifiers including decitabine, valproic acid, MS275, and SAHA, both as single agents and in combination are underway. Based on the evidence from the trials in adults, the effective application of these agents in the treatment of pediatric hematological malignancies will require careful study of the appropriate dosing and scheduling as well as a better understanding of their true mechanisms of action to aid development of markers predictive of response.

7.8 TargetingA poptosisPat hways: BCL2 Family Inhibitors, XIAP Inhibitors

7.8.1 Overview

Apoptosis is the fundamental cell death program that regulates homeostasis in many rapidly proliferating tissues, including the hematopoietic system. There is a finely regulated balance between intracellular proteins that either promote or inhibit apoptosis. In many malignant cells, including leukemias, the balance is in favor of the anti-apoptotic proteins, which promote cell survival; therefore, targeting these pathways to tip the balance toward pro-apoptotic proteins is a logical therapeutic approach (Kitada et al. 2002). The two most clinically advanced approaches target the B-cell lymphoma-2 (Bcl-2) family of anti-apoptosis proteins and XIAP, a member of the Inhibitors of Apoptosis (IAP) family of proteins. In both cases, the approaches include antisense oligonucleotides (ASO) and small molecule inhibitors and are under evaluation for the treatment of leukemias in early phase clinical trials.

7.8.2 BCL2 Family Inhibitors

There are 25 members of the Bcl-2 family regulating the intrinsic apoptosis pathway and six are anti-apoptotic: Bcl-2, Bcl-$X_{L,}$ Bcl-W, Bcl-B, Mcl-1, Bfl-1. Antisense oligonucleotides (ASO) were developed to target Bcl-2 mRNA. They result in the formation of sense-antisense hetereodimers that recruit native RNAse H, leading to degradation of the mRNA and reduction in level of Bcl-2 protein. In preclinical studies, both *in vitro* and *in vivo,* this translated to promising chemo-sensitization of B-cell malignancies. Oblimersen sodium (Genesense®) was the first of these compounds to be evaluated in clinical trials, including Phase III trials in chronic lymphocytic leukemia (CLL); however, the clinical benefit has been limited.

More recently, clinical interest has turned to small molecule inhibitor approaches targeting the Bcl-2 protein Bax and Bak binding pocket formed by the BH1-3 binding domains, thereby mimicking the pro-apoptotic activity of Bax and Bak. Clinical evaluation of pan-Bcl-2 family inhibitors (e.g., obatoclax mesylate) and Bcl-2 specific inhibitors (e.g., ABT263 and ABT737) are underway. In a Phase I study, 44 patients with refractory leukemia or MDS were treated with obatoclax mesylate. It was well tolerated with no dose-limiting toxicity up to the planned highest dose. Of note, one patient with AML, harboring the mixed lineage leukemia t(9;11) rearrangement, achieved a complete remission of 8 months duration (Schimmer et al. 2008). Clinical trials evaluating these more specific Bcl-inhibitors in leukemias are ongoing. The interim results of the Phase I/IIa trial of the oral Bcl-2 specific inhibitor ABT263 in relapsed or refractory lymphoid malignancy were recently presented (Wilson et al. 2009). It was shown that the drug-associated thrombocytopenia could be minimized using a low dose for an initial 7 days, followed by continuous dosing 21/21 days. The results of further clinical trials evaluating the use of this class of agents in leukemia, including in pediatrics, are awaited.

7.8.3 XIAP Inhibitors

The IAP family of proteins regulates the caspase activation pathway intrinsic to apoptosis. X-linked IAP (XIAP) is a member of this family and inhibits the downstream effector caspases 9 and 3. Like the Bcl-2 family, the IAP proteins are overexpressed in many malignancies, including leukemias (Tamm et al. 2000). In both adult and pediatric AML, overexpression of XIAP has been associated with poor prognosis (Tamm et al. 2004a, b; Wuchter et al. 2004). Antisense experiments targeting XIAP have demonstrated induction of Bcl-2 family independent apoptosis (LaCasse et al. 2006). The ASO directed at XIAP that is most advanced in clinical development is AEG35156. The recently reported Phase I/II trial of AEG35156 combined with cytarabine and idarubicin in relapsed refractory AML in adults (Schimmer et al. 2009) demonstrated dose-dependent knockdown of *XIAP* mRNA, with greater than 30% knockdown in patients treated at the highest dose (AEG35156 350 mg/m^2 IV over 2 h). Patients receiving this dose had the highest response rate with 15/32 (47%) achieving a CR or CRi, and notably 10/11 (91%) patients refractory to a single Induction regimen achieved a CR. AEG35156 was well tolerated in combination with chemotherapy, with only two patients developing a peripheral neuropathy that was attributed to the study drug. A further randomized study is needed to confirm the contribution of AEG35156 to this promising response rate.

In common with targeting Bcl-2 proteins, concerns relating to the potential efficiency of the ASO approach led to interest in XIAP small molecule inhibitors. The Baculovirus IAP repeat (BIR) domains 2 and 3 are believed to be the functional binding sites mediating caspase inhibition. Phenylurea compounds have been identified to target BIR 2 and induce apoptosis in a range of malignancies (Schimmer et al. 2004). In AML cell lines and primary cells, the XIAP inhibitor *N*-[(5*R*)-6-[(anilinocarbonyl)amino]-5-((anilinocarbonyl){[(2*R*)-1-(4-cyclohexylbutyl)pyrrolidin-2yl]methyl}amino) hexyl]-*N*-methyl-*N*′-phenylurea (1396-12) was most effective in cells with high baseline XIAP levels, suggesting it may be possible to target the use of these agents to subgroups of patients in whom they are most likely to be effective (Carter et al. 2005a, b). Further clinical evaluation of this promising class of drugs in hematological malignancies is awaited.

7.9 Conclusions

Childhood leukemia comprises a diverse collection of subsets defined by morphologic, phenotypic, and biological characteristics. While various subsets of ALL and AML have been known for decades, the molecular basis of these subsets and new, clinically relevant subsets have been discovered through application of burgeoning genetic technology. There is a clear and compelling rationale for developing therapies that specifically target the molecular abnormalities that may cause leukemia. Such therapies hold the promise of being more effective and less toxic than the standard approaches using chemotherapy and stem cell transplantation. The successful treatment of chronic phase CML with BCR-ABL kinase inhibitors hints at the possibilities for acute leukemia, but it is important to understand some fundamental differences between CML and acute leukemia. In its chronic phase, CML is a myeloproliferative disease caused by a single molecular abnormality. Acute leukemia, on the other hand, is a heterogeneous group of truly malignant hematopoietic tumors, each of which is caused not by one, but by multiple molecular abnormalities that differ substantially from patient to patient, and even from clone to subclone within a given patient. Thus, the development of successful molecularly targeted therapies for acute leukemia will pose tremendous challenges, and will require new paradigms of clinical and translational laboratory research.

High throughput genomics has greatly increased the complexity of the biological information available, and it is crucial that "passenger" lesions be distinguished from "driver" mutations that contribute directly to maintenance of the malignant phenotype, with the latter prioritized for targeted therapies. Similarly, agents that target molecular pathways active in bulk leukemia cells, but not in the elusive and largely quiescent population of leukemia stem cells, may prove ineffective in terms of preventing relapse and improving long-term survival. In addition, it is clear that individual patients will need to be treated with a combination of therapeutic agents. Incorporating a single molecularly targeted agent into a standard chemotherapy backbone is complex. The complexity will only increase as combinations of two or more molecularly targeted therapies are contemplated. Finally, there are particular challenges associated with clinical evaluation of molecularly targeted agents. One of these is to distinguish the toxicity attributable to the addition of a molecularly targeted agent from the toxicity of the backbone of intensive chemotherapy. Another is to determine an appropriate patient population in which to study each individual agent. Since acute leukemia is a collection of molecularly heterogeneous diseases, each agent would be expected to be effective for a subset of patients. While it seems reasonable to test a novel agent only in the patients who can be predicted to have a high likelihood of responding, clinical trials for subsets of patients with a relatively rare disease like childhood leukemia will be difficult to sufficiently power using standard trial designs. As new potential targets are identified, rapid preclinical validation is needed to select the most promising agents for therapeutic testing. New paradigms for clinical trials are needed to rapidly determine the effectiveness of new agents. The need for international collaboration will expand as well.

Despite these challenges, there has been real progress in the development of molecularly targeted agents for childhood acute leukemia. Hopefully, this progress will accelerate and will lead to improved outcomes for thesec hildren.

References

Adams J (2004) The proteasome: a suitable antineoplastic target. Nat Rev Cancer 4(5):349–360

Alsina M, Trudel S, Vallone M et al (2007) Phase I single agent antitumor activity of twice weekly-consecutive day dosing of the proteasome inhibitor carfilzomib in hematologic malignancies. Blood 110(Suppl 1):128

Aplenc R, Alonzo TA et al (2008) Safety and efficacy of gemtuzumab ozogamicin in combination with chemotherapy for pediatric acute myeloid leukemia: a report from the Children's Oncology Group. J Clin Oncol 26(14): 2390–3295

Arceci RJ, Sande J et al (2005) Safety and efficacy of gemtuzumab ozogamicin in pediatric patients with advanced CD33+ acute myeloid leukemia. Blood 106(4):1183–1188

Arico M, Valsecchi MG et al (2000) Outcome of treatment in children with Philadelphia chromosome-positive acute lymphoblastic leukemia. N Engl J Med 342(14):998–1006

Armstrong SA, Staunton JE et al (2002) MLL translocations specify a distinct gene expression profile that distinguishes a unique leukemia. Nat Genet 30(1):41–47

Armstrong SA, Kung AL et al (2003) Inhibition of FLT3 in MLL. Validation of a therapeutic target identified by gene expression based classification. Cancer Cell 3(2):173–183

Armstrong SA, Mabon ME et al (2004) FLT3 mutations in childhood acute lymphoblastic leukemia. Blood 103(9): 3544–3546

Armstrong F, Brunet de la Grange P et al (2009) NOTCH is a key regulator of human T-cell acute leukemia initiating cell activity. Blood 113(8):1730–1740

Aster JC, Pear WS et al (2008) Notch signaling in leukemia. Annu Rev Pathol 3:587–613

Attar EC, De Angelo DJ et al (2008) Phase I and pharmacokinetic study of bortezomib in combination with idarubicin and cytarabine in patients with acute myelogenous leukemia. Clin Cancer Res 14(5):1446–1454

Baldo P, Cecco S et al (2008) mTOR pathway and mTOR inhibitors as agents for cancer therapy. Curr Cancer Drug Targets 8(8):647–665

Baylin SB (2005) DNA methylation and gene silencing in cancer. Nat Clin Pract Oncol 2(Suppl 1):S4–11

Bonnet D, Dick JE (1997) Human acute myeloid leukemia is organized as a hierarchy that originates from a primitive hematopoietic cell. Nat Med 3(7):730–737

Brashem-Stein C, Flowers DA et al (1993) Ontogeny of hematopoietic stem cell development: reciprocal expression of CD33 and a novel molecule by maturing myeloid and erythroid progenitors. Blood 82(3):792–799

Brown P, Small D (2004) FLT3 inhibitors: a paradigm for the development of targeted therapeutics for paediatric cancer. Eur J Cancer 40(5):707–721, discussion 722–704

Brown P, Meshinchi S et al (2004) Pediatric AML primary samples with FLT3/ITD mutations are preferentially killed by FLT3 inhibition. Blood 104(6):1841–1849

Brown P, Levis M et al (2005) FLT3 inhibition selectively kills childhood acute lymphoblastic leukemia cells with high levels of FLT3 expression. Blood 105(2):812–820

Brown P, Levis M et al (2006) Combinations of the FLT3 inhibitor CEP-701 and chemotherapy synergistically kill infant and childhood MLL-rearranged ALL cells in a sequence-dependent manner. Leukemia: Off J Leukemia Soc Am, Leukemia Res Fund, UK 20(8):1368–1376

Cameron EE, Bachman KE et al (1999) Synergy of demethylation and histone deacetylase inhibition in the re-expression of genes silenced in cancer. Nat Genet 21(1):103–107

Carnahan J, Wang P et al (2003) Epratuzumab, a humanized monoclonal antibody targeting CD22: characterization of *in vitro* properties. Clin Cancer Res 9(10 Pt 2): 3982S–3990S

Carow CE, Levenstein M et al (1996) Expression of the hematopoietic growth factor receptor FLT3 (STK-1/Flk2) in human leukemias. Blood 87(3):1089–1096

Carter BZ, Gronda M et al (2005a) Small-molecule XIAP inhibitors derepress downstream effector caspases and induce apoptosis of acute myeloid leukemia cells. Blood 105(10): 4043–4050

Carter TA, Wodicka LM et al (2005b) Inhibition of drug-resistant mutants of ABL, KIT, and EGF receptor kinases. Proc Natl Acad Sci USA 102(31):11011–11016

Cashen AF, Schiller GJ et al (2010) Multicenter, Phase II study of Decitabine for the first-line treatment of older patients with acute myeloid leukemia. J Clin Oncol 28(4): 556–61

Castor A, Nilsson L et al (2005) Distinct patterns of hematopoietic stem cell involvement in acute lymphoblastic leukemia. Nat Med 11(6):630–637

Castoro RJ, Raynal NJ et al (2009) DNA methylation and gene expression analysis in a Phase II randomized study of Decitabine vs. Decitabine plus valproic acid in MDS and AML. ASH Annu Meeting Abstracts 114(22):3808

Chauhan D, Catley L et al (2005) A novel orally active proteasome inhibitor induces apoptosis in multiple myeloma cells with mechanisms distinct from Bortezomib. Cancer Cell 8(5):407–419

Cortes J, Thomas D et al (2004) Phase I study of bortezomib in refractory or relapsed acute leukemias. Clin Cancer Res 10(10):3371–3376

Cox CV, Evely RS et al (2004) Characterization of acute lymphoblastic leukemia progenitor cells. Blood 104(9):2919–2925

Cullion K, Draheim KM et al (2009) Targeting the Notch1 and mTOR pathways in a mouse T-ALL model. Blood 113(24):6172–6181

DeAngelo DJ (2006) A Phase I clinical trial of the notch inhibitor MK-0752 in patients with T-cell acute lymphoblastic leukemia/lymphoma (T-ALL) and other leukemias. J Clin Oncol24:6585

Dorrance AM, Liu S et al (2006) Mll partial tandem duplication induces aberrant Hox expression *in vivo* via specific epigenetic alterations. J Clin Invest 116(10):2707–2716

Douros J, Suffness M (1981) New antitumor substances of natural origin. Cancer Treat Rev 8(1):63–87

Druker BJ, Sawyers CL et al (2001a) Activity of a specific inhibitor of the BCR-ABL tyrosine kinase in the blast crisis of chronic myeloid leukemia and acute lymphoblastic leukemia with the Philadelphia chromosome. N Engl J Med 344(14):1038–1042

Druker BJ, Talpaz M et al (2001b) Efficacy and safety of a specific inhibitor of the BCR-ABL tyrosine kinase in chronic myeloid leukemia. N Engl J Med 344(14):1031–1037

Eng CP, Sehgal SN et al (1984) Activity of rapamycin (AY-22, 989) against transplanted tumors. J Antibiot (Tokyo) 37(10):1231–1237

Esteller M (2003) Cancer epigenetics: DNA methylation and chromatin alterations in human cancer. Adv Exp Med Biol 532:39–49

Esteller M (2008) Epigenetics in cancer. N Engl J Med 358(11):1148–1159

Fenaux P, Mufti GJ et al (2009) Efficacy of azacitidine compared with that of conventional care regimens in the treatment of higher-risk myelodysplastic syndromes: a randomised, open-label, phase III study. Lancet Oncol 10(3):223–232

Flotho C, Claus R et al (2009) The DNA methyltransferase inhibitors azacitidine, decitabine and zebularine exert differential effects on cancer gene expression in acute myeloid leukemia cells. Leukemia 23(6):1019–1028

Fouladi M, Laningham F et al (2007) Phase I study of everolimus in pediatric patients with refractory solid tumors. J Clin Oncol25(30):4806–4812

Franklin J, Alonzo TA et al (2008) COG AAML03P1: efficacy and safety in a pilot study of intensive chemotherapy including gemtuzumab in children newly diagnosed with acute myeloid leukemia (AML). Blood 112(11):136a

Freeman SD, Kelm S et al (1995) Characterization of CD33 as a new member of the sialoadhesin family of cellular interaction molecules. Blood 85(8):2005–2012

Friedman AD (1999) Leukemogenesis by CBF oncoproteins. Leukemia13(12):1932–1942

Gal H, Amariglio N et al (2006) Gene expression profiles of AML derived stem cells; similarity to hematopoietic stem cells. Leukemia 20(12):2147–2154

Garcia-Manero G, Assouline S et al (2008) Phase 1 study of the oral isotype specific histone deacetylase inhibitor MGCD0103 in leukemia. Blood 112(4):981–989

Giles F, Fischer T et al (2006) A phase I study of intravenous LBH589, a novel cinnamic hydroxamic acid analogue histone deacetylase inhibitor, in patients with refractory hematologic malignancies. Clin Cancer Res 12(15):4628–4635

Gojo I, Jiemjit A et al (2007) Phase 1 and pharmacologic study of MS-275, a histone deacetylase inhibitor, in adults with refractory and relapsed acute leukemias. Blood 109(7):2781–2790

Gorre ME, Sawyers CL (2002) Molecular mechanisms of resistance to STI571 in chronic myeloid leukemia. Curr Opin Hematol9(4):303–307

Graham SM, Jorgensen HG et al (2002) Primitive, quiescent, Philadelphia-positive stem cells from patients with chronic myeloid leukemia are insensitive to STI571 *in vitro*. Blood 99(1):319

Grignani F, De Matteis S et al (1998) Fusion proteins of the retinoic acid receptor-alpha recruit histone deacetylase in promyelocytic leukaemia. Nature 391(6669):815–818

Grimwade D, Enver T (2004) Acute promyelocytic leukemia: where does it stem from? Leukemia: Off J Leukemia Soc Am Leukemia Res Fund, UK 18(3):375

Gu L, Gao J et al (2008) Rapamycin reverses NPM-ALK-induced glucocorticoid resistance in lymphoid tumor cells by inhibiting mTOR signaling pathway, enhancing G1 cell cycle arrest and apoptosis. Leukemia 22(11):2091–2096

Guzman ML, Neering SJ et al (2001) Nuclear factor-kappaB is constitutively activated in primitive human acute myelogenous leukemia cells. Blood 98(8):2301–2307

Guzman ML, Swiderski CF et al (2002) Preferential induction of apoptosis for primary human leukemic stem cells. Proc Natl Acad Sci USA 99(25):16220–16225

Haarman EG, Kaspers GJ et al (2008) Circumvention of glucocorticoid resistance in childhood leukemia. Leuk Res 32(9):1417–1423

Heibert SW, Lutterbach B et al (2001) Mechanisms of transcriptional repression by the t(8;21)-, t(12;21)-, and inv(16)-encoded fusion proteins. Cancer Chemother Pharmacol 48(Suppl1):S31–3 4

Herrera L, Farah RA et al (2000) Immunotoxins against CD19 and CD22 are effective in killing precursor-B acute lymphoblastic leukemia cells *in vitro*. Leukemia 14(5):853–858

Herrera L, Yarbrough S et al (2003) Treatment of SCID/human B cell precursor ALL with anti-CD19 and anti-CD22 immunotoxins. Leukemia 17(2):334–338

Hess CJ, Errami A et al (2008) Concurrent methylation of promoters from tumor associated genes predicts outcome in acute myeloid leukemia. Leuk Lymphoma 49(6):1132–1141

Ho YK, Bargagna-Mohan P et al (2007) LMP2-specific inhibitors: chemical genetic tools for proteasome biology. Chem Biol14(4):419–430

Horton TM, Gannavarapu A et al (2006) Bortezomib interactions with chemotherapy agents in acute leukemia *in vitro*. Cancer Chemother Pharmacol 58(1):13–23

Horton TM, Pati D et al (2007) A phase 1 study of the proteasome inhibitor bortezomib in pediatric patients with refractory leukemia: a Children's Oncology Group study. Clin Cancer Res 13(5):1516–1522

Houghton PJ, Morton CL et al (2008a) Initial testing (stage 1) of the mTOR inhibitor rapamycin by the pediatric preclinical testing program. Pediatr Blood Cancer 50(4):799–805

Houghton PJ, Morton CL et al (2008b) Initial testing (stage 1) of the proteasome inhibitor bortezomib by the pediatric preclinical testing program. Pediatr Blood Cancer 50(1):37–45

Hu Y, Liu Y et al (2004) Requirement of Src kinases Lyn, Hck and Fgr for BCR-ABL1-induced B-lymphoblastic leukemia but not chronic myeloid leukemia. Nat Genet 36(5):453–461

Iwai T, Yokota S et al (1999) Internal tandem duplication of the FLT3 gene and clinical evaluation in childhood acute myeloid leukemia. The Children's Cancer and Leukemia Study Group, Japan. Leukemia: Official J Leukemia Soc Am Leukemia Res Fund, UK 13(1):38–43

Kantarjian H, Issa JP et al (2006) Decitabine improves patient outcomes in myelodysplastic syndromes: results of a phase III randomized study. Cancer 106(8):1794–1803

Khan R, Aggerholm A et al (2006) A pharmacodynamic study of 5-azacytidine in the P39 cell line. Exp Hematol 34(1):35–43

Kharas MG, Deane JA et al (2004) Phosphoinositide 3-kinase signaling is essential for ABL oncogene-mediated transformation of B-lineage cells. Blood 103(11):4268–4275

Kitada S, Pedersen IM et al (2002) Dysregulation of apoptosis genes in hematopoietic malignancies. Oncogene 21(21):3459–3474

Kiyoi H, Towatari M et al (1998) Internal tandem duplication of the FLT3 gene is a novel modality of elongation mutation which causes constitutive activation of the product. Leukemia: Off J Leukemia Soc Am Leukemia Res Fund, UK12(9):1333–1337

Klisovic MI, Maghraby EA et al (2003) Depsipeptide (FR 901228) promotes histone acetylation, gene transcription, apoptosis and its activity is enhanced by DNA methyltransferase inhibitors in AML1/ETO-positive leukemic cells. Leukemia17(2):350–358

Knapper S, Burnett AK et al (2006) A phase 2 trial of the FLT3 inhibitor lestaurtinib (CEP701) as first-line treatment for older patients with acute myeloid leukemia not considered fit for intensive chemotherapy. Blood 108(10):3262–3270

Kondo M, Horibe K et al (1999) Prognostic value of internal tandem duplication of the FLT3 gene in childhood acute myelogenous leukemia. Med Pediatr Oncol 33(6):525–529

Kopan R, Ilagan MX (2009) The canonical Notch signaling pathway: unfolding the activation mechanism. Cell 137(2): 216–233

Kottaridis PD, Gale RE et al (2002) Studies of FLT3 mutations in paired presentation and relapse samples from patients with acute myeloid leukemia: implications for the role of FLT3 mutations in leukemogenesis, minimal residual disease detection, and possible therapy with FLT3 inhibitors. Blood100(7):2393–2398

Kuang SQ, Tong WG et al (2008) Genome-wide identification of aberrantly methylated promoter associated CpG islands in acute lymphocytic leukemia. Leukemia 22(8):1529–1538

Kuhn DJ, Chen Q et al (2007) Potent activity of carfilzomib, a novel, irreversible inhibitor of the ubiquitin-proteasome pathway, against preclinical models of multiple myeloma. Blood110(9):3281–3290

LaCasse EC, Cherton-Horvat GG et al (2006) Preclinical characterization of AEG35156/GEM 640, a second-generation antisense oligonucleotide targeting X-linked inhibitor of apoptosis. Clin Cancer Res 12(17):5231–5241

Larson RA, Sievers EL et al (2005) Final report of the efficacy and safety of gemtuzumab ozogamicin (Mylotarg) in patients with CD33-positive acute myeloid leukemia in first recurrence. Cancer 104(7):1442–1452

le Viseur C, Hotfilder M et al (2008) In childhood acute lymphoblastic leukemia, blasts at different stages of immunophenotypic maturation have stem cell properties. Cancer Cell 14(1):47–58

Lee KH, Lee JH et al (2005a) Clinical effect of imatinib added to intensive combination chemotherapy for newly diagnosed Philadelphia chromosome-positive acute lymphoblastic leukemia. Leukemia: Off J Leukemia Soc Am, Leukemia Res Fund, UK 19(9):1509–1516

Lee S, Kim YJ et al (2005b) The effect of first-line imatinib interim therapy on the outcome of allogeneic stem cell transplantation in adults with newly diagnosed Philadelphia chromosome-positive acute lymphoblastic leukemia. Blood 105(9):3449–3457

Leegwater PA, Lambooy LH et al (1997) DNA methylation patterns in the calcitonin gene region at first diagnosis and at relapse of acute lymphoblastic leukemia (ALL). Leukemia 11(7):971–978

Lemaire M, Chabot GG et al (2008) Importance of dose-schedule of 5-aza-2′-deoxycytidine for epigenetic therapy of cancer. BMC Cancer 8:128

Levis M, Small D (2005) FLT3 tyrosine kinase inhibitors. Int J Hematol 82(2):100–107

Levis M, Allebach J et al (2002) A FLT3-targeted tyrosine kinase inhibitor is cytotoxic to leukemia cells *in vitro* and in vivo. Blood 99(11):3885–3891

Levis M, Pham R et al (2004) *In vitro* studies of a FLT3 inhibitor combined with chemotherapy: sequence of administration is important to achieve synergistic cytotoxic effects. Blood 104(4):1145–1150

Levis M, Murphy KM et al (2005a) Internal tandem duplications of the FLT3 gene are present in leukemia stem cells. Blood 106(2):673–680

Levis M, Smith BD et al (2005b) A Randomized, Open-Label Study of Lestaurtinib (CEP-701), an Oral FLT3 Inhibitor, administered in sequence with chemotherapy in patients with relapsed AML harboring FLT3 Activating mutations: clinical response correlates with successful FLT3 inhibition. ASH Annu Meeting Abstracts 106(11):403

Lewis HD, Leveridge M et al (2007) Apoptosis in T cell acute lymphoblastic leukemia cells after cell cycle arrest induced by pharmacological inhibition of notch signaling. Chem Biol14(2):209–219

Lin RJ, Nagy L et al (1998) Role of the histone deacetylase complex in acute promyelocytic leukaemia. Nature 391(6669): 811–814

Linenberger ML, Hong T et al (2001) Multidrug-resistance phenotype and clinical responses to gemtuzumab ozogamicin. Blood98(4):988–9 94

Lubbert M, Minden M (2005) Decitabine in acute myeloid leukemia. Semin Hematol 42(3 Suppl 2):S38–42

Marks PA, Richon VM et al (2004) Histone deacetylase inhibitors. Adv Cancer Res 91:137–168

Melki JR, Clark SJ (2002) DNA methylation changes in leukaemia. Semin Cancer Biol 12(5):347–357

Melki JR, Vincent PC et al (1999a) Cancer-specific region of hypermethylation identified within the HIC1 putative tumour suppressor gene in acute myeloid leukaemia. Leukemia 13(6):877–883

Melki JR, Vincent PC et al (1999b) Concurrent DNA hypermethylation of multiple genes in acute myeloid leukemia. Cancer Res 59(15):3730–3740

Melki JR, Vincent PC et al (2000) Hypermethylation of E-cadherin in leukemia. Blood 95(10):3208–3213

Meric-Bernstam F, Gonzalez-Angulo AM (2009) Targeting the mTOR signaling network for cancer therapy. J Clin Oncol 27(13):2278–2287

Meshinchi S, Arceci RJ (2007) Prognostic factors and risk-based therapy in pediatric acute myeloid leukemia. Oncologist 12(3):341–355

Meshinchi S, Woods WG et al (2001) Prevalence and prognostic significance of Flt3 internal tandem duplication in pediatric acute myeloid leukemia. Blood 97(1):89–94

Meshinchi S, Alonzo TA et al (2006) Clinical implications of FLT3 mutations in pediatric AML. Blood 108(12): 3654–3661

Messinger Y, Gaynon P et al (2010) Phase I study of bortezomib combined with chemotherapy in children with relapsed childhood acute lymphoblastic leukemia (ALL): a report from the therapeutic advances in childhood leukemia (TACL) consortium. Pediatr Blood Cancer Aug;55(2):254–9

Michor F, Hughes TP et al (2005) Dynamics of chronic myeloid leukaemia. Nature 435(7046):1267

Milano J, McKay J et al (2004) Modulation of notch processing by gamma-secretase inhibitors causes intestinal goblet cell metaplasia and induction of genes known to specify gut secretory lineage differentiation. Toxicol Sci 82(1):341–358

Mody R, Li S et al (2008) Twenty-five-year follow-up among survivors of childhood acute lymphoblastic leukemia: a report from the Childhood Cancer Survivor Study. Blood 111(12):5515

Momparler RL (2005) Pharmacology of 5-Aza-2′-deoxycytidine (decitabine). Semin Hematol 42(3 Suppl 2):S9–16

Momparler RL, Rivard GE et al (1985) Clinical trial on 5-aza-2′-deoxycytidine in patients with acute leukemia. Pharmacol Ther30(3):277–286

Moricke A, Reiter A et al (2008) Risk-adjusted therapy of acute lymphoblastic leukemia can decrease treatment burden and improve survival: treatment results of 2169 unselected pediatric and adolescent patients enrolled in the trial ALL-BFM 95. Blood 111(9):4477–4489

Motzer RJ, Escudier B et al (2008) Efficacy of everolimus in advanced renal cell carcinoma: a double-blind, randomised, placebo-controlled phase III trial. Lancet 372(9637): 449–456

Mulrooney DA, Dover DC et al (2008) Twenty years of follow-up among survivors of childhood and young adult acute myeloid leukemia: a report from the Childhood Cancer Survivor Study. Cancer 112(9):2071

Nguyen K, Devidas M et al (2008) Factors influencing survival after relapse from acute lymphoblastic leukemia: a Children's Oncology Group study. Leukemia: Off J Leukemia Soc Am Leukemia Res Fund, UK 22(12):2142

Nishioka C, Ikezoe T et al (2008) Blockade of mTOR signaling potentiates the ability of histone deacetylase inhibitor to induce growth arrest and differentiation of acute myelogenous leukemia cells. Leukemia 22(12):2159–2168

O'Hare T, Walters DK et al (2005) *In vitro* activity of Bcr-Abl inhibitors AMN107 and BMS-354825 against clinically relevant imatinib-resistant Abl kinase domain mutants. Cancer Res65(11):4500–4505

Oki Y, Aoki E et al (2007) Decitabine–bedside to bench. Crit Rev Oncol Hematol 61(2):140–152

Oliansky DM, Rizzo JD et al (2007) The role of cytotoxic therapy with hematopoietic stem cell transplantation in the therapy of acute myeloid leukemia in children: an evidence-based review. Biol Blood Marrow Transplant: J American Soc Blood Marrow Transplant 13(1):1

Orlowski RZ, Kuhn DJ (2008) Proteasome inhibitors in cancer therapy: lessons from the first decade. Clin Cancer Res 14(6):1649–1657

Orlowski R, Kuhn DJ, Small GW et al (2005a) Identificatin of novel inhibitors that specifically target the immunoproteasomes, and selectively induce apoptosis in multiple myeloma and other immunoproteasome-expressing model systems. Blood106: 76a

Orlowski RZ, Voorhees PM et al (2005b) Phase 1 trial of the proteasome inhibitor bortezomib and pegylated liposomal doxorubicin in patients with advanced hematologic malignancies. Blood 105(8):3058–3065

Orlowski R, Stewart K, Vallone M et al (2007) Safety and antitumor efficacy of the proteasome inhibitor carfilzomib (PR-171) dosed for five consecutive days in hematologic malignancies: phase I results. Blood Cells, Mol Dis 110: 409

Ottmann OG, Druker BJ et al (2002) A phase 2 study of imatinib in patients with relapsed or refractory Philadelphia chromosome-positive acute lymphoid leukemias. Blood 100(6): 1965–1971

Palomero T, McKenna K et al (2006) Activating mutations in NOTCH1 in acute myeloid leukemia and lineage switch leukemias. Leukemia 20(11):1963–1966

Park S, Chapuis N et al (2008) PI-103, a dual inhibitor of Class IA phosphatidylinositide 3-kinase and mTOR, has antileukemic activity in AML. Leukemia 22(9):1698–1706

Pollard JA, Alonzo TA et al (2006) FLT3 internal tandem duplication in CD34+/CD33- precursors predicts poor outcome in acute myeloid leukemia. Blood 108(8):2764–2769

Pui CH, Evans WE (2006) Treatment of acute lymphoblastic leukemia. N Engl J Med 354(2):166–178

Pui CH, Cheng C et al (2003) Extended follow-up of long-term survivors of childhood acute lymphoblastic leukemia. N Engl J Med 349(7):640

Pui CH, Relling MV et al (2004) Acute lymphoblastic leukemia. N Engl J Med 350(15):1535

Quesnel B, Fenaux P (1999) P15INK4b gene methylation and myelodysplastic syndromes. Leuk Lymphoma 35(5–6): 437–443

Raetz EA, Cairo MS et al (2008) Chemoimmunotherapy reinduction with epratuzumab in children with acute lymphoblastic leukemia in marrow relapse: a Children's Oncology Group pilot study. J Clin Oncol 26(22):3756–3762

Ravandi F, Cortes JE et al (2010) Phase I/II study of combination therapy with sorafenib, idarubicin, and cytarabine in younger patients with acute myeloid leukemia. J Clin Oncol 28(11):1856–1862

Real PJ, Ferrando AA (2009) NOTCH inhibition and glucocorticoid therapy in T-cell acute lymphoblastic leukemia. Leukemia23(8):1374–1377

Real PJ, Tosello V et al (2009) Gamma-secretase inhibitors reverse glucocorticoid resistance in T cell acute lymphoblastic leukemia. Nat Med 15(1):50–58

Rheingold SR, Sacks N, Chang YJ et al (2007) A phase I trial of Sirolimus (Rapamycin) in pediatric patients with relapsed/ refractory leukemia. Blood 110:2834

Rivard GE, Momparler RL et al (1981) Phase I study on 5-aza-2′-deoxycytidine in children with acute leukemia. Leuk Res 5(6):453–462

Rivett AJ, Hearn AR (2004) Proteasome function in antigen presentation: immunoproteasome complexes, peptide production, and interactions with viral proteins. Curr Protein Pept Sci5(3):153–161

Rizzieri DA, Feldman E et al (2008) A phase 2 clinical trial of deforolimus (AP23573, MK-8669), a novel mammalian target of rapamycin inhibitor, in patients with relapsed or refractory hematologic malignancies. Clin Cancer Res 14(9):2756–2762

Rubnitz JE (2008) Childhood acute myeloid leukemia. Curr Treat Opt Oncol 9(1):95

Saydam G, Celikkaya H, Cole P, Bertino JR, Ercikan-Abali EA (2005) mTOR inhibition leads to increased sensitivity to methotrexate. Proc Amer Assoc Cancer Res 46:3303

Schafer ES, Irizarry R et al (2009) Promoter hypermethylation in MLL-r leukemia: biology and therapeutic targeting. ASH Ann Meeting Abstracts 114(22):3472

Schimmer AD, Welsh K et al (2004) Small-molecule antagonists of apoptosis suppressor XIAP exhibit broad antitumor activity. Cancer Cell 5(1):25–35

Schimmer AD, O'Brien S et al (2008) A phase I study of the pan bcl-2 family inhibitor obatoclax mesylate in patients with advanced hematologic malignancies. Clin Cancer Res 14(24):8295–8301

Schimmer AD, Estey EH et al (2009) Phase I/II trial of AEG35156 X-linked inhibitor of apoptosis protein antisense oligonucleotide combined with idarubicin and cytarabine in patients with relapsed or primary refractory acute myeloid leukemia. J Clin Oncol 27(28):4741–4746

Scholz C, Nimmrich I et al (2005) Distinction of acute lymphoblastic leukemia from acute myeloid leukemia through microarray-based DNA methylation analysis. Ann Hematol 84(4):236–244

Schultz KR, Bowman WP et al (2009) Improved early event-free survival with imatinib in Philadelphia chromosome-positive acute lymphoblastic leukemia: a Children's Oncology Group study. J Clin Oncol 27(31):5175–5181

Shah NP, Tran C et al (2004) Overriding imatinib resistance with a novel ABL kinase inhibitor. Science (New York) 305(5682): 399–401

Sievers EL, Larson RA et al (2001) Efficacy and safety of gemtuzumab ozogamicin in patients with CD33-positive acute myeloid leukemia in first relapse. J Clin Oncol 19(13): 3244–3254

Silverman LR, Demakos EP et al (2002) Randomized controlled trial of azacitidine in patients with the myelodysplastic syndrome: a study of the cancer and leukemia group B. J Clin Oncol20(10):2429–2440

Silverman LR, McKenzie DR et al (2006) Further analysis of trials with azacitidine in patients with myelodysplastic syndrome: studies 8421, 8921, and 9221 by the Cancer and Leukemia Group B. J Clin Oncol 24(24):3895–3903

Smith BD, Levis M et al (2004) Single-agent CEP-701, a novel FLT3 inhibitor, shows biologic and clinical activity in patients with relapsed or refractory acute myeloid leukemia. Blood103(10):3669–3676

Stam RW, den Boer ML et al (2005) Targeting FLT3 in primary MLL-gene-rearranged infant acute lymphoblastic leukemia. Blood106(7):2484–2490

Stone RM, DeAngelo DJ et al (2005) Patients with acute myeloid leukemia and an activating mutation in FLT3 respond to a small-molecule FLT3 tyrosine kinase inhibitor, PKC412. Blood105(1):54–60

Taketani T, Taki T et al (2004) FLT3 mutations in the activation loop of tyrosine kinase domain are frequently found in infant ALL with MLL rearrangements and pediatric ALL with hyperdiploidy. Blood 103(3):1085–1088

Talpaz M, Shah NP et al (2006) Dasatinib in imatinib-resistant Philadelphia chromosome-positive leukemias. N Engl J Med 354(24):2531–2541

Tamm I, Kornblau SM et al (2000) Expression and prognostic significance of IAP-family genes in human cancers and myeloid leukemias. Clin Cancer Res 6(5):1796–1803

Tamm I, Richter S et al (2004a) High expression levels of x-linked inhibitor of apoptosis protein and survivin correlate with poor overall survival in childhood *de novo* acute myeloid leukemia. Clin Cancer Res 10(11):3737–3744

Tamm I, Richter S et al (2004b) XIAP expression correlates with monocytic differentiation in adult *de novo* AML: impact on prognosis. Hematol J 5(6):489–495

Taylor KH, Pena-Hernandez KE et al (2007) Large-scale CpG methylation analysis identifies novel candidate genes and reveals methylation hotspots in acute lymphoblastic leukemia. Cancer Res 67(6):2617–2625

Teachey DT, Obzut DA et al (2006) The mTOR inhibitor CCI-779 induces apoptosis and inhibits growth in preclinical models of primary adult human ALL. Blood 107(3):1149–1155

Teachey DT, Sheen C et al (2008) mTOR inhibitors are synergistic with methotrexate: an effective combination to treat acute lymphoblastic leukemia. Blood 112(5):2020–2023

Tenen DG, Hromas R et al (1997) Transcription factors, normal myeloid development, and leukemia. Blood 90(2):489–519

Thiede C, Steudel C et al (2002) Analysis of FLT3-activating mutations in 979 patients with acute myelogenous leukemia: association with FAB subtypes and identification of subgroups with poor prognosis. Blood 99(12):4326–4335

Thomas DA, Faderl S et al (2004) Treatment of Philadelphia chromosome-positive acute lymphocytic leukemia with hyper-CVAD and imatinib mesylate. Blood 103(12): 4396–4407

Tong WG, Wei Y et al (2010) Preclinical antileukemia activity of JNJ-26481585, a potent second-generation histone deacetylase inhibitor. Leuk Res 34(2):221–8

Tsellou E, Troungos C et al (2005) Hypermethylation of CpG islands in the promoter region of the p15INK4B gene in childhood acute leukaemia. Eur J Cancer 41(4):584–589

Wayne AS, Bhojwani D et al (2009) Phase I clinical trial of the anti-cd22 immunotoxin CAT-8015 (HA22) in pediatric acute lymphoblastic leukemia (abstr 838). Blood 114:345

Wei G, Twomey D et al (2006) Gene expression-based chemical genomics identifies rapamycin as a modulator of MCL1 and glucocorticoid resistance. Cancer Cell 10(4):331–342

Weng AP, Aster JC (2004) Multiple niches for Notch in cancer: context is everything. Curr Opin Genet Dev 14(1):48–54

Weng AP, Ferrando AA et al (2004) Activating mutations of NOTCH1 in human T cell acute lymphoblastic leukemia. Science306(5694):269–271

Whitman SP, Archer KJ et al (2001) Absence of the wild-type allele predicts poor prognosis in adult *de novo* acute myeloid leukemia with normal cytogenetics and the internal tandem duplication of FLT3: a cancer and leukemia group B study. Cancer Res 61(19):7233–7239

Whitman SP, Liu S et al (2005) The MLL partial tandem duplication: evidence for recessive gain-of-function in acute myeloid leukemia identifies a novel patient subgroup for molecular-targeted therapy. Blood 106(1):345–352

Wilson WH, O'Connor OA et al (2009) Phase 1/2a study of ABT-263 in relapsed or refractory lymphoid malignancies. ASH Annu Meeting Abstracts 114(22):1711

Wuchter C, Richter S et al (2004) Differences in the expression pattern of apoptosis-related molecules between childhood and adult *de novo* acute myeloid leukemia. Haematologica 89(3):363–364

Xu Q, Simpson SE et al (2003) Survival of acute myeloid leukemia cells requires PI3 kinase activation. Blood 102(3):972–980

Xu Q, Thompson JE et al (2005) mTOR regulates cell survival after etoposide treatment in primary AML cells. Blood 106(13):4261–4268

Yamamoto Y, Kiyoi H et al (2001) Activating mutation of D835 within the activation loop of FLT3 in human hematologic malignancies. Blood 97(8):2434–2439

Yao J, Huang Q et al (2009) Promoter CpG methylation of oestrogen receptors in leukaemia. Biosci Rep 29(4): 211–216

Yee KW, Zeng Z et al (2006) Phase I/II study of the mammalian target of rapamycin inhibitor everolimus (RAD001) in patients with relapsed or refractory hematologic malignancies. Clin Cancer Res 12(17):5165–5173

Zarrinkar PP, Gunawardane RN et al (2009) AC220 is a uniquely potent and selective inhibitor of FLT3 for the treatment of acute myeloid leukemia (AML). Blood 114(14):2984–2992

Zheng R, Levis M et al (2004) FLT3 ligand causes autocrine signaling in acute myeloid leukemia cells. Blood 103(1):267–274

Zugmaier G, Gokbuget N et al (2009) Report of a phase II trial of single-agent BiTE antibody Blinatumomab in patients with minimal residual disease positive B-precursor acute lymphoblastic leukemia (abstr 840). Blood 114:346

Zwaan CM, Reinhardt D et al (2003) Gemtuzumab ozogamicin: first clinical experiences in children with relapsed/refractory acute myeloid leukemia treated on compassionate-use basis. Blood101(10):3868–3871

Strategies for New Agent Development and Clinical Trial Considerations

8

Malcolm Smith, Meenakshi Devidas, Keith Wheatley, Richard B. Lock, and Sally Hunsberger

Contents

M. Smith (✉)
National Cancer Institute,
Pediatric Section, CIB, CTEP,
6130 Executive Blvd., Executive Plaza North, Rm 7025
Bethesda, MD 20892, USA
e-mail: malcolm.smith@nih.gov

M. Devidas
Children's Oncology Group - Data Center,
104 North Main Street, Suite 600,
Gainesville, FL 32601-3330, USA
e-mail: mdevidas@cog.ufl.edu

K. Wheatley
Cancer Research UK Clinical Trials Unit, School of Cancer Sciences, College of Medical and Dental Sciences,
University of Birmingham, Birmingham B15 2TT, UK
e-mail: k.wheatley@bham.ac.uk

R.B. Lock
Leukaemia Biology Program,
Children's Cancer Institute Australia for Medical Research,
PO Box 81, High Street,
Randwick, NSW 2031, Australia
e-mail: richard.lock@unsw.edu.au

S. Hunsberger
National Cancer Institute, Biometrics Research Branch,
6130 Executive Blvd., Executive Plaza North, Rm 8120
Bethesda, MD 20892, USA
e-mail: sallyh@ctep.nci.nih.gov

8.1 Introduction

Outcome for children with acute lymphoblastic leukemia (ALL) has improved dramatically, with 5-year survival rates increasing from virtually nil in the early 1960s to approaching 90% by the first decade of the twenty-first century (Horner et al. 2009). While improvements in outcome have not been as impressive for children with acute myeloid leukemia (AML), 5-year survival rates have, nonetheless, increased to approximately 60% (Horner et al. 2009). These improvements are gratifying and represent tens of thousands of children diagnosed with leukemia over the last 20–30 years who have survived to adulthood. Looking forward, there are multiple challenges in study design and conduct in moving toward the goal of curing every child diagnosed with leukemia. These include identifying ways to make sound prioritization decisions about which new treatment approaches should be studied for specific patient populations and identifying ways to develop clinical trial datasets based on limited numbers of patients that allow sufficiently reliable conclusions to be drawn about the clinical benefit that these treatment approaches afford.

Agents that are studied in the pediatric cancer setting have generally been previously studied in the adult setting. The large number of novel agents under development for adults with cancer is both an opportunity and a

G.H. Reaman and F.O. Smith (eds.), *Childhood Leukemia*,
DOI: 10.1007/978-3-642-13781-5_8, © Springer-Verlag Berlin Heidelberg 2011

challenge to pediatric oncologists involved in leukemia drug development. It is an opportunity in the sense that so many agents addressing diverse molecular targets are being studied that it increases the likelihood that targeted agents relevant in the pediatric leukemia setting will be available for clinical evaluation. However, only a small percentage of agents under evaluation in adults can be studied in children, given the constraints on the number of pediatric leukemia clinical trials of novel agents that can be performed. How, then, can rational prioritization decisions be made? The traditional approach to prioritization of identifying single-agent activity in refractory patients in conventional Phase II trials is increasingly difficult in the pediatric leukemia setting for several reasons. Effective therapy for *de novo* patients has thankfully resulted in fewer patients available for participation in clinical trials in the refractory setting. Also, practice patterns have evolved so that after initial relapse, children often proceed to one or more stem cell transplantation procedures and, therefore, do not participate in Phase II studies. Due to these issues that limit the number of patients available for single-agent Phase II leukemia trials, there is an increasing need for robust preclinical data that can allow reliable prioritization decisions to be made. As described below, *in vivo* models of pediatric leukemias are now available that faithfully recapitulate the biological and therapeutic sensitivity profiles of the leukemias from which they were established. These models will play an increasingly central role in pediatric leukemia drug development, providing "single agent" information, analogous to that previously obtained in conventional Phase II studies. The Phase II studies will then often involve the addition of novel agents to standard chemotherapy regimens, a setting in which randomized Phase II designs can play an important role.

Another challenge (and opportunity) for leukemia clinical researchers is the movement toward defining therapy based on specific biological characteristics of patients' leukemia cells. This approach is likely to lead to improvements in outcome for specific patient subsets, as evidenced by the increase in event-free survival (EFS) observed following the incorporation of imatinib into a treatment regimen for children with ALL expressing the BCR-ABL1 fusion protein (Schultz et al. 2007). The recent discovery of *JAK* family mutations in a previously unrecognized subtype of high-risk B-precursor ALL has stimulated interest in applying the same strategy by incorporating a small molecule JAK inhibitor into the treatment regimen for patients with *JAK* mutant ALL (Mullighan et al. 2009). The use of FLT3 inhibitors in children with AML whose leukemia cells have FLT3 internal tandem duplications (ITD) is another example of this approach (Brown et al. 2004). While the biological rationale for these new treatment approaches is compelling, the study design issues are substantial. The challenge of studying childhood cancers (relatively uncommon compared to adult cancers) is exacerbated by fractionation of patients into subsets that individually may represent no more than 5–10% of the whole population. The conventional approaches to reliably defining the benefit of a new treatment strategy through an adequately sized randomized Phase III trial may be difficult (or unfeasible) for some of the small, biologically defined populations. Later sections of this chapter discuss both the traditional approaches to designing Phase III trials for children with leukemia, as well as novel approaches attempting to define the benefit of new treatments in as reliable a manner as possible for patient subsets with distinctive biological characteristics.

8.2 Roleo fPr eclinicalT esting

8.2.1 Description of Ability to Establish Direct Transplant Leukemia Xenografts

Early attempts to establish transplantable experimental models of normal and malignant hematopoiesis were hampered by the relatively poor efficiency of engraftment in contemporary strains of immune-deficient mice, such as the athymic nude mouse (Nilsson et al. 1977; Luo et al. 1989), despite the ability to engraft other human tumor histotypes into this strain (Rygaard and Povlsen 1969). Consequently, syngeneic transplantable models of rapidly growing murine leukemias, such as L1210 and P388, were utilized extensively for systematic drug screening programs during the 1960s, a practice that continued well into the 1970s (Alberts and van Daalen Wetters 1976). In the 1980s, it was recognized that these murine leukemias exhibited limited predictive ability for human cancer, and that they were biased toward identifying the DNA-damaging classes of antitumor drugs (Alley et al. 2004).

A significant breakthrough in ALL xenotransplantation occurred following characterization of the severe combined immunodeficient (SCID, LtSz-scid/scid) mouse, which lacks functional B- and T-lymphocytes (McCune et al. 1988; Bosma and Carroll 1991). The

SCID strain was significantly more receptive to engraftment of ALL cell lines and directly transplanted biopsy material (Kamel-Reid et al. 1989; Uckun 1996). Moreover, intravenous inoculation of ALL cell lines or biopsies into sublethally irradiated SCID mice resulted in the manifestation of a systemic disease, with human cells detected in the peripheral blood, spleen, and bone marrow (Kamel-Reid et al. 1989, 1991). Despite the initial reports of success in utilization of the SCID mouse strain for xenografting pediatric ALL biopsy specimens and optimism that it could be used to predict clinical outcome (Uckun et al. 1995a), this was not proven to be the case in a larger follow-up study (Uckun et al. 1998). In fact, only 104/681 (15.3%) bone marrow biopsies showed evidence of engraftment (Uckun et al. 1998), possibly due to the fact that the SCID strain retains some natural killer (NK) cell, NK-T cell, macrophage, and complement system activities (Bosma and Carroll 1991).

More recently, crossing SCID mice with the non-obese diabetic (NOD) strain resulted in the even more immunodeficient NOD/SCID mouse, which harbors additional defects in NK cell, complement and macrophage function (Shultz et al. 1995). NOD/SCID mice are more receptive than SCID mice to engraftment of normal and malignant human hematopoietic cells, permitting the engraftment of pediatric ALL biopsies representative of all major disease subtypes (Baersch et al. 1997; Steele et al. 1997; Dazzi et al. 1998; Hudson et al. 1998; Wang et al. 1998; Borgmann et al. 2000; Rombouts et al. 2000; Dialynas et al. 2001; Nijmeijer et al. 2001; Lock et al. 2002). A report describing the engraftment of a series of 20 primary pediatric ALL bone marrow or peripheral blood biopsies that represented the diversity of leukemia subtypes and clinical outcomes, demonstrated that the engrafted cells retain many of the phenotypic and genotypic characteristics of the original biopsy (Borgmann et al. 2000; Lock et al. 2002). Importantly, ALL cells inoculated into NOD/SCID mice home to the bone marrow and infiltrate the hematolymphoid organs, providing an excellent orthotopic xenograft model of the disease. The NOD/SCID strain is also receptive to re-engraftment of ALL cells harvested from the bone marrows and spleens of previously engrafted mice into secondary and tertiary recipient mice in order to establish continuous xenograft lines (Liem et al. 2004). Furthermore, engraftment and leukemic burden can be monitored in real time by weekly tail-vein bleeds and flow cytometric enumeration of the proportion of human leukemia cells versus mouse mononuclear cells in the peripheral blood, allowing assessment of the antileukemic efficacy of established and novel drugs (Nijmeijer et al. 2001; Liem et al. 2004). Therefore, while some studies continue to use subcutaneously implanted xenograft models of human leukemia (Shalapour et al. 2006; Yang et al. 2007), orthotopic xenograft models of pediatric ALL should, at this time, be considered as the gold standard. This is even more apparent with the recent availability of the NOD/SCID/γ_c^{null} mouse strain (NOG or NSG), which has lower residual NK cell activity than NOD/SCID mice and is even more receptive to engraftment of human hematopoietic cells (Ito et al. 2002). Therefore, the NOD/SCID and NOG/NSG strains are likely to be receptive to engraftment of primary cells from all pediatric ALL disease subtypes and disease outcomes, thereby providing an excellent model to allow the comprehensive preclinical assessment and prioritization of new drugs for clinical trials.

8.2.2 Overview of In vivo Testing Procedures

The scientific literature reveals many examples of investigational new drugs that showed promising activity in preclinical models, but then went on to fail in clinical trials. The general consensus in the scientific community is that these preclinical models frequently overestimate drug efficacy, with the reasons for overestimation being multifactorial (Johnson et al. 2001). For example, rodents are sometimes able to tolerate higher plasma levels of many drugs compared with humans, leading to substantial activity of an agent against human tumor xenografts, but at drug levels that cannot be achieved in the clinical setting. Other reasons for claims of preclinical activity for an agent with subsequent lack of activity in the clinical setting include biological differences between the preclinical models and tumors arising in humans (e.g., faster rates of cell cycling for preclinical models compared to clinical specimens) and setting inappropriate thresholds for claiming activity in the preclinical setting. As an example of the latter, it is common for preclinical reports to pronounce an agent as showing activity when leukemia progression in treated animals occurs more slowly than in control animals, whereas in the clinic this level of activity would be termed "progressive disease" and the agent considered ineffective. For pediatric ALL, the bar for any new drug to be considered for clinical trials needs to be set extraordinarily high due to the number of established drugs that exhibit excellent clinical activity against the disease. Therefore, the setting of stringent criteria for preclinical testing may decrease the proportion of new drugs that ultimately fail in the clinic by eliminating "inactive" drugs at the preclinical stage.

Historically, the *in vivo* anti-leukemic efficacy of a broad range of new drugs has been tested using, for example, a leukemia cell line inoculated into SCID or nude mice via subcutaneous, intraperitoneal, or intravenous routes (Uckun et al. 1995a, b; Myers et al. 1996; Arguello et al. 1998; Chou et al. 1998; Yoshida et al. 1999; Gourdeau et al. 2001; Tomkinson et al. 2003; Miller et al. 2007; Uno et al. 2007; Yang et al. 2007). More recent studies have used direct explants of biopsies taken from patients with ALL and inoculated into NOD/SCID mice as subcutaneous or systemic disease (Piloto et al. 2006; Shalapour et al. 2006; Juarez et al. 2007; Teachey et al. 2008). Recognizing that pediatric ALL is a highly heterogeneous disease, the clinical activity of any new drug used as monotherapy may be better predicted by using panels of xenografts representative of that heterogeneity and derived from patients who experienced diverse treatment outcomes, rather than a single cell line or patient sample inoculated into mice; the superior predictive value of the xenograft panel has been documented for some adult tumor types (Voskoglou-Nomikos et al. 2003). Moreover, it is essential to report the results from all xenografts tested, and not only those against which significant single-agent antileukemic efficacy is observed (Gaynon 2005). In this fashion minimal criteria can be set for a particular drug to be advanced into additional preclinical testing.

As an example of the above, a systematic approach to prioritizing new drugs for clinical trials in children with cancer, including relapsed/refractory ALL, has been adopted by the NCI-funded Pediatric Preclinical Testing Program (PPTP) (Houghton et al. 2006). The ALL component of the PPTP for *in vivo* studies consists of a panel of ten molecularly characterized xenografts, representative of diverse disease subtypes and treatment outcomes, that are propagated as an orthotopic, systemic disease in NOD/SCID mice (Liem et al. 2004; Houghton et al. 2006; Neale et al. 2008). At the molecular level all PPTP xenografts were confirmed to be representative of the original tumor histiotype (Neale et al. 2008). Eight out of the panel of ten ALL xenografts are routinely used to assess the preclinical activity of a new drug (Houghton et al. 2007a, b). Since the xenograft panel for initial drug testing is representative of the heterogeneity of ALL, indications of specific drug activity against a particular ALL subtype (Lock et al. 2008a, b) can also be followed up by more extensive testing on focused xenograft subpanels representing the biological subtype of interest.

The systematic testing of new drugs against large panels of pediatric ALL xenografts poses both logistic and economic challenges. The highly efficient engraftment of human ALL cells into NOD/SCID mice, along with their reproducible rates of engraftment within any single cohort, allows experiments that are of appropriate statistical power to be carried out using only six to mice/group (Liem et al. 2004). Moreover, disease progression in each animal is conveniently, accurately, and cost-effectively monitored by weekly tail-vein bleeds (Nijmeijer et al. 2001; Liem et al. 2004). That said, systematic preclinical testing requires substantial institutional commitment and resources to support the requisite highly trained staff and to maintain the infrastructure for routinely maintaining severely immunodeficient animals for prolonged periods of testing.

Since 5-year disease-free survival rates for ALL now exceed 80% and a significant proportion of patients who relapse can be salvaged with additional therapy (Pui et al. 2008), it has been suggested that a new drug or drug regimen that elicits a 50% complete remission (CR) rate should only be considered of moderate interest to be pursued clinically (Gaynon 2005). Therefore, to maximize the likelihood that only the most active new drugs will be advanced into clinical trials, stringent objective response criteria modeled after the clinical setting should be employed to assess the single-agent efficacy of new agents against *in vivo* preclinical models (Houghton et al. 2006). For example, using criteria defined by the PPTP for the ALL xenograft panel, only a definite regression of leukemic burden elicited by a drug (decrease in human $CD45^+$ cells in the peripheral blood to <1% compared with total human plus mouse $CD45^+$ cells) results in the classification of an Objective Response (either a partial response (PR), CR, or maintained CR (MCR) depending upon the duration of human $CD45^+$ cells <1%). Classifications of stable disease (SD) or progressive disease (PD) are used if progression of the leukemia is only delayed or not contained, respectively, regardless of whether any delay in progression is significant compared with vehicle-treated control mice. Each treated mouse is scored individually, and the objective response measure (ORM) for each xenograft model is defined by the median response for that model.

Xenograft responses are further evaluated by depicting the ORM in "heat map" format, from green (PD) to red (MCR), as well as "COMPARE-like" format, both of which facilitate comparisons within and between the more than 20 new, and four established, drugs that have been evaluated to date by PPTP in Stage 1 testing (single agent at the maximum tolerated dose [MTD]) (Houghton et al. 2006, 2007a, b; Kolb et al. 2008a, b; Lock et al. 2008a, b; Maris et al. 2008a, b; Smith et al. 2008b; Tajbakhsh et al. 2008; Carol et al. 2009; Gorlick et al. 2009; Keshelava et al. 2009; Morton et al. 2009). In this fashion, only new drugs that cause objective responses in ≥50% of the panel of eight ALL xenografts, and thereby pass the Stage 1 test, are considered for additional multiple-dose and combination testing (termed Stage 2 testing). The exception to this general rule is for targeted agents for which activity is expected only for xenografts representing subsets of patients with ALL that have specific molecular characteristics, and for these agents, high level activity against the biologically relevant xenografts is sufficient. As discussed in more detail below, only a minority of the new drugs tested by PPTP have shown sufficient activity against the ALL panel xenografts to warrant Stage 2 testing.

Stage 2 testing procedures adopted by PPTP are designed to develop additional preclinical data to facilitate informed clinical prioritization decisions for agents that show promising single-agent activity in Stage 1 testing at their MTD. The additional testing may involve evaluating the agent of interest at multiple dose levels to get a sense of its therapeutic window and to determine whether activity is observed over a broad concentration range and not only at the agent's MTD. Considering that combination chemotherapy is the cornerstone of treatment, PPTP Stage 2 testing also involves evaluation of possible synergistic or antagonistic interactions of new drugs with established drugs used in the treatment of pediatric ALL. An essential component of the PPTP Stage 2 testing scheme is the comparison of pharmacokinetic parameters of active agents between mice and humans. The broad intention is to verify the clinical relevance of results demonstrating single-agent activity of any given drug against human tumor xenografts, as well as to verify that peak plasma drug concentrations and systemic exposures (measured as area under the plasma [or serum or blood] concentration versus time curve [AUC]) achieved in mice are relevant to those achievable in humans. This model has already been tested during PPTP evaluation of the DNA topoisomerase I inhibitor, topotecan (Carol et al. 2008), in which the topotecan dose and schedule was based on extensive prior knowledge of its pharmacokinetics in the pediatric cancer population (Zamboni et al. 1998). Topotecan demonstrated promising *in vivo* activity against the PPTP ALL xenograft panel (Carol et al. 2008), consistent with recent clinical observations in pediatric ALL (Furman et al. 2002; Kolb and Steinherz 2003; Hijiya et al. 2008).

8.2.3 Examples of Activity Signals

Numerous new small molecule and biological agents have shown *in vivo* anti-leukemic efficacy against ALL cell lines or patient biopsies inoculated via subcutaneous, intraperitoneal, or intravenous routes into SCID or NOD/SCID mice. However, an important characteristic of any experimental model system used for preclinical prioritization of new drugs is whether the responses to established drugs reflect the clinical experience; this characteristic is frequently overlooked. That is, can a laboratory system differentiate the activity of established drugs (e.g., vincristine or cyclophosphamide) from clinically inactive alternatives (e.g., paclitaxel or cisplatin)? While all of these drugs efficiently kill ALL cell lines *in vitro*, the clinical experience in pediatric ALL is dramatically different (Nitschke et al. 1978; Vietti et al. 1979). This challenge has been overcome, in part, by the observations that both vincristine and cyclophosphamide exceeded the criteria to pass Stage 1 testing by PPTP in its panel of ALL xenografts, whereas cisplatin was almost completely inactive (Houghton et al. 2006; Tajbakhsh et al. 2008). Therefore, having established stringent criteria for progression beyond Stage 1 testing, and validated the clinical relevance of responses of the ALL xenograft panel to established drugs, PPTP has recently identified several new drugs that exhibit significant activity, which are discussed as illustrative case studies below.

8.2.3.1 TheA uroraA Ki nasel nhibitorML N8237

Aurora A, B, and C are serine/threonine kinases that function during mitosis (Keen and Taylor 2004). Since a hallmark of cancer is inappropriate cell division, and Aurora A and B kinases are frequently overexpressed in human cancers (Marumoto et al. 2005), the development of Aurora A and B inhibitors has received much attention over the past decade (Aurora C expression appears restricted to the testes). Millennium Pharmaceuticals Inc. has developed a series of compounds that exhibit highly specific Aurora A kinase inhibitory activity compared with Aurora B (>40-fold) and other cellular kinases (Manfredi et al. 2007). The prototype compound, MLN8054, exhibited significant *in vivo* efficacy against human colorectal and prostate cancer xenografts (Manfredi et al. 2007) and its analog, MLN8237, is currently in clinical trials in adults with advanced solid and hematological malignancies (Cervantes-Ruipereze ta l. 2009).

MLN8237 was tested by the PPTP using a 20 mg/kg dose administered orally twice daily × 5 schedule that was repeated weekly. NOD/SCID mice bearing ALL xenografts were treated with MLN8237 for 3 weeks and monitored for a total of 6 weeks following the initiation of treatment. CRs or MCRs were achieved for all xenografts tested, indicating that MLN8237 is one of the most active new antileukemic drugs tested to date by the PPTP (Houghton et al. 2008). MLN8237 is currently undergoing Stage 2 testing by PPTP, which involves testing at multiple doses and assessing its *in vivo* efficacy in combination with established drugs. MLN8237 elicited objective responses in 3/3 ALL xenografts when tested at 50% of its MTD (10 mg/kg), and good leukemia control was observed in 2/3 xenografts at only 5 mg/kg (Smith et al. 2008a). A Children's Oncology Group Phase I clinical trial is evaluating MLN8237 in children with refractory solid tumors and includes an expansion cohort at the MTD for patients with relapsed/refractory ALL.

The underlying basis for the striking *in vivo* antileukemic efficacy of MLN8237 is currently unclear. An obvious analogy is that vincristine, a drug which also affects mitotic progression as its principal mechanism of action, is one of the most active single agents used in the treatment of ALL. Therefore, the *in vivo* activity of MLN8237 against ALL could be due to the rapid proliferation of the disease, although paradoxically this does not appear to be reflected in high levels of Aurora A kinase gene expression compared with xenografts representative of other common childhood cancer histiotypes (Houghton et al. 2008). On the contrary, Aurora A kinase expression in the ALL panel was markedly lower than that observed for solid tumor xenografts, suggesting that its inhibition by MLN8237 leads to acute cellular deficiency and cell death. An additional possible mechanism for the acute sensitivity of the ALL xenograft panel arises from the recent findings that a p53-dependent postmitotic G1 checkpoint is required for MLN8237-induced cell death (Kaestner et al. 2009), since all of the ALL xenografts express wild-type p53 and p53, mutations are rare in pediatric ALL (Drexler et al. 2000; Lock et al. 2002). Nevertheless, additional investigations to define the determinants of *in vivo* sensitivity of pediatric ALL to MLN8237 are warranted.

8.2.3.2 TheB cl-2I nhibitorA BT-263

One of the hallmarks of cancer is the ability to evade apoptosis (Hanahan and Weinberg 2000), and the pro- and anti-apoptotic members of the Bcl-2 family of proteins are central regulators of cell death (Adams and Cory 1998). Consequently, the development of small molecule inhibitors of Bcl-2 family members is an area of intense interest in the field of cancer research. Abbott Laboratories used a unique nuclear magnetic-resonance-based structural screening approach to develop ABT-737, a small molecule inhibitor of the anti-apoptotic proteins Bcl-2, Bcl-xL, and Bcl-w, which exhibits potent *in vitro* and *in vivo* anticancer activity (Oltersdorf et al. 2005). The orally available analog of ABT-737, ABT-263, is currently being evaluated in single-agent and combination chemotherapy clinical trials against several adult cancers, in particular chronic lymphocytic leukemia and small cell lung cancer (Tse et al. 2008; Wilson et al. 2009). Sensitivity of tumor cells to ABT-737/263 is associated with a Bcl-2-dependent phenotype (Deng et al. 2007; Del Gaizo Moore et al. 2008), while high levels of the anti-apoptotic proteins Mcl-1 and A1, to which ABT-737 exhibits low affinity binding, confer resistance (Deng eta l. 2007;Line ta l. 2007).

ABT-263 was evaluated against the PPTP panel of xenografts on a schedule of 100 mg/kg via oral gavage for 21 consecutive days, monitoring all mice for 6 weeks following the initiation of treatment, and it exhibited impressive activity against the ALL panel (Lock et al. 2008b). Three out of six ALL xenografts evaluated exhibited objective responses, including one CR and two MCRs, and two of these xenografts were derived from patients with aggressive disease who experienced fatal relapses. The sensitivity of the ALL xenograft panel to ABT-263 compared with other tumor types could be partially explained by relatively higher Bcl-2, lower Mcl-1, and higher gene expression levels of the pro-apoptotic Noxa (Lock et al. 2008b). Nevertheless, the underlying basis for the diverse responses within the ALL xenograft panel, including three PDs as well as the three objective responses noted above, was not immediately apparent and awaits additional investigation. Despite exhibiting promising single-agent activity against certain tumor types, this new class of drug may exert its most profound effects when used in rational combinations with established drugs (Oltersdorf et al. 2005; Kang et al. 2007; Trudel et al. 2007; Kuroda et al. 2008). Therefore, determining the optimal use of ABT-263 in combination with these established drugs represents a significant challenge to the pediatric oncologist.

8.2.3.3 TheA nti-CD19-DM4 Conjugated Antibody SAR3419

SAR3419 is an anti-CD19 humanized monoclonal antibody (huR4) conjugated with a maytansine derivative (N2′-deacetyl-N2′-(4-mercapto-4-methyl-1-oxopentyl) maytansine, DM4) developed by Sanofi-Aventis that has shown significant *in vivo* efficacy against xenograft models of CD19-positive human lymphoma (Al-Katib et al. 2009). SAR3419 is currently being evaluated in clinical trials for adults with relapsed/refractory B-cell non-Hodgkin's lymphoma (Younes et al. 2009).

During the course of PPTP evaluation of SAR3419, specifically against the ALL xenograft panel, two T-ALL xenografts (CD19-negative) were included as negative controls (Lock et al. 2008a). Not surprisingly, both xenografts exhibited PDs when mice were treated on a schedule of 10 mg/kg weekly × 3 via intraperitoneal injection. In contrast, using the same schedule of administration SAR3419 significantly delayed the progression of 5/5 B-lineage ALL xenografts, including three derived from patients who experienced aggressive and fatal relapses, with regressions achieved in four xenografts (one PR and three CRs). These results translate into objective responses being achieved in 80% of B-cell precursor ALL (BCP-ALL), and justify additional preclinical testing of SAR3419 (Lock et al. 2008a).

The antileukemic activity of SAR3419 is impressive considering the dosing schedule that was utilized. Nevertheless, tumor regrowth was observed following the cessation of therapy, with 3/5 xenografts reaching events prior to the end of the 6-week monitoring period (Lock et al. 2008a). Future PPTP testing will focus on optimizing the administration schedule of SAR3419 to achieve maximal antileukemic efficacy, as well as assessing its synergistic or antagonistic interactions with established drugs such as vincristine, dexamethasone, and L-asparaginase. Considering the controversy surrounding the existence and immunophenotype of leukemic stem cells (LSCs) in pediatric ALL (Bernt and Armstrong 2009), SAR3419 also represents an important tool to gain novel insights into the biology of pediatric ALL.

8.2.4 Preclinical Combination Testing

One of the most frequently posed questions when discussing the rationale for a program such as the PPTP is how one can ascertain the clinical potential of a new drug when tested as a single agent at its MTD, considering that all conventional therapy for pediatric ALL is administered as combination chemotherapy. However, all of the 10+ established drugs used in pediatric ALL treatment regimens have shown some evidence of single-agent efficacy against the disease. This observation supports the practice of initially evaluating all new drugs as single agents in the preclinical setting, and then taking the most active drugs for more detailed multiple dosing and combination testing. It can be argued that some of the "inactive" drugs would show synergistic *in vivo* efficacy if used in combination with established drugs. However, there is no clinical precedence for this, and the recent history of agents that have become part of standard treatment regimens for one or more types of hematologic malignancies suggests that substantial single-agent activity is a prerequisite for eventual clinical utility (e.g., tretinoin and arsenic trioxide for acute promyelocytic leukemia (APL), rituximab for various subtypes of non-Hodgkin lymphoma (NHL), imatinib for chronic myeloid leukemia (CML), bortezomib and lenalidomide for multiple myeloma, etc.). Thus, compelling mechanistic data are needed to support extensive preclinical evaluations of combinations involving agents that lack substantial single-agent activity.

The approach to combination testing adopted by PPTP is based on the concept of "therapeutic enhancement" (also termed "therapeutic synergy"). Therapeutic enhancement represents a therapeutic effect achieved with a tolerated regimen of a combination treatment that exceeds the optimal effect achieved at any tolerated dose of monotherapy associated with the same drugs used in the combination (Rose and Wild 2004; Houghton et al. 2010). This definition is operationalized as follows: therapeutic enhancement is considered present when the tumor growth delay (T-C) for a combination is greater than the tumor growth delay for both of the single agents tested at their MTD and when the EFS distribution for the combination treatment is significantly better ($p < 0.01$) than the EFS distributions for both of the single agents tested at their MTD. This stringent test comparing the combination activity to the activity of each single agent tested at its MTD is not followed in many published studies that claim *in vivo* synergistic interactions between novel and established drugs against various experimental leukemia models. More commonly, the efficacy of the combination is compared with the reduced doses of the single agents that are required when they are given together (Messinger et al. 1996; Uckun et al. 2002; Kuroda et al. 2003; Kang et al. 2007; Yang et al. 2007; Mason et al. 2008; Teachey et al. 2008). This has the unfortunate effect of making the combination appear more effective than the single agents, even though it may be no more effective than one or both of the single agents administered at their MTD. The preclinical and clinical experience with O6-benzylguanine, an agent that potentiates the cytotoxic effect of nitrosoureas (such as carmustine), illustrates the importance of this principle. For O6-benzylguanine, substantial reductions in nitrosourea dosing were required to safely administer it with nitrosoureas in both the preclinical and clinical setting (Keir et al. 2000; Quinn et al. 2002; Adams et al. 2008). The result in the clinical setting was that the two-drug combination using a lower carmustine dose was no more effective than carmustine used at its standard single-agent dose (Quinn et al. 2002). The potential utility of the PPTP approach to *in vivo* combination testing is supported by the PPTP's observation that the efficacy of rapamycin is enhanced when given with dexamethasone (but not vincristine) (Houghton et al. 2010), consistent with previous *in vitro* data that used a gene-expression-based chemical genomics approach to identify rapamycin as a potential glucocorticoid resistance-reversing drug in pediatric ALL (Wei et al. 2006). The efficacy of the rapamycin/glucocorticoid combination in the treatment of pediatric ALL has yet to be reported.

8.2.5 Future Directions

As conventional Phase II trials become more difficult to conduct in children with ALL, systematic approaches to preclinical testing, such as that employed by the PPTP, will play an increasingly important role in new agent prioritization. A particularly promising area for future focus is the establishment of panels of xenografts reflecting specific molecular abnormalities that have therapeutic relevance. The availability of extensive banks of viably frozen leukemia cells that have been extensively molecularly characterized makes it possible to consider establishing panels of 10–20 xenografts that have a particular molecular abnormality. These panels can then serve as a resource for identifying agents that are specifically active against ALL cases possessing the abnormality. As an example, panels of xenografts established from ALL cases that have activating *JAK* family mutations will be valuable in modeling how JAK inhibitors can be optimally used in the treatment of this distinctive subset of patients who are at high risk of treatment failure with conventional ALL therapy. Comparable preclinical models for AML may help prioritize agents for clinical evaluation against biologically definedA MLs ubtypes.

8.3 PhaseI andDo se-FindingSt udies in Children with Leukemia

Pediatric single-agent Phase I studies are generally performed in solid tumor patients, and it is now uncommon to perform a single-agent Phase I study in children with leukemia. The primary purpose of Phase I studies in the pediatric setting is to identify an appropriate dose for further evaluation of the agent in children, to determine whether the pharmacokinetic parameters for the new agent for children are relatively similar to those observed for adults, and to confirm that there are no unanticipated toxicities in children that would preclude proceeding to further clinical trials with the agent (Smith et al. 1998). While children generally tolerate anticancer agents approximately as well as adults, with the result that the recommended Phase II doses in children are highly correlated to those in adults, there are examples in which children tolerate either lower or higher doses of agents than adults (Lee et al. 2005). As an example of the former, children are particularly susceptible to the effects of tretinoin in inducing pseudotumor cerebri (Mahmoud et al. 1993).

Leukemia-specific Phase I trials are unnecessary for agents being developed for ALL, assuming that a Phase I study can be done in children with solid tumors. This is because treatment regimens for children with ALL have the same criteria for hematologic toxicity and recovery as do regimens developed for children with solid tumors. Hence, the solid-tumor-recommended Phase II dose (RP2D) is applicable to the ALL setting in which hematologic dose-limiting toxicities are also relevant. For AML, for which hematological toxicity is dose-limiting only if marrow recovery is extremely delayed, dose escalation to non-hematologic dose-limiting toxicity may be considered.

For agents for which dose escalation is required in the pediatric leukemia setting, there will generally be experience from adults with AML and dose escalation can be initiated at 70–80% of the adult MTD. A general theme in pediatric Phase I studies is that dose escalation need not extend beyond one or two dose levels above the adult MTD, an approach which has the benefit of limiting the number of patients required for study completion and also of minimizing exploration of higher, more toxic dose levels (Lee et al. 2005). The standard approach to dose escalation is the "3 + 3" design, which by convention defines the highest dose at which no more than 1 of 6 patients experience a dose-limiting toxicity (DLT) as the MTD and RP2D (Smith et al. 1998). Other approaches to dose escalation in pediatric Phase I trials include the "rolling 6 design" and the modified continual reassessment method (Skolnik et al. 2008; Onar et al. 2009). There is little experience applying these in the pediatric leukemia setting, and given the limited number of dose levels typically evaluated in pediatric leukemia Phase I trials, there has been little perceived need to pursue alternatives to the standard "3 + 3" design. Pharmacokinetic characterization in the pediatric Phase I setting should be performed to compare with data from adults and to compare with systemic exposures associated with activity in preclinical models (when available).

A dose-escalation study may be unnecessary for some agents, such as molecularly targeted agents for which an MTD was not defined in adults because of acceptable tolerability at doses that met target-effect endpoints or pharmacokinetic endpoints prior to observing dose-limiting toxicity. For agents such as this, the dose tolerated in adults can be studied as the initial dose in children, with possible exploration of one or two higher doses in case the drug disposition in children requires higher doses to match that observed in adults. When using this strategy, comparison of drug levels between children and adults at the tested dose levels is important as this allows selection of an appropriate dose for further evaluation in children. The Phase I trial of bevacizumab in children with solid tumors illustrates this approach (Bender et al. 2008).

Another clinical scenario is that of molecularly targeted agents for which clinical development occurs primarily in combination with standard agents (e.g., the BCL-2 antisense agent, oblimersen). Rather than conduct a Phase I study of the targeted agent administered alone and then a second Phase I study in which the targeted agent is used in combination with additional agents, a single Phase I study of the targeted agent in combination with other agents can be performed. For such trials, it is helpful, when possible, to initially administer the agent alone in each patient to evaluate the toxicity and pharmacokinetics of the targeted agent in isolation, followed by administration of the agent in combination with other agents. Pediatric Phase I trials of oblimersen and of erlotinib illustrate applications of this approach (Rheingold et al. 2007; Jakacki et al. 2008).

Novel agents of interest for pediatric leukemias are generally quickly moved into combination chemotherapy regimens. Novel combinations will often be tested initially in adults with leukemia. The preexisting adult experience can allow evaluation of the novel combination in children with exploration of only two or three dose levels around the doses tolerated in adults (e.g., one dose level below and one above the adult dose level). Determining appropriate doses to use in combination regimens can be very challenging, as the standard treatment regimens used for pediatric leukemias often have relatively high rates of severe and life-threatening toxicities. A general principle for novel combination regimens is that it is important to maintain the doses of the standard agents that make up the regimen, while dose-escalating the novel agent to identify the MTD that can be administered as a component of the combination. This strategy maintains the exposure of patients to known effective agents, and it was used in the development of gemtuzumab ozogamicin (GO) for children with AML (Aplenc et al. 2008). In this example, the GO dose tolerated in combination with a standard AML regimen that included mitoxantrone and cytarabine was only 3 mg/m^2 per treatment course (Aplenc et al. 2008), well below the GO single-agent dose of 6 mg/m^2 administered twice per treatment course (Arceci et al. 2005).

The ideal novel agent for use in combination regimens is one that can be added at its full single-agent dose to standard treatment regimens without substantially enhancing the toxicity of the standard regimen. A number of monoclonal antibodies directed at lymphoid antigens appear to have this property, as illustrated by experience adding rituximab to chemotherapy regimens used for treating NHL and ALL (Coiffier et al. 2002; Thomas et al. 2006). The pediatric experience in adding epratuzumab to standard re-Induction therapy is another example of the tolerability of combination regimens that include naked antibodies targeting lymphoid-specific antigens (Raetz et al. 2008). Some small molecule kinase inhibitors can be used at their single-agent dose when combined with standard chemotherapy regimens, as illustrated by the addition of imatinib to intensive chemotherapy regimens for children and adults with Ph$^+$ ALL (Thomas et al. 2004).

For some investigational agents, it is either not possible or not appropriate to maintain the single-agent dose of the novel agent in combination regimens and/or to maintain the conventional doses of the agents in the standard regimen. It may be necessary to either develop a regimen that maximizes the dose intensity of one component of the combination or to develop a regimen that accepts lower than standard doses of all components of the regimen. The likelihood for success for these types of combinations is decreased, and they are generally not pursued in the absence of convincing rationale for leukemia-specific synergy for the combination. There can also be cases in which the novel agent is so active in a particular patient population that it is appropriate to maximize its delivery while reducing doses or deleting standard agents from the novel combination regimen. This strategy has been applied for imatinib for elderly adults with Ph$^+$ ALL, for which the combination of imatinib with vincristine and dexamethasone appears to be more effective than standard Induction therapy (Rea et al. 2006; Nishii et al. 2007).

Correct attribution of adverse events to a new agent that is added to a standard drug regimen can be difficult. This task is made easier when the standard regimen has a well-defined pattern of toxicity and when the new agent and the standard regimen have nonoverlapping toxicity profiles. A key element of successful conduct of these studies is a clear delineation of adverse events that truly limit dose escalation, as the background toxicity for standard leukemia treatment regimens generally exceeds that conventionally accepted in Phase I trials. A conceptual approach for assessing the clinical significance of adverse events is to focus on both their severity and their reversibility, with either excessive severity or slow reversibility being sufficient to consider an adverse event dose-limiting (Horton et al. 2010). This approach can be operationalized by considering life-threatening Grade 4 toxicities and non-resolving Grade 3 toxicities that result in delay of administration of planned treatment beyond a defined period as dose-limiting (Horton et al. 2010).

8.4 PhaseI ISt udies

The primary objective of Phase II studies is to screen an agent for antitumor activity in order to prioritize it for further testing and to reduce the number of negative large Phase III studies that are conducted. Effective prioritization leading to positive Phase III studies limits the number of patients who are exposed to potentially inferior and/or highly toxic therapy and allows quicker progress in identifying more effective treatments. Another objective of Phase II studies is to learn more about the toxicity of the new agent being tested. Pharmacokinetic and pharmacodynamic objectives are often incorporated to develop additional data to guide further development of the agent. A positive Phase II study results in the identification of an agent that has acceptable toxicity and promising efficacy.

The primary population for Phase II studies is patients who have relapsed one or more times after initial standard therapy. The primary endpoint used in Phase II leukemia trials is typically complete remission (CR) after 4 weeks of treatment. This endpoint is used in Phase II testing because it is observed early in the course of treatment and because it connotes a level of anti-leukemia activity associated with agents that have been shown to improve outcome in the acute leukemia setting. Examples from the leukemia/lymphoma setting show that agents with substantial remission-inducing activity in resistant/refractory patient populations are able to improve outcome when evaluated in Phase III trials for patients with earlier stages of disease. Examples include tretinoin and arsenic trioxide for APL, imatinib for CML, and rituximab for follicular lymphoma and diffuse large B-cell lymphoma.

In the 1990s and before, there were a limited number of agents to be studied and few known active agents. Studies were designed under the assumption that spontaneous CRs after recurrence were very unlikely (i.e., would occur in less than 5% of patients). Since very few CRs occurred, biases that could influence CR rates such as patient selection and differences in patient care across institutions did not need to be accounted for. This led to the use of single-arm studies, the design of which will be described in detail later.

Currently, there are a wide variety of active drugs to treat leukemia, and it is of interest to study combinations of active agents. Since some of the new molecularly targeted agents have little or no overlapping toxicities with standard agents, it is often of particular interest to add these agents to known active combinations. Studying combination treatment regimens that include active agents raises new issues. When treated with an active agent(s), not all patients achieve CR. The characteristics of patients who achieve CR are different from those that do not achieve CR. Therefore the CR rate in a sample of patients treated with an active agent will vary based on the composition of the patient characteristics. If a single-arm study design is used to determine whether a combination including an active agent has increased activity over the active agent alone, it is difficult to attribute the increase in activity to the combination rather than to other biases such as the composition of the patient characteristics in the sample. Designs that are used to address these issues are the randomized controlled screening design and the selection design (described below).

The single-arm Simon 2 stage design is a useful design to consider when single agents are being studied and the patient characteristics do not influence CR (Simon 1989). The design provides a mechanism for screening for active agents with relatively small sample sizes. With this design an uninteresting level of activity (p_0) is specified and is typically set to 5%. A promising level of activity (p_a) is also specified and is typically set to 20%. Historically, the idea has been that an agent that could not produce a CR rate of 20% was not likely to produce a clinically meaningful overall survival benefit in subsequent Phase III testing. A criterion based on the number of observed CRs needed to consider the agent promising is specified. The sample size and CR criterion are established so that the type I error rate (probability of concluding an inactive agent is active, i.e., a false positive error) is no greater than a specified level α and the type II error rate (the probability of concluding an active agent is inactive, i.e., a false negative error) is no greater than a specified level β. The type I and II error rates are typically set to 0.1 to balance the probability of missing an active agent and moving forward with an inactive agent. A futility analysis is performed after a portion of the patients have been accrued and evaluated for CR. If the futility criteria is met (i.e., the agent has a low probability of being considered active at the end of the study), the study is stopped early so that fewer patients will be exposed to a toxic agent that has little likelihood of benefiting them. So, with $p_0 = 0.05$, $p_a = 0.2$, $\alpha = 0.1$, and $\beta = 0.1$ a study would accrue 12 patients and if no CRs were observed, the study would stop for uninteresting activity; otherwise, accrual would continue until 37 total patients had been entered onto the study. At the end of accrual, four or more CRs would be evidence of interesting activity. The development of nelarabine for T-cell ALL illustrates this general approach. In the pediatric Phase II study of nelarabine, a two-stage design was used with α and β, both set at approximately 0.1 and with an "interesting" response rate of 35% ($p_a = 0.35$) and an "uninteresting" response rate of 15% ($p_0 = 0.15$) targeted.

As discussed earlier, the current Phase II paradigm for leukemia is changing, and single-agent Phase II studies are increasingly difficult to perform. When studying combinations that include an active agent(s), the null CR rate or uninteresting rate is no longer 5%. The null rate is the background CR rate of patients treated with the active agent(s). It is of interest to determine whether the new agent or combination has a CR rate higher than the CR rate of the active agent(s). Unfortunately the true CR rate of the active agent(s) is unknown and observed rates typically have wide variability associated with them. The variability is due to the fact that the estimates often come from small studies and in small studies the characteristics of the patient population accrued to the study will strongly influence the observed CR rate. In a single-arm study, misspecifying the null rate of activity can have major implications on the probability of concluding that there is interesting activity when in fact the new agent is not active (type I error) and on the probability of concluding there is uninteresting activity when in fact the agent does have activity (type II error).

As an example, consider the addition of a novel agent to standard re-Induction therapy for children with an early first relapse, for whom the standard re-Induction therapy is effective in inducing remission in approximately 70% of patients. Table 8.1 shows the probability of the errors in conclusions in a single-arm study when the null rate p_0 is either specified too low or too high. The error in the specification of the null rate could be due to accruing patients with a different mix of prognostic factors than the observed historical data, or to the known active treatment working better or worse than it did in the population that was previously accrued. As can be seen from the table, when the true rate is less than 70% (the specified null response rate has been set too high) and the agent truly has activity, the probability of concluding that the agent is interesting is lower than the desired level of 0.90. This means that a promising agent could be missed. When the true rate is larger than 70% (i.e., the specified rate has been set too low) the probability of concluding activity is larger than the desired level of 0.1. This means that Phase III studies will be conducted when there is no true activity signal more often than desired, leading to many patients being exposed to an inactive toxic agent with little hope for benefit and resulting in lost opportunities to improve outcome for the patient population being studied.

In this new age of drug development, other types of Phase II studies are required. An important component of these Phase II study designs involves randomization so that the influence of patient characteristics or population biases is minimized. Randomization is also important when supportive care or other clinical factors may change the expected outcome in the population being studied. For studies in which one or more experimental agents are added to a standard regimen, randomizing patients to the standard arm and the standard plus new agent(s) is a solution. The difficulty in these types of studies is that some patients who are at high risk for disease progression will be randomized to the standard of care. Although from a research perspective this is appropriate since it not known whether the new agent is beneficial, from the patient/family perspective it may be unappealing to not receive a new agent. Successful conduct of these studies therefore requires that investigators have equipoise for the question being addressed and that the investigators be able to communicate this effectively to patients/families.

Rubinstein et al. proposed a screening design in which the type I error, or probability of concluding an experimental agent is active when it is not, is set to 0.15 or 0.2 and the type II error, or probability of concluding an active agent is not active, is set to 0.2 (Rubinstein et al. 2005). Both of these errors are larger than the 0.1 level commonly used in single-arm Phase II studies. Since randomized studies require more patients than single-arm studies, the error rates were increased to allow for smaller sample size. Although it may appear that the error rates are smaller with a single-arm study design, in the example of Table 8.1 the type II error rate is larger than 0.2 when the null rate has been specified too high by a difference of 2.4% and the type I error rate is larger than 0.2 when the true null rate has been specified too low by a difference of 3%. Therefore, although the suggested error rates of 0.2 for a randomized screening design appear to be inflated over those of a single-arm study, in practice when studying a combination of agents it is very likely that the single-arm study error rates will be larger than 0.2. In the example presented in Table 8.1, a randomized study with type I error set at 0.2 and power of 80% would require 56 patients per arm. With the randomized design, the type I error rate will always be maintained irrespective of how the population of the sample compares to historical studies and the power will be known for specified alternatives. However, as can be seen in Table 8.1, this is not true for the single-arm study.

Table 8.1 The probability of concluding that the activity of an agent is uninteresting or interesting when the null response rate is either specified too low, correctly, or too high. With an assumed null response rate of 70% and an alternative rate of 85% (absolute difference of 15%), a sample size of 59 patients is needed to have 90% power and a type I error rate of 0.1

	Truenul l rate (%)	Type I error (probability of concluding inactive agent is active)	Type II error (probability of concluding active agent is inactive)[a]
P_0 is specified too high	60%	<0.01	0.69
	65%	0.02	0.35
	67.6%	0.05	0.20
	70%	0.10	0.10
P_0i s specified too low	73%	0.20	0.03
	75%	0.31	0.01
	80%	0.64	<0.99

[a]The agent increases activity by 15% over the true null rate

For the randomized screening design, it is important to consider the implications of a positive or negative study on the ability to conduct a Phase III study. A positive randomized Phase II study with EFS as the endpoint may jeopardize the ability to perform a well-designed Phase III study; hence, it is appropriate to use an intermediate endpoint (e.g., CR rate) as the primary endpoint of the study. Additionally, conducting the randomized Phase II study in a patient population (e.g., patients in relapse) that is distinctive from the eventual population in which a Phase III study will be conducted (e.g., newly diagnosed patients) can help maintain the ability to conduct a definitive study.

A selection design is another randomized design that is appropriate for some combination Phase II studies (Simon et al. 1985). This design is appropriate when it is of interest to prioritize regimens with a core therapy and several experimental agents individually added to the core therapy or to select among different dosing schedules. In this design, the arms will not be compared formally but the arm with the "best" activity will be chosen for further study. With this design the regimens or schedules must have similar levels of toxicity and some previous promising activity data.

The sample size for the selection design is chosen to ensure that if one of the regimens or schedules (arms in the study) has a superior response rate by a specified margin then this arm will be selected as the best arm with high probability. For example, if there were two new promising agents with similar toxicity, then randomizing 26 patients to each arm would ensure that the probability of correctly selecting the best arm was 0.9 when the true response rate of the best arm is 85% and the true response rate of the lowest arm is 70%. At the end of the study the arm with the most responses is chosen as the best arm. An unappealing feature of the design is that an arm will be chosen as the best arm even if the observed CR rate in the "winning" arm is very low. A modification of the design to address this issue is to incorporate a test for activity of each arm using the standard criteria for single-arm studies. This ensures that an arm that is chosen to move forward will have met at least a minimum requirement for activity.

The advantages of the randomized selection design over separate single-arm studies include decreasing the effects of selection bias, any differences in patient evaluation criteria, and differences in patient care across centers. It is important to note that this design is not appropriate when the arms under study are a standard regimen and the standard plus a new agent. If these were the two arms of interest, then the arm with the new agent would be selected with probability 0.5 even if the new agent was adding nothing. Even including the requirement for a minimum activity level would not be appropriate as the standard arm is the most appropriate control and the arms should be compared with a statistically appropriate design.

There may be instances when an agent has shown so much promise in either the adult setting or the preclinical setting that moving directly from Phase I to the *de novo* setting with a Phase III study (thus skipping the Phase II development component) would be of interest once safe doses of the agent had been determined in children. The benefit of this approach is that the final answer of clinical benefit would potentially be obtained sooner. The drawback is that a large study would be launched with no Phase II data so that if the agent is not beneficial and this could have been predicted with Phase II data, then more patients would be exposed to the new, but ineffective, agent than needed to be. Therefore, this approach should only be used when there is sufficient evidence of activity from sources other than a Phase II study, and aggressive monitoring rules for futility should be incorporated into the study.

8.5 Phasel IISt udies

8.5.1 Rationale for Randomized Trials

It is rare for new treatments for leukemia, or indeed in any field of medicine, to produce large benefits. Even when they have, randomized trials have generally been performed to confirm that these treatments are effective (e.g., imatinib in CML [O'Brien et al. 2003] and tretinoin in APL [Fenaux et al. 1993]). It is more likely that a new treatment will lead to either a moderate, but nevertheless clinically worthwhile, benefit or will be ineffective. In order to distinguish between these two possibilities, it is necessary to ensure that potential errors are eliminated, or at least minimized. Errors fall into two categories: systematic errors, or biases, and random errors, which are due to the play of chance (the latter will be considered later) (Gray et al. 2008). Biases can be introduced as a result of confounding factors that differ between the group of patients being given a new treatment and the control group receiving the standard treatment. If a nonrandomized study is performed using historical controls, other factors in addition to the introduction of a new treatment may have changed over time, including improvements in other aspects of patient management such as supportive care, changes in diagnostic methods, modifications of disease classification and staging systems, and a general improvement in clinical standards through increased experience, both at the individual clinician level and communally. It is not possible to quantify many of these potential confounders and, hence, they cannot be adequately adjusted for in the analyses. Examples of the likely impact of improved supportive care include a halving in the number of treatment-related deaths in children during Induction and Consolidation chemotherapy in the MRC AML10 trial in the second half of the study compared to the first, down from 14% to 7% ($p = 0.03$) (Stevens et al. 1998), and a two-thirds reduction in such events in children with Down syndrome AML between the MRC AML10 and AML12 trials (44% vs 15%, $p = 0.04$), with treatment being similar in the two studies (B. Gibson, personal communication 2010). A pertinent example from older AML patients demonstrated results in the opposite direction in historical and randomized comparisons of the same treatments, i.e., a significant benefit in CR rate for the experimental regimen in the historical comparison, but a significantly worse CR rate in the valid randomized comparison (Wheatley 2002). Outcome of patients with AML entered into the UK MRC trials improved substantially in the 30 years from 1970 to 1999 (Fig. 8.1) (Gibson et al. 2005), yet none of the randomized comparisons with these trials demonstrated benefit for the novel treatment arms; the large increase in survival from 1970 to 1985 is most likely related to improvements in supportive care enabling effective intensive chemotherapy to be given more safely. The failure of these trials to identify effective new therapies might be perceived as a failing in the rationale for using randomized controlled trials (RCTs). However, "negative" trials can be just as informative as positive ones, leading to the elimination from practice of ineffective, but possibly toxic and expensive, treatments that might otherwise have become widely used on the basis of poor-quality nonrandomized evidence.

Since there is evidence that nonrandomized studies tend to overestimate treatment effects (Schulz et al. 1995), and it may not be possible to predict either the extent or direction of bias in nonrandomized studies (Kunz and Oxman 1998), RCTs are widely recognized as the best method for obtaining reliable evidence on treatment efficacy (i.e., "randomization is the only way to control for confounders that are not known or not measured" [Higgins and Green 2008]). The process of randomization ensures that the groups being compared are similar in all respects other than the treatments being evaluated, with any differences being due to chance. A proviso is that RCTs must be performed to a high standard to ensure that biases are not introduced by poor methodology, including factors that will be considered below such as allocation concealment, the need for follow-up to be as complete as possible, and use of intention-to-treat (ITT) analysis.

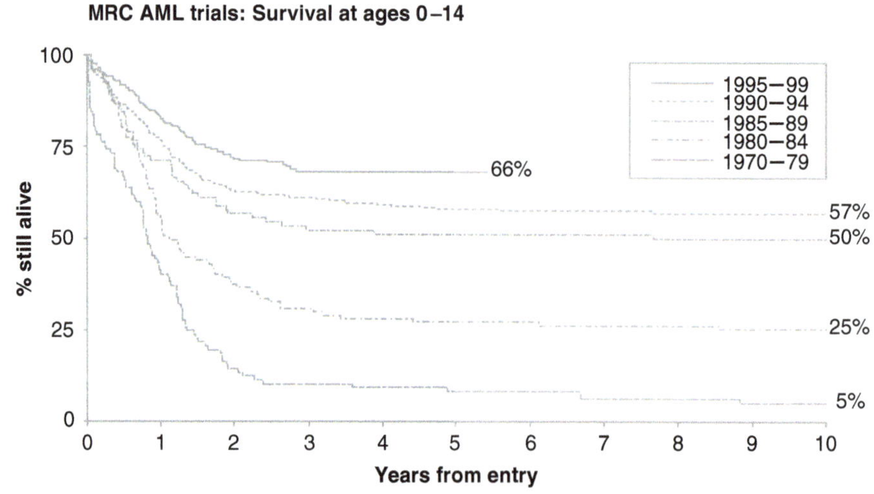

Fig.8.1 Improveds urvival in children in MRC AML trials over time, 1970–1999 (Gibsone ta l. 2005)

The effects demonstrated by RCTs have been more positive in ALL than in AML, with multiple trials identifying more effective treatments over the years. These have defined current standard therapy for ALL patients. Some examples include the following:

1. Study 106 of the Children's Cancer Group (CCG) proved the advantage of Berlin-Frankfurt-Münster (BFM)-based regimens for high-risk ALL (Gaynon eta l. 1993).
2. CCG-105 showed that more effective systemic therapy might spare CNS negative standard-risk patients from receiving whole-brain irradiation, established delayed Intensification as a standard for standard-risk ALL, but also showed that four-drug Induction and intensive Consolidation are not needed(T ubergene ta l. 1993a, b).
3. CCG-1882 established that "Augmented BFM (ABFM) regimen," consisting of longer and stronger post-Induction Intensification, resulted in superior outcomes for high-risk patients with slow day 7 response to Induction (Fig. 8.2) (Nachman et al. 1998).
4. The advantage of dexamethasone in Induction and Maintenance over prednisone for standard-risk ALL was established on CCG-1922 (Fig. 8.3) (Bostrom et al. 2003). This advantage was also supported by results of recent Medical Research Council (MRC) and BFM trials (Mitchell et al. 2005;Sc hrappee ta l. 2009).
5. The benefit of stronger, but not longer, post-Induction Intensification (ABFM regimen without second delayed Intensification) for high-risk patients with a rapid day 7 response to Induction therapy was shown in CCG-1961 (Fig. 8.4) (Seibel et al. 2008).

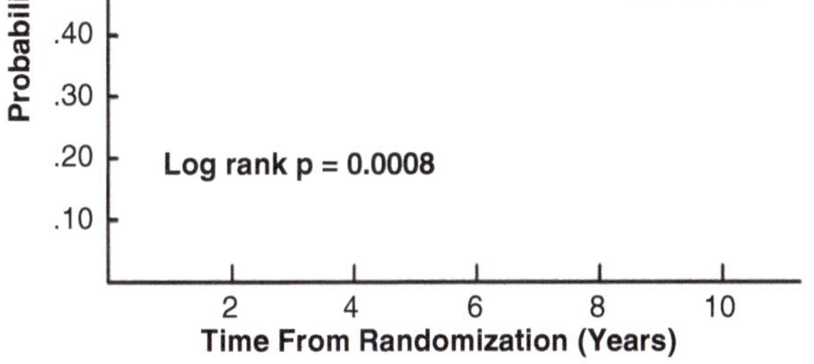

Fig. 8.2 CCG-1882 event-free survival by systemic chemotherapeutic regimen for higher-risk slow early response (M3 on induction day 7) patients (Nachman et al. 1998). 5-Year event-free survival (EFS) was significantly better in the augmented-therapy group than in the standard-therapy group (72.6 ± 3.9% vs 57.0 ± 4.2%, p=0.0008)

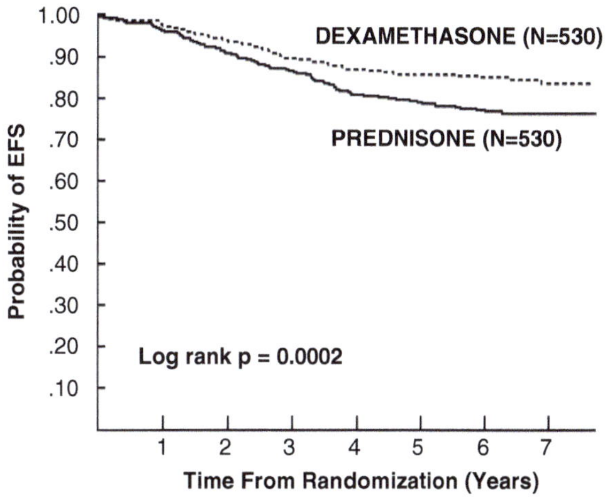

Fig. 8.3 CCG-1922 event-free survival by systemic chemotherapy regimen (dexamethasone vs. prednisone) for standard-risk patients (Bostrom et al. 2003). The 6-year event-free survival (EFS) ± standard error is 85.5 ± 1.7% in patients randomized to dexamethasone and 79.1 ± 1.9% in patients randomized to prednisone (p= 0.002)

8.5.2 Design

8.5.2.1 Eligibility

For trials to have relevance to routine clinical practice, they should include the types of patients who would receive the treatment under investigation if it were shown to be effective. Hence, eligibility criteria should be broad to enable accrual of a representative population. Restrictive entry criteria can also limit the number of patients entered, leading to lower power and less reliable results.

8.5.2.2 Endpoints

The main events in Phase III leukemia trials are response, relapse, second malignant neoplasms, and

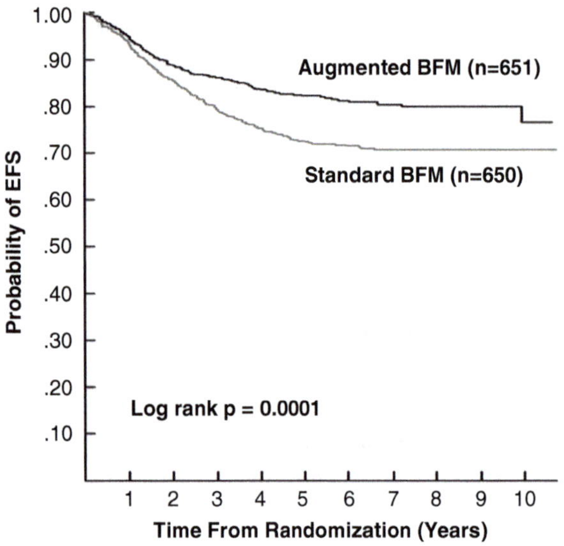

Fig. 8.4 CCG-1961 event-free survival (EFS) for high-risk patients with a rapid day 7 response to Induction therapy according to the type of post-induction chemotherapy (Seibel et al. 2008). Results show a significant benefit for stronger versus standard post-induction intensification (5-year EFS 82.2 ± 1.6% and 72.5 ± 1.9%, respectively, p=0.0001)

death. Depending upon the therapeutic question to be addressed, several endpoints may be relevant in leukemia clinical trials:

- Event-free survival (EFS) is defined as the time from on study to Induction failure, relapse, second malignant neoplasm, or death as a firste vent.
- Disease-free survival (DFS) is defined as the time from achievement of remission to death in remission, relapse, or second malignant neoplasm.
- Overall survival (OS) may be measured from diagnosis or from a later time point (e.g., the time of attaining remission), depending upon the study question.
- Complete remission (CR) rate measures the percentage of patients achieving remission, with causes for failure to achieve remission being classified into Induction deaths (i.e., related to the treatment and the resulting hypoplasia, e.g., infection, hemorrhage, or other adverse events) and resistant disease (i.e., failure of the therapy to eradicate the disease). CR rate is generally not a primary endpoint in Phase III trials in newly diagnosed acute leukemia patients, since the impact of changes in remission therapy on EFS or OS have greater clinical meaning.

While OS provides the "bottom line" result as to whether a new treatment actually results in fewer deaths, EFS is usually preferred as the primary endpoint in pediatric cancer trials. Use of OS as an endpoint may not be practical for evaluating therapies in leukemias (especially ALL) for which the OS rates are high (90–95%), since death from disease may occur a long time after start of therapy and other events may occur in the interim (e.g., allogeneic transplantation after relapse), influencing the result of the trial. Subsequent therapies for these events could then have an effect on OS, the primary endpoint for the first study. Since the event rate is higher, use of EFS leads to better power (and hence lower sample sizes) to detect a difference. However, it cannot necessarily be assumed that EFS is perfectly correlated with OS. For example, meta-analyses in ALL have shown that Intensification improves both EFS and OS, but that an improvement in EFS with longer maintenance does not translate into a survival benefit (1996). When selecting EFS rather than OS as a primary endpoint, an implicit assumption is that relapse has such severe clinical sequelae (e.g., the need for allogeneic stem cell transplantation) that treatment interventions that provide incremental reductions in relapse rate are desirable even if they may add some additional treatment-related morbidity.

Short-term surrogate endpoints (e.g., post-Induction blast count and minimal residual disease [MRD]) are less useful as endpoints for RCTs because of the limited evidence to support their predictive (as opposed to their prognostic) value. The current COG ALL risk classification system uses cytogenetics, day 15 marrow blast count, and end of Induction MRD levels to assign patients to appropriate risk-based post-Induction therapy as they have been found to be strong prognostic factors. However, these early endpoints have not been proven to be true surrogates for long-term endpoints like survival.

Treatment toxicity needs to be assessed and balanced against clinical outcome for both acute, short-term effects and late effects (e.g., infertility and intellectual impairment). As prognosis improves and patients live longer, health-related quality of life (HRQOL) increases in importance, providing justification for the incorporation of HRQOL secondary endpoints (particularly those that address long-term effects) into clinical trials. However, in the pediatric setting, short-term toxicities that resolve relatively quickly are considered acceptable in order to achieve better long-term survival rates with high quality of survivorship. This should be kept in mind when considering reduction in therapy questions for patient subgroups identified to have a very low risk of relapse, and the potential benefits in terms of reduced toxicities should be carefully weighed against the risk of increased relapse rates.

8.5.2.3 SampleSi zeC alculation

Conventionally, sample sizes for RCTs have been determined based on relatively standard, albeit somewhat arbitrary, considerations with respect to type I error (α) and power. A two-sided 0.05 level test is commonly used to compare treatment arms studied in RCTs. Alternatively, a one-sided test may be selected if it is not of interest to prove that a new treatment is worse than the standard of care. Under the latter scenario, the level of significance for the one-sided test in adult cancer clinical trials is often reduced to 0.025, but due to the smaller number of pediatric patients it is conventional in the pediatric setting to accept that a one-sided alpha of 0.05 provides sufficiently strong evidence to be convincing and to change clinical practice.

Power is typically set at 80–90%, meaning that large trials are needed in order to detect the realistically moderate treatment effects that are likely to occur, i.e., large numbers reduce random errors due to the play of chance. A common problem is an overly optimistic expectation of what a new treatment will achieve, leading to small underpowered trials; ideally trials should be designed to detect the smallest difference that would be considered clinically meaningful. For example, to detect a 10% absolute improvement in survival from 40% in the control group to 50% with the new treatment requires about 370 patients per arm at 80% power and 500 per arm at 90% power, both at an alpha of 5% (two-sided test). In poorer prognosis disease, the numbers needed will be smaller; e.g., to detect an increase in survival from 20% to 30% requires 250 patients per arm at 80% power. Conversely, when prognosis is very good, larger numbers are needed in order to be able to detect the smaller absolute differences that are likely to occur; e.g., 730 patients per arm are needed to detect a 4% improvement from 90% to 94%, and this rises to 1,360 per arm for a 3% increase. It also needs to be borne in mind that sample size considerations vary depending on the endpoint being evaluated (e.g., time to event data, dichotomous outcomes such as response rates, or continuous parameters).

An issue that can arise when dealing with rare diseases (including infant ALL, BCR-ABL fusion positive ALL, *JAK* mutation positive ALL, DS ALL or AML, APL) is whether a RCT is possible. The conventional view, based on the above considerations, would be that a RCT should not be undertaken if it does not have enough power to provide reliable answers, resulting in nonrandomized historical comparison (without necessarily much better power) that may be subject to the biases described earlier. An alternative is to undertake a randomized trial, accepting that it has less power and hence requires more cautious interpretation. Such a trial could still be based on conventional sample size calculations, but using higher alpha (e.g., 0.2) or lower power (e.g., 0.7) (Sposto and Stram 1999). As an example, outcome for infants with MLL rearranged ALL (MLL-R) is poor (3-year EFS rates less than 50%). COG is testing the FLT3 inhibitor lestaurtinib (a strategy with a strong biological rationale) in infants with MLL-R. Patients found to have MLL-R are randomized to ± lestaurtinib and a common backbone therapy at the end of Induction. Given that the annual accrual rate for infants, and specifically for MLL-R infants, is low (~50/year), it would not be feasible to design a two-arm randomized trial with the usual parameters. Using a one-sided test with a relaxed type I error rate (15%), the study is powered (80%) to look for an improvement in 3-year EFS from 50% to 65%. An alternative is to present the results as a probability distribution, and give the probabilities that, for example, treatment is more than 10% or 20% better than control. This approach provides less certainty about the benefit of a new treatment and puts a greater onus on clinical interpretation, balancing possible benefits against counterbalancing factors such as toxicity and financial cost. This suggestion that alternative criteria might apply under certain circumstances should not be seen as an excuse to perform smaller trials when patient numbers do permit large RCTs to be undertaken using conventional sample size considerations.

The above discussion relates to trials that aim to show superiority of a new treatment over standard therapy. As outcome of acute leukemia improves, questions arise as to whether reductions in treatment may be appropriate, i.e., is outcome maintained but with less toxicity? Trials aimed at determining the equivalence, or non-inferiority, of treatments have different sample size and interpretative considerations, as well as clinical ones, from superiority trials (Piaggio et al. 2006). Sample sizes are larger for equivalence trials, though the use of one-sided tests can help reduce the number of patients somewhat. This can mean that the margin needed to demonstrate equivalence may have to be large in order to meet conventional sample size considerations, raising issues of whether this is clinically acceptable. Hence, the alternative approach to sample sizes considered above may be particularly relevant to equivalence and non-inferiority trials; e.g., non-inferiority trials (e.g., looking at therapy reduction questions for subgroups at low risk for relapse) can be designed to achieve higher (e.g., 90%) power, while allowing for a higher type I error rate (e.g., 10%) (Chan 2002; Wanga ndH ung 2003).

8.5.2.4 Accrual

ALL is sufficiently frequent for many national groups to be able to run their own trials, at least for the major subtypes. For AML, and for the rarer subtypes of ALL (infants, BCR-ABL fusion positive, relapsed disease), patient numbers preclude large national trials based on conventional sample size considerations in all but the largest countries. COG accrues over 2,500 B-precursor ALL patients annually, making the use of RCTs feasible in large subgroups including NCI standard-risk (1,200/year) and high-risk (600/year) patients; however, subgroups including infants and rare biologically defined subsets have low annual accrual rates. Hence, alternative strategies are required. One strategy is to undertake international trials, such as those performed by the BFM group (Creutzig et al. 2001), as illustrated by a recent successful trial in relapsed AML that accrued 360 patients from 20 countries (Kaspers et al. 2009). Such trials can be politically challenging (e.g., getting several groups to agree on the questions and design can be difficult) as well as logistically challenging (e.g., varying regulatory requirements), although the use of electronic data collection forms and on-line data entry has made the practicalities of multinational trials easier. Another strategy is to collaborate with adult hematologists, an approach taken in the UK for newly diagnosed AML since 1988 (trials AML10, AML12, AML15). Although a heterogeneous disease, there is no clear-cut distinction between AML in children and younger adults; for instance, cytogenetic prognostic factors apply across the age groups (Grimwade et al. 1998). Treatment has varied between children and adults, but mainly in minor respects (and sometimes not based on clear evidence) that do not impact upon the randomized questions being addressed (e.g., children in the MRC trials receive intrathecal therapy, and receive daunorubicin over a longer period). Flexibility has also been permitted with pediatricians electing to take part in only some of the multiple available randomizations within AML12 (Burnett et al. 2010) or continuing randomizing once the randomization closed in adults. Finally, the accrual and follow-up periods may need to be extended to obtain the numbers of patients and events needed to give reliable results (e.g., accrual to recent MRC trials has been in process for 6 or 7 years (Gibson et al. 2005; Burnett et al. 2010)), although in general it is preferable to complete accrual within 5 years.

8.5.2.5 Single-ArmT rials

Identifying the contributions of molecularly targeted new agents in rare biologic subgroups may create challenges with the use of standard RCTs, even with the alternatives for reducing sample size presented in earlier sections. Single-arm trials using comparison to historical control populations have been used in this setting when data for controls are available (for the standard therapy), or in situations in which outcomes on past trials have been consistently very poor for the patient subgroup. For example, the COG trial AALL0031 for BCR-ABL fusion positive ALL was designed as a single-arm trial in which imatinib was given in combination with an intensive backbone chemotherapy. The study had short-term endpoints looking at MRD before and after imatinib administration in the first two blocks of Consolidation therapy. In addition, EFS was to be compared with historical controls from prior COG trials. Outcome on past trials for these patients was so poor (3-year EFS 35%) compared to that seen on AALL0031 (3-year EFS 80%, $p < 0.0001$) that the AALL0031 results provided strong evidence that imatinib contributes to improved outcome when added to standard therapy. However, it is important to realize that most interventions will not produce such pronounced effects. As described in the discussion of randomized Phase II trials, with smaller treatment effects there is benefit for randomization even when type I and II error rates need to be adjusted beyond those traditionally used.

8.5.2.6 Randomization

The term "randomization" is actually something of a misnomer, since the method used to allocate patients to one arm or another is frequently not random (e.g., a coin toss, or based on a random number list), instead being constrained to ensure that approximately equal numbers of patients are allocated to each group, both overall and within prognostically important groups. Two stratification methods are commonly used to achieve this balance: block randomization and minimization (Peto 1982). The essential aspect of any randomization procedure is not whether the process is random, but whether allocation concealment is achieved, i.e., the randomizing clinician must not be able to predict which treatment his/her patient will be assigned, since this could lead to selective entry into the trial. In multicenter trials, it has been shown that the use of block stratification and minimization do not lead to predictability of the next allocation, though in single-center trials or those stratified by center (if open label) use of these methods can lead to the possibility of predicting the next allocation (Brown et al. 2005; Hills et al. 2009).

The timing of randomization is critical in that it should occur as close to the point when the therapeutic interventions on the randomized arms begin. If the randomization occurs well in advance of this time point, the likelihood of patients not receiving the randomized therapy becomes higher; some patients may refuse therapy, some may experience events (adverse events, progression, relapse, death) prior to the point of change in therapy between the two arms. Exclusion of such patients from the randomized comparison can introduce bias. Hence, obtaining informed consent and randomization should ideally occur just prior to the therapy change on the randomized arms. Although some patients may refuse the randomization, this is unlikely to introduce problems such as can happen with too early randomization (Hills et al. 2003).

In contrast to balanced randomization, adaptive allocation methods, in which randomization probabilities are changed as outcome information is collected, have also been proposed (Berry and Eick 1995; Karrison et al. 2003; Berry 2006; Cheung et al. 2006), though there are caveats about their application in the pediatric setting as described below. With these adaptive methods, patients are allocated in a manner that increases their likelihood of assignment to the treatment(s) that is performing better. Adaptive allocation methods based on both conventional frequentist approaches and on Bayesian methods have been described, but greatest attention has been given to using Bayesian methods (Berry and Eick 1995; Karrison et al. 2003; Cheung et al. 2006). Clinical trials employing these Bayesian designs may have multiple treatment arms, and arms may be added or dropped based on emerging outcome results (Berry 2006). A disadvantage of this approach is its inefficiency, as balanced randomization provides the greatest ability to distinguish between the effects of compared treatments for any given sample size. An additional risk of this approach is that an inconclusive answer may be obtained, if there is question or controversy about the prior distribution of the treatment effect assumed for the Bayesian design (Howard et al. 2005). Another important issue is that the presence of a time trend (e.g., the improved outcome over time described above for MRC AML trials) can result in incorrect conclusions about the relative effectiveness of compared treatments when adaptive allocation is employed (Chappell and Karrison 2007). The ethical issue of minimizing the number of patients receiving an inferior treatment can be addressed in trials using conventional frequentist designs through protocol-prescribed interim analyses of efficacy data with stopping rules for both superiority and for futility, as appropriate (Smith et al. 1997).

8.5.2.7 FactorialDes igns

If there is more than one question of clinical interest that needs to be addressed, factorial designs are an efficient method to use. In a factorial design, patients are entered into more than one randomization. Hence, if there are two questions being addressed, patients are randomized to A versus B and to X versus Y, leading to four possible allocations: AX, BX, AY, and BY. This is called a 2 × 2 factorial design. The design can be extended to incorporate more than two randomizations. Use of a factorial design is dependent on the treatments being evaluated being compatible with each other (i.e., they can be given together within the same trial). Factorial designs may involve allocation to more than one randomization at the same time (e.g., two Induction questions) or at different time points (e.g., one Induction and one Consolidation randomization). Factorial designs are used routinely in ALL trials, allowing the available patient resources to be used to answer two study questions at the same time. For example, the COG high-risk ALL trial AALL0232 has a factorial design with a steroid randomization in Induction (dexamethasone vs. prednisone) and a randomization between Capizzi and high-dose methotrexate in Interim Maintenance. In the MRC AML15 trial, children could be entered into up to five randomizations.

In the absence of interactions between the factors, the sample size for a factorial design is similar to that for a single-question trial. If there is a negative interaction between treatments (i.e., the benefit of the combination is less than the sum of the individual benefits), the sample size is increased, but not to the size that would be needed if two separate trials were conducted. It is recommended that factorial designs be used only when *a priori* it is believed (based on the mechanism of action of the two interventions) that there is no interaction between the two interventions. Interactions can be qualitative (when the direction of the treatment differences for one randomization varies among the treatments of another randomization), as illustrated by a study evaluating A versus B and X versus Y, when treatment B is beneficial when used with treatment X but is harmful when used with treatment Y. Alternatively, interactions can be quantitative (i.e., when the magnitude of the treatment effects for one randomization varies among the treatments of another randomization, but the direction of the treatment effects is the same). Quantitative interactions are generally more common than qualitative interactions (Peto 1982). If there is no interaction, a stratified analysis is used to estimate the main effects. If there is significant interaction, then various subset analyses can be done to compare the individual treatments, recognizing that the study was not powered for such comparisons (Green 2001).

8.5.2.8 CorrelativeSt udies

Trials make an excellent backbone for the addition of laboratory studies. Correlative studies on biology or health-related quality of life endpoints can either be embedded in the therapeutic trial for the population of interest or be set up as separate companion trials to the therapeutic trial. Embedded studies usually are more successful in getting the required number of biologic samples/patients for the correlative studies. Refusal rates tend to be lower as compared to enrolling on a separate correlative study, which would also require separate regulatory (e.g., Institutional Review Board) approvals. Banking of leukemia specimens from patients enrolled on Phase III clinical trials can be particularly valuable, as the banked cases will have extensive clinical annotation (eventually including outcome data). Collections of banked specimens have played central roles in identifying key biological characteristics of childhood leukemias and in identifying biological factors associated with prognosis. While prognostic factors are of interest, they become more interesting if they are also predictive factors (i.e., they can be used to predict response to treatment and potentially be used to direct therapy) (Taube et al. 2009). Large RCTs, evaluating the contribution of a novel molecularly targeted agent to standard therapy, represent an ideal setting in which to define the contribution of putative predictive biomarkers (Taube et al. 2009).

8.5.3 Analysis

8.5.3.1 Intention-to-Treat

As discussed, randomization eliminates differences between the arms due to patient selection and other confounding factors. Hence, it is important not to introduce biases subsequent to the randomization process (e.g., by selectively excluding patients from one arm but not the other). The intention-to-treat principle means that all patients are analyzed in the arm to which they were allocated irrespective of whether they received the allocated treatment or not.

8.5.3.2 StatisticalT ests

The statistical methodology for RCTs is well-established. In most circumstances, a limited number of statistical tests are needed: Fisher exact or chi-square for dichotomous data (e.g., response rates), log-rank for time-to-event data (e.g., EFS, OS), t-tests or Wilcoxon tests for continuous parameters depending on the distribution of the data. Multivariate methods to adjust for covariates are often useful: logistic regression for dichotomous data, Cox regression for time-to-event data. As endpoints such as quality of life become more important, more novel methods for dealing with the analysis of data collected at several time points (e.g., repeated measures analysis) are likely to become more widely used.

8.5.3.3 InterimA nalysis

During the course of a Phase III trial, it is important for ethical reasons to monitor for early convincing evidence of efficacy (i.e., that a new treatment is better than the control arm) and safety (Beauchamp and Childress 1994). Stopping a study early for efficacy allows future patients to get the more efficacious treatment more quickly. In some settings, it is also appropriate to monitor for futility (i.e., evidence that the new treatment is not better than the control by a minimally important amount). Stopping a study early for futility reduces the number of patients receiving a treatment that provides little benefit and that potentially causes substantial toxicity.

As treating physicians are blinded to emerging outcome results for Phase III trials, interim monitoring is the responsibility of independent data and safety monitoring committees (DSMC) (Beauchamp and Childress 1994; Smith et al. 1997). A study DSMC has the role of stopping (or recommending stopping) a trial if accumulated data indicate that the initial equipoise surrounding the study question has shifted and uncertainty no longer prevails (Beauchamp and Childress 1994). Protocols for Phase III clinical trials generally include detailed interim analysis plans that provide guidance to the study statistician and to the DSMC about the timing of interim monitoring and about the stopping boundaries to be used at each monitoring point. Repeatedly testing interim data for efficacy can inflate false positive error rates. Standard statistical approaches to interim monitoring that preserve type I error have been developed and are widely used (Friedman et al. 1999; Jennison and Turnbull 2000). Repeated testing for futility can affect the study power, and approaches to futility monitoring that maintain study power have been developed (Lan et al. 1982; Jennison and Turnbull 2000).

8.5.3.4 SubgroupA nalyses

It is of considerable clinical interest to investigate whether certain types of patients benefit more or less from a new therapy than others. In some protocols, subgroup analyses are prospectively specified, and appropriate statistical analysis plans are included in the protocol for defining the treatment effect for these subgroups. More commonly, however, subgroup analyses are unplanned and performed *post hoc*. Such subgroup analyses are subject to misinterpretation since, when a trial is broken down into smaller sections for analysis and multiple analyses are performed, the likelihood that spurious effects will be seen by chance is increased. Testing for interaction (heterogeneity or trend as appropriate) to address whether there is evidence that the treatment effect differs across subgroups is a more conservative analytic approach than inspection of subgroup p-values (Assmann et al. 2000; Wheatley and Hills 2001). Regardless of the analysis method employed, results from unplanned subgroup analyses should be interpreted cautiously and generally presented as exploratory analyses requiring independent confirmation.

8.5.4 Reporting of Results

It is important that the results of a trial are reported objectively, with presentation of all protocol-specified endpoints and avoidance of selective reporting of, or emphasis on, the more positive results (Moher et al. 2001). Results should be presented primarily as an estimate of the treatment's effect (e.g., relative risk, hazard ratio), with a measure of the degree of uncertainty surrounding the estimate (e.g., 95% confidence interval, standard error) (Gardner and Altman 1986). Results should not be reported simply as p-values, and interpretation should not be based simply on whether a result is conventionally statistically significant (i.e., $p < 0.05$ means it works; $p > 0.05$ means it does not).

From a clinical perspective, reporting of absolute benefits, such as absolute risk reduction (ARR), or harms, may be more informative than reporting of proportional differences, such as relative risks and hazard ratios. Giving a number needed to treat (NNT) or harm (NNH) can be a useful way of presenting the result in a way that is readily understandable for clinicians, i.e., how many patients do I need to treat to prevent one death or one relapse?

8.5.5 Meta-analysis

Meta-analysis involves the quantitative synthesis of the results from several trials addressing the same, or a similar, question. It can provide more reliable evidence than any individual trial by including larger numbers of patients and events and by avoiding selective emphasis on the results of specific studies (e.g., the more positive ones). It may be especially useful in rare diseases, for which the individual trials are too small to be really reliable when taken on their own. For example, a published data meta-analysis has summarized the evidence for autologous transplantation in children with AML (Bleakley et al. 2002), while individual patient data (IPD) meta-analyses have been performed on trials of Intensification and Maintenance therapies. Childhood ALL Collaborative Group 1996, CNS-directed therapy (Clarke et al. 2003), and anthracycline usage in ALL. Childhood ALL Collaborative Group 2009.

8.6 Summary

A key factor for success in improving outcome for children with leukemia in the coming years is the appropriate prioritization of new treatments for evaluation in Phase III clinical trials. Given the challenges in conducting single-agent Phase II trials in the pediatric leukemia setting, the application of reliable preclinical models will be increasingly important in selecting novel agents and combinations of agents on which to focus in the clinic. These preclinical data, combined with the genomic and epigenomic characterization of childhood leukemias, will provide the underpinnings for future clinical success.

Randomized trials have provided (and continue to provide) a robust methodology for the evaluation of new treatments for pediatric leukemia. Through these trials, both effective and ineffective interventions have been reliably identified, leading to improved outcomes for patients. As the underlying mechanisms of leukemia become better-understood, leading to further disease subdivisions, new challenges for trial design with smaller numbers of patients will need to be addressed.

Acknowledgments This work was supported by NO1CM42216 from the National Cancer Institute (USA) and by Children's Cancer Institute Australia for Medical Research. Children's Cancer Institute Australia for Medical Research is affiliated with the University of New South Wales and Sydney Children's Hospital. It was also supported in part by Children's Cancer Group grant CA 13539, Pediatric Oncology Group grants CA 29139, 30969, and Children's Oncology Group grants CA 98413,98543.

References

Adams JM, Cory S (1998) The Bcl-2 protein family: arbiters of cell survival. Science 281:1322–1326

Adams DM, Zhou T et al (2008) Phase 1 trial of O6-benzylguanine and BCNU in children with CNS tumors: a Children's Oncology Group study. Pediatr Blood Cancer 50(3): 549–553

Alberts DS, van Daalen Wetters T (1976) The effect of phenobarbital on cyclophosphamide antitumor activity. Cancer Res36(8):2785–2789

Al-Katib AM, Aboukameel A et al (2009) Superior antitumor activity of SAR3419 to rituximab in xenograft models for non-Hodgkin's lymphoma. Clin Cancer Res 15(12):4038–4045

Alley M, Hollingshead M et al (2004) Human tumor xenograft models in NCI drug development. In: Teicher B, Andrews P (eds) Anticancer drug development guide: preclinical screening, clinical trials, and approval. Humana Press, Totowa, NJ, pp125–152

Aplenc R, Alonzo TA et al (2008) Safety and efficacy of gemtuzumab ozogamicin in combination with chemotherapy for pediatric acute myeloid leukemia: a report from the Children's Oncology Group. J Clin Oncol 26(14): 2390–3295

Arceci RJ, Sande J et al (2005) Safety and efficacy of gemtuzumab ozogamicin in pediatric patients with advanced CD33+ acute myeloid leukemia. Blood 106(4):1183–1188

Arguello F, Alexander M et al (1998) Flavopiridol induces apoptosis of normal lymphoid cells, causes immunosuppression, and has potent antitumor activity *In vivo* against human leukemia and lymphoma xenografts. Blood 91(7):2482–2490

Assmann SF, Pocock SJ et al (2000) Subgroup analysis and other (mis)uses of baseline data in clinical trials. Lancet 355(9209):1064–1069

Baersch G, Mollers T et al (1997) Good engraftment of B-cell precursor ALL in NOD-SCID mice. Klin Padiatr 209:178–185

Beauchamp TL, Childress JF (1994) Principles of biomedical ethics. Oxford University Press, New York

Bender JL, Adamson PC et al (2008) Phase I trial and pharmacokinetic study of bevacizumab in pediatric patients with refractory solid tumors: a Children's Oncology Group Study. J Clin Oncol 26(3):399–405

Bernt KM, Armstrong SA (2009) Leukemia stem cells and human acute lymphoblastic leukemia. Semin Hematol 46(1):33–38

Berry DA (2006) Bayesian clinical trials. Nat Rev Drug Discov 5(1):27–36

Berry DA, Eick SG (1995) Adaptive assignment versus balanced randomization in clinical trials: a decision analysis. Stat Med14(3):231–246

Bleakley M, Lau L et al (2002) Bone marrow transplantation for paediatric AML in first remission: a systematic review and meta-analysis. Bone Marrow Transplant 29(10):843–852

Borgmann A, Baldy C et al (2000) Childhood ALL blasts retain phenotypic and genotypic characteristics upon long-term serial passage in NOD/SCID mice. Pediatr Hematol Oncol 17(8):635–650

Bosma MJ, Carroll AM (1991) The SCID mouse mutant: definition, characterization, and potential uses. Annu Rev Immunol 9:323–350

Bostrom BC, Sensel MR et al (2003) Dexamethasone versus prednisone and daily oral versus weekly intravenous mercaptopurine for patients with standard-risk acute lymphoblastic leukemia: a report from the Children's Cancer Group. Blood101(10):3809–3817

Brown P, Meshinchi S et al (2004) Pediatric AML primary samples with FLT3/ITD mutations are preferentially killed by FLT3 inhibition. Blood 104(6):1841–1849

Brown S, Thorpe H et al (2005) Minimization–reducing predictability for multi-centre trials whilst retaining balance within centre. Stat Med 24(24):3715–3727

Burnett AK, Hills R et al (2010) Attempts to optimize induction and consolidation chemotherapy in acute myeloid leukaemia: results of the MRC AML12 trial. J Clin Oncol 28(4): 586–595

Carol H, Morton C et al (2008) Pediatric Preclinical Testing Program (PPTP) evaluation of the topoisomerase I inhibitor topotecan. AACR Meeting Abstracts 2008(1_Annual_Meeting): 2996

Carol H, Lock R et al (2009) Initial testing (stage 1) of the kinesin spindle protein inhibitor Ispinesib by the pediatric preclinical testing program. Pediatr Blood Cancer 53(7):1255–1263

Cervantes-Ruiperez A, Elez ME et al (2009) Phase I pharmacokinetic (PK) and pharmacodynamic (PD) study of MLN8237, a novel selective aurora A kinase (AAK) inhibitor, in patients (pts) with advanced solid tumors. J Clin Oncol 27:15s (Suppl; abstr 2565)

Chan IS (2002) Power and sample size determination for noninferiority trials using an exact method. J Biopharm Stat 12(4):457–469

Chappell R, Karrison T (2007) Continuous Bayesian adaptive randomization based on event times with covariates by Cheung et al. Stat Med 25:55–70, Stat Med 2006;26(15): 3050–3052; author reply 3052–3054

Cheung YK, Inoue LY et al (2006) Continuous Bayesian adaptive randomization based on event times with covariates. Stat Med 25(1):55–70

Childhood Acute Lymphoblastic Leukaemia Collaborative Group (CALLCG) (2009) Beneficial and harmful effects of anthracyclines in the treatment of childhood acute lymphoblastic leukaemia: a systematic review and meta-analysis. Br J Haematol 145(3):376–388

Childhood ALL Collaborative Group (1996) Duration and intensity of maintenance chemotherapy in acute lymphoblastic leukaemia: overview of 42 trials involving 12 000 randomised children. Lancet 347(9018):1783–1788

Chou TC, Zhang XG et al (1998) Desoxyepothilone B is curative against human tumor xenografts that are refractory to paclitaxel. Proc Natl Acad Sci USA 95(26):15798–15802

Clarke M, Gaynon P et al (2003) CNS-directed therapy for childhood acute lymphoblastic leukemia: Childhood ALL Collaborative Group overview of 43 randomized trials. J Clin Oncol 21(9):1798–1809

Coiffier B, Lepage E et al (2002) CHOP chemotherapy plus rituximab compared with CHOP alone in elderly patients with diffuse large-B-cell lymphoma. N Engl J Med 346(4):235–242

Creutzig U, Ritter J et al (2001) Idarubicin improves blast cell clearance during induction therapy in children with AML: results of study AML-BFM 93. AML-BFM Study Group. Leukemia15(3):348–354

Dazzi F, Capelli D et al (1998) The kinetics and extent of engraftment of chronic myelogenous leukemia cells in non-obese diabetic/severe combined immunodeficiency mice reflect the phase of the donor's disease: an *in vivo* model of chronic myelogenous leukemia biology. Blood 92(4):1390–1396

Del Gaizo Moore V, Schlis KD et al (2008) BCL-2 dependence and ABT-737 sensitivity in acute lymphoblastic leukemia. Blood111(4):2300–2309

Deng J, Carlson N et al (2007) BH3 profiling identifies three distinct classes of apoptotic blocks to predict response to ABT-737 and conventional chemotherapeutic agents. Cancer Cell12(2):171–185

Dialynas DP, Lee M-J et al (2001) Preconditioning with fetal cord blood facilitates engraftment of primary childhood T-cell acute lymphoblastic leukemia in immunodeficient mice. Blood 97(10):3218–3225

Drexler HG, Fombonne S et al (2000) p53 alterations in human leukemia-lymphoma cell lines: *in vitro* artifact or prerequisite for cell immortalization? Leukemia 14(1):198–206

Fenaux P, Le Deley MC et al (1993) Effect of all transretinoic acid in newly diagnosed acute promyelocytic leukemia. Results of a multicenter randomized trial. European APL 91 Group. Blood 82(11):3241–3249

Friedman LM, Furberg CD et al (1999) Fundamentals of clinical trials. Springer, New York

Furman WL, Stewart CF et al (2002) Protracted intermittent schedule of topotecan in children with refractory acute leukemia: a pediatric oncology group study. J Clin Oncol 20(6): 1617–1624

Gardner MJ, Altman DG (1986) Confidence intervals rather than P values: estimation rather than hypothesis testing. Br Med J (Clin Res Ed) 292(6522):746–750

Gaynon PS (2005) Childhood acute lymphoblastic leukaemia and relapse. Br J Haematol 131:579–587

Gaynon PS, Steinherz PG et al (1993) Improved therapy for children with acute lymphoblastic leukemia and unfavorable presenting features: a follow-up report of the Childrens Cancer Group Study CCG-106. J Clin Oncol 11(11): 2234–2242

Gibson BE, Wheatley K et al (2005) Treatment strategy and long-term results in paediatric patients treated in consecutive UK AML trials. Leukemia 19(12):2130–2138

Gorlick R, Kolb EA et al (2009) Initial testing (stage 1) of Lapatinib by the pediatric preclinical testing program. Pediatr Blood Cancer 53(4):594–598

Gourdeau H, Bibeau L et al (2001) Comparative study of a novel nucleoside analogue (Troxatyl, troxacitabine, BCH-4556) and AraC against leukemic human tumor xenografts expressing high or low cytidine deaminase activity. Cancer Chemother Pharmacol 47(3):236–240

Gray R, Collins R et al (2008) Large-scale randomized evidence: trials and overviews. In: Price P, Sikora K, Illidge T (eds) Treatment of cancer. Oxford University Press, London

Green S (2001) Factorial designs with time-to-event end points. In: Crowley J (ed) Handbook of statistics in clinical oncology. Marcel Dekker, New York, pp 161–171

Grimwade D, Walker H et al (1998) The importance of diagnostic cytogenetics on outcome in AML: analysis of 1, 612 patients entered into the MRC AML 10 trial. The Medical Research Council Adult and Children's Leukaemia Working Parties. Blood 92(7):2322–2333

Hanahan D, Weinberg RA (2000) The hallmarks of cancer. Cell 100(1):57–70

Higgins J, Green S (2008) Cochrane handbook for systematic reviews of interventions. Wiley, Chichester

Hijiya N, Stewart CF et al (2008) Phase II study of topotecan in combination with dexamethasone, asparaginase, and vincristine in pediatric patients with acute lymphoblastic leukemia in first relapse. Cancer 112(9):1983–1991

Hills RK, Richards SM et al (2003) Corner cutting compromises clinical trials: the inherent problems with up-front randomisation and a common standard arm. Leuk Res 27(12): 1071–1073

Hills RK, Gray R et al (2009) Balancing treatment allocations by clinician or centre in randomised trials allows unacceptable levels of treatment prediction. J Evidence-Based Med 2(3):196–204

Horner MJ, Ries LAG et al (2009) "Cancer Statistics Review, 1975–2006." http://seer.cancer.gov/csr/1975_2006/

Horton TM, Sposto R et al (2010) Toxicity assessment of molecularly targeted drugs incorporated into multiagent chemotherapy regimens for pediatric acute lymphocytic leukemia (ALL): review from an international consensus conference. Pediatr Blood Cancer 54(7):872–878

Houghton PJ, Morton CL et al (2006) The pediatric preclinical testing program: Description of models and early testing results. Pediatr Blood Cancer 49:928–940

Houghton PJ, Morton CL et al (2007a) Initial testing (stage 1) of the mTOR inhibitor rapamycin by the pediatric preclinical testing program. Pediatr Blood Cancer 50:799–805

Houghton PJ, Morton CL et al (2007b) Initial testing (stage 1) of the proteasome inhibitor bortezomib by the pediatric preclinical testing program. Pediatr Blood Cancer 50:37–45

Houghton P, Morton C et al (2008) Pediatric preclinical testing program (PPTP) evaluation of the Aurora A kinase inhibitor MLN8237. AACR Meeting Abstracts 2008 (1_Annual_Meeting):2997

Houghton PJ, Morton CL et al (2010) Stage 2 combination testing of rapamycin with cytotoxic agents by the Pediatric Preclinical Testing Program. Molecular cancer therapeutics 9(1):101–112

Howard G, Coffey CS et al (2005) Is Bayesian analysis ready for use in phase III randomized clinical trials? Beware the sound of the sirens. Stroke 36(7):1622–1623

Hudson WA, Li Q et al (1998) Xenotransplantation of human lymphoid malignancies is optimized in mice with multiple immunologic defects. Leukemia 12:2029–2033

Ito M, Hiramatsu H et al (2002) NOD/SCID/gamma(c)(null) mouse: an excellent recipient mouse model for engraftment of human cells. Blood 100(9):3175–3182

Jakacki RI, Hamilton M et al (2008) Pediatric phase I and pharmacokinetic study of erlotinib followed by the combination of erlotinib and temozolomide: a Children's Oncology Group Phase I Consortium Study. J Clin Oncol 26(30):4921–4927

Jennison C, Turnbull BW (2000) Group sequential methods with applications to clinical trials. Chapman & Hall/CRC Press, BocaR aton/London

Johnson JI, Decker S et al (2001) Relationships between drug activity in NCI preclinical *in vitro* and *in vivo* models and early clinical trials. Br J Cancer 84(10):1424–1431

Juarez J, Dela Pena A et al (2007) CXCR4 antagonists mobilize childhood acute lymphoblastic leukemia cells into the peripheral blood and inhibit engraftment. Leukemia 21(6):1249–1257

Kaestner P, Stolz A et al (2009) Determinants for the efficiency of anticancer drugs targeting either Aurora-A or Aurora-B kinases in human colon carcinoma cells. Mol Cancer Ther 8(7):2046–2056

Kamel-Reid S, Letarte M et al (1989) A model of human acute lymphoblastic leukemia in immune-deficient SCID mice. Science246(4937):1597–1600

Kamel-Reid S, Letarte M et al (1991) Bone marrow from children in relapse with pre-B acute lymphoblastic leukemia proliferates and disseminates rapidly in *scid* mice. Blood 78:2973–2981

Kang MH, Kang YH et al (2007) Activity of vincristine, L-ASP, and dexamethasone against acute lymphoblastic leukemia is enhanced by the BH3-mimetic ABT-737 *in vitro* and *in vivo*. Blood110(6):2057–2066

Karrison TG, Huo D et al (2003) A group sequential, response-adaptive design for randomized clinical trials. Control Clin Trials24(5):506–522

Kaspers GJ, Zimmermann M et al (2009) Addition of Liposomal Daunorubicin (DaunoXomer) to FLAG Significantly Improves Treatment Response in Pediatric Relapsed AML: Final Results From the International Randomised Phase III Study Relapsed AML 2001/01. Blood (ASH Annual Meeting Abstracts) Abstr #18

Keen N, Taylor S (2004) Aurora-kinase inhibitors as anticancer agents. Nat Rev Cancer 4(12):927–936

Keir ST, Dolan ME et al (2000) O6-benzylguanine-mediated enhancement of nitrosourea activity in Mer-central nervous system tumor xenografts – implications for clinical trials. Cancer Chemother Pharmacol 45(6):437–440

Keshelava N, Houghton PJ et al (2009) Initial testing (stage 1) of vorinostat (SAHA) by the pediatric preclinical testing program. Pediatr Blood Cancer 53(3):505–508

Kolb EA, Steinherz PG (2003) A new multidrug reinduction protocol with topotecan, vinorelbine, thiotepa, dexamethasone, and gemcitabine for relapsed or refractory acute leukemia. Leukemia 17(10):1967–1972

Kolb EA, Gorlick R et al (2008a) Initial testing (stage 1) of a monoclonal antibody (SCH 717454) against the IGF-1 receptor by the pediatric preclinical testing program. Pediatr Blood Cancer 50(6):1190–1197

Kolb EA, Gorlick R et al (2008b) Initial testing of dasatinib by the pediatric preclinical testing program. Pediatr Blood Cancer50(6):1198–1206

Kunz R, Oxman AD (1998) The unpredictability paradox: review of empirical comparisons of randomised and non-randomised clinical trials. BMJ 317(7167):1185–1190

Kuroda J, Kimura S et al (2003) The third-generation bisphosphonate zoledronate synergistically augments the anti-Ph+ leukemia activity of imatinib mesylate. Blood 102(6): 2229–2235

Kuroda J, Kimura S et al (2008) ABT-737 is a useful component of combinatory chemotherapies for chronic myeloid leukaemias with diverse drug-resistance mechanisms. Br J Haematol140(2):181–190

Lan G, Simon R et al (1982) Stochastically curtailed tests in long-term clinical trials. Sequent Anal 1(3):207–219

Lee DP, Skolnik JM et al (2005) Pediatric phase I trials in oncology: an analysis of study conduct efficiency. J Clin Oncol 23(33):8431–8441

Liem NL, Papa RA et al (2004) Characterization of childhood acute lymphoblastic leukemia xenograft models for the preclinical evaluation of new therapies. Blood 103(10): 3905–3914

Lin X, Morgan-Lappe S et al (2007) "Seed" analysis of off-target siRNAs reveals an essential role of Mcl-1 in resistance to the small-molecule Bcl-2/Bcl-XL inhibitor ABT-737. Oncogene 26(27):3972–3979

Lock RB, Liem N et al (2002) The nonobese diabetic/severe combined immunodeficient (NOD/SCID) mouse model of childhood acute lymphoblastic leukemia reveals intrinsic differences in biologic characteristics at diagnosis and relapse. Blood 99(11):4100–4108

Lock R, Carol H et al (2008a) Pediatric Preclinical Testing Program (PPTP) evaluation of the anti-CD19-DM4 conjugated antibody SAR3419. Eur J Cancer Suppl 6(12):61

Lock R, Carol H et al (2008b) Initial testing (stage 1) of the BH3 mimetic ABT-263 by the pediatric preclinical testing program. Pediatr Blood Cancer 50(6):1181–1189

Luo Y, Hara H et al (1989) Establishment of ascitic tumor of human pre-B acute lymphoblastic leukemia in nonconditioned nude mice. Cancer Res 49(3):706–710

Mahmoud HH, Hurwitz CA et al (1993) Tretinoin toxicity in children with acute promyelocytic leukaemia. Lancet 342(8884):1394–1395

Manfredi MG, Ecsedy JA et al (2007) Antitumor activity of MLN8054, an orally active small-molecule inhibitor of Aurora A kinase. Proc Natl Acad Sci USA 104(10): 4106–4111

Maris JM, Courtright J et al (2008a) Initial testing of the VEGFR inhibitor AZD2171 by the pediatric preclinical testing program. Pediatr Blood Cancer 50(3):581–587

Maris JM, Courtright J et al (2008b) Initial testing (stage 1) of sunitinib by the pediatric preclinical testing program. Pediatr Blood Cancer 51(1):42–48

Marumoto T, Zhang D et al (2005) Aurora-A – a guardian of poles. Nat Rev Cancer 5(1):42–50

Mason KD, Vandenberg CJ et al (2008) *In vivo* efficacy of the Bcl-2 antagonist ABT-737 against aggressive Myc-driven lymphomas. Proc Natl Acad Sci USA 105(46): 17961–17966

McCune JM, Namikawa R et al (1988) The SCID-hu mouse: murine model for the analysis of human hematolymphoid differentiation and function. Science 241(4873):1632–1639

Messinger Y, Yanishevski Y et al (1996) Treatment of human B-cell precursor leukemia in SCID mice using a combination of the investigational biotherapeutic agent B43-PAP with cytosine arabinoside. Clin Cancer Res 2(9): 1533–1542

Miller CP, Ban K et al (2007) NPI-0052, a novel proteasome inhibitor, induces caspase-8 and ROS-dependent apoptosis alone and in combination with HDAC inhibitors in leukemia cells. Blood 110(1):267–277

Mitchell CD, Richards SM et al (2005) Benefit of dexamethasone compared with prednisolone for childhood acute lymphoblastic leukaemia: results of the UK Medical Research Council ALL97 randomized trial. Br J Haematol 129(6):734–745

Moher D, Schulz KF et al (2001) The CONSORT statement: revised recommendations for improving the quality of reports of parallel-group randomized trials. JAMA 285(15): 1987–1991

Morton CL, Houghton PJ et al (2009) Initial testing of Aplidin by the pediatric preclinical testing program. Pediatr Blood Cancer53:509–512

Mullighan CG, Zhang J et al (2009) JAK mutations in high-risk childhood acute lymphoblastic leukemia. Proc Natl Acad Sci USA 106(23):9414–9418

Myers DE, Chandan-Langlie M et al (1996) *In vitro* and *in vivo* anti-leukemic efficacy of cyclic AMP modulating agents against human leukemic B-cell precursors. Leuk Lymphoma 22(3–4):259–264

Nachman JB, Sather HN et al (1998) Augmented post-induction therapy for children with high-risk acute lymphoblastic leukemia and a slow response to initial therapy. N Engl J Med 338(23):1663–1671

Neale G, Su X et al (2008) Molecular characterization of the pediatric preclinical testing panel. Clin Cancer Res 14(14):4572–4583

Nijmeijer BA, Mollevanger P et al (2001) Monitoring of engraftment and progression of acute lymphoblastic leukemia in individual NOD/SCID mice. Exp Hematol 29:322–329

Nilsson K, Giovanella BC et al (1977) Tumorigenicity of human hematopoietic cell lines in athymic nude mice. Int J Cancer 19(3):337–344

Nishii K, Sakakura M et al (2007) Successful treatment with imatinib combined with less intensive chemotherapy (vincristine and dexamethasone) as induction therapy in a very elderly patient with Philadelphia chromosome-positive acute lymphoblastic leukemia. Int J Hematol 85(3): 273–274

Nitschke R, Starling KA et al (1978) Cis-diamminedichloroplatinum (NSC-119875) in childhood malignancies: a Southwest Oncology Group study. Med Pediatr Oncol 4(2):127–132

O'Brien SG, Guilhot F et al (2003) Imatinib compared with interferon and low-dose cytarabine for newly diagnosed chronic-phase chronic myeloid leukemia. N Engl J Med 348(11):994–1004

Oltersdorf T, Elmore SW et al (2005) An inhibitor of Bcl-2 family proteins induces regression of solid tumours. Nature 435(7042):677–681

Onar A, Kocak M et al (2009) Continual reassessment method vs. traditional empirically based design: modifications motivated by Phase I trials in pediatric oncology by the Pediatric Brain Tumor Consortium. J Biopharm Stat 19(3):437–455

Peto R (1982) Statistical aspects of cancer trials. In: Halnan KE (ed) Treatment of cancer. Chapman & Hall, London, pp867–871

Piaggio G, Elbourne DR et al (2006) Reporting of noninferiority and equivalence randomized trials: an extension of the CONSORT statement. JAMA 295(10):1152–1160

Piloto O, Nguyen B et al (2006) IMC-EB10, an anti-FLT3 monoclonal antibody, prolongs survival and reduces nonobese diabetic/severe combined immunodeficient engraftment of some acute lymphoblastic leukemia cell lines and primary leukemic samples. Cancer Res 66(9):4843–4851

Pui CH, Robison LL et al (2008) Acute lymphoblastic leukaemia. Lancet 371(9617):1030–1043

Quinn JA, Pluda J et al (2002) Phase II trial of carmustine plus O(6)-benzylguanine for patients with nitrosourea-resistant recurrent or progressive malignant glioma. J Clin Oncol 20(9):2277–2283

Raetz EA, Cairo MS et al (2008) Chemoimmunotherapy reinduction with epratuzumab in children with acute lymphoblastic leukemia in marrow relapse: a Children's Oncology Group Pilot Study. J Clin Oncol 26(22):3756–3762

Rea D, Legros L et al (2006) High-dose imatinib mesylate combined with vincristine and dexamethasone (DIV regimen) as induction therapy in patients with resistant Philadelphia-positive acute lymphoblastic leukemia and lymphoid blast crisis of chronic myeloid leukemia. Leukemia 20(3):400–403

Rheingold SR, Hogarty MD et al (2007) Phase I Trial of G3139, a bcl-2 antisense oligonucleotide, combined with doxorubicin and cyclophosphamide in children with relapsed solid tumors: a Children's Oncology Group Study. J Clin Oncol 25(12):1512–1518

Rombouts WJC, Martens ACM et al (2000) Identification of variables determining the engraftment potential of human acute myeloid leukemia in the immunodeficient NOD/SCID human chimera model. Leukemia 14:889–897

Rose WC, Wild R (2004) Therapeutic synergy of oral taxane BMS-275183 and cetuximab versus human tumor xenografts. Clin Cancer Res 10(21):7413–7417

Rubinstein LV, Korn EL et al (2005) Design issues of randomized phase II trials and a proposal for phase II screening trials. J Clin Oncol 23(28):7199–7206

Rygaard J, Povlsen CO (1969) Heterotransplantation of a human malignant tumour to "Nude" mice. Acta Pathol Microbiol Scand77(4):758–760

Schrappe M, Zimmermann M et al (2009) Dexamethasone in induction can eliminate one third of all relapses in childhood acute lymphoblastic leukemia (ALL): results of an International Randomized Trial in 3655 patients (Trial AIEOP-BFM ALL 2000). Blood (ASH Annual Meeting Abstracts) 112:Abstr#7

Schultz KR, Bowman WP et al (2007) Improved early event free survival (EFS) in children with Philadelphia chromosome-positive (Ph+) acute lymphoblastic leukemia (ALL) with intensive Imatinib in combination with high dose chemotherapy: Childrens Oncology Group (COG) Study AALL0031. Blood 110(11):Abstr #4

Schulz KF, Chalmers I et al (1995) Empirical evidence of bias. Dimensions of methodological quality associated with estimates of treatment effects in controlled trials. JAMA 273(5): 408–412

Seibel NL, Steinherz PG et al (2008) Early postinduction intensification therapy improves survival for children and adolescents with high-risk acute lymphoblastic leukemia: a report from the Children's Oncology Group. Blood 111(5): 2548–2555

Shalapour S, Zelmer A et al (2006) The thalidomide analogue, CC-4047, induces apoptosis signaling and growth arrest in childhood acute lymphoblastic leukemia cells *in vitro* and *in vivo*. Clin Cancer Res 12(18):5526–5532

Shultz LD, Schweitzer PA et al (1995) Multiple defects in innate and adaptive immunologic function in NOD/LtSz-scid mice. J Immunol 154(1):180–191

Simon R (1989) Optimal two-stage designs for phase II clinical trials. Control Clin Trials 10(1):1–10

Simon R, Wittes RE et al (1985) Randomized phase II clinical trials. Cancer Treat Rep 69(12):1375–1381

Skolnik JM, Barrett JS et al (2008) Shortening the timeline of pediatric phase I trials: the rolling six design. J Clin Oncol 26(2):190–195

Smith MA, Ungerleider RS et al (1997) Role of independent data-monitoring committees in randomized clinical trials sponsored by the National Cancer Institute. J Clin Oncol 15(7):2736–2743

Smith M, Bernstein M et al (1998) Conduct of phase I trials in children with cancer. J Clin Oncol 16(3):966–978

Smith MA, Houghton PJ et al (2008a) Pediatric Preclinical Testing Program (PPTP) stage 2 testing of the Aurora A kinase inhibitor MLN8237. Eur J Cancer Suppl 6(12):92

Smith MA, Morton CL et al (2008b) Stage 1 testing and pharmacodynamic evaluation of the HSP90 inhibitor alvespimycin (17-DMAG, KOS-1022) by the pediatric preclinical testing program. Pediatr Blood Cancer 51(1):34–41

Sposto R, Stram DO (1999) A strategic view of randomized trial design in low-incidence paediatric cancer. Stat Med 18(10):1183–1197

Steele JPC, Clutterbuck RD et al (1997) Growth of human T-cell lineage acute leukemia in severe combined immunodeficiency (SCID) mice and non-obese diabetic SCID mice. Blood90(5):2015–2019

Stevens RF, Hann IM et al (1998) Marked improvements in outcome with chemotherapy alone in paediatric acute myeloid leukemia: results of the United Kingdom Medical Research Council's 10th AML trial. MRC Childhood Leukaemia Working Party. Br J Haematol 101(1):130–140

Tajbakhsh M, Houghton PJ et al (2008) Initial testing of cisplatin by the pediatric preclinical testing program. Pediatr Blood Cancer 50(5):992–1000

Taube SE, Clark GM et al (2009) A perspective on challenges and issues in biomarker development and drug and biomarker codevelopment. J Natl Cancer Inst 101(21): 1453–1463

Teachey DT, Sheen C et al (2008) mTOR inhibitors are synergistic with methotrexate: an effective combination to treat acute lymphoblastic leukemia. Blood 112(5):2020–2023

Thomas DA, Faderl S et al (2004) Treatment of Philadelphia chromosome-positive acute lymphocytic leukemia with hyper-CVAD and imatinib mesylate. Blood 103(12): 4396–4407

Thomas DA, Faderl S et al (2006) Chemoimmunotherapy with hyper-CVAD plus rituximab for the treatment of adult Burkitt and Burkitt-type lymphoma or acute lymphoblastic leukemia. Cancer 106(7):1569–1580

Tomkinson B, Bendele R et al (2003) OSI-211, a novel liposomal topoisomerase I inhibitor, is active in SCID mouse models of human AML and ALL. Leuk Res 27(11):1039–1050

Trudel S, Stewart AK et al (2007) The Bcl-2 family protein inhibitor, ABT-737, has substantial antimyeloma activity and shows synergistic effect with dexamethasone and melphalan. Clin Cancer Res 13(2 Pt 1):621–629

Tse C, Shoemaker AR et al (2008) ABT-263: a potent and orally bioavailable Bcl-2 family inhibitor. Cancer Res 68(9): 3421–3428

Tubergen DG, Gilchrist GS et al (1993a) Improved outcome with delayed intensification for children with acute lymphoblastic leukemia and intermediate presenting features: a Childrens Cancer Group phase III trial. J Clin Oncol 11(3): 527–537

Tubergen DG, Gilchrist GS et al (1993b) Prevention of CNS disease in intermediate-risk acute lymphoblastic leukemia: comparison of cranial radiation and intrathecal methotrexate and the importance of systemic therapy: a Childrens Cancer Group report. J Clin Oncol 11(3):520–526

Uckun FM (1996) Severe combined immunodeficient mouse models of human leukemia. Blood 88(4):1135–1146

Uckun FM, Sather H et al (1995a) Leukemic cell growth in SCID mice as a predictor of relapse in high-risk B-lineage acute lymphoblastic leukemia. Blood 85(4):873–878

Uckun FM, Stewart CF et al (1995b) *In vitro* and *in vivo* activity of topotecan against human B-lineage acute lymphoblastic leukemia cells. Blood 85(10):2817–2828

Uckun FM, Sather HN et al (1998) Prognostic significance of B-lineage leukemic cell growth in SCID mice: a Children's Cancer Group Study. Leuk Lymphoma 30(5–6): 503–514

Uckun FM, Zheng Y et al (2002) *In vivo* pharmacokinetic features, toxicity profile, and chemosensitizing activity of alpha-cyano-beta-hydroxy-beta- methyl-N-(2, 5-dibromophenyl) propenamide (LFM-A13), a novel antileukemic agent targeting Bruton's tyrosine kinase. Clin Cancer Res 8(5): 1224–1233

Uno S, Kinoshita Y et al (2007) Antitumor activity of a monoclonal antibody against CD47 in xenograft models of human leukemia. Oncol Rep 17(5):1189–1194

Vietti TJ, Nitschke R et al (1979) Evaluation of cis-dichlorodiammineplatinum(II) in children with advanced malignant diseases: Southwest Oncology Group Studies. Cancer Treat Rep63(9–10):1611 –1614

Voskoglou-Nomikos T, Pater JL et al (2003) Clinical predictive value of the *in vitro* cell line, human xenograft, and mouse allograft preclinical cancer models. Clin Cancer Res 9(11): 4227–4239

Wang SJ, Hung HM (2003) Assessing treatment efficacy in non-inferiority trials. Control Clin Trials 24(2):147–155

Wang JCY, Lapidot T et al (1998) High level engraftment of NOD/SCID mice by primitive normal and leukemic hematopoietic cells from patients with chronic myeloid leukemia in chronic phase. Blood 91(7):2406–2414

Wei G, Twomey D et al (2006) Gene expression-based chemical genomics identifies rapamycin as a modulator of MCL1 and glucocorticoid resistance. Cancer Cell 10(4):331–342

Wheatley K (2002) SAB–a promising new treatment to improve remission rates in AML in the elderly? Br J Haematol 118(2):432–433

Wheatley K, Hills RK (2001) Inappropriate reporting and interpretation of subgroups in the AML-BFM 93 study. Leukemia 15(11):1803–1804

Wilson WH, O'Connor OA et al (2009) Phase 1/2a Study of ABT-263 in Relapsed or Refractory Lymphoid Malignancies. Blood (ASH Annual Meeting Abstracts) 114:Abstr #1711

Yang J, Ikezoe T et al (2007) AZD1152, a novel and selective aurora B kinase inhibitor, induces growth arrest, apoptosis, and sensitization for tubulin depolymerizing agent or topoisomerase II inhibitor in human acute leukemia cells *in vitro* and *in vivo*. Blood 110(6):2034–2040

Yoshida N, Ishii E et al (1999) The laminin-derived peptide YIGSR (Tyr-Ile-Gly-Ser-Arg) inhibits human pre-B leukaemic cell growth and dissemination to organs in SCID mice. Br J Cancer 80(12):1898–1904

Younes A, Gordon L et al (2009) Phase I Multi-dose escalation study of the anti-CD19 Maytansinoid immunoconjugate SAR3419 administered by intravenous (IV) infusion every 3 weeks to patients with relapsed/ refractory B-cell non-Hodgkin's lymphoma (NHL). Blood (ASH Annual Meeting Abstracts) 114:Abstr #585

Zamboni WC, Stewart CF et al (1998) Relationship between topotecan systemic exposure and tumor response in human neuroblastoma xenografts. J Natl Cancer Inst 90(7): 505–511

Part VI

Late Effects of Leukemia and Its Therapy

Late Sequelae in Children with Acute Lymphoblastic Leukemia: Impact onL ong-TermSur vivalandQual ityo fL ife

9

Joseph P. Neglia, Maura O'Leary, and Smita Bhatia

Contents

J.P. Neglia
Department of Pediatrics, University of Minnesota, Minneapolis, MN, USA

M.O 'Leary
Children'sO ncologyG roup, Bethesda, MD,U SA

S.B hatia (✉)
Department of Population Sciences, City of Hope National Medical Center, 1500 E. Duarte Road, Duarte, CA 91010, USA
e-mail:s bhatia@coh.org

9.1 Introduction

Acute lymphoblastic leukemia (ALL) is the most common childhood malignancy, with an annual incidence rate of three to four cases per 100,000 children (Horner et al. 2009). As shown in Fig. 9.1, there has been a tremendous progress in survival rates over the past several decades. Among patients treated with

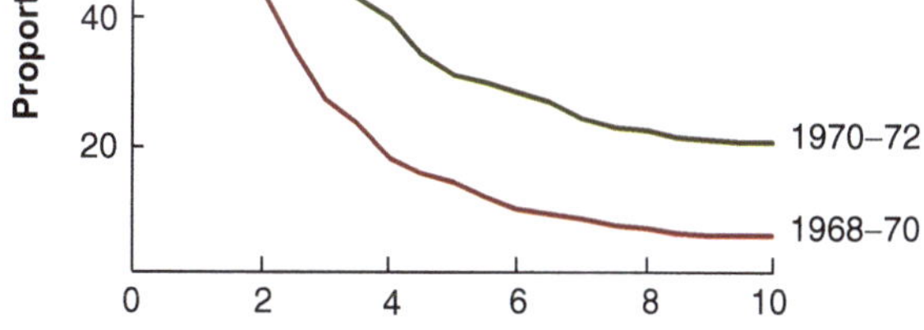

Fig. 9.1 Overall survival of children diagnosed with acute lymphoblastic leukemia and treated on legacy Children's Oncology Grouppr otocols(1968–1997)

G.H. Reaman and F.O. Smith (eds.), *Childhood Leukemia*,
DOI: 10.1007/978-3-642-13781-5_9, © Springer-Verlag Berlin Heidelberg 2011

contemporary risk-based therapy, the overall 5-year survival rates exceed 85% (Brenner et al. 2001; Ries et al. 2001) and the event-free survival (EFS) rates exceed 80% (Pui and Evans 1998; Schrappe et al. 2000; Silverman et al. 2001). With this success has come the need to consider the long-term morbidity and mortality associated with treatments responsible for the improvement in survival, as well as the quality of thiss urvival.

Unlike adults, the growing child tolerates the acute side effects of therapy relatively well. However, the use of cancer therapy at an early age can produce complications that may not become apparent until years later as the child matures; hence the term "late-effect" for a late-occurring or chronic outcome, either physical or psychological, that persists or develops beyond 5 years from diagnosis of ALL. Because of the relatively young age of the cancer survivors and the potential for longevity, the delayed consequences of therapy may have a significant impact on their lives, and on society at large. Long-term sequelae of treatment, such as impaired intellectual and psychomotor functioning (Jankovic et al. 1994a, b), endocrine abnormalities (Hameed and Zacharin 2005), cardiotoxicity (Lipshultz et al. 1991), and second malignancies (Pui et al. 1989; Neglia et al. 1991; Nygaard et al. 1991; Loning et al. 2000) are now being reported with increasing frequency in this growing population of survivors. Topics that are reviewed in this chapter are summarized in Table 9.1 and include issues related to the specific late-effects faced by ALL survivors and the future research opportunities that need to be explored.

Table9.1 Commonly occurring late-effects in survivors of childhood acute lymphoblastic leukemia (ALL)

Adverse outcome	Therapeutic exposures associated with increased risk	Factors associated with highest risk
Neurocognitive deficits	Cranial irradiation, intrathecal methotrexate, cytarabine	Female sex, younger age (<5 years) at treatment, cranial irradiation, and intrathecal chemotherapy
Cardiomyopathy/congestiveh eart failure	Anthracyclines	High cumulative doses, females, younger than 5 years at treatment, mediastinal radiation
Therapy-related myelodysplasia	Alkylating agents, topoisomerase II inhibitors, anthracyclines	Increasing dose of chemotherapeutic agents, older age at therapeutic exposure
Thyroid cancer	Radiation to the thyroid gland	Increasing dose up to 29 Gy, female sex, younger age at radiation
Skin cancer (basal cell, squamous cell, melanoma)	Radiation therapy	Orthovoltage radiation (prior to 1970) – delivery of greater dose to skin, additional excessive exposure to sun, tanning booths
Secondary brain tumor	Cranial irradiation	Increasing dose, younger age at treatment
Hypothyroidism	Radiation to the thyroid gland	Increasing dose, female sex, age at treatment
Hypogonadism	Alkylatinga gents,c raniospinal irradiation, abdomino-pelvic irradiation, gonadal irradiation	Male sex, treatment during peripubertal or postpubertal period in girls, higher cumulative doses of alkylators
Precocious puberty	Cranial irradiation	Female sex, younger age at treatment, radiation dose >18 Gy
Chronic hepatitis C virus (HCV) infection and HCV-related sequelae	Transfusions before 1993	Living in hyperendemic area
Short stature	Cranial irradiation, corticosteroids, total body irradiation	Younger age at treatment, cranial radiation dose >18 Gy, unfractionated (10 Gy) total body irradiation
Obesity	Cranial irradiation	Younger age at treatment (<8 years), female sex, cranial irradiation dose >20 Gy
Osteopenia/osteoporosis	Corticosteroids,c raniospinal irradiation, total body irradiation	Associated hypothyroidism, hypogonadism, growth hormone deficiency
Osteonecrosis	Corticosteroids,hi gh-dose radiation to any bone	Dexamethasone, adolescence, female sex

9.2 Burdeno f Morbidity

Investigators have described the burden of morbidity by quantifying the chronic medical problems experienced by ALL survivors (Pui et al. 1989; Mody et al. 2008). Mody et al. (2008) reported one or more chronic medical conditions in 50% of survivors, compared with 37.8% of siblings ($p < 0.001$). Survivors were found to be 3.7 times more likely than siblings to report a severe or life-threatening chronic medical condition and 2.8 times more likely to report multiple chronic medical conditions, after adjusting for age at interview, sex, and ethnicity. Highest risks were seen for musculoskeletal conditions (e.g., major joint replacements), cardiac conditions (e.g., congestive heart failure [CHF]), and neurologic conditions (e.g., cognitive deficits). Among ALL survivors, the cumulative incidence of any chronic medical condition 25 years from diagnosis was 64.9%, while that of a severe, life-threatening condition was 21.3%. Of note, 92% of the nonirradiated survivors who remained in complete continuous remission reported no severe or life-threatening chronic medical conditions.

These studies demonstrate quite conclusively that the implications of cure are not trivial, and that the burden of morbidity carried by ALL survivors is substantial. Furthermore, these data support a critical need for follow-up of ALL survivors into adult life. There is also an urgent need for healthcare providers to be aware of "at risk" populations in order to develop appropriate surveillance strategies, and for survivors to participate in that surveillance.

9.3 Cardiotoxicity

Anthracyclines are widely used for the treatment of childhood ALL, and may result in cardiotoxicity. Chronic cardiotoxicity usually manifests itself as subclinical cardiomyopathy that may eventually lead to clinically overt congestive heart failure (CHF) (Fig. 9.2). Reported incidences of CHF vary from 0% to 16% in measurements ranging from 0.9 to 4.6 years following treatment (Kremer et al. 2002). The incidence of anthracycline-induced cardiomyopathy is dose-dependent, and a cumulative dose of anthracyclines greater than 300 mg/m^2 has been associated with an 11-fold increased risk of CHF when compared

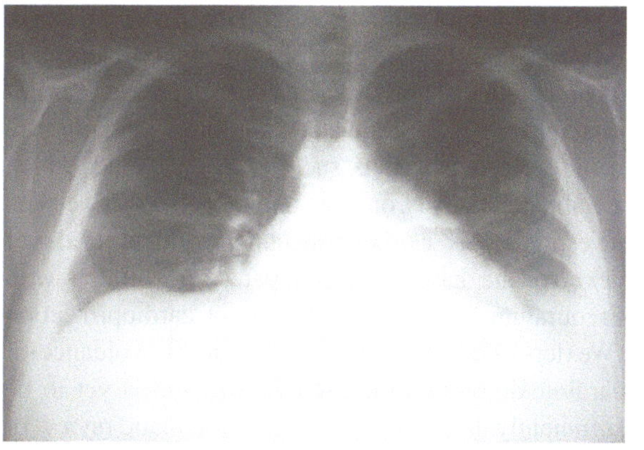

Fig. 9.2 Plain chest radiograph depicting anthracycline-related congestivehe artf ailure

with a dose less than 300 mg/m^2; the risk of CHF continues to increase with time from exposure and approaches 5% after 15 years (Kremer et al. 2001).

Abnormalities of left ventricular structure and function are found in up to 60% of anthracycline-treated survivors of childhood ALL (Lipshultz et al. 1991). Cardiotoxicity has been shown to have two forms: the first is characterized by depressed contractility and is associated with higher cumulative anthracycline dose and female sex, and the second is characterized by increased afterload and decreased left ventricular mass and wall thickness. The latter form of cardiotoxicity is related to time since treatment, age at treatment, and anthracycline dosage (Lipshultz et al. 1995). These cardiac abnormalities are persistent and progressive after anthracycline therapy (Lipshultz et al. 2005). The abnormalities are most severe after highest cumulative doses of anthracyclines, but may appear even after low doses. More follow-up is needed to determine the natural history and clinical significance of these abnormalities (Lipshultz 2000).

Among anthracycline-exposed patients, the risk for cardiotoxicity can be increased by mediastinal radiation (Fajardo et al. 1968), uncontrolled hypertension (Prout et al. 1977), exposure to nonanthracycline chemotherapeutic agents (especially cyclophosphamide, dactinomycin, mitomycin C, dacarbazine, vincristine, bleomycin, and methotrexate) (Smith et al. 1977; Von Hoff et al. 1982), female gender (Lipshultz et al. 1995), younger age, and electrolyte imbalances such as hypokalemia and hypomagnesemia. The evidence regarding the association between anthracycline-induced cardiotoxicity and the method of administration is insufficient to draw meaningful conclusions (Legha et al. 1982; Shapira et al. 1990; Lipshultz et al. 2002).

Prevention of cardiotoxicity is a focus of active investigation. Certain analogs of doxorubicin and daunomycin that are associated with decreased cardiotoxicity, but have equivalent antitumor activity, are being explored. Agents such as dexrazoxane, which are able to remove iron from anthracyclines, have been investigated as cardioprotectants. Clinical trials of dexrazoxane have been conducted in children with encouraging evidence of short-term cardioprotection (Wexler 1998); however, the long-term avoidance of cardiotoxicity with the use of this agent is yet to be sufficiently determined. A recent systematic review of published data found some limited evidence of the effectiveness of cardioprotectants (Bryant et al. 2007). Dexrazoxane (Lipshultz et al. 2004) and coenzyme Q10 (Iarussi et al. 1994) were both reported to protect cardiac function during anthracycline therapy. In fact, dexrazoxane was reported to have prevented or reduced cardiac injury, as reflected by less elevation of troponin T levels during doxorubicin treatment, without compromising the antileukemic efficacy of the doxorubicin. However, longer follow-up is needed to determine the influence of dexrazoxane on cardiac function.

9.3.1 Recommended Screening and Follow-Up

Patients exposed to anthracyclines need ongoing monitoring for late-onset cardiomyopathy using physical examination and serial noninvasive testing (echocardiogram, electrocardiogram) (Shankar et al. 2008). The frequency of echocardiograms can range from yearly to every 5 years, depending on cumulative anthracycline dose, age at exposure, and treatment with mediastinal radiation. Aerobic exercise is generally safe and should be encouraged for most patients. However, intensive isometric activities (e.g., heavy weight lifting, wrestling) should be avoided. Pregnant women previously treated with anthracyclines should be closely monitored, as changes in volume during the third trimester could add significant stress to a potentially compromised myocardium (van Dalen et al. 2006). Specific recommendations for monitoring, based on age and therapeutic exposure, are delineated within the Children's Oncology Group (COG) *Long-Term Follow-Up Guidelines* available at www.survivorshipguidelines.org.

9.4 NeurocognitiveEf fects

Treatment for any childhood cancer can result in damaging effects on the central nervous system (CNS). Survivors of ALL may experience decline in intellectual function, learning problems, behavior disorders, school failure, and impaired employability. Though neurocognitive effects were originally described for children who underwent cranial radiation, subsequent studies have suggested that children treated with chemotherapy alone may also be at risk for neurobehavioral deficits, although of a less severe nature.

9.4.1 Radiation

The use of either prophylactic or therapeutic cranial radiation has been clearly associated with late neurocognitive impairment in children with ALL. Although the mechanism is not entirely clear, radiation therapy can impair short-term memory, visual spatial ability, somatosensory functioning, and executive function, all of which can manifest as intellectual impairment (Meadows et al. 1981; Cousens et al. 1988; Mulhern et al. 1988; Stehbens et al. 1991; Brown and Madan-Swain 1993). These deficits are often not apparent during the treatment period, but manifest years later when children are referred for special education services (Rubenstein et al. 1990; Mulhern et al. 1991; Jankovic et al. 1994a, b). Children treated with radiotherapy at younger ages are particularly at risk (Robison et al. 1984; Cousens et al. 1988), as are females (Bleyer et al. 1990; Waber et al. 1990). Radiation dose is a strong predictor of neurocognitive deficits, with cranial radiation doses equal to or exceeding 2,400 centigray (cGy) resulting in greater impairment(Fus se ta l. 2000).

9.4.2 Chemotherapy

Recognition of the neurocognitive late-effects of radiation has made the need for effective chemotherapy in ALL even more important. Currently, most children with ALL do not receive radiation therapy and new research suggests that the population of children requiring radiation may continue to decrease over time (Pui et al. 2009). Radiation has been supplanted by the use of intrathecal (IT) chemotherapy accompanied by higher doses of systemic chemotherapy, which have given rise to new concerns in the ALL survivor population.

Methotrexate has been the mainstay of ALL therapy for many years and while effective, has clear acute and chronic risks associated with its use. Acute neurotoxic events have been shown to occur significantly more often among those children who received intravenous methotrexate in addition to IT methotrexate during Consolidation therapy (Mahoney et al. 1998). The presenting acute event was most commonly seizures, which occurred in approximately 80% of patients with acute neurotoxicity. Other observed acute neurotoxicities included paresthesias, weakness, headaches, aphasia, ataxia, dysarthria, arachnoiditis, and choreoathetosis. Computed tomography and magnetic resonance imaging (MRI) findings among those children with acute neurotoxicity were most commonly white matter changes characterized as hypodense areas with or without microangiopathic calcifications. Overall, approximately 10% of children in this trial who were treated with combined intermediate dose systemic methotrexate and IT methotrexate developed neurotoxicity. Ongoing follow-up of this group is continuing. Children treated with IT methotrexate in the absence of systemic methotrexate have shown less acute toxicity. In a large investigation conducted by the Childhood Cancer Survivor Study (CCSS), 4,151 5+ year survivors of ALL who had not been irradiated and had never experienced a relapse of ALL reported no more chronic neurologic conditions than a sibling control group (Mody et al. 2008).

Concern has been expressed about the long-term neurocognitive effects of glucocorticoid exposure in children with ALL. Glucocorticoids may result in CNS toxicity as evidenced by both animal experiments and clinical observation. Rat studies demonstrate that glucocorticoids disrupt the energy metabolism of neurons in the hippocampus, an important organ for memory processing, rendering them more vulnerable to toxic insults (Sapolsky 1993). This finding is worrisome in the childhood cancer population because these patients are given steroids concurrently with other toxic agents (Waber et al. 2000). Because of recent data suggesting that dexamethasone is less likely than prednisone to result in CNS relapse, increased scrutiny has been given to survivor populations exposed to either dexamethasone or prednisone as their primary glucocorticoid therapy. In a sequential study, children who were treated with dexamethasone were noted to have poorer neurocognitive outcomes than children treated with prednisone (Waber et al. 2000). More recently, the COG has investigated neurocognitive outcomes among children randomized to either dexamethasone or prednisone on a therapeutic trial. In that study, almost 100 patients were evaluated with a standard neurocognitive battery, and no group differences were found in the distribution of neurocognitive or academic performance after adjustment for age, gender, and time from diagnosis (Kadan-Lottick et al. 2009).

Children who experience a neurocognitive late-effect often present with limitations in age-appropriate activities of daily living, including school performance, independent living, and some domains of quality of life (QOL) (Mulhern and Palmer 2003). Global declines in IQ and performance, characteristic of many children who have received CNS-directed therapy, are secondary effects resulting from "core" changes in a child's ability to attend to and process new information. This difficulty with information acquisition underlies the challenges these children face, and explains why, without proactive investigation, these effects may not become evident for years.

Interventions to improve cognitive performance are receiving increased attention. Cognitive rehabilitation is an intervention "intended to restore lost cognitive functions or to teach the patient skills to compensate for cognitive losses that cannot be restored" (Mulhern and Palmer 2003). Butler and colleagues have developed an outpatient rehabilitation program targeted at disorders of attention and associated processes (Butler and Copeland 2002). Stimulant medications, such as methylphenidate hydrochloride may also be effective for ALL survivors with neurocognitive sequelae and have shown benefit in early research (Daly and Brown 2007;B utlere ta l. 2008).

9.4.3 Recommended Screening and Follow-Up

All physicians engaged in the care of ALL survivors should be aware of the possible neurocognitive complications of the patient's prior therapy. Health providers should monitor the patient at clinic visits with a history that includes questions, tailored to the age of the patient, about developmental milestones, school performance, peer relations, need for special education services, and neurological abnormalities (e.g., weakness, seizures). More detailed questions should assess domains of neurocognitive functioning that tend to be impaired specifically in ALL survivors, such as executive functioning. As deficits in neurocognitive functioning often do not present until several years after treatment and can be subtle and/or subclinical, presymptomatic neuropsychological assessment should be strongly considered. The timing of this assessment depends on the individual patient, but may be particularly helpful at school reentry to facilitate transition.

9.5 Endocrine Late-Effects

Survivors of all childhood cancers, and in particular childhood ALL, have long been recognized to be at risk for endocrine late-effects. These endocrine late-effects can be subtle or overt and may have substantial impact on a survivor's health and quality of life. There is no aspect of the endocrine system that cannot be affected by ALL therapy. Impairment of growth, thyroid function, gonadal function, bone mineralization, and pancreatic and adrenal function have all been described in survivors of childhood ALL (Hameed and Zacharin 2005; Pizzo and Poplack 2006; Geenen et al. 2007; Mody et al. 2008; Nandagopal et al. 2008; Steffens et al. 2008). Importantly, many of these late-effects are predictable by prior therapy and amenable to medical intervention.

9.5.1 Growth

Impairment of growth is one of the major late-effects of childhood ALL therapy (Sklar et al. 1993; Huma et al. 1995; Sklar 1995; Chemaitilly et al. 2007). Cranial radiation can have a significant impact on growth and may lead to final height reductions of 5–10 cm in children treated with 2,400 cGy of radiation (Robison et al. 1985; Schriock et al. 1991). Reductions in final height are less severe among children treated with 1,800 cGy or no radiation at all (Sklar et al. 1993; Chow et al. 2007a, b). In a recent investigation in the CCSS, self-reported adult height was compared between 2,434 ALL survivors and 3,009 sibling controls. The risk for adult short stature (defined as a high standard deviation score of ≥2) was up to 3.4-fold greater among the ALL survivors (Chow et al. 2007a, b). Among survivors treated with greater than 2,000 cGy of cranial radiation, females and those diagnosed at an early age were at greatest risk of adult short stature. Radiation received in the course of hematopoietic cell transplantation has also been associated with a reduction in adult height (Chemaitilly et al. 2007). Radiation of the spine in the course of ALL therapy may reduce adult height through impairment of spinal growth as well as the inability of the irradiated spine to respond to growth hormone therapy (Brownstein et al. 2004). Furthermore, thyroid dysfunction and the early onset of puberty observed in girls treated for ALL with cranial radiation may also reduce final height (Groot-Loonen et al. 1996; Chow et al. 2008).

Treatment of children with recognized growth hormone deficiency is effective in improving adult height. Therefore, early recognition of growth hormone deficiency and the correction of other endocrinopathies are important in obtaining maximal response (Brown-stein et al. 2004). A small, but statistically significant, increase in the risk of secondary cancers has been reported from the CCSS in association with growth hormone therapy and therefore must be considered in the decision to start growth hormone therapy (Ergun-Longmire eta l. 2006).

9.5.2 Thyroid Function

Both hyper- and hypothyroidism have been reported among survivors of childhood ALL and have clearly been associated with the use of radiation as part of cranial prophylaxis or hematopoietic cell transplantation (Steffens et al. 2008; Chow et al. 2009). The risk of hypothyroidism following ALL therapy increases with increasing dose of radiation to the thyroid region. The risk appears to be greater among women than men, but is clearly elevated in both groups. The onset of thyroid dysfunction may be several years after treatment of childhood leukemia and lifelong surveillance is important (Pasqualini et al. 1991; Mohn et al. 1997; Chow eta l. 2009).

9.5.3 Gonadal Function

The majority of male and female long-term survivors of childhood ALL who were treated without radiotherapy will have normal gonadal function and reproductive outcomes (Byrne et al. 2004; Green et al. 2009). However, there are specific, predictable late-effects that are therapy-specific and unique for males and females.

In men, germ cell damage is much more common in response to gonadotoxic therapeutic exposure than Leydig cell damage, and as a result, men may have reduced fertility without any overt evidence of testicular damage. Exposure of the testes to radiation doses as low as 400–600 cGy may result in permanent azoospermia (Pizzo and Poplack 2006; Sarafoglou et al. 1997). ALL survivors who were treated with high doses of alkylating agents may also be at risk for germ cell damage, in particular, those survivors treated with high doses of cyclophosphamide. In contrast, Leydig cell function is generally very well preserved in leukemia survivors, although careful monitoring of Leydig cell function in boys following testicular radiation is strongly recommended (Sklar 1999). Radiotherapy doses in excess of 30 Gy are known to induce Leydig cell failure.

In contrast, loss of germ cell function in women usually accompanies loss of hormone production. Women who are exposed to pelvic radiation are recognized to be at increased risk, as are women who are exposed to high doses of alkylating agents. Premature menopause has also been recognized as a risk of childhood cancer therapy; however, most patients successfully treated for ALL are not exposed to the high doses of radiation and/or alkylating agents associated with the greatest risk of these events (Byrne 1999; Sklar 2005;Skla re ta l. 2006;G reene ta l. 2009).

9.5.4 Obesity/Metabolic Syndrome

As survivors of childhood ALL age, they will experience the same health risks as the general American population. Among these risks, cardiovascular disease is of great concern because of the unique health history of this population early in life. As many of the risk factors for cardiovascular disease are modifiable, attention has been focused to determine the prevalence of cardiovascular disease risk factors among the ALL survivors.

Obesity has been increasingly recognized as a late complication of therapy among childhood ALL survivors (Oeffinger et al. 2003; Chow et al. 2007a, b; Asner et al. 2008; Miyoshi et al. 2008). Of particular concern is that the prevalence of obesity appears to rise with increasing time from completion of therapy. In a longitudinal study conducted by the CCSS, changes in body mass index from baseline enrollment into the CCSS to a second time point (a mean of 7.8 years later) were analyzed for 1,451 ALL survivors and 2,167 sibling controls. The body mass index of the ALL survivors who had been treated with cranial radiation therapy showed a significantly greater increase than the sibling control group. Younger age at the time of radiation therapy and female gender significantly increased the risk of obesity (Garmey et al. 2008). It is important to note that in this investigation the children who had not received cranial radiation had a weight gain similar to that of the control group; however, the association between obesity and cranial radiation has not been observed by all investigators (Razzouk et al. 2007).

The mechanisms underlying weight gain in ALL survivors are now being investigated. For example, specific polymorphisms of the leptin receptor gene were found to be associated with obesity in female survivors of childhood ALL exposed to cranial radiation (Ross et al. 2004). Other treatment-related factors may also increase the likelihood of obesity in ALL survivors, including impairments of strength and mobility (Ness et al. 2007) and neuropathy (van Brussel et al. 2006). Interventions to decrease obesity in ALL survivors are now underway and have predominantly focused on the initiation of exercise during therapy (Arroyave et al. 2008; Moyer-Mileur et al. 2009).

Metabolic syndrome is a clinical entity characterized by abdominal obesity, elevated plasma glucose, dyslipidemia, hypertension, and a prothrombotic and proinflammatory state (Grundy et al. 2005). In the general population, metabolic syndrome is an important risk factor for later onset of diabetes and cardiovascular disease (Grundy et al. 2005). Central to metabolic syndrome is the occurrence of insulin resistance. Accumulating evidence suggests that children treated for ALL may have a greater risk of developing metabolic syndrome than the general population. A small case-control study showed that 16% of the childhood cancer survivors had evidence of obesity, hyperinsulinemia, and low HDL cholesterol, as compared to none of the controls (Talvensaari et al. 1996). Other investigators have noted similar findings. Sixty percent of ALL survivors who had been treated with cranial radiation had two or more components of the metabolic syndrome, as compared to 20% of those not treated with cranial radiation (Gurney et al. 2006). Increased levels of insulin resistance have also been reported in a recent cross-sectional study of 118 survivors of childhood ALL. Female ALL survivors, especially those who had been treated with cranial radiation, were at greatest risk (Oeffinger 2008).

In addition, untreated growth hormone deficiency was observed in 85% of ALL survivors who had received prior cranial radiation; these patients, particularly the females, also tended to have higher fasting insulin, abdominal obesity, and dyslipidemia (Gurney et al. 2006). Untreated growth hormone deficiency is a frequent finding among those children previously irradiated. Treatment with growth hormone has been shown to reduce the prevalence of metabolic syndrome in growth hormone-deficient survivors of childhood ALL(F olline ta l. 2006).

9.6 BoneHeal th

While children are undergoing treatment for ALL and immediately afterward, some may experience bone pain, gait changes, or fractures in addition to the better-known complication of osteonecrosis (ON). These changes have been linked to alterations in the metabolism of vitamin D, magnesium, and calcium; this altered metabolism leads to altered bone turnover and weakened bone (Atkinson et al. 1989). Further research by the same investigators found that symptoms of bone pain were common (36% at initial presentation) and linked to a longer presentation period before the ALL was diagnosed. They found that most of the children with ALL already had alterations in bone mass and bone metabolism when they were diagnosed with ALL, suggesting that the defective mineralization and decreased bone mass are a result of the leukemic process as opposed to the chemotherapy (Halton et al. 1995). Other investigators have detailed significant bony alterations that occur while on therapy and lead to ongoing sequelae posttherapy (Strauss et al. 2001). The 5-year cumulative incidence of fractures and ON in patients treated for ALL has been reported to be 30% overall and as high as 51% in patients older than 9 years of age at diagnosis. Patients exposed to dexamethasone have been noted to have a higher rate of bone morbidity than those treated with prednisone.

ON has become increasingly prominent as a major long-term complication of ALL treatment. It is associated with progressive joint damage, pain, arthritis, and eventual joint replacement in some cases. With the increased use of dexamethasone in the newer generation of treatment protocols, the incidence has increased and the age of onset has decreased. The Children's Cancer Group (CCG) published a retrospective analysis of ON from the CCG-1882 study for high-risk ALL (Mattano et al. 2000). In the 1,409 children with ALL, the overall risk of ON was 9.3%. The incidence was 0.9% in patients less than 10 years, 13.5% in 10–15-year olds, and 18% in 16–20-year olds. Females were at higher risk than males. The patients with ON tended to be older at diagnosis than those without ON. Patients treated with two delayed intensifications (DI) (with two 21-day courses of continuous dexamethasone) as part of augmented therapy for slow response were more likely to develop ON. The predominant joints affected included hips and knees (24% and 31%, respectively).

A subsequent COG study found the incidence of ON to be 10.8% in patients who received a single DI that included a continuous 21-day course of dexamethasone and 5.5% in patients who received two DIs with discontinuous dexamethasone (alternate weeks of therapy) in each of the two cycles. In the highest-risk patients (10–20-year olds), the incidence of ON among patients who received continuous dexamethasone was 13.4%, while it was 7.5% among those exposed to discontinuous dexamethasone (Seibel et al. 2008; Reaman 2009).

Other international groups have reported only a modest increase in the risk of ON among patients treated for ALL. Arico et al. reported the overall incidence of ON to be 1.1% in patients treated with a BFM-type intensive chemotherapy; yet, when patients from the 10–17 year age-group were evaluated, the incidence was 7.4%. Females over the age of 10 were at particularly high risk (Arico et al. 2003). The ALL-BFM-95 trial had an overall incidence of ON of 1.8%. Patients over 10 years of age had an 8.9% rate and patients over 15 had a rate of 16.7% (Burger et al. 2005).

Relling and colleagues utilized a candidate gene approach to examine genetic risk factors for ON in children with ALL (Van Veldhuizen et al. 1993). They identified polymorphisms in genes *TYMS* and *VDR* that were associated with an increased risk of ON; both of these genes are associated with the pharmacodynamics of methotrexate and prednisone, commonly used to treat ALL. A recent study found plasminogen activator inhibitor (*PAI 1*) gene polymorphism to be associated with ON in patients previously treated for ALL. PAI-1 serum levels have been associated with thrombosis, and a thrombotic etiology has been implicated in the pathogenesis of ON (Relling et al. 2004). This study reinforces the premise that genetic factors contribute to sequelae of treatment for malignancies (Frenche ta l. 2008).

The 20-year incidence of ON is significantly higher among all cancer survivors, approaching 0.43% compared to 0.03% for siblings. Furthermore, the incidence of ON is higher among those diagnosed with ALL after 16 years of age (2.8%), as compared with those diagnosed at a younger age (0.2%). Other risk factors include exposure to dexamethasone and radiation therapy(K adan-Lotticke ta l. 2008).

The outcome of patients with ON depends on the severity of functional compromise and pain, as well as the joints involved. Due to the young age of the patients and the potential for bone growth, these patients should be evaluated by orthopedists to determine the best plan of care (Marchese et al. 2008). Surgical intervention such as core decompression, bone grafting, and joint replacement have been utilized to decrease pain and improve mobility (Werner et al. 2003; Karimova et al. 2007).

9.7 Hepatotoxicity

While abnormalities of liver function are common among patients actively receiving ALL therapy, chronic liver disease as a result of therapy is rare. Routine donor screening for hepatitis C virus (HCV) began in 1993; therefore, patients who were treated for childhood cancer prior to donor screening for HCV are at a higher risk of having acquired HCV from the blood product transfusions they received. The prevalence of HCV infection in this population approaches ~10% (Fioredda et al. 2005). Patients treated before blood products were routinely screened for HCV are also more likely to have issues with chronic liver sequelae such as cirrhosis, hepatic failure, and hepatocellular carcinoma(B hatia 2003).

Characteristically, patients on Maintenance regimens including 6-mercaptopurine (6MP) and methotrexate experience transient fluctuations in transaminases and bilirubin, which is more exaggerated among patients with a deficiency of thiopurine *S*-methyltransferase (TPMT) enzyme activity (Relling eta l. 1999a, b).

More recently, with the attempt to replace 6-mercaptopurine (6MP) with 6-thioguanine (6TG) in two large trials in the United States and the UK, a new disease process was observed. Patients who were on the 6TG arm developed portal hypertension, thrombocytopenia, and splenomegaly (Broxson et al. 2005; Lennard et al. 2006). Microscopically, the patients had occlusive venopathy and nodular regenerative hyperplasia (De Bruyne et al. 2006). While it resolved with cessation of the drug in some patients, in others, it became a progressive condition now identified as hepatic sinusoidal obstruction syndrome (SOS) (Murri et al. 2004). Additional complications have occurred during the natural history of SOS, including esophageal varices with associated bleeding. Physical symptoms related to this toxicity have developed months to years after exposure and indicate that patients who were treated on these regimens will require screening even off therapy (Reaman 2009), reinforcing the need for close follow-up of patients who received 6TG.

Recent studies have determined that using escalating dose methotrexate for Interim Maintenance increases EFS (Matloub et al. 2008). However, patients with decreased methylenetetrahydrofolate reductase (MTHFR) activity have been noted to be at risk for increased methotrexate toxicity; in addition, *MTHFR C677T* polymorphism has been linked to liver toxicity. Chronic conditions have not been reported to date, but screening of patients for this mutation and other gene polymorphisms, including glutathione S-transferase genes, could predict hepatic toxicity during therapy (Chiusolo et al. 2002; Imanishi et al. 2007).

Screening guidelines in patients who have received 6MP, 6TG, or methotrexate should include a yearly physical exam with transaminases and bilirubin screening. For patients with complications from 6TG, more extensive initial evaluations with abdominal ultrasound, MRI, and liver biopsy may be indicated. In patients with portal hypertension, screening for esophageal varices should be considered after consultation with a gastroenterologist. Persistence of liver function abnormalities may warrant further evaluation for infectious causes of hepatic dysfunction, especially in patients treated before 1993.

9.8 SecondMa lignantN eoplasms

Second malignant neoplasms (SMNs) are defined as histologically distinct neoplasms that develop 2 or more months after the diagnosis of the primary cancer. For survivors of childhood ALL, the risk of SMNs is modest at best. The estimated actuarial risk of developing an SMN has been reported at 2.5% (Neglia et al. 1991) and 3.3% at 15 years (Loning et al. 2000) and, among those treated with contemporary, risk-based therapy, the risk is lower at 1.2% at 10 years (Fig. 9.3) (Bhatia et al. 2002). This represents a sevenfold to 14-fold increased risk compared with an age and sex-matched general population. Hijiya et al. described the cumulative incidence of SMNs in children treated for ALL who were followed for over 30 years; they found the cumulative incidence to be 4.2% at 15 years and 10.9% at 30 years, representing a 13.5-fold increased risk compared with the general population (Hijiya et al. 2007). A second cohort with extended follow-up demonstrated the cumulative incidence to be 5.3% at 25 years, and the excess risk to be fivefold when compared with the general population (Mody et al. 2008).

Variables associated with an increased risk of SMNs include female sex (relative risk [RR] = 1.8), radiation to the craniospinal axis (RR = 1.6), and relapse of primary disease (RR = 3.5) (Bhatia et al. 2002). Unique associations with specific therapeutic exposures have resulted in the classification of SMNs into two distinct groups: (1) chemotherapy-related myelodysplasia and acute myeloid leukemia (t-MDS/AML); and (2) radiation-related solid SMNs. Characteristics of t-MDS/AML include a short latency (<3 years from primary cancer diagnosis) and association with alkylating agents and topoisomerase II inhibitors. Solid SMNs have a strong and well-defined association with radiation, and are characterized by a latency that exceeds 10 years.

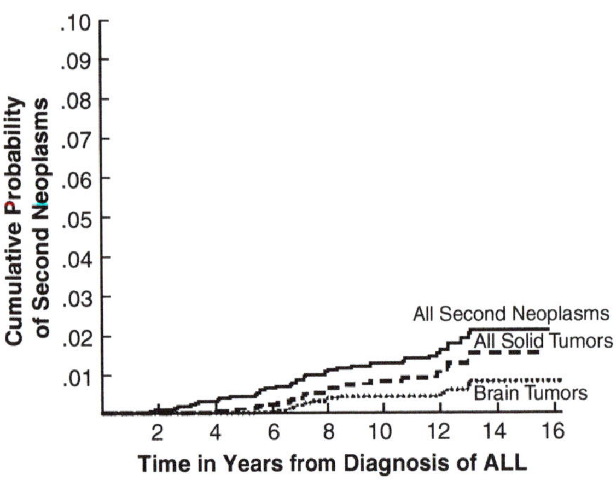

Fig. 9.3 Cumulative risk of second malignant neoplasms in children treated for acute lymphoblastic leukemia on legacy Children'sO ncologyG rouppr otocols(Bhatiae ta l. 2002)

9.8.1 Therapy-Related Myelodysplasia and Acute Myeloid Leukemia

t-MDS/AML is a clonal disorder characterized by distinct chromosomal changes (Smith et al. 2003; Schoch et al. 2004; Pedersen-Bjergaard et al. 2006). Two types are recognized by the WHO classification: alkylating agent-related type, and topoisomerase II inhibitor-related type (Vardiman et al. 2002).

9.8.1.1 AlkylatingA gent-Relatedt -MDS/AML

Mutagenicity is related to the ability of alkylating agents to form crosslinks and/or transfer alkyl groups to form DNA monoadducts. Alkylation results in inaccurate base pairing during replication and single and double-strand breaks in the double helix as the alkylated bases are repaired. The risk of alkylating agent-related t-MDS/AML is dose-dependent, and has a latency of 3–5 years after exposure; it is associated with abnormalities involving chromosomes 5 (−5/del[5q]) and 7 (−7/del[7q]) (Michels et al. 1985; Karp and Sarkodee-Adoo 2000).

9.8.1.2 Topoisomerasel II nhibitor-Related t-MDS/AML

Topoisomerase II catalyzes the relaxation of supercoiled DNA by covalently binding and transiently cleaving and religating both strands of the DNA helix. DNA topoisomerase II inhibitors stabilize the enzyme-DNA covalent intermediate, decrease the religation rate, and cause chromosomal breakage. These events initiate apoptosis, required for antineoplastic activity.

Occasionally, repair of chromosomal damage results in chromosomal translocations, leading to leukemogenesis. Most of the translocations disrupt a breakpoint cluster region between exons 5 and 11 of the band 11q23 and fuse mixed lineage leukemia (MLL) with a partner gene (Bower et al. 1994; Felix et al. 1995; Broeker et al. 1996). Topoisomerase II inhibitor-related t-AML presents as overt leukemia after a latency of 6 months to 3 years; it is associated with balanced translocations involving chromosome bands 11q23 or 21q22.

Epipodophyllotoxins have also been associated with the development of t-AML. Pui et al. (1989) reported the risk of epipodophyllotoxin-related t-AML in patients with ALL to be 3.8% at 6 years. They also demonstrated that the risk depends largely on the schedule of drug administration. This risk is significantly higher than that reported by others, in part because epipodophyllotoxins were not used in the therapeutic protocols used to treat the other cohorts.

Among childhood ALL survivors, t-MDS/AML occurs after a relatively short latency. The vast majority of events occur within the first 10 years, with a plateau thereafter, and the magnitude of long-term risk is usually less than 0.5% (Bhatia et al. 2002).

9.8.2 Therapy-Related Solid Second Malignancies

Therapy-related solid second malignancies demonstrate a strong relation with ionizing radiation. The risk of solid second malignancies is highest when the exposure occurs at a younger age, increases with the total dose of radiation, and with time after radiation (Neglia et al. 2001). Radiation-related solid SMNs account for the largest burden of second malignancies (~80%). Some of the well-established radiation-related solid SMNs include thyroid cancer, brain tumors, sarcomas, and basal cell carcinomas.

9.8.2.1 Second Brain Tumors

An increased risk of brain tumors has been observed among long-term survivors of childhood ALL (Neglia et al. 1991; Kimball Dalton et al. 1998; Jenkinson and Hawkins 1999; Loning et al. 2000; Bhatia et al. 2002). The cumulative incidence of brain tumors approaches 0.5% at 10 years from diagnosis of ALL (Bhatia et al. 2002). Brain tumors are more likely to develop among patients who have received radiation, and the risk increases with radiation dose (Neglia et al. 1991; Loning et al. 2000; Bhatia et al. 2002). An increased risk of brain tumors has been reported among those younger than 5 years of age at radiation (Neglia et al. 1991; Loning et al. 2000). Two primary histologic types of second brain tumors have been identified. These include slow growing meningiomas and more rapidly growing gliomas. While the meningiomas generally respond to surgical resection, gliomas have a significantly worse outcome, with the need for multimodality therapy.

An unusually high incidence of second brain tumors was reported among children treated on a therapeutic protocol at St. Jude Children's Research Hospital (Relling et al. 1999a, b). The St. Jude protocol differed from previous protocols in that more intensive systemic antimetabolite therapy was given before and during radiation therapy. An assessment of clinical, biologic, and pharmacokinetic features revealed higher erythrocyte concentrations of thioguanine nucleotide metabolites and a higher proportion of defective thiopurine methyl transferase phenotype among patients with brain tumors compared with those without brain tumors, indicating that underlying genetic characteristics and treatment variables may have contributed to the excess of brain tumors in this population.

9.8.2.2 Second Thyroid Cancers

When second thyroid cancer occurs, it usually develops 10–15 years after treatment and is associated with an excellent long-term outcome (Bhatia et al. 2002). The risk of developing second thyroid cancer is highest in younger children, and it is associated with craniospinal radiation in a dose-dependent fashion. The two most common types of radiation-related thyroid cancer include papillary cancer and follicular cancer. Papillary cancer is more common and has a better outcome.

9.8.2.3 Soft Tissue Sarcomas

ALL survivors have also been observed to be at an increased risk of soft tissue sarcoma, with the survivors cohort reported to be at a ninefold increased risk when compared with the general population. The risk of soft tissue sarcomas has not been correlated with therapeutic exposures.

Li–Fraumeni syndrome is a familial syndrome in which patients have an exceptionally high risk of developing multiple primary cancers. Brain tumors, sarcomas, and leukemias are all characteristic cancers in the familial Li–Fraumeni syndrome. The excess risk of additional primary cancers is mainly for cancers that are characteristic of Li–Fraumeni syndrome, with the highest risk observed for survivors of childhood cancer (Hisada et al. 1998). Therefore, cancer survivors in these families need to be monitored closely, especially for the development of SMNs.

9.8.3 Pathogenesis of Second Malignancies

Carcinogenesis is a multistep process in which somatic cells acquire a series of stable genetic mutations in a specific clonal lineage. Finette et al. (2000) tested the hypotheses that genetic instability develops early to produce an increased rate of mutations in a distant clone, and that multiple mutations simply accumulate as a consequence of extensive clonal proliferation. They postulated that genetic instability likely involves cellular changes that affect the expression and/or function of cell cycle, cell death, and DNA repair pathways.

Since SMNs remain a significant threat to the health of ALL survivors, vigilant screening is important for those at risk. Because t-MDS/AML usually manifests within 10 years following exposure, monitoring with an annual complete blood count for 10 years after exposure to alkylating agents or topoisomerase II inhibitors is recommended. Most other second cancers are associated with radiation exposure. Screening recommendations include careful annual physical examination of the skin and underlying tissues in the radiation field with radiographic or other cancer screening evaluationsa sindic ated.

9.9 LateMo rtality

Survivors of ALL are at risk for late-effects that can result in premature death, although the incidence of these deaths is decreasing. The CCSS followed a cohort of 5,760 children with ALL who had survived at least 5 years after diagnosis (Mody et al. 2008). Cumulative mortality was 13% at 25 years from diagnosis, with recurrent ALL and second malignancies being the major causes of death. Overall survival was 96.1% at 25 years for survivors treated without radiation therapy and 87.3% for survivors treated with radiation. Twenty-year survival improved from 82% for patients treated in 1970–1974 to 90% for those treated in 1980–1986. Overall survival for nonirradiated, nonrelapsed survivors was 97.8%.

Pui et al. described the long-term survival of 10-year survivors treated on St. Jude Children's Research Hospital therapeutic protocols. The death rate for the irradiated group slightly exceeded the expected rate in the general US population (standardized mortality ratio [SMR] = 1.9), whereas that for the nonirradiated group did not differ from the population norm (SMR = 1.75) (Pui et al. 2003). Continued observation is needed to define lifetime cause-specific risk, and to determine modifiable causes of premature deaths, so that targeted interventions can be developed.

9.10 Qualityo fL ife

With 5-year survival estimates for children with ALL approaching 85%, health-related quality of life (HRQOL) in the survivors has become a focus of many studies (te Winkel et al. 2008). When ALL patients in Maintenance therapy were tested, results detailed that these children had decreased physical, social, and emotional health compared to controls. Parental reports in this study indicated that they felt their child's physical deficiencies affected their overall health (Waters eta l. 2003).

While preadolescent ALL survivors do not appear to have quality of life (QOL) concerns when compared with healthy comparison groups, adolescent survivors, in particular females, are at an increased risk for reporting compromised QOL in many domains, such as physical functioning, cognitive functioning, and intimate relations (Wu et al. 2007).

Fatigue is prevalent in ALL patients, with incidence rates approaching 30%. Factors that have been associated with fatigue are female gender, Hispanic ethnicity, unemployment, and disease recurrence. Further analyses have linked fatigue to having children, sleep disorders, pain, obesity, cognitive problems, and exercise-induced symptoms. The lowest QOL scores were noted in patients who were fatigued or depressed (Meeske et al. 2005). The CCSS explored the issues of fatigue, sleep disturbance (Mulrooney et al. 2008), social outcomes (Gurney et al. 2009), and psychological status (Zeltzer et al. 2009). They noted that adolescent leukemia survivors have a higher rate of depression and anxiety than the general population, and leukemia patients on more aggressive therapy are also at increased risk of somatization. The incidence of fatigue in this survivor cohort was 15% (Mulrooney et al. 2008). These reports emphasize the importance of fatigue, an often overlooked symptom, as a significant predictor of poor QOL and indicate the importance of screening for fatigue and depression in ALL survivors.

9.10.1 Challenges with Delivering Survivorship Care

Providing age and developmental-stage appropriate healthcare to ALL survivors is emerging as a significant challenge in medicine. ALL survivors seek and receive care from a wide variety of healthcare professionals, including oncologists, specialists, surgeons, primary care physicians, gynecologists, nurses, psychologists, and social workers. The Institute of Medicine has recognized the need for a systematic plan for lifelong surveillance that incorporates risks based on therapeutic exposures, genetic predisposition, health-related behaviors, and comorbid health conditions (Hewitte ta l. 2003).

Optimal healthcare delivery to this unique population requires the establishment of necessary infrastructure including several key components: (1) longitudinal care utilizing a comprehensive multidisciplinary team approach, (2) continuity, with a single healthcare provider coordinating needed services, and (3) an emphasis on the whole person, with sensitivity to the cancer experience and its impact on the entire family. The COG has developed a resource guide to assist institutions in establishing and enhancing long-term follow-up programs and services for survivors. The Long-Term Follow-Up Program Resource Guide offers a broad perspective from a variety of long-term follow-up programs within the COG and can be downloaded from www.survivorshpguidelines.org.

Although the number of ALL survivors is rapidly increasing, healthcare professionals outside academic centers are likely to see only a small number in their practice, and due to the heterogeneity of treatments received, there will likely be little similarity in their required follow-up care. It is thus predictable that primary care physicians are generally unfamiliar with the health risks of childhood ALL survivors. There is a veritable absence of information regarding this population in the primary care-based literature. This is driven in part by the fact that adult survivors of childhood ALL represent a small fraction of a primary care physician's practice.

Regardless of the setting for follow-up, the first step in any evaluation is to have at hand an outline of the patient's medical history, including a treatment summary. Once completed, the treatment summary allows the survivor or their healthcare provider to interface with the COG *Long-Term Follow-Up Guidelines* to determine recommended follow-up care (Table 9.2). Before the long-term survivor graduates from a pediatric oncologist's care, this treatment record and possible long-term problems should be reviewed with the family and, in the case of adolescents or young adults, with the patient. Correspondence between the pediatric oncologist and subsequent caretakers should address the same issues.

9.11 CancerSur vivorship:Fut ure Research Opportunities

The growing survivor population provides remarkable opportunities for research relating to the etiopathogenesis of cancer and to early detection and prevention of adverse outcomes. Studying outcomes in ALL survivors is facilitated by detailed knowledge of the therapeutic exposures, coupled with close follow-up after these exposures; this enables researchers to study testable hypotheses and determine the effects of host and therapy-related factors in the development of adverse outcomes ranging from carcinogenesis and organ dysfunction to psychosocial consequences. Opportunities also exist to explore gene--environment interactions that may modify individual responses to treatment, as well as susceptibility to developing adverse outcomes, thus providing insights into the identification of high-risk populations.

Table9.2 Selected exposure-based screening recommendations[a]

Therapeutic exposure	Potential late effect	Recommended screening
Neurocognitive dysfunction		
Cranial radiation (including total body irradiation)	Neurocognitivede ficit	Baseline neuropsychological assessment, repeated as clinically indicated and at key educational transition points
Intrathecal methotrexate		Yearly assessment of vocational/educational progress
Intermediate/high-doseI V methotrexate or cytarabine		
Cardiac compromise		
Anthracycline chemotherapy	Cardiomyopathy	Yearly history and physical exam
	Subclinical left ventricular dysfunction	Baselinee lectrocardiogram
		Periodic echocardiogram as indicated based on dose and age at exposure
		Cardiac consultation as indicated for symptomatic patients, for patients with subclinical abnormalities on screening evaluations, and for patients who are pregnant or considering pregnancy who have received cumulative anthracycline doses of ≥300m g/m^2 or <300 mg/m^2i f combined, with radiation potentially impacting the heart
Endocrine dysfunction		
Radiation impacting thyroid	Hypothyroidism (primary or central)	Yearly history and physical exam
Radiation impacting hypothalamic-pituitary axis	Hyperthyroidism	Yearly thyroid function test (free T4, TSH)
	Growth hormone deficiency	8 am serum cortisol if radiation to HP axis ≥40 Gy – test yearly for at least 15 years
	Central adrenal insufficiency	
	Hyperprolactinemia	Prolactin level if positive history for galactorrhea, amenorrhea (females), or decreased libido (males)
Gonadal function		
Alkylating chemotherapy	Hypogonadism	Yearly history and physical exam including evaluation of secondary sexual characteristics and sexual function
Surgical removal of both gonads	Gonadal failure	
Radiationin volving gonads	Infertility	Baseline (females – age 13; males – age 14) assessment of gonadal function (LH, FSH, estradiol, or testosterone); repeat as clinically indicated in patients with delayed puberty or signs/symptoms of hormonal deficiency
	Prematurem enopause (females)	
		Additional evaluations as indicated (e.g., semen analysis)
Second cancers		
Etoposide	Acute myeloid leukemia	CBC, platelet, differential, yearly for 10 years following exposure
Anthracyclines		
Alkylating chemotherapy	Acute myeloid leukemia/ myelodysplasia	
Radiation	SMN in radiation field (skin, bone, soft tissue, thyroid)	Yearly history and physical exam with inspection and palpation of tissues in radiation field

[a]Screening recommendations adapted from the *Children's Oncology Group Long-Term Follow-Up Guidelines;* available at www.survivorshipguidelines.org

The growing population of ALL survivors carries a significant burden of morbidity, necessitating comprehensive long-term follow-up of these survivors. This follow-up should ideally begin at the completion of active therapy, with a documented summarization of therapeutic exposures that dictates following recommendations within the long-term follow-up guidelines, thus ensuring standardization of care received by the survivors. However, many barriers prevent effective follow-up, with the most fundamental barrier being the lack of knowledge regarding survivorship issues demonstrated by both the long-term survivors and the primary care physicians caring for them. Shortcomings of the healthcare system also pose potential barriers, and include logistical issues such as a lack of capacity within centers, training and educational deficiencies, and inadequate communication between pediatric oncologists and primary care physicians who provide the bulk of follow-up. Finally, a major obstacle faced by ALL survivors in the United States is the difficulty in obtaining affordable health insurance, which makes it impossible for some survivors to seek and obtain appropriate long-term care, even if they are aware and willing.

Attention also needs to be focused on development of interventional strategies, such as behavior modification, educational interventions, and chemoprevention. Execution of these intervention strategies in the setting of clinical trials would facilitate understanding of the impact of the specific interventions in early detection, with an overall reduction in morbidity and mortality and an ultimate improvement in the overall quality of life of ALL survivors.

Notwithstanding these unique opportunities, conduct of survivorship research faces several challenges. Survivorship research is an evolving issue. With more than 20% of ALL patients in need of better treatment options, new agents and combinations of agents are being developed. Targeted therapies such as imatinab mesylate and other growth factor inhibitors will likely contribute to increased survivorship. Evaluation of their late-effects will need to keep in step with their increased usage. Evidence-based research will need to be performed to determine whether they will live up to the expectation of a lower prevalence of side effects. Furthermore, the influence of genetic profiles on susceptibility to late-effects, as well as their interaction with lifestyle exposures such as tobacco, alcohol, and diet, is of growing interest and has not been fully explored. However, the biggest challenge in conducting sound survivorship research remains the multifactorial etiology of the adverse effects, which necessitates large sample sizes of well-characterized cohorts with complete long-term follow-up.

References

Arico M, Boccalatte MF et al (2003) Osteonecrosis: an emerging complication of intensive chemotherapy for childhood acute lymphoblastic leukemia. Haematologica 88(7): 747–753

Arroyave WD, Clipp EC et al (2008) Childhood cancer survivors' perceived barriers to improving exercise and dietary behaviors. Oncol Nurs Forum 35(1):121–130

Asner S, Ammann RA et al (2008) Obesity in long-term survivors of childhood acute lymphoblastic leukemia. Pediatr Blood Cancer 51(1):118–122

Atkinson SA, Fraher L et al (1989) Mineral homeostasis and bone mass in children treated for acute lymphoblastic leukemia. J Pediatr 114(5):793–800

Bhatia S (2003) Late effects among survivors of leukemia during childhood and adolescence. Blood Cells Mol Dis 31(1): 84–92

Bhatia S, Sather HN et al (2002) Low incidence of second neoplasms among children diagnosed with acute lymphoblastic leukemia after 1983. Blood 99:4257–4264

Bleyer WA, Fallavollita J et al (1990) Influence of age, sex, and concurrent intrathecal methotrexate therapy on intellectual function after cranial irradiation during childhood: a report from the Children's Cancer Study Group. Pediatr Hematol Oncol7(4):329–338

Bower M, Parry P et al (1994) Trithorax gene rearrangements in therapy-related acute leukemia after etoposide treatment. Leukemia8: 226–229

Brenner H, Kaatsch P et al (2001) Long-term survival of children with leukemia achieved by the end of the second millennium. Cancer 92(7):1977–1983

Broeker PLS, Super HG et al (1996) Distribution of 11q23 breakpoints within MLL breakpoint cluster region in *de novo* acute leukemia and therapy-related acute myeloid leukemia: correlation with scaffold attachment regions and topoisomerase II consensus binding sites. Blood 87:1912–1922

Brown RT, Madan-Swain A (1993) Cognitive, neuropsychological, and academic sequelae in children with leukemia. J Learn Disabil 26(2):74–90

Brownstein CM, Mertens AC et al (2004) Factors that affect final height and change in height standard deviation scores in survivors of childhood cancer treated with growth hormone: a report from the childhood cancer survivor study. J Clin Endocrinol Metab 89(9):4422–4427

Broxson EH, Dole M et al (2005) Portal hypertension develops in a subset of children with standard risk acute lymphoblastic leukemia treated with oral 6-thioguanine during maintenance therapy. Pediatr Blood Cancer 44(3):226–231

Bryant J, Picot J et al (2007) Clinical and cost-effectiveness of cardioprotection against the toxic effects of anthracyclines

given to children with cancer: a systematic review. Br J Cancer96(2):226–230
Burger B, Beier R et al (2005) Osteonecrosis: a treatment related toxicity in childhood acute lymphoblastic leukemia (ALL) – experiences from trial ALL-BFM 95. Pediatr Blood Cancer 44(3):220–225
Butler RW, Copeland DR (2002) Attentional processes and their remediation in children treated for cancer: a literature review and the development of a therapeutic approach. J Int Neuropsychol Soc 8(1):115–124
Butler RW, Sahler OJ et al (2008) Interventions to improve neuropsychological functioning in childhood cancer survivors. Dev Disabil Res Rev 14(3):251–258
Byrne J (1999) Infertility and premature menopause in childhood cancer survivors. Med Pediatr Oncol 33(1):24–28
Byrne J, Fears TR et al (2004) Fertility of long-term male survivors of acute lymphoblastic leukemia diagnosed during childhood. Pediatr Blood Cancer 42(4):364–372
Chemaitilly W, Boulad F et al (2007) Final height in pediatric patients after hyperfractionated total body irradiation and stem cell transplantation. Bone Marrow Transplant 40(1): 29–35
Chiusolo P, Reddiconto G et al (2002) Preponderance of methylenetetrahydrofolate reductase C677T homozygosity among leukemia patients intolerant to methotrexate. Ann Oncol 13(12):1915–1918
Chow EJ, Friedman DL et al (2007a) Decreased adult height in survivors of childhood acute lymphoblastic leukemia: a report from the Childhood Cancer Survivor Study. J Pediatr 150(4):370–375, 375 e371
Chow EJ, Pihoker C et al (2007b) Obesity and hypertension among children after treatment for acute lymphoblastic leukemia. Cancer 110(10):2313–2320
Chow EJ, Friedman DL et al (2008) Timing of menarche among survivors of childhood acute lymphoblastic leukemia: a report from the Childhood Cancer Survivor Study. Pediatr Blood Cancer 50(4):854–858
Chow EJ, Friedman DL et al (2009) Risk of thyroid dysfunction and subsequent thyroid cancer among survivors of acute lymphoblastic leukemia: a report from the Childhood Cancer Survivor Study. Pediatr Blood Cancer 53(3):432–437
Cousens P, Waters B et al (1988) Cognitive effects of cranial irradiation in leukaemia: a survey and meta-analysis. J Child Psychol Psychiatry 29(6):839–852
Daly BP, Brown RT (2007) Scholarly literature review: management of neurocognitive late effects with stimulant medication. J Pediatr Psychol 32(9):1111–1126
De Bruyne R, Portmann B et al (2006) Chronic liver disease related to 6-thioguanine in children with acute lymphoblastic leukaemia. J Hepatol 44(2):407–410
Ergun-Longmire B, Mertens AC et al (2006) Growth hormone treatment and risk of second neoplasms in the childhood cancer survivor. J Clin Endocrinol Metab 91(9): 3494–3498
Fajardo LF, Stewart JR et al (1968) Morphology of radiation-induced heart disease. Arch Pathol 86(5):512–519
Felix CA, Lange BJ et al (1995) Chromosome band 11q23 translocation breakpoints are DNA topoisomerase II cleavage sites. Cancer Res 55:4287–4292
Finette BA, Homans AC et al (2000) Emergence of genetic instability in children treated for leukemia. Science 288(5465): 514–517
Fioredda F, Gigliotti AR et al (2005) HCV infection in very-long-term survivors after cancer chemotherapy and bone marrow transplantation. a single-center experience. J Pediatr Hematol Oncol 27:481–485
Follin C, Thilen U et al (2006) Improvement in cardiac systolic function and reduced prevalence of metabolic syndrome after two years of growth hormone (GH) treatment in GH-deficient adult survivors of childhood-onset acute lymphoblastic leukemia. J Clin Endocrinol Metab 91(5): 1872–1875
French D, Hamilton LH et al (2008) A PAI-1 (SERPINE1) polymorphism predicts osteonecrosis in children with acute lymphoblastic leukemia: a report from the Children's Oncology Group. Blood 111(9):4496–4499
Fuss M, Poljanc K et al (2000) Full Scale IQ (FSIQ) changes in children treated with whole brain and partial brain irradiation. A review and analysis. Strahlenther Onkol 176(12): 573–581
Garmey EG, Liu Q et al (2008) Longitudinal changes in obesity and body mass index among adult survivors of childhood acute lymphoblastic leukemia: a report from the Childhood Cancer Survivor Study. J Clin Oncol 26(28): 4639–4645
Geenen MM, Cardous-Ubbink MC et al (2007) Medical assessment of adverse health outcomes in long-term survivors of childhood cancer. JAMA 297(24):2705–2715
Green DM, Sklar CA et al (2009) Ovarian failure and reproductive outcomes after childhood cancer treatment: results from the Childhood Cancer Survivor Study. J Clin Oncol 27(14): 2374–2381
Groot-Loonen JJ, van Setten P et al (1996) Shortened and diminished pubertal growth in boys and girls treated for acute lymphoblastic leukaemia. Acta Paediatr 85(9):1091–1095
Grundy SM, Cleeman JI et al (2005) Diagnosis and management of the metabolic syndrome: an American Heart Association/ National Heart, Lung, and Blood Institute Scientific Statement. Circulation 112(17):2735–2752
Gurney JG, Ness KK et al (2006) Metabolic syndrome and growth hormone deficiency in adult survivors of childhood acute lymphoblastic leukemia. Cancer 107(6):1303–1312
Gurney JG, Krull KR et al (2009) Social outcomes in the Childhood Cancer Survivor Study cohort. J Clin Oncol 27(14):2390–2395
Halton JM, Atkinson SA et al (1995) Mineral homeostasis and bone mass at diagnosis in children with acute lymphoblastic leukemia. J Pediatr 126(4):557–564
Hameed R, Zacharin MR (2005) Long-term endocrine effects of cancer treatment: experience of the Royal Children's Hospital, Melbourne. J Paediatr Child Health 41(1–2): 36–42
Hewitt M, Weiner SL et al (2003) Childhood cancer survivorship: improving care and quality of life: Institute of Medicine. The National Academy Press, Washington, DC
Hijiya N, Hudson MM et al (2007) Cumulative incidence of secondary neoplasms as a first event after childhood acute lymphoblastic leukemia. JAMA 297(11):1207–1215
Hisada M, Garber JE et al (1998) Multiple primary cancers in families with Li-Fraumeni syndrome. J Natl Cancer Inst 90(8):606–611
Horner MJ, Ries LAG et al (2009) SEER Cancer Statistics Review, 1975–2006, based on November 2008 SEER data submission. National Cancer Institute, Bethesda, MD

Huma Z, Boulad F et al (1995) Growth in children after bone marrow transplantation for acute leukemia. Blood 86(2): 819–824

Iarussi D, Auricchio U et al (1994) Protective effect of coenzyme Q10 on anthracyclines cardiotoxicity: control study in children with acute lymphoblastic leukemia and non-Hodgkin lymphoma. Mol Aspects Med 15(Suppl): s207–212

Imanishi H, Okamura N et al (2007) Genetic polymorphisms associated with adverse events and elimination of methotrexate in childhood acute lymphoblastic leukemia and malignant lymphoma. J Hum Genet 52(2):166–171

Jankovic M, Brouwers P et al (1994) Association of 1800 cGy cranial irradiation with intellectual function in children with acute lymphoblastic leukaemia. ISPACC. International Study Group on Psychosocial Aspects of Childhood Cancer. Lancet344:224–22 7

Jenkinson H, Hawkins M (1999) Secondary brain tumours in children with ALL. Lancet 354(9184):1126

Kadan-Lottick NS, Dinu I et al (2008) Osteonecrosis in adult survivors of childhood cancer: a report from the childhood cancer survivor study. J Clin Oncol 26(18):3038–3045

Kadan-Lottick NS, Brouwers P et al (2009) A comparison of neurocognitive functioning in children previously randomized to dexamethasone or prednisone in the treatment of childhood acute lymphoblastic leukemia. Blood 114(9): 1746–1752

Karimova EJ, Rai SN et al (2007) Femoral head osteonecrosis in pediatric and young adult patients with leukemia or lymphoma. J Clin Oncol 25(12):1525–1531

Karp JE, Sarkodee-Adoo CB (2000) Therapy-related acute leukemia. Clin Lab Med 20(1):71–81

Kimball Dalton VM, Gelber RD et al (1998) Second malignancies in patients treated for childhood acute lymphoblastic leukemia. J Clin Oncol 16(8):2848–2853

Kremer LCM, van Dalen EC et al (2001) Anthracycline-induced clinical heart failure in a cohort of 607 children: long-term follow-up study. J Clin Oncol 19:191–196

Kremer LC, van Dalen EC et al (2002) Frequency and risk factors of anthracycline-induced clinical heart failure in children: a systematic review. Ann Oncol 13(4):503–512

Legha SS, Benjamin RS et al (1982) Reduction of doxorubicin cardiotoxicity by prolonged continuous intravenous infusion. Ann Intern Med 96(2):133–139

Lennard L, Richards S et al (2006) The thiopurine methyltransferase genetic polymorphism is associated with thioguanine-related veno-occlusive disease of the liver in children with acute lymphoblastic leukemia. Clin Pharmacol Ther 80(4): 375–383

Lipshultz SE (2000) Ventricular dysfunction clinical research in infants, children and adolescents. Prog Pediatr Cardiol 12(1): 1–28

Lipshultz SE, Colan SD et al (1991) Late cardiac effects of doxorubicin therapy for acute lymphoblastic leukemia in childhood. N Engl J Med 324(12):808–815

Lipshultz SE, Lipsitz SR et al (1995) Female sex and drug dose as risk factors for late cardiotoxic effects of doxorubicin therapy for childhood cancer. N Engl J Med 332(26): 1738–1743

Lipshultz SE, Giantris AL et al (2002) Doxorubicin administration by continuous infusion is not cardioprotective: the Dana-Farber 91-01 Acute Lymphoblastic Leukemia protocol. J Clin Oncol 20(6):1677–1682

Lipshultz SE, Rifai N et al (2004) The effect of dexrazoxane on myocardial injury in doxorubicin-treated children with acute lymphoblastic leukemia. N Engl J Med 351:145–153

Lipshultz SE, Lipsitz SR et al (2005) Chronic progressive cardiac dysfunction years after doxorubicin therapy for childhood acute lymphoblastic leukemia. J Clin Oncol 23(12): 2629–2636

Loning L, Zimmermann M et al (2000) Secondary neoplasms subsequent to Berlin-Frankfurt-Munster therapy of acute lymphoblastic leukemia in childhood: significantly lower risk without cranial radiotherapy. Blood 95(9): 2770–2775

Mahoney DH Jr, Shuster JJ et al (1998) Acute neurotoxicity in children with B-precursor acute lymphoid leukemia: an association with intermediate-dose intravenous methotrexate and intrathecal triple therapy – a Pediatric Oncology Group study. J Clin Oncol 16(5):1712–1722

Marchese VG, Connolly BH et al (2008) Relationships among severity of osteonecrosis, pain, range of motion, and functional mobility in children, adolescents, and young adults with acute lymphoblastic leukemia. Phys Ther 88(3): 341–350

Matloub Y, Bostrom B et al (2008) Escalating dose intravenous methotrexate without leucovorin rescue during interim maintenance is superior to oral methotrexate for children with standard risk acute lymphoblastic leukemia (SR-ALL): Children's Oncology Group study 1991. ASH Abstract #9

Mattano LA, Sather HN et al (2000) Osteonecrosis as a complication of treating acute lymphoblastic leukemia in children: a report from the Children's Cancer Group. J Clin Oncol 18: 3262–3272

Meadows AT, Gordon J et al (1981) Declines in IQ scores and cognitive dysfunctions in children with acute lymphocytic leukaemia treated with cranial irradiation. Lancet 2(8254): 1015–1018

Meeske KA, Siegel SE et al (2005) Prevalence and correlates of fatigue in long-term survivors of childhood leukemia. J Clin Oncol23(24):5501–5510

Michels SD, McKenna RW et al (1985) Therapy-related acute myeloid leukemia and myelodysplastic syndrome: a clinical and morphologic study of 65 cases. Blood 65(6): 1364–1372

Miyoshi Y, Ohta H et al (2008) Endocrinological analysis of 122 Japanese childhood cancer survivors in a single hospital. Endocr J 55(6):1055–1063

Mody R, Li S et al (2008) Twenty-five-year follow-up among survivors of childhood acute lymphoblastic leukemia: a report from the Childhood Cancer Survivor Study. Blood 111(12):5515–5523

Mohn A, Chiarelli F et al (1997) Thyroid function in children treated for acute lymphoblastic leukemia. J Endocrinol Invest20(4):215–219

Moyer-Mileur LJ, Ransdell L et al (2009) Fitness of children with standard-risk acute lymphoblastic leukemia during maintenance therapy: response to a home-based exercise and nutrition program. J Pediatr Hematol Oncol 31(4):259–266

Mulhern RK, Palmer SL (2003) Neurocognitive late effects in pediatric cancer. Curr Probl Cancer 27(4):177–197

Mulhern RK, Wasserman AL et al (1988) Memory function in disease-free survivors of childhood acute lymphocytic leukemia given CNS prophylaxis with or without 1, 800 cGy cranial irradiation. J Clin Oncol 6(2):315–320

Mulhern RK, Fairclough D et al (1991) A prospective comparison of neuropsychologic performance of children surviving leukemia who received 18-Gy, 24-Gy, or no cranial irradiation. J Clin Oncol 9(8):1348–1356

Mulrooney DA, Ness KK et al (2008) Fatigue and sleep disturbance in adult survivors of childhood cancer: a report from the childhood cancer survivor study (CCSS). Sleep 31(2): 271–281

Murri R, Ammassari A et al (2004) Patient-reported and physician-estimated adherence to HAART: social and clinic center-related factors are associated with discordance. J Gen Intern Med 19(11):1104–1110

Nandagopal R, Laverdiere C et al (2008) Endocrine late effects of childhood cancer therapy: a report from the Children's Oncology Group. Horm Res 69(2):65–74

Neglia JP, Meadows AT et al (1991) Second neoplasms after acute lymphoblastic leukemia in childhood. N Engl J Med 325:1330–1336

Neglia JP, Friedman DL et al (2001) Second malignant neoplasms in five-year survivors of childhood cancer: childhood cancer survivor study. J Natl Cancer Inst 93:618–629

Ness KK, Baker KS et al (2007) Body composition, muscle strength deficits and mobility limitations in adult survivors of childhood acute lymphoblastic leukemia. Pediatr Blood Cancer49(7):975–981

Nygaard R, Garwicz S et al (1991) Second malignant neoplasms in patients treated for childhood leukemia. A population-based cohort study from the Nordic countries. The Nordic Society of Pediatric Oncology and Hematology (NOPHO). Acta Paediatr Scand 80(12):1220–1228

Oeffinger KC (2008) Are survivors of acute lymphoblastic leukemia (ALL) at increased risk of cardiovascular disease? Pediatr Blood Cancer 50(2 Suppl):462–467, discussion 468

Oeffinger KC, Mertens AC et al (2003) Obesity in adult survivors of childhood acute lymphoblastic leukemia: a report from the Childhood Cancer Survivor Study. J Clin Oncol 21(7):1359–1365

Pasqualini T, McCalla J et al (1991) Subtle primary hypothyroidism in patients treated for acute lymphoblastic leukemia. Acta Endocrinol (Copenh) 124(4):375–380

Pedersen-Bjergaard J, Christiansen DH et al (2006) Alternative genetic pathways and cooperating genetic abnormalities in the pathogenesis of therapy-related myelodysplasia and acute myeloid leukemia. Leukemia 20(11):1943–1949

Pizzo PA, Poplack DG (2006) Principles and practice of pediatric oncology. Lippincott Williams & Wilkins, Philadelphia, PA

Prout MN, Richards MJ et al (1977) Adriamycin cardiotoxicity in children: case reports, literature review, and risk factors. Cancer39(1):62–65

Pui CH, Evans WE (1998) Acute lymphoblastic leukemia. N Engl J Med 339(9):605–615

Pui CH, Behm FG et al (1989) Secondary acute myeloid leukemia in children treated for acute lymphoid leukemia. N Engl J Med 321(3):136–142

Pui CH, Cheng C et al (2003) Extended follow-up of long-term survivors of childhood acute lymphoblastic leukemia. N Engl J Med 349(7):640–649

Pui CH, Campana D et al (2009) Treating childhood acute lymphoblastic leukemia without cranial irradiation. N Engl J Med 360(26):2730–2741

Razzouk BI, Rose SR et al (2007) Obesity in survivors of childhood acute lymphoblastic leukemia and lymphoma. J Clin Oncol25(10):1183–1189

Reaman GH (2009). Personal communication

Relling MV, Hancock ML et al (1999a) Mercaptopurine therapy intolerance and heterozygosity at the thiopurine S-methyltransferase gene locus. J Natl Cancer Inst 91(23): 2001–2008

Relling MV, Rubnitz JE et al (1999b) High incidence of secondary brain tumours after radiotherapy and antimetabolites. Lancet354(9172):34–39

Relling MV, Yang W et al (2004) Pharmacogenetic risk factors for osteonecrosis of the hip among children with leukemia. J Clin Oncol 22(19):3930–3936

Ries LAG, Eisner MP et al (2001). SEER Cancer Statistics Review, 1973–1999. National Cancer Institute, Bethesda, MD. http://seer.cancer.gov/csr/1975-2002

Robison LL, Nesbit ME Jr et al (1984) Factors associated with IQ scores in long-term survivors of childhood acute lymphoblastic leukemia. Am J Pediatr Hematol Oncol 6(2): 115–121

Robison LL, Nesbit ME Jr et al (1985) Height of children successfully treated for acute lymphoblastic leukemia: a report from the Late Effects Study Committee of Childrens Cancer Study Group. Med Pediatr Oncol 13(1):14–21

Ross JA, Oeffinger KC et al (2004) Genetic variation in the leptin receptor gene and obesity in survivors of childhood acute lymphoblastic leukemia: a report from the Childhood Cancer Survivor Study. J Clin Oncol 22(17):3558–3562

Rubenstein CL, Varni JW et al (1990) Cognitive functioning in long-term survivors of childhood leukemia: a prospective analysis. J Dev Behav Pediatr 11(6):301–305

Sapolsky RM (1993) Potential behavioral modification of glucocorticoid damage to the hippocampus. Behav Brain Res 57(2):175–182

Sarafoglou K, Boulad F et al (1997) Gonadal function after bone marrow transplantation for acute leukemia during childhood. J Pediatr 130(2):210–216

Schoch C, Kern W et al (2004) Karyotype is an independent prognostic parameter in therapy-related acute myeloid leukemia (t-AML): an analysis of 93 patients with t-AML in comparison to 1091 patients with *de novo* AML. Leukemia 18(1):120–125

Schrappe M, Reiter A et al (2000) Improved outcome in childhood acute lymphoblastic leukemia despite reduced use of anthracyclines and cranial radiotherapy: results of trial ALL-BFM 90. German-Austrian-Swiss ALL-BFM Study Group. Blood95(11):3310–3322

Schriock EA, Schell MJ et al (1991) Abnormal growth patterns and adult short stature in 115 long-term survivors of childhood leukemia. J Clin Oncol 9(3):400–405

Seibel NL, Steinherz PG et al (2008) Early postinduction intensification therapy improves survival for children and adolescents with high-risk acute lymphoblastic leukemia: a report from the Children's Oncology Group. Blood 111(5): 2548–2555

Shankar SM, Marina N et al (2008) Monitoring for cardiovascular disease in survivors of childhood cancer: report from the Cardiovascular Disease Task Force of the Children's Oncology Group. Pediatrics 121:e387–396

Shapira J, Gotfried M et al (1990) Reduced cardiotoxicity of doxorubicin by a 6-hour infusion regimen. A prospective randomized evaluation. Cancer 65(4):870–873

Silverman LB, Gelber RD et al (2001) Improved outcome for children with acute lymphoblastic leukemia: results of Dana-Farber Consortium protocol 91-01. Blood 97(5):1211–1218

Sklar C (1995) Growth and endocrine disturbances after bone marrow transplantation in childhood. Acta Paediatr Suppl 411:57–61, discussion 62

Sklar C (1999) Reproductive physiology and treatment-related loss of sex hormone production. Med Pediatr Oncol 33(1):2–8

Sklar C (2005) Maintenance of ovarian function and risk of premature menopause related to cancer treatment. J Natl Cancer Inst Monogr 34:25–27

Sklar C, Mertens A et al (1993) Final height after treatment for childhood acute lymphoblastic leukemia: comparison of no cranial irradiation with 1800 and 2400 centigrays of cranial irradiation. J Pediatr 123(1):59–64

Sklar CA, Mertens AC et al (2006) Premature menopause in survivors of childhood cancer: a report from the childhood cancer survivor study. J Natl Cancer Inst 98(13):890–896

Smith PJ, Ekert H et al (1977) High incidence of cardiomyopathy in children treated with adriamycin and DTIC in combination chemotherapy. Cancer Treat Rep 61(9):1736–1738

Smith SM, Le Beau MM et al (2003) Clinical-cytogenetic associations in 306 patients with therapy-related myelodysplasia and myeloid leukemia: the University of Chicago series. Blood102(1):43–52

Steffens M, Beauloye V et al (2008) Endocrine and metabolic disorders in young adult survivors of childhood acute lymphoblastic leukaemia (ALL) or non-Hodgkin lymphoma (NHL). Clin Endocrinol (Oxf) 69(5):819–827

Stehbens JA, Kaleita TA et al (1991) CNS prophylaxis of childhood leukemia: what are the long-term neurological, neuropsychological, and behavioral effects? Neuropsychol Rev 2(2):147–177

Strauss AJ, Su JT et al (2001) Bony morbidity in children treated for acute lymphoblastic leukemia. J Clin Oncol 19(12): 3066–3072

Talvensaari KK, Lanning M et al (1996) Long-term survivors of childhood cancer have an increased risk of manifesting the metabolic syndrome. J Clin Endocrinol Metab 81(8): 3051–3055

te Winkel ML, Appel IM et al (2008) Impaired dexamethasone-related increase of anticoagulants is associated with the development of osteonecrosis in childhood acute lymphoblastic leukemia. Haematologica 93(10):1570–1574

van Brussel M, Takken T et al (2006) Physical function and fitness in long-term survivors of childhood leukaemia. Pediatr Rehabil9(3):267–274

van Dalen EC, van der Pal HJ et al (2006) Clinical heart failure during pregnancy and delivery in a cohort of female childhood cancer survivors treated with anthracyclines. Eur J Cancer42(15):2549–2553

Van Veldhuizen PJ, Neff J et al (1993) Decreased fibrinolytic potential in patients with idiopathic avascular necrosis and transient osteoporosis of the hip. Am J Hematol 44(4): 243–248

Vardiman JW, Harris NL et al (2002) The World Health Organization (WHO) classification of the myeloid neoplasms. Blood 100(7):2292–2302

Von Hoff DD, Rozencweig M et al (1982) The cardiotoxicity of anticancer agents. Semin Oncol 9(1):23–33

Waber DP, Gioia G et al (1990) Sex differences in cognitive processing in children treated with CNS prophylaxis for acute lymphoblastic leukemia. J Pediatr Psychol 15(1): 105–122

Waber DP, Carpentieri SC et al (2000) Cognitive sequelae in children treated for acute lymphoblastic leukemia with dexamethasone or prednisone. J Pediatr Hematol Oncol 22(3): 206–213

Waters EB, Wake MA et al (2003) Health-related quality of life of children with acute lymphoblastic leukaemia: comparisons and correlations between parent and clinician reports. Int J Cancer 103(4):514–518

Werner A, Jager M et al (2003) Joint preserving surgery for osteonecrosis and osteochondral defects after chemotherapy in childhood. Klin Padiatr 215(6):332–337

Wexler L (1998) Ameliorating anthracycline cardiotoxicity in children with cancer: clinical trials with dexrazoxane. Semin Oncol25: 86–92

Wu E, Robison LL et al (2007) Assessment of health-related quality of life of adolescent cancer patients using the Minneapolis-Manchester Quality of Life Adolescent Questionnaire. Pediatr Blood Cancer 48(7):678–686

Zeltzer LK, Recklitis C et al (2009) Psychological status in childhood cancer survivors: a report from the Childhood Cancer Survivor Study. J Clin Oncol 27(14):2396–2404

Acute Toxicities, Late Sequelae, and Quality of Survivorship in Children with Acute Myeloid Leukemia: The Impact of Allogeneic Stem Cell Transplant

10

Julianne Byrne, John Horan, and H. Stacy Nicholson

Contents

J. Byrne (✉)
Boyne Research Institute, Duke House, Duke Street, Drogheda, Ireland
e-mail: jbyrne@boyneresearch.ie

J. Horan
Emory School of Medicine/Children's Healthcare of Atlanta, AFLAC Cancer Center and Blood Disorders Service, 1405 Clifton Road NE, Atlanta, Georgia 30322, USA
e-mail: john.horan@choa.org

H. S. Nicholson
Pediatric Hematology/Oncology, Doernbecher Childrens Hospital – OHSU, 3181 SW Sam Jackson Park Rd., Portland, OR 97239-3098, USA
e-mail: nicholss@ohsu.edu

10.1 Introduction

Acute myeloid leukemia (AML) is a heterogeneous group of hematological malignancies that arise within bone marrow precursors of the myeloid, monocyte, erythroid, and megakaryocytic lineages (Pizzo and Poplack 2005). It comprises between 15% and 20% of all leukemias occurring during childhood. The incidence of new cases varies during childhood by year of age; the highest incidence is in early childhood, with about 12 cases per million in children up to age 2, declining steadily thereafter to its lowest incidence of about 4 per million at age 9, then climbing again during adolescence (Fig. 10.1). AML affects male and female children and black and white children in the US about equally (Ries and Smith 1999). Survival after AML (5-year relative survival) has increased steadily in the US over the period 1975–2005, from a rate of 18.8% in 1975–1977 to 60.2% in the period 1999–2005 for children diagnosed from 0 to 14 years of age (Fig. 10.2). It is likely that the growth and refinement of allogeneic hematopoietic stem cell transplant (HSCT) from related and unrelated donors since the 1970s has contributed to this improvement. However, survival after AML still lags considerably behind acute lymphoblastic leukemia (ALL), for which survival had

G.H. Reaman and F.O. Smith (eds.), *Childhood Leukemia*,
DOI: 10.1007/978-3-642-13781-5_10, © Springer-Verlag Berlin Heidelberg 2011

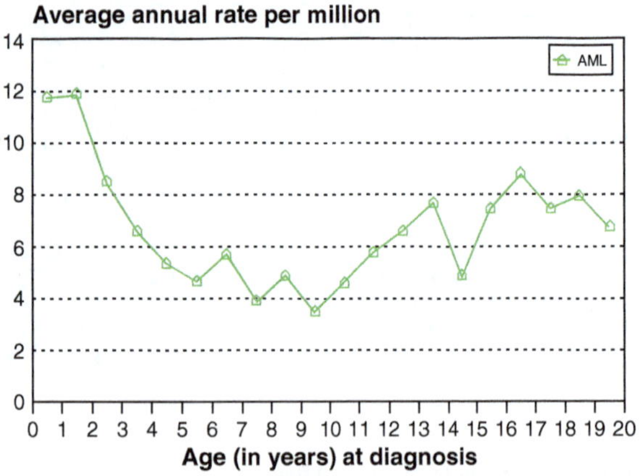

Fig. 10.1 AML age-specific incidence rates, all races, both sexes, SEER, 1976–1984 and 1986–1994 combined. (NCI Pediatric Monograph, 1999)

reached 89.0% in the interval 1999–2005 (Ries and Smith 1999). Again in contrast to ALL, survival after AML was slightly better for females than for males with AML, but there were no detectable differences between blacks and whites (Ries and Smith 1999). Within Europe from 1988 to 1997, regional differences in survival after AML in children were pronounced from North to East, where survival was significantly poorer.

In the 1980s, several single center studies demonstrated that HLA-matched related bone marrow transplantation (BMT) was an effective treatment for children with AML (Kersey et al. 1982; Santos et al. 1983; Sanders et al. 1985; Brochstein et al. 1987). This experience was subsequently corroborated by multicenter studies (Horowitz and Bortin 1993; Nesbit et al. 1994). The use of HCST for pediatric AML has grown since then and has expanded to include the use of alternative donor sources, especially unrelated adult bone marrow grafts and unrelated cord blood grafts (Kernan eta l. 1993;R ubinsteine ta l. 1998).

10.2 TimingandA ppropriateness of Transplant in Pediatric AML

Despite the vast experience in transplantation for pediatric AML, uncertainty exists regarding its optimal place in therapy. This is especially true for patients with newly diagnosed disease. With improvements in chemotherapy, most cooperative groups have abandoned the use of HSCT for patients in first complete remission (CR1) with favorable prognoses, patients with acute promyelocytic leukemia (APL) and more recently, patients with favorable cytogenetic factors, including inv(16) and t(8;21). Disagreement exists, however, for patients with less favorable prognoses. Some investigators contend that given the recent advances in chemotherapy, transplant should be reserved largely for treatment of relapsed disease

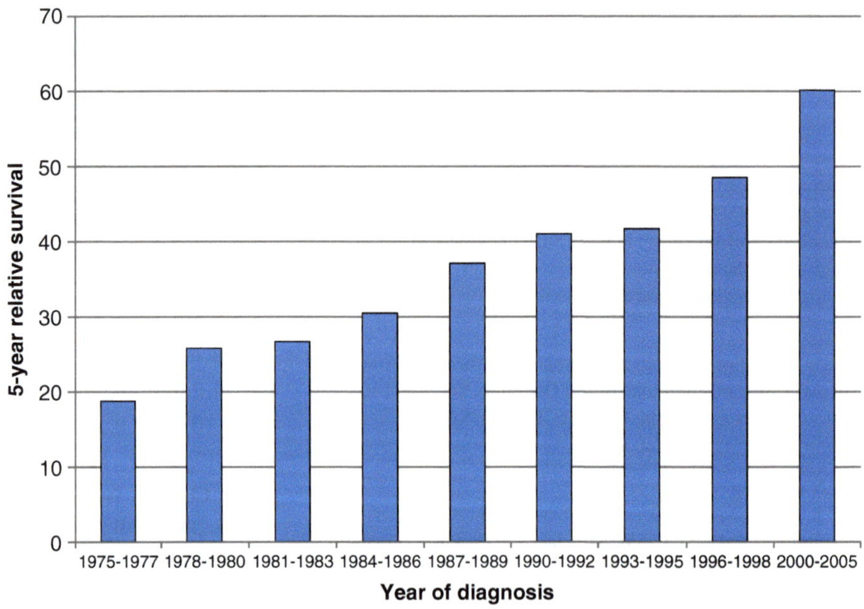

Fig.10.2 Five-yearr elative survival rates (%) for children diagnosed at ages 0–14 with AML by grouped years of diagnosis. (Adapted from SEER Cancer Statistics Review, 1975–2006; http://seer.cancer.gov/csr/1975_2006/browse_csr.php?section=28&page=sect_28_table.08.html#table1)

(Creutzig and Reinhardt 2002). Others, citing the superior outcomes that have been attained with matched related donor BMT in Children's Oncology Group (COG) trials, argue that the optimal timing of transplant for most patients is CR1 (Chen et al. 2002). A recent meta-analysis shed some light on this controversy (Horan et al. 2008). This study, which assessed the impact of disease risk on the relative efficacy of BMT, included 1,373 patients from four cooperative group trials that compared HLA-matched related donor BMT to chemotherapy alone: Children's Cancer Group (CCG) 2891 (Woods et al. 2001), Pediatric Oncology Group (POG) 8821 (Ravindranath et al. 1996), CCG 2961 (Lange et al. 2008), and Medical Research Council (MRC) 10 (Hann et al. 1998; Stevens et al. 1998). Using cytogenetics and the percentage of marrow blasts after the first course of chemotherapy, patients were stratified into favorable, intermediate, and poor-risk disease groups. Patients who could not be risk classified were analyzed separately. Patients with APL, Down syndrome, or secondary leukemia were excluded. In the intermediate-risk group, the estimated disease-free survival (DFS) at 8 years for nontransplant patients was 39%, while it was 58% for BMT patients. The estimated overall survival (OS) for nontransplant intermediate-risk patients was 51%, while it was 62% for BMT patients. Both differences were significant ($p < 0.01$). There were no significant differences for survival in the other two risk groups or in the nonrisk stratifiedpa tients(Fig. 10.3).

A limitation of this study is that the data was drawn predominantly from Children's Oncology Group (COG) studies. Given the lack of data from cooperative groups in Europe, Asia, and elsewhere, caution should be used in generalizing the results. The possibility that the findings of the study may not be universally applicable is raised by the results of the Berlin-Frankfurt-Muenster 98 (BFM) and the MRC 12 trials; both studies demonstrated survival rates in intermediate-risk patients treated with chemotherapy alone that were similar to the rate that was observed for patients receiving BMT in the meta-analysis (Gibson et al. 2005; Creutzig et al. 2006). However, a straightforward comparison with the BFM experience is difficult, because it employed a dichotomous, rather than tripartite, prognostic system.

The lack of benefit observed in this pediatric meta-analysis in poor-risk disease patients stands in contrast to the results of a recent meta-analysis in adult patients that demonstrated that patients with poor-risk disease

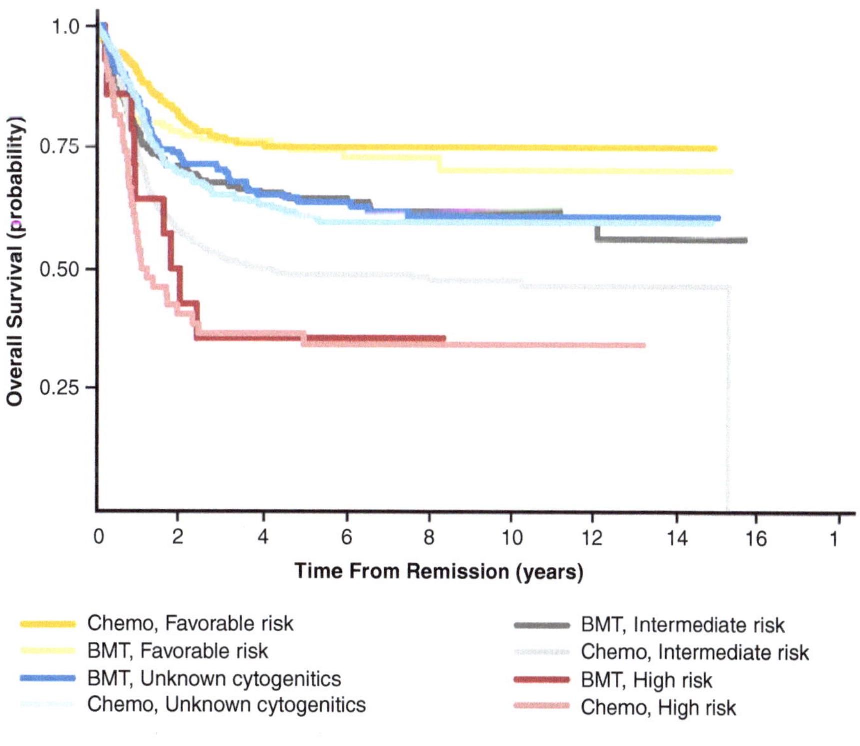

Fig.10.3 Estimatedo verall survival stratified by risk group and postremission treatment. Chemo, chemotherapy; BMT, bone marrow transplantation. (From Horane ta l.2008)

benefit from HLA-matched related donor HSCT in CR1 (Koreth et al. 2009). The pediatric meta-analysis included a very small number of poor-risk patients and, therefore, the efficacy of HSCT in these patients needs to be studied further. As risk stratification schemes are refined through the identification of new prognostic markers, the population of patients that will benefit from BMT will need to be redefined. For example, a retrospective analysis performed by COG indicated that pediatric patients whose leukemia has an FLT3 internal tandem duplication, a relatively recently identified marker of poor-risk disease, appear to benefit greatly from allogeneic HSCT (Meshinchi et al. 2006)(Fig. 10.4).

The role of allogeneic HSCT is more clearly defined in patients whose leukemia relapses after receiving chemotherapy alone as initial therapy, since these patients generally have a very poor outcome (Stahnke et al. 1998; Webb et al. 1999). In this setting, the use of an unrelated donor graft is nearly as effective as a HLA-matched related donor graft. A Center for International Blood and Marrow Transplant Research (CIBMTR) analysis of HLA-matched related donor HSCTs performed after myeloablative conditioning between 1998 and 2006 demonstrated a 3-year overall survival rate of 57% in patients younger than 20 years who were transplanted in a second clinical remission (CR2) (CIBMRT 2008). A recent study from the U.S. National Marrow Donor Program demonstrated a slightly poorer overall survival rate, 47% at five years, in pediatric patients who underwent unrelated donor bone marrow transplants in CR2 (Bunin et al. 2008).

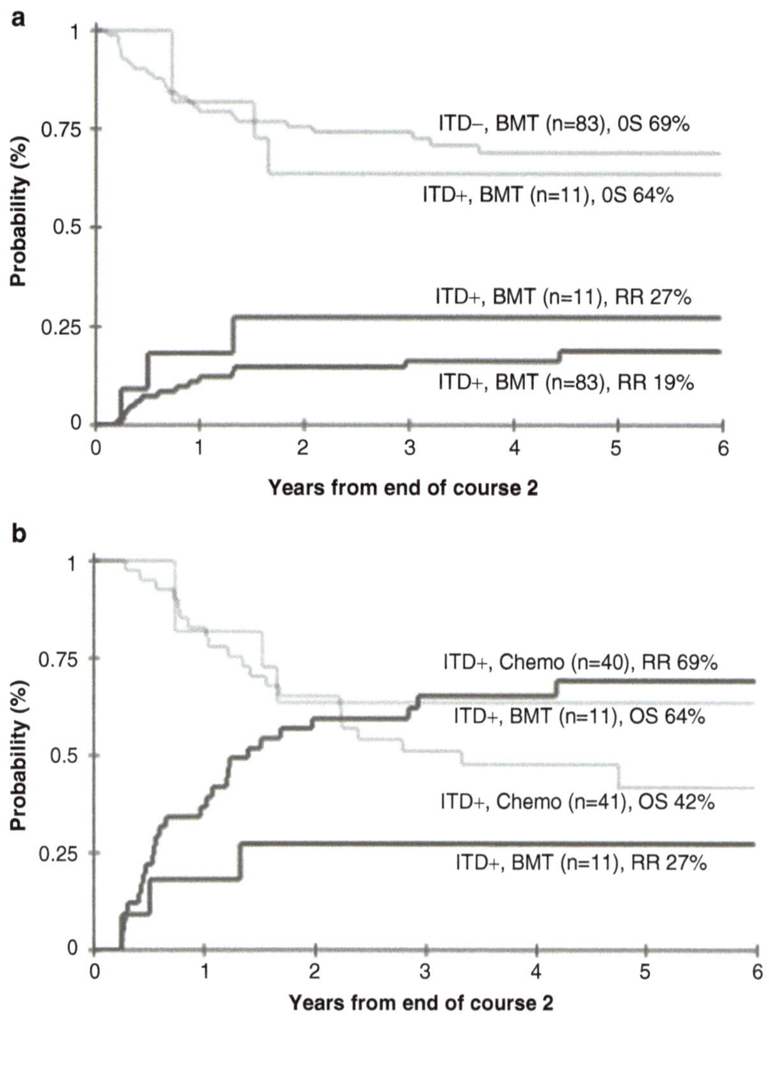

Fig.10.4 Efficacy of allogeneic HSCT in FLT3/ITD-positive AML. (**a**) Relapse risk (*solid lines*)a nd overall survival (*shaded lines*)i n recipients of matched related donor stem cell transplant with and without FLT3/ITD. (**b**) Relapse risk (*solid lines*) and overall survival (*shaded lines*) in patients with FLT3/ITD treated with Consolidation chemotherapy vs. matched related donor stem cell transplant. HSCT, hematopoietic stem cell transplant; ITD, internal tandem duplication. (From Meshinchi et al. 2006, with permission)

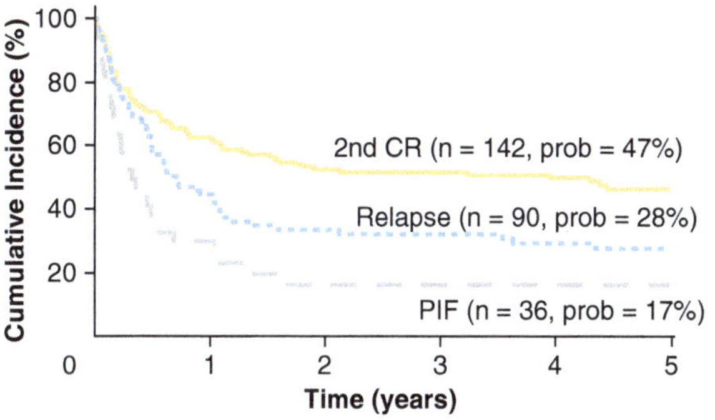

Fig. 10.5 The five-year probabilities of overall survival after unrelated donor bone marrow transplantation by disease status at transplantation. PIF, primary Induction failure; CR, complete remission.(FromB unine ta l. 2008,w ithpe rmission)

Similarly, a Eurocord (a European registry of cord blood transplants that operates on behalf of the EBMT, the European Group for Blood and Marrow Transplants) study showed a two-year leukemia-free survival rate of 50% in pediatric patients who received unrelated cord blood transplants in CR2 (Michel et al. 2003). Patients with more advanced disease, especially those whose disease is not in remission at the time of transplant, fare worse, regardless of whether they receive a matched related donor, unrelated marrow donor, or unrelated cord blood transplant (CIBMRT 2008; Bunin eta l. 2008)(Fig. 10.5).

10.3 HematopoieticSt emC ellSo urces and Donor Types

Autologous HSCT has been utilized to treat patients with AML in CR1 as well as patients with more advanced disease (Godder et al. 2004). Several cooperative-group randomized controlled trials (RCT), however, have demonstrated that for patients with AML in CR1, autologous transplantation appears to offer no advantage over chemotherapy alone (Ravindranath et al. 1996; Stevens et al. 1998; Woods et al. 2001).

The three sources of hematopoietic stem cells (bone marrow, cytokine-mobilized peripheral blood, and umbilical cord blood) have all been utilized for allogeneic transplantation in pediatric AML. While there are no large-scale studies specifically comparing the efficacy in this setting, comparative studies in children with hematological malignancies have been performed, and this research has guided the utilization of the three sources in pediatric AML. A CIBMTR study comparing HLA-identical peripheral blood stem cell transplantation (PBSCT) and BMT demonstrated that, unlike in adults, PBSCT in children is associated with poorer survival, probably because recipients of PBSCT are more likely to develop chronic graft-vs.-host disease (GVHD) (Eapen et al. 2004).

Studies conducted by Eurocord and the CIBMTR comparing single umbilical cord blood grafts to bone marrow grafts, have demonstrated similar efficacy in unrelated donor and HLA-matched related donor transplantation (Rocha et al. 2000; Rocha et al. 2001; Eapen et al. 2007). Until recently, the high risk for delayed and failed engraftment stemming from the small cell dose of most cord blood units has limited the use of cord blood transplantation in older children and adolescents, like adults (Rubinstein et al. 1998). This limitation has been overcome with the recent advent of double unit cord blood transplants; single center experience suggests that this approach more frequently causes GVHD, but has a potent graft-vs.-leukemia (GVL) effect (Barker et al. 2005). Because of its seemingly stronger GVL effect, double unit cord blood transplantation may be advantageous in smaller children, even though engraftment after single unit transplants is not usually a problem in these patients. To answer this question, a randomized-controlled trial comparing one vs. two unit transplants in pediatric patients with acute leukemia is currently being conducted by the COG and the U.S. Blood and Marrow Transplant Clinical Trials Network.

Haploidentical family donor grafts have also been used for pediatric AML. While they are utilized far less often than unrelated donor grafts, encouraging results have been reported in small series of patients (Goddere ta l. 2000;La nge ta l. 2004).

10.4 ConditioningR egimens

Most centers employ myeloablative conditioning for pediatric AML. In cooperative group trials for newly diagnosed AML, several combinations have been used prior to HLA-matched related donor BMT, including total body irradiation (TBI) and cyclophosphamide

(Cy), the combination of high-dose busulfan and Cy, and the combination of TBI and etoposide (Ravindranath et al. 1996; Stevens et al. 1998; Woods et al. 2001; Becton et al. 2006; Lange et al. 2008). The comparative efficacy of these regimens in this setting has not been well studied. A small case series from the Société Française de Greffe de Moelle demonstrated similar outcomes in children with AML who received busulfan and four 50 mg/kg doses of cyclophosphamide (BuCy4) and those who received TBI-based conditioning. Busulfan combined with two 60 mg/kg doses of cyclophosphamide (BuCy2), however, was associated with inferior survival (Michel et al. 1994). A much larger study of adults from the CIBMTR, in contrast, demonstrated comparable outcomes with TBICy, BuCy4, and BuCy2 (Litzow et al. 2002). Importantly, both of these studies utilized experience that largely predates the widespread adoption of pharmacokinetic testing-based busulfan dosing and the introduction of the intravenous formulation of busulfan (Yeager et al. 1992; Kletzel et al. 2006). While the effectiveness of TBI-based conditioning and BuCy appear to be similar, BuCy may be more appropriate for children, as it has been associated with fewer late effects (Michel eta l. 1997).

Emerging data in adults suggests that reduced-intensity conditioning may represent an effective alternative to myeloablative conditioning in AML (Aoudjhane et al. 2005). While reduced-intensity conditioning would be expected to lessen the late effects of HSCT in children and therefore could be advantageous, experience with reduced-intensity conditioning for pediatric AML remains limited. The results of a recent multicenter trial of reduced-intensity conditioning that included children and adolescents with a variety of hematological malignancies, a small number of whom had AML, has provided a foundation for further work in this area (Pulsipher et al. 2009).

10.5 Graftvs .H ostDi seasePr ophylaxis

In transplant for AML, as with other types of leukemia, a delicate balance exists between the beneficial GVL and the harmful GVH reactions (Horowitz et al. 1990; Neudorf et al. 2004). In a seminal study performed by the CIBMTR of over two thousand children and adults who received HLA-matched related donor BMT for ALL or AML in CR1 or chronic myelogenous leukemia (CML) in 1st chronic phase, the severity of acute and chronic GVHD was inversely related to relapse risk (Horowitz et al. 1990). Because of the deleterious effects of GVHD, though, only mild GVHD was associated with improved survival (Horowitz et al. 1990). A smaller study performed by the COG of children who received matched related donor BMT as part of the CCG 2981 trial specifically highlights the importance of the relationship between GVHD and the GVL effect in pediatric AML (Neudorf et al. 2004). In this study, patients who developed mild to moderate acute GVHD had the best DFS rate; then came patients who did not develop acute GVHD, followed by patients who developed severe acute GVHD (Fig. 10.6). In the multivariate analysis, the relative risk of relapse or death associated with mild to moderate acute GVHD was 0.66, although this result did not achieve statistical significance in this relatively small study ($p = 0.165$).

In BMT for pediatric AML, as in many other settings, the combination of cyclosporine (or tacrolimus) and four doses of methotrexate are typically employed for GVHD prophylaxis, whether a related or an unrelated donor is used (Storb et al. 1989a, b; Ratanatharathorn et al. 1998; Nash et al. 2000).

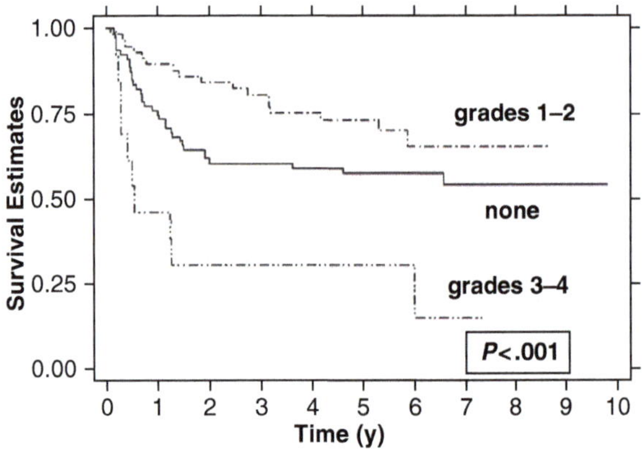

Fig. 10.6 Disease-free survival according to acute GVHD status: none ($n = 79$), grades 1–2 ($n = 58$), and grades 3–4 ($n = 13$). Estimates at 6 years are 58%, 65%, and 15%, respectively. P-value compares patients with grades 3–4 acute GVHD to patients without GVHD or with grades 1–2. (From Neudorf eta l. 2004,w ithpe rmission)

A CIBMTR study, however, suggests that in matched related donor BMT for pediatric leukemia, where the risk for severe GVHD is low, this combination is no better, as measured in terms of survival, than the less potent regimens of cyclosporine alone or methotrexate alone (Ringden et al. 1993). A more recent Italian multicenter RCT in pediatric patients with leukemia which compared low-dose cyclosporine to standard-dose cyclosporine, in fact, demonstrated a strong trend toward improved DFS, largely attributable to a lower rate of relapse, in the group that received the lower dose regimen (Locatelli et al. 2000). In unrelated donor cord blood transplantation, in which the pace of engraftment is slow in comparison to bone marrow, the myelosuppressive effects of methotrexate are usually avoided and, instead, cyclosporine is used either alone or in combination with methylprednisolone or mycophenolate mofetil (Rocha et al. 2000; Barker et al. 2005; Kurtzberg et al. 2008; MacMillan et al. 2009). Ex-vivo T-cell depletion, once a commonly employed means of preventing GVHD from unrelated donor bone marrow transplants, has been abandoned by many centers after a multicenter RCT in unrelated donor transplantation demonstrated that while T-cell depletion greatly reduces the risk for acute GVHD, this benefit is outweighed by an increased risk for infection and leukemic relapse (Wagner et al. 2005).

10.6 Transplant-RelatedMo rbidity and Mortality

The transplant process can cause serious and sometimes fatal complications, which stem primarily from infection (Engelhard et al. 1986), conditioning regimen-related organ injuries, such as veno-occlusive disease of the liver (sinusoidal obstruction syndrome), or acute lung injury (Weiner et al. 1986; Bearman 1995), and GVHD (Glucksberg et al. 1974; Gale et al. 1987). Risk for treatment-related mortality (TRM) is influenced by age, type of donor, and disease status. Children up to the age of 10 years who undergo matched related donor BMT in CR1 have less than a 10% risk of TRM (Horan et al. unpublished data from meta-analysis of MRC 10, POG 8821, CCG 2891, and CCG 2961 trials). By contrast, patients over the age of 10 receiving an unrelated donor BMT for AML with advanced disease (CR2, primary refractory or in relapse) have a 40% risk of TRM (Bunin et al. 2008). Importantly, a recent analysis by the CIBMTR of children and adults with AML who underwent matched related donor or unrelated donor HSCT after myeloablative conditioning demonstrated that the risk for TRM has declined since the 1980s (Horan et al. 2008). Table 10.1 shows the results for matched related donor transplants. It is unclear, though, whether there has been a similar reduction in nonfatal morbidities.

Table 10.1 Multivariate analyses of treatment-related mortality and overall mortality after matched related donor hematopoietic stem cell transplant in first and second complete remission by period of diagnosis, adjusted for differences in patient and disease characteristics over time (Horan 2009, unpublished data)

Period	*N*	Treatment-related mortality RR (95% CI)	*P*	Overall mortality RR (95% CI)	*P*
First complete remission					
1985–1989	1,111	1.0		1.0	
1990 1994	1,265	0.8 (0.7–0.1)	<0.01	0.9 (0.8–1.1)	0.15
1995–1999	871	0.7 (0.6–0.8)	<0.01	0.8 (0.7–0.9)	<0.01
2000–2004	457	0.5 (0.4–0.7)	<0.01	0.7 (0.6–0.9)	<0.01
Second complete remission					
1985–1989	202	1.0		1.0	
1990–1994	228	0.8 (0.6–1.1)	0.14	0.9 (0.7–1.1)	0.28
1995–1999	199	0.6 (0.4–0.8)	<0.01	0.9 (0.7–1.2)	0.44
2000–2004	121	0.3 (0.2–0.5)	<0.01	0.6 (0.4–0.9)	<0.01

RR relative risk, *CI* confidencei nterval

10.7 Quality of Life During the Peritransplant Period

For most pediatric patients who receive allogeneic HSCT for AML, like children who receive transplants for other indications, the peritransplant period is characterized by anxiety and sadness, partly from prolonged isolation, nausea from high-dose chemotherapy or TBI, and pain from mucositis. Those patients who develop serious complications, such as infection, veno-occlusive disease or GVHD, have added stress, pain, and discomfort. A prospective Austrian study showed the early negative effects of HSCT on the physical, emotional, and social well-being of children undergoing HSCT. The cohort, which was primarily comprised of patients with acute leukemia, most of whom received unrelated donor or mismatched related donor transplants, demonstrated that the general quality of life (QOL) of pediatric transplant recipients declined greatly in the first month after transplant before recovering to its pretransplant baseline in most patients by day 100 (Felder-Puig et al. 2006).

10.8 Late Graft vs. Host Disease

In transplant for pediatric AML, as in other transplant settings, persistent or late-occurring GVHD can negatively impact long-term quality of life. Although previously, any case of GVHD that persisted or occurred beyond transplant day 100 was referred to as chronic GVHD, a recent U.S. National Institutes of Health (NIH) consensus conference put forth new diagnostic criteria, which distinguish chronic GVHD from late-occurring acute GVHD, that is, GVHD that presents with findings typical of acute GVHD, but develops more than 100 days from transplant and which often evolves into chronic GVHD (Filipovich et al. 2005). These criteria rely on a comprehensive organ-based scoring system to classify severity of chronic GVHD as mild, moderate, or severe, rather than limited and extensive as had been conventional previously (Shulman et al. 1980). The impact on functional impairment is emphasized in this system. Thus, mild disease causes little impairment, while severe disease causes significant disability.

In children receiving HSCT for AML, the risk for chronic GVHD, which is typically preceded by early acute GVHD, is influenced by several factors, especially donor type. In the CCG 2891 trial, for instance, the incidence after matched related donor transplants was 21% (Neudorf et al. 2004), while in the aforementioned CIBMTR study of unrelated donor transplant for advanced pediatric AML, it was 31% (Bunin et al. 2008). A significant proportion of pediatric patients who develop chronic GVHD will have mild cases (previously referred to as limited chronic GVHD) (Shulman et al. 1980), which typically require little to no treatment (Parsons et al. 1999; Neudorf et al. 2004); however, many children who develop late GVHD will require prolonged systemic immune suppression and some will ultimately die from it (Vigorito et al. 2009).

10.9 Late Deaths

Deaths from second malignancies during long-term follow-up after allogeneic HSCT for AML in childhood contribute a small proportion to late mortality. The International Bone Marrow Transplant Registry (IBMTR, now merged with the National Marrow Donor Program and renamed the Center for International Blood and Marrow Transplant Research, CIBMTR), a group of more than 300 transplant centers worldwide that pool their data on allogeneic transplants, reported on long-term survival and late deaths among children and adults in 1999 (Socie et al. 1999). Among 2,058 AML survivors who were disease-free 2 years after transplant at an average age of 27 years (range <1–57), 214 (10.4%) had died by the time of follow-up. Median follow-up time was 80 months. The most common causes of death among the 214 AML survivors were relapse (56%), GVHD (23%), new cancers (7%), infection without GVHD (5%), and organ failure (3%). Risk factors for late deaths in AML survivors were: transplant while not in remission or in second or subsequent remission (vs. in CR1) and active chronic GVHD at 2 years (vs. no GVHD). The total excess mortality for patients with AML relative to the general population after matching for sex, age, and nationality decreased steadily with time from transplant from 19.2% at 2 years to less than 5% at 9 years (Table 10.2). Since this study included mostly adults at diagnosis, it is not clear how well these findings apply to children and young adults.

Table 10.2 Relative mortality among AML survivors who lived at least two years after allogeneic transplant (matched to the general population for age, sex, and nationality). (Adapted from Sociee ta l. 1999)

Yearss ince transplant	Relative mortality	95%C I
Two	19.2	12.7–25.7
Five	10.2	7.0–13.4
Nine	4.5	1.0–8.0

CI confidence interval

10.10 Second Cancers

In general, second malignancies after allogeneic BMT follow a specific sequence of clinical events. Initially, posttransplant lymphoproliferative disorders (PTLD) occur mostly within the first posttransplant year at a rate of 1–2% (Deeg and Socie 1998; Socie et al. 2000; Majhail 2008). These lymphoid proliferations mostly involve B-lymphocytes, which result from Epstein-Barr infection. Other risk factors include T-cell depletion of the graft, acute or chronic GVHD, and use of grafts from unrelated or mismatched related donors. Myelodysplastic syndrome (MDS)/leukemia as a second malignancy is rare after allogeneic HCT.

A number of large studies in children have shown that the increased risk of developing a second solid tumor varies from 2% to 6% at 10 years from transplant (Kolb et al. 1999; Socie et al. 2000; Bhatia et al. 2001; Baker et al. 2003; Curtis et al. 2005; Shimada et al. 2005; Leisenring et al. 2006; Gallagher and Forrest 2007; Friedman et al. 2008). Significant risk factors include TBI, GVHD, primary disease, male sex, and pretransplantation therapies. Rizzo et al (Rizzo et al. 2009) published results from 28,874 transplant patients from the CIBMTR, updating a 1997 report (Curtis et al. 1997). Of all the transplanted patients, 25% had been treated for AML and 34% had been transplanted before the age of 20 years. The overall relative risk (observed-to-expected ratio, O/E) for a new invasive solid cancer was 2.09, and rose from 1.3 at less than 1 year to 3.28 at 15 years or longer. Although numbers were small, relative risks tended to rise over time for cancers of the oral cavity, liver, and thyroid, and for sarcomas of the bone and soft tissue as well. Among very long-term survivors (>10 years), a three-fold increase in breast cancer, significantly elevated risks of bone sarcomas and cancers of the oral cavity and liver, and a six-fold excess risk of melanoma were seen.

Socie et al. (2000), in a study based on patients identified through the IBMTR and the Fred Hutchinson Cancer Research Center, looked at second malignancies in children after transplant for leukemia. A total of 3,182 children with acute leukemia included 35.5% with AML. The excess risk (O/E) after AML was 48 (95% CI 29-74), not different from the excess risk after ALL (O/E = 44). Children who were less than 5 years at transplant had the highest risk for new malignancies with a relative risk of 115; the relative risk declined to 75 during ages 5–10 years and to 18 during the ages 10–16 years ($p = 0.001$). Among all acute leukemias, posttransplant lymphoproliferative disease (PTLD) predominated during the first posttransplant year and declined thereafter. Melanoma and CNS tumors were more common within the first 10 years after transplant compared to greater than 10 years from transplant. Nearly half (12/25) of the second solid malignancies occurred in children treated for AML. These included mucoepidermoid carcinoma of the salivary gland ($n = 2$), osteosarcoma ($n = 2$), malignant fibrous histiocytoma ($n = 1$), melanoma ($n = 3$), papillary carcinoma of the thyroid ($n = 1$), and brain cancers ($n = 3$). The excess risk for solid tumors as a function of time since transplant increased, as was shown for adults, from 12 (O/E) during the first year after transplant to 46 during the 5–9 years posttransplant. Significant risk factors for second malignancies, overall, were younger age at transplant, high-dose TBI, and moderate to severe chronic GVHD. When the authors assessed risk factors for brain and thyroid cancers only, younger age at transplant was the strongest risk factor with a relative risk of 12.2, suggesting that the brain and thyroid gland are highly sensitive to the effects of radiotherapy at a very young age. All PTLD cases occurred before the age of 5 years. Risk factors included moderate/severe GVHD with a relative risk of 6.5, and transplantation from an unrelated donor or >2 HLA-antigen disparate family donor (relative risk = 4.8).

A series of 3,372 consecutive HSCTs performed at the University of Minnesota included 44.9% patients transplanted before the age of 20 years; 17.6% of patients had AML as their primary cancer (Baker et al. 2003). Among survivors, overall, solid tumors occurred

2.8 times more often than expected and the risk was significantly elevated for melanoma and tumors of the brain and oral cavity. Nearly half of patients died from their posttransplant solid tumor and overall median survival was 4.5 years.

A number of tumor-specific second cancer studies after HSCT for malignancies have been published in the last decade. Cancers of the thyroid are among the most frequent posttransplant second malignancies (Curtis et al. 1997; Kolb et al. 1999; Socie et al. 2000; Baker et al. 2003; Rizzo et al. 2009). In a study from the European Group for Blood and Marrow Transplantation (EBMT) consortium of 78,914 patients (81.9% had hematologic malignancies, mean follow-up was 12.7 years, 26.7% were aged less than 20), Cohen et al (Cohen et al. 2007) reported an overall excess risk of 3.26 for second thyroid carcinoma. The highest independent risk factor was young age at transplant; transplant before age 11 conferred a 24.6-fold excess risk compared to transplant after the age of 20 years. Other significant factors were chronic GVHD, TBI, and female gender, each of which conferred independent relative risks of approximately three-fold. Of the 32 cases of thyroid cancer, four occurred in patients with a primary AML. For thyroid cancer, the opportunities for early detection seem limited. In this study, 6 of 32 individuals with thyroid cancer as a second malignancy had neither clinically detectable signs of thyroid disease nor laboratory thyroid test dysfunction. Cancer was most usually detected during routine yearly ultrasound examination. A single institution long-term follow-up study from the G. Gaslini Hospital in Genoa of children treated with fractionated TBI reported that six thyroid carcinomas (14%) were detected between 8 and 17.3 years following transplant (Faraci et al. 2005).

While AML survivors posttransplant have not been specifically studied, increasing risks for breast cancer with time elapsed since transplant, up to 10.8-fold greater than expected at ≥20 years in a large international series, is of great concern (Friedman et al. 2008).

Both basal cell carcinoma (BCC) and squamous cell carcinoma (SCC) incidences were elevated during long-term follow-up of 4,810 patients treated with HSCT (Leisenring et al. 2006). Risk for SCC, but not for BCC, seemed to increase with time elapsed since transplant. TBI and white race were significant risk factors for BCC but not for SCC. Young age at exposure and clinical chronic GVHD increased the risk for both types of skin cancer. Clearly, opportunities exist for screening and secondary prevention of skin cancer, especially in young patients who have been treated for malignancy with HSCT and TBI and who have experienced GVHD.

In smaller series from single institutions, a number of second cancers have been observed. Two survivors (7%) with thyroid malignancies (original primary cancer not stated) were noted in a series of 30 pediatric survivors of HSCT and hyperfractionated TBI (Chemaitilly et al. 2007). A single AML patient treated with allogeneic BMT for relapse developed a mucoepidermoid carcinoma at 4.1 years posttransplant; preparatory regimen included TBI with 15 Gy (Leung et al. 2001). A long-term follow-up study of children treated with HSCT for AML or ALL before 3 years of age found that two survivors developed second malignancies, one a breast cancer at 22 years posttransplant and the second a chest wall melanoma 8 years posttransplant. Whether these two survivors had ALL or AML as their primary cancer was not stated (Perkins et al. 2007). A single breast cancer developed in one of 200 survivors with MDS in a large study of breast cancer as a second primary following HSCT (Friedman et al. 2008).

In the absence of detailed data concerning AML survivors treated with BMT and other modalities during childhood, it would be prudent to assume that trends detected among older survivors with other cancers apply. That is, AML survivors treated with BMT and other modalities have a continuing risk for second malignancies; early age at diagnosis, severe chronic GVHD, TBI and increasing radiation dose, and gender (specific for some tumors) place AML survivors at increased risk for a new malignancy, and the site-specific risk changes with the survivor's age. Since some risks increase with elapsed time, continued medical attention following established guidelines is warranted.

10.11 CardiopulmonaryT oxicity

Though cardiac and pulmonary late effects have been studied after transplant, there is little information on children transplanted for AML. It may be misleading to extrapolate from late effects experienced by survivors of other types of cancer diagnosed in adulthood. Survivors of lymphoma would have had high-dose radiotherapy and chemotherapy in addition to their transplant regimen, while leukemia survivors may not have had the same *de novo* treatment. In addition, cardiac and cardiovascular problems may arise years after treatment. The impact of interactions between aging and treatment exposures, as well as lifestyle issues, such as smoking, on the health of long-term survivors of cancer remains to be investigated. In the same way, the potential for a cascade of cardiovascular and other symptoms in women who experience ovarian ablation after transplant for cancer during childhood is a concern.

The U.S. Bone Marrow Transplantation Survivors Study, a collaboration between the City of Hope and the University of Minnesota, evaluated morbidity in adult survivors of adult cancer by self-report. Without specific mention of AML survivors, Baker found that survivors were twice as likely to report hypertension as siblings. No other cardiovascular outcomes were more frequent; arterial disease, myocardial infarction, and stroke occurred in less than 2% of survivors (Baker et al. 2007). Another negative study from a European clinical trial of pediatric AML BMT reported a transient decrease of the cardiac shortening fraction after Consolidation and Intensification treatment phases, but echographic monitoring of the cardiac function after at least 3 years of follow-up failed to reveal any significant cardiotoxicity (Entz-Werle et al. 2005). While improvement in pulmonary function was observed in some, most showed no change after a median interval of 4.2 years. Most survivors in this single-institution study received autologous transplants, but some had allogeneic transplants; possible differences in clinical status were not evaluated. Mild restrictive pulmonary disease was found in one study (Faraci et al. 2005). Dyslipidemias were found in half of a series of children who were treated in infancy with HSCT, possibly associated with early development of the metabolic syndrome, leading to increased risk for later cardiac disease and diabetes (Perkins et al. 2007). A prospective 5-year clinical study of 58 children who underwent autologous HSCT for cancer (types not mentioned) found that the cumulative incidence of asymptomatic lung and heart sequelae after 5 years was 21%; however, at 5 years none of the fully evaluated patients had pulmonary restrictive or obstructive abnormalities and all had a normal QOL score, indicating some degree of recovery in this group (Uderzo et al. 2009). Studies of older patients in the Bone Marrow Transplant Survivor Study of all types of childhood and adult cancers reported that among deaths in AML (>2 year) survivors, none were attributable to cardiac or pulmonary causes (Bhatia et al. 2005). A nested case-control study of late congestive heart failure (CHF) after HSCT implicated pretransplant exposure to anthracyclines and presence of comorbidities as primary risk factors for late CHF after transplant (Armenian et al. 2008). A report from the EBMT (Tichelli et al. 2008) evaluated late cardiovascular events after transplant for a number of cancers, including acute leukemia, in 1-year survivors, including some children. The cumulative incidence of an arterial event was 6% at 15 years posttransplant. The established cardiovascular risk factors, including smoking, physical activity, and diabetes, significantly increased their risk. Young age at transplant may be protective; older age at transplant (≥30) conferred a six-fold higher risk for arterial complications.

In summary, studies of cardiopulmonary late effects in children treated with allogeneic HSCT for AML are limited and contradictory, indicating the need for larger, more focused studies to improve medical surveillance and counseling for families and survivors.

10.12 Fertility and Offspring After BMT for AML

Gonadal failure is a frequent consequence of HSCT. Impairment is exacerbated by increasing doses of alkylating agents, TBI, and older age of both women and men (Carter et al. 2006). Both preservation and recovery of gonadal function are possible in some cases, particularly in younger women and men, and in those treated with lower doses of alkylating agent chemotherapy and TBI (Sanders et al. 1996; Schechter et al. 2005; Chemaitilly et al. 2006). Time since transplant and lack of chronic GVHD also appear to improve the likelihood of gonadal recovery (Rovo et al. 2006). Preservation of fertility and successful pregnancy may be possible if reduced-intensity conditioning precedes transplant (Fuchs et al. 2009). Some degree of gonadal damage is present even in prepubertal children receiving transplants with TBI (Bakker and Massa 2000).

In one series of children transplanted for AML, Michel (Michel et al. 1997) and colleagues found that both girls in the study had primary ovarian failure, while all of five assessable boys appeared to have normal Leydig cell function. Some degree of pubertal delay was found in three of 17 (18%) boys treated for acute leukemia during childhood with high-dose chemotherapy and hyperfractionated TBI (Sarafoglou et al. 1997), while 7 of 16 girls (44%) had clinical and biochemical evidence of ovarian failure. One has recovered ovarian function after 5 years. Similar results were shown in a series of children that included five girls and five boys with AML (Couto-Silva et al. 2001), with more girls than boys having gonadal damage.

Outcome of pregnancy among BMT survivors may be less favorable than expected. There is some evidence from relatively small studies of survivors of adverse pregnancy outcomes. Preterm delivery seems to occur more often than expected (Sanders et al. 1996; Salooja et al. 2001). Miscarriages were more common in pregnancies of female TBI recipients after cyclophosphamide preparation (Sanders et al. 1996). Offspring of women treated during childhood for BMT with TBI and alkylating agents could be at higher risk of germ cell mutation manifesting as genetic disease (birth defects) in the offspring. However, relatively small studies have documented no excess rates of birth defects to males or females after BMT (Salooja et al. 2001; Carter et al. 2006; Rovo et al. 2006). Negative studies in long-term survivors of non-BMT therapies provide reassurance that the risk, if present, is at least not large (Byrne et al. 1998; Winther et al. 2009).

Preservation and/or restoration of fertility remain special problems in pediatric oncology and in long-term follow-up care. A summary of the literature and available options are discussed in the American Society of Clinical Oncology (ASCO) recommendations for fertility preservation (Lee et al. 2006), and further elaborated by Jeruss (Jeruss and Woodruff 2009; Woodruff 2009). New methods of ovarian shielding may protect against loss of fertility in women undergoing TBI for HSCT (Nakagawa et al. 2008); premature ovarian failure may be prevented by adjuvant gonadotropin-releasing hormone agonist analogue (Blumenfeld et al. 2008). Banking sperm is becoming more effective as a way to preserve male fertility, though not an option for prepubertal boys.

10.13 OtherOr ganT oxicities

Other endocrine problems that occur after transplant include thyroid dysfunction and growth abnormalities. Thyroid dysfunction mainly consists of hypothyroidism due to direct damage to the thyroid gland (Socie et al. 2003), and remains a problem for children for at least 30 years posttransplant (Sanders et al. 2009). Impaired linear growth and reductions in final height may accompany transplant preceded by either single-dose or hyperfractionated TBI. Modifying factors include gender, age at treatment, prior cranial radiotherapy, preparative regimens based on chemotherapy, or TBI (Woolfrey et al. 1998; Cohen et al. 1999; Sanders et al. 2005). Explanations for growth impairment could include growth hormone deficiency, actual damage to growing bone, or both. One issue of concern is whether single-dose TBI or hyperfractionated TBI causes less damage to growing bone. In a study of 30 adults treated at or before the age of 12 years, Chemaitilly et al. (2007) demonstrated no difference in final height between the two radiotherapy (RT) modalities. Final height, both standing and to a greater extent, sitting, were significantly reduced, more so if survivors were treated at a younger age. The addition of TBI after cranial RT seemed to be associated with the greatest reduction in final height, with no RT associated with the least or no reduction (Cohen et al. 1999). Although not all studies including multiple types of malignancies tested the independent contribution of cancer type, one study that did (Cohen et al. 1999) did not find a difference in final height between ALL, AML, and CML, suggesting that the primary disease itself does not predict growth. There is some evidence that conditioning regimens using busulfan compared to TBI may produce less organ toxicity (Afify et al. 2000; Bernard et al. 2009).

Other late complications following transplant for AML in childhood include bony abnormalities such as decreased bone mineral density, osteochondromas (Bordigoni et al. 2002; Taitz et al. 2004), and osteonecrosis, dental anomalies, including absence of teeth and abnormally shaped teeth (Vaughan et al. 2005), dyslipidemias and metabolic syndrome (Taskinen et al. 2000; Faraci et al. 2005; Perkins et al. 2007), eye problems, including cataracts and dry eye syndrome (Tichelli 1994; Michel et al. 1997; Fahnehjelm et al. 2008), and possibly impaired physical performance in some proportion of children and young adults (Hovi et al. 2010).

10.14 Quality ofL ifeand Neuropsychometric Outcomes

Few studies of health-related quality of life (HRQOL) have been performed in survivors of childhood and adolescent AML, although studies of HRQOL following BMT are somewhat more common and usually include survivors of AML. However, many studies have small sample sizes and are uncontrolled or compare results only to normative data.

HRQOL was studied in 52 Swedish children who had been treated with allogeneic HSCT (Forinder et al. 2005); 8 had AML. The Swedish version of the Child Health Questionnaire (CHQ) was used to measure the QOL outcomes, and the authors found that the overall QOL scores in survivors were not different from U.S. norms. However, the survivors did have lower subscale scores in the following domains: bodily pain, general health, and self-esteem.

As noted earlier in this chapter, there is an adverse impact upon QOL early following BMT (Felder-Puig et al. 2006). A longitudinal study measured HRQOL at five time points during the first year following transplantation. In general, QOL was most impacted at 10 days following BMT and steadily improved during the first six months after BMT; however, some individuals did not experience this degree of improvement. At 1 year after BMT, lower scores persisted in emotional functioning, pain, and communication.

Barrera and Atenafu studied QOL in 46 survivors of pediatric BMT and compared their results to those of a group of sibling controls (Barrera and Atenafu 2008). They found that the physical summary score was significantly lower for survivors, but the psychosocial summary score was not different. Multivariable analysis did not show any variable other than treatment that explained the difference in QOL scores. This study also included neuropsychological outcomes (see below).

Younger age at treatment often portends a higher burden regarding late effects. In a study of 17 survivors of BMT before age three (Perkins et al. 2007), using the age-appropriate CHQ questionnaires, the authors found no adverse QOL outcomes compared to normative data. However, the neuropsychometric outcomes from this group were more informative (see below).

In the largest study to date of HRQOL in survivors of childhood and adolescent AML (Nicholson et al. 2005), 180 survivors of AML diagnosed before 21 years of age were studied using the CHQ and SF-36 instruments. This study included 100 survivors who had been treated with chemotherapy, 26 who had had an autologous BMT, and 54 who had had an allogeneic BMT. Survivors were 20 years of age, on average (range, 8–39), and had been diagnosed at a median age of 4 years (range 0–20); 47% were male and 88% were Caucasian. The overall QOL scores did not differ by treatment group, although those treated with allogeneic BMT had a lower physical summary score when compared to those treated with chemotherapy. The transplant survivors also had a higher burden of more frequent and more severe chronic health conditions; 76% of those treated with allogeneic BMT, 58% of those treated with autologous BMT, and 44% of those treated with chemotherapy reported a chronic health condition. Ninety five percent reported that their health was excellent, very good, or good. Five percent reported cancer-related pain, and 13% reported cancer-related anxiety.

In a cross-sectional study of HRQOL outcomes in 214 adults survivors of HSCT, survivors were found to generally have a good quality of life (Sanders et al. 2010), although significantly lower than a control group in terms of the SF-36 physical summary score as well as the physical function, role physical, and general health domains. In this study, the 68 survivors of AML were more likely to have poorer physical functioning than survivors of the other diseases that made up this cross-sectional study (nonmalignant, ALL, CML). However, they did not differ from the other survivors in terms of overall psychological or cognitive functioning. AML survivors were 27 years of age on average, had a mean time since transplant of 14.7 years, and were evenly split between males and females.

All these studies taken together suggest that HRQOL in survivors is generally good; however, individual survivors may experience late effects or symptoms that negatively impact their QOL, and variations in QOL may occur in individuals.

IQ and other neuropsychometric parameters may also be impacted by anticancer therapy. In a study of 102 BMT survivors that included 32 treated for AML and was powered to detect a 3 point drop in global measures of intelligence (IQ), Phipps et al. (2000) found no difference in IQ or in academic achievement at either 1 or 3 years following BMT. Furthermore, use of TBI in the conditioning regimen was not associated with a drop in IQ; however, those children treated with BMT prior to three years of age had a fall in IQ at both one and three years following BMT.

In a more detailed, but small, study of 17 survivors of acute leukemia (including 14 with AML) treated with BMT prior to the age of three years (Perkins et al. 2007), Perkins found that IQ scores did not differ from population norms. However, survivors performed more poorly on measures of sustained attention, inhibition, response speed, and consistency of attentional effort. Measures of fine motor speed /dexterity and visual-motor integration skills were also inferior to normative data. Academic achievement was not impacted, but measures of adaptive functioning were inferior. In this study, all but 4 had had an allogeneic transplant (76%), and TBI was given to 11 patients (65%). These survivors had been transplanted at a mean age of 1.67 years and the mean follow-up time was 11.5 years (range, 3.25–22.33). Interestingly, none had had chronic GVHD.

In a study of 46 survivors of BMT during childhood, Barrera et al found that survivors did not have significant differences in IQ compared to a group of 33 siblings (Barrera and Atenafu 2008). However, survivors had significantly lower spelling scores and somewhat lower scores in arithmetic and reading (not statistically significant). Psychological adjustment was similar for survivors and siblings, and both were within normal ranges. The QOL outcomes for this study were noteda bove.

10.15 Conclusion

Effective treatments with HSCT for AML in childhood continue to evolve and will contribute to improvements in survival. As survival improves, surveillance and intervention for late effects take on greater roles in management of childhood cancer. However, much remains to be understood as children become adults; specific questions include: what are the predictive factors that can be used to determine who is most in need of follow-up; what comorbidities occur; and which survivors can benefit from intervention studies. As survival after transplant for AML continues to improve, issues of concern include care, management, surveillance, detection, and prevention of adverse outcomes by the late effects care team. The medical surveillance experts, the survivor, and the family should practice effective cooperation with the goal of achieving a good health-relatedqua lityoflife .

References

Afify Z, Shaw PJ et al (2000) Growth and endocrine function in children with acute myeloid leukaemia after bone marrow transplantation using busulfan/cyclophosphamide. Bone Marrow Transplant 25(10):1087–1092

Aoudjhane M, Labopin M et al (2005) Comparative outcome of reduced intensity and myeloablative conditioning regimen in HLA identical sibling allogeneic haematopoietic stem cell transplantation for patients older than 50 years of age with acute myeloblastic leukaemia: a retrospective survey from the Acute Leukemia Working Party (ALWP) of the European group for Blood and Marrow Transplantation (EBMT). Leukemia19(12):2304–2312

Armenian SH, Sun CL et al (2008) Late congestive heart failure after hematopoietic cell transplantation. J Clin Oncol 26(34):5537–5543

Baker KS, DeFor TE et al (2003) New malignancies after blood or marrow stem-cell transplantation in children and adults: incidence and risk factors. J Clin Oncol 21(7):1352–1358

Baker KS, Ness KK et al (2007) Diabetes, hypertension, and cardiovascular events in survivors of hematopoietic cell transplantation: a report from the bone marrow transplantation survivor study. Blood 109(4):1765–1772

Bakker B, Massa GG (2000) Pubertal development and growth after total-body irradiation and bone marrow transplantation for haematological malignancies. Eur J Pediatr 159(1–2): 31–37

Barker JN, Weisdorf DJ et al (2005) Transplantation of 2 partially HLA-matched umbilical cord blood units to enhance engraftment in adults with hematologic malignancy. Blood 105(3):1343–1347

Barrera M, Atenafu E (2008) Cognitive, educational, psychosocial adjustment and quality of life of children who survive hematopoietic SCT and their siblings. Bone Marrow Transplant42(1):15–21

Bearman SI (1995) The syndrome of hepatic veno-occlusive disease after marrow transplantation. Blood 85(11):3005–3020

Becton D, Dahl GV et al (2006) Randomized use of cyclosporin A (CsA) to modulate P-glycoprotein in children with AML in remission: Pediatric Oncology Group Study 9421. Blood 107(4):1315–1324

Bernard F, Bordigoni P et al (2009) Height growth during adolescence and final height after haematopoietic SCT for childhood acute leukaemia: the impact of a conditioning regimen with BU or TBI. Bone Marrow Transplant 43(8):637–642

Bhatia S, Louie AD et al (2001) Solid cancers after bone marrow transplantation. J Clin Oncol 19(2):464–471

Bhatia S, Robison LL et al (2005) Late mortality in survivors of autologous hematopoietic-cell transplantation: report from the Bone Marrow Transplant Survivor Study. Blood 105(11): 4215–4222

Blumenfeld Z, Avivi I et al (2008) Gonadotropin-releasing hormone agonist decreases chemotherapy-induced gonadotoxicity and premature ovarian failure in young female patients with Hodgkin lymphoma. Fertil Steril 89(1):166–173

Bordigoni P, Turello R et al (2002) Osteochondroma after pediatric hematopoietic stem cell transplantation: report of eight cases. Bone Marrow Transplant 29(7):611–614

Brochstein JA, Kernan NA et al (1987) Allogeneic bone marrow transplantation after hyperfractionated total-body irradiation and cyclophosphamide in children with acute leukemia. N Engl J Med 317(26):1618–1624

Bunin NJ, Davies SM et al (2008) Unrelated donor bone marrow transplantation for children with acute myeloid leukemia beyond first remission or refractory to chemotherapy. J Clin Oncol26(26):4326–4332

Byrne J, Rasmussen SA et al (1998) Genetic disease in offspring of long-term survivors of childhood and adolescent cancer. Am J Hum Genet 62(1):45–52

Carter A, Robison LL et al (2006) Prevalence of conception and pregnancy outcomes after hematopoietic cell transplantation: report from the Bone Marrow Transplant Survivor Study. Bone Marrow Transplant 37(11):1023–1029

Chemaitilly W, Mertens AC et al (2006) Acute ovarian failure in the childhood cancer survivor study. J Clin Endocrinol Metab91(5):1723– 1728

Chemaitilly W, Boulad F et al (2007) Final height in pediatric patients after hyperfractionated total body irradiation and stem cell transplantation. Bone Marrow Transplant 40(1): 29–35

Chen AR, Alonzo TA et al (2002) Current controversies: which patients with acute myeloid leukaemia should receive a bone marrow transplantation? – an American view. Br J Haematol 118(2):378–384

CIBMRT (2008) CIBMTR summary slides. CIBMTR Newsletter 14(1):8

Cohen A, Rovelli A et al (1999) Final height of patients who underwent bone marrow transplantation for hematological disorders during childhood: a study by the Working Party for Late Effects-EBMT. Blood 93(12):4109 4115

Cohen A, Rovelli A et al (2007) Risk for secondary thyroid carcinoma after hematopoietic stem-cell transplantation: an EBMT Late Effects Working Party Study. J Clin Oncol 25(17):2449–2454

Couto-Silva AC, Trivin C et al (2001) Factors affecting gonadal function after bone marrow transplantation during childhood. Bone Marrow Transplant 28(1):67–75

Creutzig U, Reinhardt D (2002) Current controversies: which patients with acute myeloid leukaemia should receive a bone marrow transplantation? – a European view. Br J Haematol 118(2):365–377

Creutzig U, Zimmermann M et al (2006) Less toxicity by optimizing chemotherapy, but not by addition of granulocyte colony-stimulating factor in children and adolescents with acute myeloid leukemia: results of AML-BFM 98. J Clin Oncol24(27):4499–4506

Curtis RE, Rowlings PA et al (1997) Solid cancers after bone marrow transplantation. N Engl J Med 336(13):897–904

Curtis RE, Metayer C et al (2005) Impact of chronic GVHD therapy on the development of squamous-cell cancers after hematopoietic stem-cell transplantation: an international case-control study. Blood 105(10):3802–3811

Deeg HJ, Socie G (1998) Malignancies after hematopoietic stem cell transplantation: many questions, some answers. Blood 91(6):1833–1844

Eapen M, Horowitz MM et al (2004) Higher mortality after allogeneic peripheral-blood transplantation compared with bone marrow in children and adolescents: the Histocompatibility and Alternate Stem Cell Source Working Committee of the International Bone Marrow Transplant Registry. J Clin Oncol22(24):4872–4880

Eapen M, Rubinstein P et al (2007) Outcomes of transplantation of unrelated donor umbilical cord blood and bone marrow in children with acute leukaemia: a comparison study. Lancet 369(9577):1947–1954

Engelhard D, Marks MI et al (1986) Infections in bone marrow transplant recipients. J Pediatr 108(3):335–346

Entz-Werle N, Suciu S et al (2005) Results of 58872 and 58921 trials in acute myeloblastic leukemia and relative value of chemotherapy vs allogeneic bone marrow transplantation in first complete remission: the EORTC Children Leukemia Group report. Leukemia 19(12):2072–2081

Fahnehjelm KT, Tornquist AL et al (2008) Dry-eye syndrome after allogeneic stem-cell transplantation in children. Acta Ophthalmol86(3):253–258

Faraci M, Barra S et al (2005) Very late nonfatal consequences of fractionated TBI in children undergoing bone marrow transplant. Int J Radiat Oncol Biol Phys 63(5):1568–1575

Felder-Puig R, di Gallo A et al (2006) Health-related quality of life of pediatric patients receiving allogeneic stem cell or bone marrow transplantation: results of a longitudinal, multicenter study. Bone Marrow Transplant 38(2):119–126

Filipovich AH, Weisdorf D et al (2005) National Institutes of Health consensus development project on criteria for clinical trials in chronic graft-versus-host disease: I Diagnosis and staging working group report. Biol Blood Marrow Transplant 11(12):945–956

Forinder U, Lof C et al (2005) Quality of life and health in children following allogeneic SCT. Bone Marrow Transplant 36(2):171–176

Friedman DL, Rovo A et al (2008) Increased risk of breast cancer among survivors of allogeneic hematopoietic cell transplantation: a report from the FHCRC and the EBMT-Late Effect Working Party. Blood 111(2):939–944

Fuchs EJ, Luznik L et al (2009) Successful pregnancy and childbirth after reduced-intensity conditioning and partially HLA-mismatched BMT. Bone Marrow Transplant 43(12): 969–970

Gale RP, Bortin MM et al (1987) Risk factors for acute graft-versus-host disease. Br J Haematol 67(4):397–406

Gallagher G, Forrest DL (2007) Second solid cancers after allogeneic hematopoietic stem cell transplantation. Cancer 109(1):84–92

Gibson BE, Wheatley K et al (2005) Treatment strategy and long-term results in paediatric patients treated in consecutive UK AML trials. Leukemia 19(12):2130–2138

Glucksberg H, Storb R et al (1974) Clinical manifestations of graft-versus-host disease in human recipients of marrow from HL-A-matched sibling donors. Transplantation 18(4): 295–304

Godder KT, Hazlett LJ et al (2000) Partially mismatched related-donor bone marrow transplantation for pediatric patients with acute leukemia: younger donors and absence of peripheral blasts improve outcome. J Clin Oncol 18(9): 1856–1866

Godder K, Eapen M et al (2004) Autologous hematopoietic stem-cell transplantation for children with acute myeloid leukemia in first or second complete remission: a prognostic factor analysis. J Clin Oncol 22(18):3798–3804

Hann IM, Richards SM et al (1998) Analysis of the immunophenotype of children treated on the Medical Research Council United Kingdom Acute Lymphoblastic Leukaemia Trial XI (MRC UKALLXI). Medical Research Council Childhood Leukaemia Working Party. Leukemia 12(8): 1249–1255

Horan JT, Alonzo TA et al (2008) Impact of disease risk on efficacy of matched related bone marrow transplantation for pediatric acute myeloid leukemia: the Children's Oncology Group. J Clin Oncol 26(35):5797–5801

Horowitz MM, Bortin MM (1993) Results of bone marrow transplants from human leukocyte antigen-identical sibling donors for treatment of childhood leukemias. A report from the International Bone Marrow Transplant Registry. Am J Pediatr Hematol Oncol 15(1):56–64

Horowitz MM, Gale RP et al (1990) Graft-versus-leukemia reactions after bone marrow transplantation. Blood 75(3): 555–562

Hovi L, Kurimo M et al (2010) Suboptimal long-term physical performance in children and young adults after pediatric allo-SCT. Bone Marrow Transplant 45(4):738–745

Jeruss JS, Woodruff TK (2009) Preservation of fertility in patients with cancer. N Engl J Med 360(9):902–911

Kernan NA, Bartsch G et al (1993) Analysis of 462 transplantations from unrelated donors facilitated by the National Marrow Donor Program. N Engl J Med 328(9):593–602

Kersey JH, Ramsay NK et al (1982) Allogeneic bone marrow transplantation in acute nonlymphocytic leukemia: a pilot study. Blood 60(2):400–403

Kletzel M, Jacobsohn D et al (2006) Pharmacokinetics of a test dose of intravenous busulfan guide dose modifications to achieve an optimal area under the curve of a single daily dose of intravenous busulfan in children undergoing a reduced-intensity conditioning regimen with hematopoietic stem cell transplantation. Biol Blood Marrow Transplant 12(4):472–479

Kolb HJ, Socie G et al (1999) Malignant neoplasms in long-term survivors of bone marrow transplantation. Late Effects Working Party of the European Cooperative Group for Blood and Marrow Transplantation and the European Late Effect Project Group. Ann Intern Med 131(10):738–744

Koreth J, Schlenk R et al (2009) Allogeneic stem cell transplantation for acute myeloid leukemia in first complete remission: systematic review and meta-analysis of prospective clinical trials. JAMA 301(22):2349–2361

Kurtzberg J, Prasad VK et al (2008) Results of the Cord Blood Transplantation Study (COBLT): clinical outcomes of unrelated donor umbilical cord blood transplantation in pediatric patients with hematologic malignancies. Blood 112(10): 4318–4327

Lang P, Greil J et al (2004) Long-term outcome after haploidentical stem cell transplantation in children. Blood Cells Mol Dis33(3):281–287

Lange BJ, Smith FO et al (2008) Outcomes in CCG-2961, a children's oncology group phase 3 trial for untreated pediatric acute myeloid leukemia: a report from the children's oncology group. Blood 111(3):1044–1053

Lee SJ, Schover LR et al (2006) American Society of Clinical Oncology recommendations on fertility preservation in cancer patients. J Clin Oncol 24(18):2917–2931

Leisenring W, Friedman DL et al (2006) Nonmelanoma skin and mucosal cancers after hematopoietic cell transplantation. J Clin Oncol 24(7):1119–1126

Leung W, Sandlund JT et al (2001) Second malignancy after treatment of childhood non-Hodgkin lymphoma. Cancer 92(7):1959–1966

Litzow MR, Perez WS et al (2002) Comparison of outcome following allogeneic bone marrow transplantation with cyclophosphamide-total body irradiation versus busulphan-cyclophosphamide conditioning regimens for acute myelogenous leukaemia in first remission. Br J Haematol 119(4):1115–1124

Locatelli F, Zecca M et al (2000) Graft versus host disease prophylaxis with low-dose cyclosporine-A reduces the risk of relapse in children with acute leukemia given HLA-identical sibling bone marrow transplantation: results of a randomized trial. Blood 95(5):1572–1579

MacMillan ML, Weisdorf DJ et al (2009) Acute graft-versus-host disease after unrelated donor umbilical cord blood transplantation: analysis of risk factors. Blood 113(11): 2410–2415

Majhail NS (2008) Old and new cancers after hematopoietic-cell transplantation. Hematology Am Soc Hematol Educ Program142–149

Meshinchi S, Alonzo TA et al (2006) Clinical implications of FLT3 mutations in pediatric AML. Blood 108(12): 3654–3661

Michel G, Gluckman E et al (1994) Allogeneic bone marrow transplantation for children with acute myeloblastic leukemia in first complete remission: impact of conditioning regimen without total-body irradiation – a report from the Societe Francaise de Greffe de Moelle. J Clin Oncol 12(6): 1217–1222

Michel G, Socie G et al (1997) Late effects of allogeneic bone marrow transplantation for children with acute myeloblastic leukemia in first complete remission: the impact of conditioning regimen without total-body irradiation – a report from the Societe Francaise de Greffe de Moelle. J Clin Oncol 15(6):2238–2246

Michel G, Rocha V et al (2003) Unrelated cord blood transplantation for childhood acute myeloid leukemia: a Eurocord Group analysis. Blood 102(13):4290–4297

Nakagawa K, Kanda Y et al (2008) Ovarian shielding allows ovarian recovery and normal birth in female hematopoietic SCT recipients undergoing TBI. Bone Marrow Transplant 42(10):697–699

Nash RA, Antin JH et al (2000) Phase 3 study comparing methotrexate and tacrolimus with methotrexate and cyclosporine for prophylaxis of acute graft-versus-host disease after marrow transplantation from unrelated donors. Blood 96(6): 2062–2068

Nesbit ME Jr, Buckley JD et al (1994) Chemotherapy for induction of remission of childhood acute myeloid leukemia followed by marrow transplantation or multiagent chemotherapy: a report from the Childrens Cancer Group. J Clin Oncol12(1):127–135

Neudorf S, Sanders J et al (2004) Allogeneic bone marrow transplantation for children with acute myelocytic leukemia in first remission demonstrates a role for graft versus leukemia in the maintenance of disease-free survival. Blood 103(10): 3655–3661

Nicholson HS, Zhou T et al (2005) "Quality of life in survivors of childhood and adolescent acute myelogenous leukemia (AML) does not differ by treatment (bone marrow transplant (BMT) vs. chemotherapy). A report from the Children"s Oncology Group (COG) Blood (ASH Annual Meeting Abstracts) 106:701

Parsons SK, Gelber S et al (1999) Quality-adjusted survival after treatment for acute myeloid leukemia in childhood: A Q-TWiST analysis of the Pediatric Oncology Group Study 8821. J Clin Oncol 17(7):2144–2152

Perkins JL, Kunin-Batson AS et al (2007) Long-term follow-up of children who underwent hematopoeitic cell transplant (HCT) for AML or ALL at less than 3 years of age. Pediatr Blood Cancer 49(7):958–963

Phipps S, Dunavant M et al (2000) Cognitive and academic functioning in survivors of pediatric bone marrow transplantation. J Clin Oncol 18(5):1004–1011

Pizzo P, Poplack DA (2005) Principles and practice of pediatric oncology. Lippincott, Boston

Pulsipher MA, Boucher KM et al (2009) Reduced-intensity allogeneic transplantation in pediatric patients ineligible for myeloablative therapy: results of the Pediatric Blood and Marrow Transplant Consortium Study ONC0313. Blood 114(7):1429–1436

Ratanatharathorn V, Nash RA et al (1998) Phase III study comparing methotrexate and tacrolimus (prograf, FK506) with methotrexate and cyclosporine for graft-versus-host disease prophylaxis after HLA-identical sibling bone marrow transplantation. Blood 92(7):2303–2314

Ravindranath Y, Yeager AM et al (1996) Autologous bone marrow transplantation versus intensive consolidation chemotherapy for acute myeloid leukemia in childhood. Pediatric Oncology Group. N Engl J Med 334(22):1428–1434

Ries LA, Smith MA (1999) Cancer incidence and survival among children and adolescents: United States SEER Program 1975–1995. National Cancer Institute, SEER Program, Bethesda

Ringden O, Horowitz MM et al (1993) Methotrexate, cyclosporine, or both to prevent graft-versus-host disease after HLA-identical sibling bone marrow transplants for early leukemia? Blood 81(4):1094–1101

Rizzo JD, Curtis RE et al (2009) Solid cancers after allogeneic hematopoietic cell transplantation. Blood 113(5): 1175–1183

Rocha V, Wagner JE Jr et al (2000) Graft-versus-host disease in children who have received a cord-blood or bone marrow transplant from an HLA-identical sibling. Eurocord and International Bone Marrow Transplant Registry Working Committee on Alternative Donor and Stem Cell Sources. N Engl J Med 342(25):1846–1854

Rocha V, Cornish J et al (2001) Comparison of outcomes of unrelated bone marrow and umbilical cord blood transplants in children with acute leukemia. Blood 97(10):2962–2971

Rovo A, Tichelli A et al (2006) Spermatogenesis in long-term survivors after allogeneic hematopoietic stem cell transplantation is associated with age, time interval since transplantation, and apparently absence of chronic GvHD. Blood 108(3):1100–1105

Rubinstein P, Carrier C et al (1998) Outcomes among 562 recipients of placental-blood transplants from unrelated donors. N Engl J Med 339(22):1565–1577

Salooja N, Szydlo RM et al (2001) Pregnancy outcomes after peripheral blood or bone marrow transplantation: a retrospective survey. Lancet 358(9278):271–276

Sanders JE, Thomas ED et al (1985) Marrow transplantation for children in first remission of acute nonlymphoblastic leukemia: an update. Blood 66(2):460–462

Sanders JE, Hawley J et al (1996) Pregnancies following high-dose cyclophosphamide with or without high-dose busulfan or total-body irradiation and bone marrow transplantation. Blood87(7):3045–3052

Sanders JE, Guthrie KA et al (2005) Final adult height of patients who received hematopoietic cell transplantation in childhood. Blood 105(3):1348–1354

Sanders JE, Hoffmeister PA et al (2009) Thyroid function following hematopoietic cell transplantation in children: 30 years' experience. Blood 113(2):306–308

Sanders JE, Hoffmeister PA et al (2010) The quality of life of adult survivors of childhood hematopoietic cell transplant. Bone Marrow Transplant 45(4):746–754

Santos GW, Tutschka PJ et al (1983) Marrow transplantation for acute nonlymphocytic leukemia after treatment with busulfan and cyclophosphamide. N Engl J Med 309(22): 1347–1353

Sarafoglou K, Boulad F et al (1997) Gonadal function after bone marrow transplantation for acute leukemia during childhood. J Pediatr 130(2):210–216

Schechter T, Finkelstein Y et al (2005) Pregnancy after stem cell transplantation. Can Fam Physician 51:817–818

Shimada K, Yokozawa T et al (2005) Solid tumors after hematopoietic stem cell transplantation in Japan: incidence, risk factors and prognosis. Bone Marrow Transplant 36(2): 115–121

Shulman HM, Sullivan KM et al (1980) Chronic graft-versus-host syndrome in man. A long-term clinicopathologic study of 20 Seattle patients. Am J Med 69(2):204–217

Socie G, Stone JV et al (1999) Long-term survival and late deaths after allogeneic bone marrow transplantation. Late Effects Working Committee of the International Bone Marrow Transplant Registry. N Engl J Med 341(1):14–21

Socie G, Curtis RE et al (2000) New malignant diseases after allogeneic marrow transplantation for childhood acute leukemia. J Clin Oncol 18(2):348–357

Socie G, Salooja N et al (2003) Nonmalignant late effects after allogeneic stem cell transplantation. Blood 101(9): 3373–3385

Stahnke K, Boos J et al (1998) Duration of first remission predicts remission rates and long-term survival in children with relapsed acute myelogenous leukemia. Leukemia 12(10): 1534–1538

Stevens RF, Hann IM et al (1998) Marked improvements in outcome with chemotherapy alone in paediatric acute myeloid leukemia: results of the United Kingdom Medical Research Council's 10th AML trial. MRC Childhood Leukaemia Working Party. Br J Haematol 101(1):130–140

Storb R, Deeg HJ et al (1989a) Methotrexate and cyclosporine versus cyclosporine alone for prophylaxis of graft-versus-host disease in patients given HLA-identical marrow grafts for leukemia: long-term follow-up of a controlled trial. Blood 73(6):1729–1734

Storb R, Deeg HJ et al (1989b) Graft-versus-host disease prevention by methotrexate combined with cyclosporin compared to methotrexate alone in patients given marrow grafts for severe aplastic anaemia: long-term follow-up of a controlled trial. Br J Haematol 72(4):567–572

Surveillance, Epidemiology, and End Results (SEER) Program (www.seer.cancer.gov) SEER*Stat Database: Incidence – SEER 9 Regs Limited-Use, Nov 2008 Sub (1973-2006) <Katrina/Rita Population Adjustment> – Linked To County Attributes – Total U.S., 1969–2006 Counties, National Cancer Institute, DCCPS, Surveillance Research Program, Cancer Statistics Branch, released April 2009, based on the November 2008 submission

Taitz J, Cohn RJ et al (2004) Osteochondroma after total body irradiation: an age-related complication. Pediatr Blood Cancer42(3):225–229

Taskinen M, Saarinen-Pihkala UM et al (2000) Impaired glucose tolerance and dyslipidaemia as late effects after bone-marrow transplantation in childhood. Lancet 356(9234): 993–997

Tichelli A (1994) Late ocular complications after bone marrow transplantation. Nouv Rev Fr Hematol 36(Suppl 1): S79–S82

Tichelli A, Passweg J et al (2008) Late cardiovascular events after allogeneic hematopoietic stem cell transplantation: a retrospective multicenter study of the Late Effects Working Party of the European Group for Blood and Marrow Transplantation. Haematologica 93(8):1203–1210

Uderzo C, Pillon M et al (2009) Cardiac and pulmonary late effects do not negatively influence performance status and non-relapse mortality of children surviving five yr after autologous hematopoietic cell transplantation: report from the EBMT Paediatric Diseases and Late Effects Working Parties. Pediatr Transplant 13(6):719–724

Vaughan MD, Rowland CC et al (2005) Dental abnormalities after pediatric bone marrow transplantation. Bone Marrow Transplant36(8):725–729

Vigorito AC, Campregher PV et al (2009) Evaluation of NIH consensus criteria for classification of late acute and chronic GVHD. Blood 114(3):702–708

Wagner JE, Thompson JS et al (2005) Effect of graft-versus-host disease prophylaxis on 3-year disease-free survival in recipients of unrelated donor bone marrow (T-cell Depletion Trial): a multi-centre, randomised phase II-III trial. Lancet 366(9487):733–741

Webb DK, Wheatley K et al (1999) Outcome for children with relapsed acute myeloid leukaemia following initial therapy in the Medical Research Council (MRC) AML 10 trial. MRC Childhood Leukaemia Working Party. Leukemia 13(1):25–31

Weiner RS, Bortin MM et al (1986) Interstitial pneumonitis after bone marrow transplantation. Assessment of risk factors. Ann Intern Med 104(2):168–175

Winther JF, Boice JD Jr et al (2009) Radiotherapy for childhood cancer and risk for congenital malformations in offspring: a population-based cohort study. Clin Genet 75(1):50–56

Woodruff TK (2009) Preserving fertility during cancer treatment. Nat Med 15(10):1124–1125

Woods WG, Neudorf S et al (2001) A comparison of allogeneic bone marrow transplantation, autologous bone marrow transplantation, and aggressive chemotherapy in children with acute myeloid leukemia in remission: a report from the Children's cancer group [In Process Citation]. Blood 97(1):56–62

Woolfrey AE, Gooley TA et al (1998) Bone marrow transplantation for children less than 2 years of age with acute myelogenous leukemia or myelodysplastic syndrome. Blood 92(10): 3546–3556

Yeager AM, Wagner JE Jr et al (1992) Optimization of busulfan dosage in children undergoing bone marrow transplantation: a pharmacokinetic study of dose escalation. Blood 80(9): 2425–2428

Part VII

Psychosocial Implications of Acute Leukemia Diagnosis and Treatment for Children and Families

11 Appreciation and the Interdisciplinary Management of the Psychosocial Impact of Leukemia on Children and Their Families

Anne L. Angiolillo, Momcilo Jankovic, Riccardo Haupt, Kathleen Ruccione, E. Anne Lown, and Robert B. Noll

Contents

A.L. Angiolillo (✉)
Division of Oncology, Center for Cancer and Blood Disorders, Children's National Medical Center, Washington, DC, USA
e-mail: aangioli@cnmc.org

M. Jankovic
Department of Pediatrics, University of Milano-Bicocca, San Gerardo Hospital, Monza, Italy

R. Haupt
Epidemiology and Biostatistics Section, Scientific Directorate & Department of Hematology/Oncology, Gaslini Children's Hospital, Genova, Italy

K. Ruccione
Children's Hospital, Los Angeles, CA, USA

E.A. Lown
Alcohol Research Group, Emeryville, CA, USA

R.B. Noll
Developmental and Behavioral Pediatrics, Department of Pediatrics, Children's Hospital of Pittsburgh, Pittsburgh, PA, USA

11.1 Models of Psychosocial Health Services

Because of the life-altering and potentially lingering psychosocial effects of leukemia on children and families, pediatric health professionals have developed a variety of interventions to mitigate family distress. Psychosocial health services are psychological and social services and interventions that enable patients, their families, and health care providers to optimize biomedical health care and to manage the psychological/behavioral and social aspects of illness and its consequences so as to promote better health (IOM 2008). Interventions are shaped by, informed by, and/or delivered by psychologists, psychiatrists, social workers, nurses, and chaplains, as well as by oncology subspecialists, ethicists, patients and their families, and advocacy organizations (Holland 2003). These interventions vary in their target population (patients, siblings, and/or parents and other family caregivers), settings, and characteristics. For example, a recent review of psychosocial health services for cancer patients and their families by the United States Institute of Medicine (IOM) found some interventions that were derived from a theoretical framework, some that were based on research evidence,

G.H. Reaman and F.O. Smith (eds.), *Childhood Leukemia*,
DOI: 10.1007/978-3-642-13781-5_11, © Springer-Verlag Berlin Heidelberg 2011

and some that had undergone empirical testing; few evidenced all three characteristics (IOM 2008). Nevertheless, the IOM identified five common elements of models for the effective delivery of psychosocial health services: (1) identifying psychosocial health needs, (2) connecting patients and families to needed services, (3) supporting them in managing the illness, (4) coordinating psychosocial care with biomedical care, and (5) following up on care delivery to evaluate the effectiveness of these services (Fineberg 2008).

Effective patient–provider communication, as described elsewhere in this chapter (IOM 2008), is central to all the components of psychosocial health services models. The change in attitudes toward open communication about cancer with children and their families was instrumental in the evolution of psychosocial health services. Patenaude and Kupst note that mental health professionals first began to have a role within pediatric oncology treatment teams to assist with the emotional issues related to open communication. With their presence, mental health professionals fostered awareness of behavioral challenges faced by children with cancer, and the impact of cancer on the whole family (Patenaude et al. 2005).

An early example of a comprehensive pediatric cancer psychosocial health services program, based at Children's Hospital Los Angeles in the mid-1970s, was purposively designed to be a part of the biomedical treatment team and was comprised of mental health professionals with pediatric oncology training (clinical psychologists, social worker, oncology nurse coordinator, and child life specialists); the program had a nonpathologic short-term psychosocial rehabilitation emphasis, with the family viewed as the adaptive unit (Kellerman 1980). Twenty years later, a multidisciplinary panel, convened by an American Cancer Society initiative, developed a psychosocial protocol for childhood cancer to offer clinical practice guidelines for all disciplines through the phases of cancer treatment (Lauria et al. 1996). The protocol's components include use of a multidisciplinary team of specialists, availability of essential programs and resources, multidisciplinary and integrated assessment, identification of common psychosocial issues and clinical interventions, and use of outcome evaluations.

The most recent update of the American Academy of Pediatrics' Guidelines for Pediatric Cancer Centers states that oncologic care should be provided in a pediatric center that meets defined criteria for personnel, facilities, and capabilities. The criteria include pediatric oncology nurses, social workers, pediatric psychologists, child life specialists, and access to family support services, as well as a formal program for cancer education for the family and instruction on self-management (Corrigan and Feig 2004). Another relevant source of standards and guidelines is the National Comprehensive Cancer Network (NCCN), a US organization of comprehensive cancer centers. Although primarily directed toward adult cancer patients, the NCCN developed consensus standards for psychosocial care centered on distress management (Table 11.1), as well as guidelines for evaluating and treating patients with severe distress that can be adapted for use with families of young people with cancer.

Table 11.1 NCCN Standards of care for distress management v.12010

Distress should be recognized, monitored, documented, and treated promptly at all stages of disease and in all settings.
Screening should identify the level and nature of the distress.
All patients should be screened for distress at their initial visit, at appropriate intervals, and as clinically indicated, especially with changes in disease status (i.e., remission, recurrence, progression).
Distress should be assessed and managed according to clinical practice guidelines.
Interdisciplinary institutional committees should be formed to implement standards for distress management.
Educational and training programs should be developed to ensure that health care professionals and certified chaplains have knowledge and skills in the assessment and management of distress.
Licensed mental health professionals and certified chaplains experienced in psychosocial aspects of cancer should be readily available as staff members or by referral.
Medical care contracts should include reimbursement for services provided by mental health professionals.
Clinical health outcomes measurement should include assessment of the psychosocial domain (for example, quality of life and patient and family satisfaction).
Patients, families, and treatment teams should be informed that management of distress is an integral part of total medical care and provided with appropriate information about psychosocial services in the treatment center and the community.
Quality distress management programs/services should be included in institutional continuous quality improvement projects.

The development of models, standards, clinical guidelines, and publications such as the IOM report, "*Cancer Care for the Whole Patient: Meeting Psychosocial Health Needs*," indicates that psychosocial health services are being recognized as an essential aspect of quality care for children with cancer and their families. How patients and families are linked to psychosocial health services will vary. Methods include using local resources, referral to remote providers, or on-site collocation/clinical integration of services (IOM 2008). However, the IOM asserts that it is possible for all cancer care providers to meet the standard of care (Table 11.2) in some way. The report made three recommendations that underscore (1) the need for health care providers to ensure that their patients receive care that meets the standard; (2) the need for patient education and advocacy organizations to educate patients and families about what psychosocial health services to expect, and (3) the need for evaluation of approaches to efficiently provide psychosocial health services that meet the standard (IOM 2008). Translating these recommendations into practice represents a major challenge. Few pediatric cancer treatment centers have been able to develop and sustain a comprehensive program of psychosocial health services. One exemplar is the HOPE Program at Children's Hospital Los Angeles, which has implemented a model with interdigitated components for patient and family education, school and social reintegration, age/developmental stage and role-specific support groups, neuropsychology services, a clinical psychology referral service, outcomes research, and student/staff training. This program relies entirely on philanthropic support and grant funding.

Table 11.2 A recommended standard of care (Adapted from IOM 2008)

All parties establishing or using standards for the quality of cancer care should adopt the following as a standard:
All cancer care should ensure the provision of appropriate psychosocial health services by:
Facilitating effective communication between patients[a] and care providers
Identifying each patient's psychosocial health needs
Designing and implementing a plan that
Links the patient with needed psychosocial services
Coordinates biomedical and psychosocial care
Engages and supports patients in managing their illness and health
Systematically following up on, reevaluating, and adjusting plans

[a]The term "patients" refers to both patients and families when the patient is a child

A number of resources are available for health care providers to use as adjuncts to psychosocial health services, such as the American Psychosocial Oncology Society (APOS) on-line multidisciplinary training modules available at http://www.apos-society.org/professionals/meetings-ed/webcasts/webcasts-multidisciplinary.aspx, which include a module on the challenges and strategies in establishing a psychosocial program. Other resources include the APOS "*Quick Reference for Pediatric Oncology Clinicians: The Psychiatric and Psychological Dimensions of Pediatric Cancer Symptom Management*" (Wiener et al. 2009), and public web portals and websites (such as searchHOPE.org and CureSearch.org). A resource recommended by the IOM report, but not yet extant is a directory of pediatric cancer programs that have psychosocial health services; such a listing would contribute to the ability of providers everywhere to consult operating programs, share lessons learned, and collaborate to implement today's standards and guidelines.

Finally, there is a growing body of scientific publications related to psychosocial health services and interventions that should form the foundation for empirically supported psychosocial health services. The literature is filled with research-based conclusions on which type of psychosocial intervention is best (Masera et al. 1993), including when and how to communicate with the child about the diagnosis (Jankovic et al. 1994; Masera et al. 1997a, b), how to help parents maintain some sense of normality in their family life (Horwitz and Kazak 1990; Birenbaum 1991), how to help the child return to school (Masera et al. 1995), how to keep the siblings informed (Chesler et al. 1991), how to start parent groups (Chesler and Barbarin 1987), how to involve parents in medical decision-making (Chesler and Barbarin 1987), how to prepare for the terminal phase of the disease when it occurs for some unfortunate children (Spinetta et al. 1981), and how to continue to monitor long-term survivors (Speechley and Noh 1992; Masera et al. 1996). However, based on excellent recent review articles and meta-analyses, it has become evident that there are significant challenges to be addressed in this area. Many studies to date have been descriptive and correlational

(Kazak 2005) and there has been limited ability to compare results across studies. A meta-analysis of 12 intervention studies found only modest support for the effectiveness of current interventions, with the most notable positive findings for parents' distress and adjustment; no significant effect sizes were found for child distress (Pai et al. 2006).

There is a need for more intervention research that ties together intervention elements, outcomes, and measures to theoretical models, as well as research that reports effect sizes, identifies specific subsets of patients for targeted interventions (or possibly no needed interventions), includes participants with ethnic and linguistic diversity, tests brief deliverable interventions that mesh with pediatric biomedical practice, utilizes longitudinal and control group designs, addresses both issues of survivorship and palliative care, and identifies correlates or predictors of positive adaptation and adjustment (Kazak 2005; Patenaude and Kupst 2005; Phipps 2005; Pai et al. 2006). In addition, interdisciplinary research that taps the varying perspectives of psychology, nursing, social work, and others should be the norm in a field as interdisciplinary in nature as psycho-oncology. The empirical underpinnings of psychosocial health services are a fertile area for ongoing research and collaboration. Findings from this research will guide the implementation and refinement of the services provided to help patients and families cope with the formidable challenges of childhood leukemia.

11.2 Communicationo fDi agnosis

Helping a family whose child has been diagnosed with a life-threatening illness is a daunting task. Communication technique is the most basic skill that must be mastered when the diagnosis of leukemia, or any other cancer, has to be reported to the patient and family. The technique and skill one uses becomes the first step in a communicative process between the medical team and the family that allows for growth and change over time. Initial communication of the diagnosis to the family is the most important physician interaction, crucial for a family that is in shock from the information that their child has a potentially fatal disease. Keeping in mind that communication is an ongoing effort that will be continued for many days and weeks to come, the following is a well-accepted approach.

As soon as possible, when laboratory and clinical results are confirmed, the senior physician or the director of the clinic (when available) communicates the diagnosis to both parents together and tells them about the "program of care." This should be communicated in a private room in the presence of a nurse from the inpatient clinic where the child is being treated. The treatment program, the prognosis, and roles of each team member should be carefully explained. The family should be told how it might confront the difficult experience, and attention should be paid to particular family needs, especially regarding the school and other siblings. With the consent of the parents, the meeting can be audio taped, and a copy of the tape given to the parents (Tattersall et al. 1994; Masera et al. 2003). The primary care physician or family physician should have the option of attending this meeting; in addition, the primary physician should be frequently updated on the patient's status through periodic letters or telephone calls. An opportunity for contact with the treating clinic's physician should be offered to the primary physician.

In past years, evidence mounted that children, siblings, and parents would be best served by being encouraged to bring their anxieties about the illness and its possible consequences into the open. Therefore, studies were developed that focused greater attention on how parents and medical personnel communicated with the child (Masera et al. 1997a, b). Parents most often manage what and how their children are told about leukemia. Adolescents or young adults vary in their preferences as to how much information should be disclosed to them. Some adolescents and young adults with cancer prefer to be fully informed about their disease, but approximately one-third of those surveyed declared their preference not to know (Masera et al. 1997a, b; Spinetta et al. 2003). The active process of seeking and obtaining information about leukemia/cancer appears to be related to improved self-confidence, and young survivors who preferred and received open communication about their diagnosis and prognosis at the initial stage of the disease also showed significantly less anxiety and depression later on. Attitudes about information seeking may change over time, and the extent to which survivors and their family members perceive risks of relapse or a "need to know" may also influence information seeking (Olechnowicz et al. 2002; Zwaanswijk et al. 2007; Coyne 2008). Thus, communication continues to be a dynamic process.

There are, at the present, no hard and fast rules about when, how, and what should be explained to a child regarding the diagnosis of cancer, and at what age (Mulhern et al. 1981; Spinetta et al. 1981; Chesler et al. 1986). How this issue is managed, especially for the young child, depends upon the parents' child-rearing values in conjunction with their views regarding the child's level of development and capacity to understand. Cultural norms and expectations enter heavily into this issue of communication (Spinetta 1978; Slavin et al. 1982; Chesler et al. 1991; Jankovic et al. 1994; Masera et al. 1997a, b). Many parents find it difficult to talk to young children about issues as serious as the diagnosis of leukemia. Without proper communication, the child's reaction to the disease, treatment, and new or altered life situations can cause additional stress for the parents.

Parents want what is best for the child, but are often at a loss as to how to tell the child about the illness. By the time parents are told of the diagnosis, many children are already aware that something is wrong with their health. Despite this awareness by the child, parents find it very difficult to begin the dialogue. Communication of the diagnosis, especially to the young child, is often done in the presence of the parents, and even by the parents themselves. In some cases, the physician may communicate with the child directly without the parents being present, thereby opening the dialogue so that the parents and the child can then speak freely about the illness (Jankovic et al. 1994). By having the physician speak directly to the child from the beginning, trust, rapport, and confidence are established between the child and the physician, making subsequent discussions and decision sharing more feasible and more effective. This will ensure, on the part of the child, a more ready and willing compliance with the treatment regimen.

Problems occur when the communication approach must be modified to meet the needs and cultural expectations of particular children and their families. This is especially true when conclusions that are appropriate for one familial setting or culture are applied to another familial situation and/or culture. The communication of a diagnosis to the child can become problematic in a culture not accustomed to such openness with children. In such a culture, the family must be counseled regarding the importance of such open communication. In addition, they must be shown how to communicate at the child's level of development. Involving the parents in the decision-making process regarding their child's treatment, especially at the terminal phase, is very difficult in a culture that is used to a physician making all such decisions. Any movement in the direction of greater parental involvement must be tailored not only to cultural expectations, but also to the individual family's level of preparedness for such involvement. Sending a child back to school as soon as possible after initial treatment might not be acceptable to many parents or teachers. Nevertheless, these individuals must be educated on the value of an early return to school for the patient. Asking a parent to discipline their child in a manner consistent with family history may be problematic for parents who are culturally expected to give special treatment to a sick child (Masera et al. 1997a, b).

It is a challenge for pediatric hematologists to modify their approach to the children and their families for maximal success, in a manner most appropriate to and respectful of the needs of the families within their own culturals etting.

11.3 Sociall mpacto ft he Child–Schooll ssue

As treatment for childhood leukemia became more widely effective, studies began to focus on children treated as outpatients. Although these studies demonstrated that the children continued to be aware of the seriousness of their illness (Spinetta and Maloney 1975), they dwelled less and less on their illness and were able, while in remission, to live a relatively normal life, somewhat free of concerns about their illness. Survival, on the other hand, means that the children have to continue to be educated toward eventually becoming fully functioning adult members of the society. Therefore, it is important to focus attention on the normalizing influence of school. Programs should be developed to help the children to return to their typical life as school children, and teachers should be trained to treat the children as normally as possible. Depending on medical conditions, and the wishes of the child, channels of communication should be open between the hospital personnel and the teachers at the school of origin. This could begin with a letter to the principal and informational booklets sent to the teachers. Telephone calls would follow this preliminary contact, inviting the teacher to visit the cancer treatment center (Lansky et al. 1983; Jankovic et al. 1994; Masera et al. 1995).

A physician from the cancer treatment center could go to the school of origin to explain the medical aspects of leukemia to the teachers and to the child's classmates. The leukemic child should attend the explanation and should be actively involved. An annual meeting between in-hospital teachers and teachers from the child's school of origin should be encouraged (Masera et al. 1997a, b). This approach helps the leukemic child return to the usual school routines. It also helps classmates in their psychosocial growth by helping them avoid discrimination of colleagues who are "different" and by addressing their fear of the unknown.

11.4 Discussiono ft heT reatment Plan and Informed Consent

Compliance with medical regimens is an unquestioned assumption, but do the children have a right to participate in medical decisions regarding their own treatment? Clearly, the answer to this question depends on the developmental level of the child, as well as on the particular culture's view of the rights of the child (Blusteina ndM oreno 1999;B ragadottir 2000).

It is important to distinguish "informed consent" from "valid informed consent" (Syse 2000). "Informed consent" by itself has often come to mean legally signed documentation, without necessarily incorporating understanding on the part of the signer. "Valid informed consent" emphasizes the patient's understanding of that to which consent is being given. The understanding must include the reasonable as well as irrational thoughts and emotions associated with the proposed treatment program. Valid informed consent comes first and foremost with human interaction, and not only with standardized models and formalized written documentation. Physicians should be encouraged to share developmentally relevant and culturally appropriate medical information with the child, so that the child can actively participate in the decision-making process for health-related interventions.

For adolescents of legal age, there should be a full and legally mandated power to make their own decisions regarding medical treatment, with all of the rights and privileges accorded to adult patients, which in fact they are (Spinetta et al. 2002). Younger children should be accorded full respect for their capacity to understand and for their desire, at an appropriate age level, to participate in decisions regarding medical interventions (Jankovic et al. 2004). Each clinic should take it upon itself to put in writing, procedures for informed consent to be followed at that particular clinic (Spinetta et al. 2003, 2006, 2009).

11.5 FamilyDi stressandR esilience in the Face of a Childhood Cancer Diagnosis

A diagnosis of leukemia in a child is a profoundly challenging event for parents and other family members. While most families adjust well to the demands of an ill child, substantial distress is widely reported initially, especially depression and anxiety. Increasingly complex treatments and extended care of a sick child in the home can compel parents to shift their daily routine resulting in employment changes, difficulty caring for other siblings, and loss of social and personal time. The extended length of cancer treatment means these changes can be enduring and sometimes accompanied by employment instability, shifts in support networks, and financial challenges (Eiser and Upton 2007). Though distress is often reported, parents also exhibit resilience, find new meaning in life, experience appreciation for the help from friends and family for their child's care and support, and note personal benefits of the cancer experience, including increased self-confidence, renewed family closeness, and greater clarity about meaningful elements of their lives. Relatively stable families tend to remain stable during treatment despite its challenges.

The following section will present a framework for understanding parent and sibling distress and resilience during and after the treatment of an ill child, describe the adjustment of mothers, fathers, and siblings to childhood cancer, and describe resilience in coping with the experience. It will also provide recommendations, based on current evidence, to improve, support, and enhance coping.

11.5.1 A Framework for Understanding Distress

A social-ecological model can be applied to better understand the distress of the family in the context of childhood illness. The illness impacts the entire family system including parents, siblings, grandparents, and so on (Kazak 1989). As such, it is important that the treatment environment takes into account and supports key elements of each child's family. The importance of addressing parental distress cannot be overemphasized. Their healthy adjustment leads to better overall family functioning and benefits the survivors' and siblings' well-being (Massimo and Caprino 2007; Noll andK upst 2007).

The social-ecological perspective extends the examination of factors beyond individual characteristics and coping behaviors to include family functioning, neighborhood resources, and community conditions (Kazak 2001). This model for understanding stress and adaptation was first proposed by Bronfenbrenner (1979) and later applied to childhood chronic illness by Kazak (1992). This model (Fig. 11.1) examines the child with cancer, parents, and siblings in relation to their environment through a series of concentric circles. The central circle contains individual characteristics (demographic, health status, coping, and cancer). The next ring includes the immediate family environment, reflecting parental psychological and social adjustment. This is followed by three more circles that include: (1) the neighborhood (health care settings, local agencies, schools, and peers); (2) systems beyond the immediate family (parents' workplaces and social networks or siblings' schools); and (3) policy (for instance, protections from the American Disabilities Act) or culture (which can impact on attitudes and prejudices towards cancer). All of these factors play a role in determining the adjustment of the child, parents, and siblings.

The model points to the need for support and care of parents of children with cancer to come from multiple levels and suggests that the burden should not fall

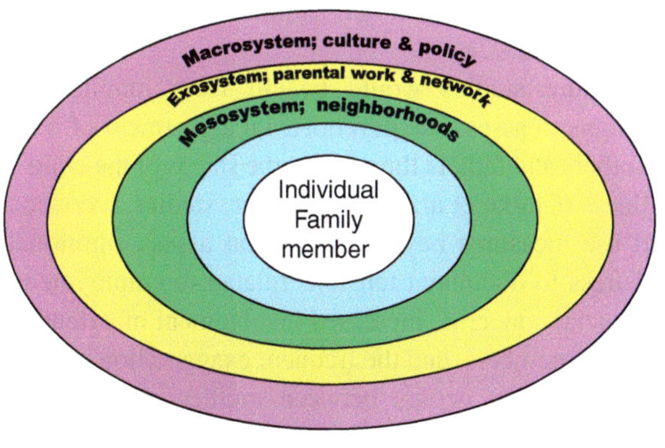

Fig.11.1 Thes ociale cologicalm odel

solely on the health care organization. The introduction of websites for families with a child with cancer helps create momentum for family, friend, and neighborhood support that can complement programs provided by the health care setting. Because families commonly seek information on the web, providing parents with recommended sites has the potential to ensure support and minimize risk.

11.5.2 Mothers

Mothers of children with cancer often report anxiety and depression (Sloper 2000a, b; Landolt et al. 2003; Barrera et al. 2004; Steele et al. 2004) when their child is initially diagnosed. There is some evidence that they also experience other symptoms of posttraumatic stress syndrome (PTSS) and posttraumatic stress disorder (PTSD) (Pelcovitz et al. 1996; Stuber et al. 1996; Brown et al. 2003; Kazak et al. 2004a, b, 2005). The period following the child's diagnosis and the start of treatment is often especially challenging as mothers adjust to the reality of their child's illness. During this time, over half the mothers meet criteria for acute stress disorder (Patino-Fernandez et al. 2008). As mothers begin to focus on treatment-related concerns, the acute symptoms diminish over the next 6 months. However, there is evidence that a relatively small subset of mothers remain highly distressed for longer periods of time. These mothers tend to have poorer personal and coping resources (Dolgin et al. 2007). While mothers of children with cancer experience significant distress, psychopathology does not appear to occur more frequently than what is reported for parents of typically developing children (Brown et al. 1992).

Nearly 30% of mothers of adolescents with cancer meet the criteria for PTSD (Kazak et al. 2004a, b), and 68% of mothers whose children are in treatment have moderate to severe symptoms (Kazak et al. 2005). Rates remain high (44%) by the end of treatment (Stuber et al. 1996; Manne et al. 1998, 2001; Kazak et al. 2004a, b). However, not all studies report rates of PTSD being higher than norms. PTSD rates have been noted to be lower or similar to controls in mothers of children with cancer being treated as outpatients and in mothers whose children have completed treatment (Jurbergs et al. 2009). It is worth noting that there has been some controversy about PTSD rates among parents of children with cancer.

Rates of PTSD vary greatly between studies due to different methods of measurement of PTSD, measurement of distress at different time points during the treatment or survivorship, and variable use of controls. While it is clear that a subset of parents have higher stress responses to the childhood cancer experience, a broader perspective should be adopted, including measurement of subclinical PTSS and other psychological problems and the use of longitudinal methods to study adjustment over time (Jurbergs et al. 2009; Manne 2009; Werba and Kazak 2009).

A number of risk factors for distress have been identified. Trait anxiety (long-term anxiety that preceded the cancer) appears to be the strongest predictor of PTSS (Hoekstra-Weebers et al. 1999), along with perceived life threat and perceived treatment intensity for the child, lack of social support (Kazak et al. 1998), and poor coping skills (Kupst et al. 1995). Social support is widely described as improving mothers' adjustment (Speechley and Noh 1992; Noll et al. 1995; Dahlquist et al. 1996; Kazak et al. 1997; Manne et al. 2000; Best et al. 2001). However, not all social support is equally effective. Support from close family members buffers distress more than social support from the wider community, though mothers of children with cancer do mobilize larger social networks than comparison mothers (Gerhardt et al. 2007).

Problem Solving Skills Training has shown promise in reducing negative affect and increasing mothers' ability to cope with the complex needs of a family affected by pediatric cancer. The training involves eight individualized sessions emphasizing six steps: having a positive orientation, identifying the problem, determining possible options, evaluating options and choosing the best one, implementing the option and determining if it worked (Sahler et al. 2005). This training was studied using a large sample of 430 English, Spanish, and Hebrew speaking mothers from eight sites in the USA and Israel. While the training was found to be effective for all mothers, it was particularly effective for single mothers, Spanish speaking mothers, and young mothers.

A second interventional study has provided preliminary data on 49 parents (primarily mothers) of children newly diagnosed with cancer and also focused on teaching coping skills. This intervention included six face-to-face sessions, telephone calls, and a web-based component. The intervention was most effective in reducing symptoms of distress among mothers who reported low social support at the time of diagnosis (Ewinge ta l. 2009).

11.5.3 Fathers

A smaller body of research describes adaptation among fathers of children with cancer, showing that they report similar levels of distress compared to norms or controls (Overholser and Fritz 1990; Noll et al. 1995), as well as similar levels of anxiety, family conflict, and social support as comparisons (Gerhardt et al. 2007). In a review study, few differences were described between mothers' and fathers' perceptions of marital, family, and child functioning, though traditional gender roles in parenting tasks were reported (Clarke et al. 2009). While fathers' anxiety appears to be lower than that of mothers' at diagnosis, fathers' anxiety is less likely to decrease over the treatment period (Dahlquist eta l. 1996).

Despite depression and anxiety rates comparable to controls, PTSD (at some point since their child's diagnosis) is more common among fathers (11.5%) of children with cancer compared to controls, although it is lower than the rate among mothers (29.5%) of children with cancer (Kazak et al. 2004a, b). While some fathers experience PTSS, a majority of fathers of adolescent survivors also reported posttraumatic growth (Barakat et al. 2006). Predictors of distress often differ between mothers and fathers. Mothers tend to seek out more social support and use more emotion-focused coping (Clarke et al. 2009) compared to fathers, who focus their attention on employment or financial concerns (Frank et al. 2001). Resources that help fathers to adapt and remain positive about their child's cancer include support from health care professionals, extended family members, and church communities (Brody and Simmons 2007).

Future studies would benefit from longitudinal designs to assess the psychosocial adjustment of both mothers and fathers throughout the stages of the child's illness (Clarke et al. 2009). Further, studies may need to use measures beyond those that assess emotional distress to document tensions related to employment, financial concerns, increased involvement of extended family members, and the frequent exaggeration of gender roles that occurs between mothers and fathers. While some work has demonstrated that distress in mothers can be alleviated utilizing straightforward behavioral strategies, similar evidence has not been reported for fathers.

11.5.4 Siblings

The often long and complex treatment protocols for patients with leukemia have the potential to take a toll on siblings, whose needs can become a low priority for family, relatives, and oncology care teams. Treatments often involve many visits to the hospital, prolonged hospitalizations, preoccupation of parents, disruptions in home life, and loss of company and companionship of the sister or brother with cancer. In this context, some research has reported that siblings experience anxiety, depression, academic problems, loneliness, conflicted feelings, isolation, physical health problems (Zeltzer et al. 1996; Houtzager et al. 1999) and family, school and social problems (Alderfer et al. 2010). Posttraumatic stress symptoms are common among siblings, with 29–38% reporting moderate to severe symptoms (Alderfer et al. 2003; Kazak et al. 2004a, b; Packmane ta l. 2004).

Findings related to sibling distress are not consistent and some studies find no emotional adjustment differences in siblings compared to norms or controls. In a review of 65 studies of siblings of children with cancer, 68% of the studies described no differences in depression and 78% reported no difference in anxiety compared to norms (Alderfer et al. 2010). Psychopathology is unusual (Barrera et al. 2002; Houtzager et al. 2004a, b). While most siblings adjust well, those who have difficulties are often older, females (Alderfer et al. 2003), have chaotic families (Houtzager et al. 2004a, b), and are closer to the time of diagnosis (Houtzager et al. 2004a, b; Lahteenmaki et al. 2004). Of note, positive outcomes related to emotional, family and school/social adjustment have also been reported by siblings. Increased closeness between family members is often described as a benefit (Sloper 2000a, b;M acLeode ta l. 2003;W ienere ta l. 2008).

Interventions to support siblings include individualized programs, camps, and support groups aimed at increasing medical knowledge and coping skills. There is some suggestion that, as a whole, these types of interventions result in significant decreases in symptoms of depression (Prchal and Landolt 2009). Further work using randomized clinical trials is badly needed to ensure that evidence-based interventions can be provided. Current recommendations encourage the inclusion of siblings in support groups and hospital visits, but are not yet supported by empirical studies. Inclusion of siblings is difficult when treatment occurs at a distance from the home. In these situations, camps and national sibling support programs are recommended.

The presence of the family in the treatment setting facilitates identification and prevention of psychosocial problems among siblings. Because of high demands in oncology treatment settings, there is a clear need for sibling support to come from nonmedical settings, particularly from the community of people and institutions surrounding the survivor and family. Interventions based in school, religious communities, neighborhoods, and sports or afterschool programs may provide a natural basis for sibling support. While pediatric oncology teams often lack the resources to manage these issues for each sibling, they can serve as a resource to the broader community that provides behavioral health support to children.

In summary, there is considerable evidence that parents and family caregivers experience significant distress when children are initially diagnosed with cancer. There is evidence suggesting that specific interventions can alleviate distress for family caregivers with the potential to facilitate child's care. Work needs to be done to identify empirically supported interventions that might facilitate the adjustment of siblings, so that treatment teams can tailor care to best meet the needsoff amilies.

11.6 Diagnosiso fDep ressiveo rA nxiety Disorders and Serotonin Reuptake Inhibitor Prescription Practices

The improved rates of survival for children with cancer are a result of increasingly aggressive and complex protocols. During therapy, there has been a significant focus on children's behavioral health. Specifically, there has been considerable focus on distress, anxiety, and depression that may occur in children who are receiving treatment for cancer. Several recent review articles (Marsland et al. 2006; Dolgin et al. 2007; Noll and Kupst 2007) have examined the evidence for increased rates of psychiatric disorders (specifically depression or anxiety) in children with cancer during treatment. Despite the obvious challenges and stress, the prevalence of psychosocial dysfunction (i.e., psychopathology or social dysfunction) is similar to that found in the general population or appropriate comparison groups, such as age and gender-matched peers. While many behavioral health specialists and members of pediatric oncology treatment teams hold the view that depression and/or anxiety in children with cancer is underrecognized, the data from numerous studies using a wide range of measurement strategies (observations, questionnaires, interviews) and sources of data (patients, parents, professional observations), show modest evidence for an increased prevalence of internalizing disorders in children receiving treatment for cancer. Noll and Kupst (Noll and Kupst 2007) present Human EvolutionAry Response to Trauma/Stress (HEART), a framework with which to examine human responses to randomly occurring traumatic or stressful life events in pediatric behavioral health, not pediatric psychology (Fig. 11.2). This theoretical position predicts that children with cancer should not become dysfunctional unless the treatment or disease has an adverse affect on the child's central nervous system. Despite evidence that rates of depression or anxiety in children with cancer are not greater than those of healthy peers, the 10.2% rate of medication for depression greatly exceeds the 1% documented in the general pediatricpopula tion(Ems liee ta l. 2004).

While depression and anxiety may not be more common in children receiving treatment for cancer than for typically developing children, identification of depression or anxiety in children with cancer is extremely important. These behavioral health problems are commonly associated with poorer medical outcomes and increased disability for children who are receiving treatment for medical illness (Shemesh et al. 2002). Unfortunately, two of the three main symptoms of depression in children (loss of interest and loss of energy) and several of the additional symptoms of depressive disorders (decreased concentration, low self confidence, sleep disturbance, decrease in appetite) overlap with common symptoms experienced by children during treatment for their disease (Reuter and Harter 2004). This overlap of symptoms makes the diagnosis of depressive disorder or anxiety disorder in a child who is physically sick and hospitalized an exceptionally challenging enterprise, even for the most experienced pediatric oncology or behavioral health specialist. Recent work (Hedstrom et al. 2006) demonstrates that estimates of distress by physicians and nurses compared to adolescents' self-reports are reasonably acceptable for ratings of physical distress, but staff ratings for psychosocial problems, such as anxiety and depression, show poor correspondence to the self-reports of adolescents. Of importance, physicians and nurses consistently overestimated levels of anxiety and depression.

As stated, evidence suggests that psychiatric disorders in children with cancer are not more common than in typically developing children, and it is challenging to differentiate symptoms of depression or anxiety from side effects of cancer and its treatment. However, it still seems

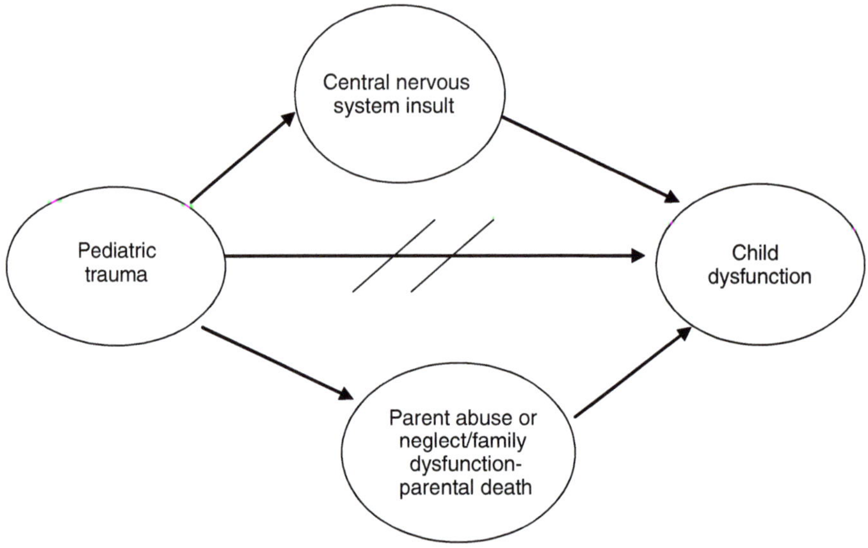

Fig. 11.2 Human EvolutionAry Response to Trauma/Stress(HEART)

likely that some children with cancer will experience these problems, given the base rates of these disorders in typically developing children and teenagers. The National Institutes of Health have recently sponsored two multisite randomized controlled trials exploring treatment options for anxiety (Walkup et al. 2008) and depressive disorders (March et al. 2004) in children and adolescents. Both investigations used medications, cognitive behavioral therapy, or the combination of both to treat these children. The conclusion from both studies was similar, showing that a combination of medication and cognitive behavioral therapy offers the most effective treatment for these disorders. Of note, both of these multisite trials excluded children with a chronic illness, such as cancer. Little has been published concerning the impact of psychotropic medications for children who are also receiving chemotherapy. Based on these data, a prudent recommendation for children with cancer who are experiencing symptoms of anxiety or depression is an initial trial of cognitive behavioral therapy, and if this is not immediately effective, psychotropic medications can be added. The aim of this recommendation is to reduce potential drug interactions and adverse events. Additionally, this recommendation is made within the context of recent work suggesting that published evidence based on antidepressant trials may be biased (that is, there has been selective publication of positive results) (Turner et al. 2008).

Some recent work has closely examined the Selective Serotonin Reuptake Inhibitor (SSRI) prescription practices of pediatric oncologists. This topic is of particular interest due to lack of data supporting the efficacy and safety of these medications in pediatric populations, as well as the 2004 conclusion of the FDA that SSRIs can increase suicidal thoughts and behaviors in children and adolescents (Leslie et al. 2005), resulting in a "black box warning" label for all SSRIs. A single site study performed by Kersun and Kazak (2006) surveyed 28 pediatric oncology attendings and 12 fellows. Half of the respondents reported prescribing SSRIs to oncology patients; of the half that did not report prescribing these medications, only four reported not doing so based on the FDA black box warning.

An additional study used a similar brief questionnaire to examine the SSRI prescribing practices of pediatric oncologists at nine institutions (Weiner et al. 2010). One hundred and fifty-three of 193 (79%) attendings and fellows (99 attendings, 54 fellows) responded to the 17-item survey. The survey asked how often the physicians prescribed SSRIs for their pediatric cancer patients and how physicians monitored patients in accordance with the FDA black box warning. Seventy-one percent of the respondents confirmed prescribing SSRIs to children with cancer. Of those prescribing, 50% prescribed to their patients less than 5% of the time, 36% prescribed 5–10% of the time, 12% prescribed 10–25% of the time, and 2% prescribed over 50% of the time. Physicians were also asked to describe their comfort levels with prescribing specific psychotropic medications, with interesting results. For fluoxetine (Prozac), the only SSRI indicated for pediatric populations, 63% of respondents felt uncomfortable prescribing. Conversely, paroxetine (Paxil), which is contraindicated for children under 18 years, was preferred by 56% of prescribers.

In response to a "yes or no" item in the questionnaire asking whether the FDA black box warning had affected their practices, 51% of respondents answered that it had not. Startlingly, while 71% of the pediatric oncologists surveyed prescribed SSRIs to their patients, the awareness of monitoring procedures associated with the black box warning was minimal. Prescribers did not report following FDA guidelines for follow-up after being prompted with an open-ended question; there was no mention of follow-up for clinical worsening or suicidal ideation/risk, they did not profess to provide a written medical guide for parents, specific guidelines for monitoring beginning with weekly face-to-face meetings were not mentioned, and there was no acknowledgement of the need to watch for specific signs of behavioral activation. Of note, 11% of respondents reported always consulting a psychiatrist before prescribing these medications and 13% stated that they always consulted a psychologist before prescribing. It is feasible that the monitoring was done by these consultants.

In summary, there is considerable evidence from peer-reviewed journals that the prevalence of depressive or anxiety disorders for children with any type of cancer is not increased compared to typically developing children. Making a diagnosis of a depressive or anxiety disorder in children with cancer is exceptionally complex as a result of overlap of symptoms. Current evidence-based treatment recommendations for treating depressive or anxiety disorders in children include the concurrent use of medications and cognitive behavioral therapy. Despite these facts and the FDA's black box warning, a large number of children receiving treatment for pediatric malignancies receive SSRIs from their treating oncologist. The disparity between the peer-reviewed literature and the current clinical practices bears further investigation.

11.7 Issues Around the Death of a Child

The death of a child is devastating for parents and families. Although bereavement is a highly complex and delicate process affected by social, cultural, religious, and spiritual context, some common themes emerge. It is important to identify practices that are helpful to parents and families who experience this loss. Although an intervention to change the ultimate outcome might not exist , health care providers can have a profound impact on the framing of events for parents and families experiencing such a loss.

Compassionate, informative, and attentive health care staff can have an enormous impact on parents coping with this overwhelming situation. Rini's study (Rini and Loriz 2007) demonstrated the need for a member of the health care staff to function as a coach to assist, describe, and guide parents through this process. Interviewed parents did not want to be alone and expressed a desire to be guided through the process. In addition, the actual setting where death occurs influenced the perception and experience of those parents studied. The parents felt a need to be in a soothing, comfortable environment where there was freedom to grieve and complete tasks deemed important to that family unit (Rini et al. 2007).

Clerici et al (2006) assessed the psychological needs of parents after the death of their child from cancer both in a retrospective and prospective fashion. Retrospectively, the study found that more than 50% of parents spontaneously contacted the medical staff. Prospectively, the staff contacted families by telephone about 4 weeks after the patient's death in order to invite them to a meeting; 17 families were contacted and the majority of them decided to come back to the department for a conference. Overall, this study demonstrated that parents have a need to have further contact with the team that took care of their children with cancer (Clerici et al. 2006). This study should raise awareness that the medical team needs to offer psychological support for parents through continued communication after the child's death, as this can be an integral part of the bereavement process.

Jankovic et al. (1989) described their 7-year experience with physicians contacting parents who lost their child secondary to leukemia. Physicians contacted the parents within the first few months after the death. Sixty-four of 72 couples (89%) agreed to a meeting. This study concluded that most parents needed to talk to their physician at least once as many of them still had unanswered questions. In addition, parents benefited from the reassurance that all that could be done for the child was done. This work suggests that the opportunity to speak with the attending staff should be routinely provided to these parents (Jankovic et al. 1989).

Similarly, Kreicbergs et al. (2007) suggested that closing sessions with the attending staff after the death of a child are beneficial, especially for mothers. In addition, closure talks with a psychologist or social worker involved in the child's care were found to provide the best support for mothers over the long term.

The death of a child due to cancer can also pose important bereavement problems for the professional staff. It is unimaginable for the physician not to be touched by the inevitable pain and distress associated with a patient's death, especially a child with cancer. Redinbaugh et al examined doctors' emotional reactions to recent death of a patient. They found that doctors who developed long-term relationships with their patients got to know them better and this was associated with a more satisfying experience; however, this also made them more vulnerable to feelings of loss when those patients died (Redinbaugh et al. 2003).

After a patient's death, the physician may question whether to attend the memorial, wake, and/or funeral services, and if so, whether to be concerned about blurring professional and personal boundaries. Peters has suggested that "a physician's presence at a visitation or funeral can be an important last act of care and a first step toward coming to terms with the death of a patient for the medical provider and the family (Peters 2004)." The physician's presence at these services is a natural extension of the art of healing as it serves to comfort and assist the survivors (Hood 2003). According to Peters, if the physician--patient--family relationship progressed from clinical to close friendship, then it is beneficial for the care provider to say farewell or grieve the death of a patient/friend (Peters 2004). When Peters asked colleagues, most expressed benefits from attending a funeral, although some described concerns. The first concern related to the mixing of personal and professional boundaries and the second to the risk of being asked clinical questions by family members or friends of the deceased (Peters 2004). However, the benefits of enriching one's life, helping one in the healing process and strengthening the relationship with the family members seemed to override the concerns.

The physician cannot always cure, but can always care. In pediatric oncology, most physician--patient relationships are long-term, leading to fond friendships, and attending a funeral illustrates this important connectedness. The choice of attendance properly remains with the individual. Each individual member of the core team needs to decide what method of offering condolences works best in each case. Arroll confirms that regular funeral attendance does not fit all; however, experience indicates that there are personal and family benefits to be gained and little to be lost (Arrolla ndF alloon 2007).

11.8 IssuesR elatedt oSur vivorship

The use of effective multimodal therapies has resulted in a dramatic increase in survival for children and adolescents with leukemia. In turn, the improved survival rate has made it imperative to study both the physical and psychological long-term effects of leukemia and its treatment. The cancer treatment experience can be potentially disruptive to patients' academic, emotional, and social development. Patients are susceptible to these adverse effects not only during the acute treatment, but throughout their lives. Hence, upon the completion of the therapy, the cancer survivor can rightly experience a myriad of feelings including happiness, joy, panic, anxiety, uncertainty, and transformation.

Although every patient's experience with cancer and its treatment is different, some common concerns exist. These include potentially impaired neurocognitive, reproductive, endocrine, cardiovascular, and pulmonary function, poor educational attainment, posttraumatic stress, altered self-image/esteem, altered interpersonal relationships and social outcomes, employment and insurance issues, second malignancies, and the threat of disease recurrence, just to name a few.

Barrera et al conducted a large population-based cohort study of the long-term educational and social outcomes of young survivors of childhood cancer. In this multicenter retrospective study, 800 survivors aged 17 years or younger were matched by age and gender with a group of 923 control participants. Based on parental report, they found that child and adolescent survivors of cancer, especially those with central nervous system (CNS) tumors and leukemia, were more likely to experience educational difficulties and were less likely to have close friends compared to population controls (Barrera et al. 2005). Survivors who were treated with cranial radiation therapy alone or in combination with intrathecal methotrexate had the poorest educational outcomes and were the most likely not to have close friends (Barrera et al. 2005). In addition, young childhood cancer survivors reportedly had lower self-esteem when compared to controls. The authors concluded that children and adolescents who survived cancer, particularly those who had CNS tumors, leukemia, and neuroblastoma, required close monitoring for early educational and social difficulties.

The Childhood Cancer Survivor Study (CCSS) was started in 1993 to better understand the late effects experienced by childhood cancer survivors originally diagnosed between 1970 and 1986 (Robison et al. 2002). More than 14,000 childhood cancer survivors were identified for this long-term, retrospective cohort study taking place at 27 participating research centers in North America and Canada. Researchers who have studied the CCSS data have identified a number of potential late effects which include risk of second malignancies, endocrine and reproductive outcome, cardiopulmonary complications, and psychosocial implications. However, when examining the long-term toxicities described below, one should keep in mind that most patients diagnosed with acute lymphoblastic leukemia are now treated quite differently than those that constituted the CCSS patient cohort.

Gurney's review of the literature from the CCSS suggested that childhood cancer survivors generally had similar high school graduation rates, but were more likely to require special education services when compared to sibling groups (Gurney et al. 2009). In addition, the review found that survivors were slightly less likely to attend college, and were more likely to be unemployed and not married as young adults. Compared with siblings, leukemia survivors demonstrated elevated rates of psychological distress (Thornton and Carmody 2005; Zeltzer et al. 2008). During the adolescent period, parents reported that leukemia survivors experienced increased rates of depression, anxiety, and social skills deficits compared with sibling controls (Schultz et al. 2007). The findings of these studies have important implications for long-term follow-up care targeting early educational rehabilitation and social skills training programs in order to maximize the survivors' academic and social success.

Schultz et al. evaluated 2,979 adolescent survivors of childhood cancer from the CCSS and 649 siblings in order to determine the incidence of depression/anxiety, headstrong behavior, attention deficits, peer conflict/social withdrawal, antisocial behaviors, and social competence (Schultz et al. 2007). Overall, multivariate analyses showed that survivors were 1.5 times more likely than siblings to have symptoms of depression/anxiety and 1.7 times more likely to have antisocial behaviors. Scores in the depression/anxiety, attention deficit, and antisocial domains were significantly elevated in adolescents treated for leukemia or CNS tumors when compared with siblings. Treatments with cranial radiation and/or intrathecal methotrexate were specific risk factors (Schultz et al. 2007). Hence, adolescent survivors of childhood cancer, especially those with a history of leukemia, may be at increased risk for adverse behavioral and social outcomes.

Also using data from the CCSS, Zebrack et al. examined the clinical psychological outcome in long-term survivors of childhood leukemia, Hodgkin disease and non-Hodgkin lymphoma. They found that these survivors were significantly more likely than sibling controls to report symptoms of depression and somatic depression (Zebrack et al. 2002). Therefore, increased surveillance of the leukemia population should be a priority.

Overall, these results facilitate understanding of the difficulties that leukemia survivors encounter integrating into society. Having a heightened awareness and better understanding of the relationship between childhood cancer survivorship and educational/social outcomes is paramount to assisting in the development of preventive intervention and rehabilitation to ensure that these patients become productive adults leading fulfilling lives.

References

Alderfer MA, Labay LE et al (2003) Brief report: does posttraumatic stress apply to siblings of childhood cancer survivors? J Pediatr Psychol 28(4):281–286

Alderfer MA, Long KA et al (2010) Psychosocial adjustment of silbings of children with cancer: a systematic review. Psycho-Oncology (in press) 2010 Aug; 19(8): 789–805

Arroll B, Falloon K (2007) Should doctors go to patients' funerals? BMJ 334(7607):1322

Barakat LP, Alderfer MA et al (2006) Posttraumatic growth in adolescent survivors of cancer and their mothers and fathers. J Pediatr Psychol 31(4):413–419

Barrera M, Chung JYY et al (2002) Preliminary investigation of a group intervention for siblings of pediatric cancer patients. Children's Health Care 31:131–142

Barrera M, D'Agostino NM et al (2004) Predictors and mediators of psychological adjustment in mothers of children newly diagnosed with cancer. Psychooncology 13(9): 630–641

Barrera M, Shaw AK et al (2005) Educational and social late effects of childhood cancer and related clinical, personal, and familial characteristics. Cancer 104(8):1751–1760

Best M, Streisand R et al (2001) Parental distress during pediatric leukemia and posttraumatic stress symptoms (PTSS) after treatment ends. J Pediatr Psychol 26(5):299–307

Birenbaum LK (1991) Measurement of family coping. J Pediatr Oncol Nurs 8(1):39–42

Blustein J, Moreno JD (1999) Valid consent to treatment and the unsupervised adolescent. In: Blustein J, Levine C, Dubler NN (eds) The adolescent alone: decision making in health care in the United States. Cambridge University Press, Cambridge/New York, pp 100–110

Bragadottir H (2000) Children's rights in clinical research. J Nurs Scholarsh 32(2):179–184

Brody AC, Simmons LA (2007) Family resiliency during childhood cancer: the father's perspective. J Pediatr Oncol Nurs 24(3):152–165

Bronfenbrenner U (1979) The ecology of human development. Harvard University Press, Cambridge, MA

Brown RT, Kaslow NJ et al (1992) Psychiatric and family functioning in children with leukemia and their parents. J Am Acad Child Adolesc Psychiatry 31(3):495–502

Brown RT, Madan-Swain A et al (2003) Posttraumatic stress symptoms in adolescent survivors of childhood cancer and their mothers. J Trauma Stress 16(4):309–318

Chesler MA, Barbarin OA (1987) Childhood cancer and the family: meeting the challenge of stress and support. Brunner/Mazel, New York

Chesler MA, Paris J et al (1986) "Telling" the child with cancer: parental choices to share information with ill children. J Pediatr Psychol 11(4):497–516

Chesler MA, Allswede J et al (1991) Voices from the margin of the family: siblings of children with cancer. J Psychosoc Oncol9: 19–42

Clarke NE, McCarthy MC et al (2009) Gender differences in the psychosocial experience of parents of children with cancer: a review of the literature. Psychooncology 18(9):907–915

Clerici CA, Ferrari A et al (2006) Assistance to parents who have lost their child with cancer. Tumori 92(4):306–310

Corrigan JJ, Feig SA (2004) Guidelines for pediatric cancer centers. Pediatrics 113(6):1833–1835

Coyne I (2008) Children's participation in consultations and decision-making at health service level: a review of the literature. Int J Nurs Stud 45(11):1682–1689

Dahlquist LM, Czyzewski DI et al (1996) Parents of children with cancer: a longitudinal study of emotional distress, coping style, and marital adjustment two and twenty months after diagnosis. J Pediatr Psychol 21(4):541–554

Dolgin MJ, Phipps S et al (2007) Trajectories of adjustment in mothers of children with newly diagnosed cancer: a natural history investigation. J Pediatr Psychol 32(7):771–782

Eiser C, Upton P (2007) Costs of caring for a child with cancer: a questionnaire survey. Child Care Health Dev 33(4):455–459

Emslie GJ, Heiligenstein JH et al (2004) Fluoxetine treatment for prevention of relapse of depression in children and adolescents: a double-blind, placebo-controlled study. J Am Acad Child Adolesc Psychiatry 43(11):1397–1405
Ewing LJ, Marsland AL et al (2009) Social support moderates the impact of a stress management intervention on depression symptoms in parents of pediatric cancer patients (submitted)
Fineberg HV (2008) Cancer care for the whole patient. Medscape J Med 10(9):213
Frank NC, Brown RT et al (2001) Predictors of affective responses of mothers and fathers of children with cancer. Psychooncology10 (4):293–304
Gerhardt CA, Gutzwiller J et al (2007) Parental adjustment to childhood cancer: a replication study. Families, Systems Health25:263–275
Gurney JG, Krull KR et al (2009) Social outcomes in the Childhood Cancer Survivor Study cohort. J Clin Oncol 27(14):2390–2395
Hedstrom M, Kreuger A et al (2006) Accuracy of assessment of distress, anxiety, and depression by physicians and nurses in adolescents recently diagnosed with cancer. Pediatr Blood Cancer46(7):773–7 79
Hoekstra-Weebers JE, Jaspers JP et al (1999) Risk factors for psychological maladjustment of parents of children with cancer. J Am Acad Child Adolesc Psychiatry 38(12): 1526–1535
Holland JC (2003) American Cancer Society Award lecture. Psychological care of patients: psycho-oncology's contribution. J Clin Oncol 21(23 Suppl):253s–265s
Hood GA (2003) Why I go to patients' funerals. Med Econ 80(12):88
Horwitz WA, Kazak AE (1990) Family adaptation to childhood cancer: sibling and family system variables. J Clin Child Psychol19:221–22 8
Houtzager BA, Grootenhuis MA et al (1999) Adjustment of siblings to childhood cancer: a literature review. Support Care Cancer7(5):302–320
Houtzager BA, Grootenhuis MA et al (2004a) Quality of life and psychological adaptation in siblings of paediatric cancer patients, 2 years after diagnosis. Psychooncology 13(8): 499–511
Houtzager BA, Oort FJ et al (2004b) Coping and family functioning predict longitudinal psychological adaptation of siblings of childhood cancer patients. J Pediatr Psychol 29(8):591–605
IOM (2008) Cancer care for the whole patient: Meeting psychosocial health needs. The National Academies Press, Washington,D C
Jankovic M, Masera G et al (1989) Meetings with parents after the death of their child from leukemia. Pediatr Hematol Oncol6(2):155–160
Jankovic M, Loiacono NB et al (1994) Telling young children with leukemia their diagnosis: the flower garden as analogy. Pediatr Hematol Oncol 11(1):75–81
Jankovic M, Spinetta JJ et al (2004) Non-conventional therapies in childhood cancer: guidelines for distinguishing non-harmful from harmful therapies: a report of the SIOP Working Committee on Psychosocial Issues in Pediatric Oncology. Pediatr Blood Cancer 42(1):106–108
Jurbergs N, Long A et al (2009) Symptoms of posttraumatic stress in parents of children with cancer: are they elevated relative to parents of healthy children? J Pediatr Psychol 34(1):4–13
Kazak AE (1989) Families of chronically ill children: a systems and social-ecological model of adaptation and challenge. J Consult Clin Psychol 57(1):25–30
Kazak AE (1992) The social context of coping with childhood chronic illness: family systems and social support. In: La Greca A, Siegel L, Wallander J, Walker C (eds) Stress and coping in child health. Guilford, New York, pp 262–278
Kazak AE (2001) Comprehensive care for children with cancer and their families: a social ecological framework buiding research, practice and policy. Children's Services 4(4): 217–233
Kazak AE (2005) Evidence-based interventions for survivors of childhood cancer and their families. J Pediatr Psychol 30(1):29–39
Kazak AE, Barakat LP et al (1997) Posttraumatic stress, family functioning, and social support in survivors of childhood leukemia and their mothers and fathers. J Consult Clin Psychol65(1):120–129
Kazak AE, Stuber ML et al (1998) Predicting posttraumatic stress symptoms in mothers and fathers of survivors of childhood cancers. J Am Acad Child Adolesc Psychiatry 37(8): 823–831
Kazak A, Alderfer M et al (2004a) Posttraumatic stress disorder (PTSD) and posttraumatic stress symptoms (PTSS) in families of adolescent childhood cancer survivors. J Pediatr Psychol29(3):211–219
Kazak AE, Alderfer MA et al (2004b) Treatment of posttraumatic stress symptoms in adolescent survivors of childhood cancer and their families: a randomized clinical trial. J Fam Psychol18(3):493–504
Kazak AE, Boeving CA et al (2005) Posttraumatic stress symptoms during treatment in parents of children with cancer. J Clin Oncol 23(30):7405–7410
Kellerman J (1980) Comprehensive psychosocial care of the child with cancer: description of a program. In: Kellerman J (ed) Psychological aspects of childhood cancer. Charles C. Thomas, Springfield, IL, pp 195–214
Kersun LS, Kazak AE (2006) Prescribing practices of selective serotonin reuptake inhibitors (SSRIs) among pediatric oncologists: a single institution experience. Pediatr Blood Cancer47(3):339–342
Kreicbergs UC, Lannen P et al (2007) Parental grief after losing a child to cancer: impact of professional and social support on long-term outcomes. J Clin Oncol 25(22):3307–3312
Kupst MJ, Natta MB et al (1995) Family coping with pediatric leukemia: ten years after treatment. J Pediatr Psychol 20(5):601–617
Lahteenmaki PM, Sjoblom J et al (2004) The siblings of childhood cancer patients need early support: a follow up study over the first year. Arch Dis Child 89(11):1008–1013
Landolt MA, Vollrath M et al (2003) Incidence and associations of parental and child posttraumatic stress symptoms in pediatric patients. J Child Psychol Psychiatry 44(8):1199–1207
Lansky SB, Cairns NU et al (1983) School attendance among children with cancer: a report from two centers. J Psychosoc Oncol1: 75–82
Lauria MM, Hockenberry-Eaton M et al (1996) Psychosocial protocol for childhood cancer. A conceptual model. Cancer 78(6):1345–1356
Leslie LK, Newman TB et al (2005) The Food and Drug Administration's deliberations on antidepressant use in pediatric patients. Pediatrics 116(1):195–204

MacLeod KD, Whitsett SF et al (2003) Pediatric sibling donors of successful and unsuccessful hematopoietic stem cell transplants (HSCT): a qualitative study of their psychosocial experience. J Pediatr Psychol 28(4):223–230

Manne S (2009) Commentary: adopting [corrected] a broad perspective on posttraumatic stress disorders, childhood medical illness and injury. J Pediatr Psychol 34(1):22–26

Manne SL, Du Hamel K et al (1998) Posttraumatic stress disorder among mothers of pediatric cancer survivors: diagnosis, comorbidity, and utility of the PTSD checklist as a screening instrument. J Pediatr Psychol 23(6):357–366

Manne S, DuHamel K et al (2000) Association of psychological vulnerability factors to post-traumatic stress symptomatology in mothers of pediatric cancer survivors. Psychooncology 9(5):372–384

Manne S, Nereo N et al (2001) Posttraumtic stress symptoms and stressful life events predict the long-term adjustment of survivors of childhood cancer and their mothers. J Consult Clin Psychol 69:1037–1047

March J, Silva S et al (2004) Fluoxetine, cognitive-behavioral therapy, and their combination for adolescents with depression: treatment for adolescents with depression study (TADS) randomized controlled trial. JAMA 292(7):807–820

Marsland AL, Ewing LJ et al (2006) Psycological and social effects of surviving childhood cancer. In: Comprehensive handbook of childhood cancer and sickle cell disease: a biopsychosocial approach. Oxford University Press, Oxford/ New York, pp 237–261

Masera G, Spinetta JJ et al (1993) SIOP Working Committee on psychosocial issues in pediatric oncology. Med Pediatr Oncol21(9):627–628

Masera G, Jankovic M et al (1995) SIOP Working Committee on psychosocial issues in pediatric oncology: guidelines for school/education. Med Pediatr Oncol 25(6):429–430

Masera G, Chesler M et al (1996) SIOP Working Committee on psychosocial issues in pediatric oncology: guidelines for care of long-term survivors. Med Pediatr Oncol 27(1):1–2

Masera G, Chesler MA et al (1997a) SIOP Working Committee on psychosocial issues in pediatric oncology: guidelines for communication of the diagnosis. Med Pediatr Oncol 28(5):382–385

Masera G, Jankovic M et al (1997b) The psychosocial program for childhood leukemia in Monza, Italy. Ann N Y Acad Sci 824:210–220

Masera G, Beltrame F et al (2003) Audiotaping communication of the diagnosis of childhood leukemia: parents' evaluation. J Pediatr Hematol Oncol 25(5):368–371

Massimo LM, Caprino D (2007) The truly healthy adult survivor of childhood cancer: inside feelings and behaviors. Minerva Pediatr59(1):43–4 7

Mulhern RK, Crisco JJ et al (1981) Patterns of communication among pediatric patients with leukemia, parents, and physicians: prognostic disagreements and misunderstandings. J Pediatr 99(3):480–483

Noll RB, Kupst MJ (2007) Commentary: the psychological impact of pediatric cancer hardiness, the exception or the rule? J Pediatr Psychol 32(9):1089–1098

Noll R, Garstein MA et al (1995) Comparing parental distress for families with chldren who have cancer and matched comparison families without children with cancer. Family Syst Med 13:11–28

Olechnowicz JQ, Eder M et al (2002) Assent observed: children's involvement in leukemia treatment and research discussions. Pediatrics 109(5):806–814

Overholser JC, Fritz GK (1990) The impact of childhood cancer on the family. J Psychosoc Oncol 8:71–85

Packman WL, Crittenden MR et al (2004) Camp Okizu: preliminary investigation of a psychological intervention for siblings of pediatric cancer patients. Children's Health Care 33:201–215

Pai AL, Drotar D et al (2006) A meta-analysis of the effects of psychological interventions in pediatric oncology on outcomes of psychological distress and adjustment. J Pediatr Psychol31(9):978–988

Patenaude AF, Kupst MJ (2005) Psychosocial functioning in pediatric cancer. J Pediatr Psychol 30(1):9–27

Patino-Fernandez AM, Pai AL et al (2008) Acute stress in parents of children newly diagnosed with cancer. Pediatr Blood Cancer50(2):289–292

Pelcovitz D, Goldenberg B et al (1996) Posttraumatic stress disorder in mothers of pediatric cancer survivors. Psychosomatics 37(2):116–126

Peters J (2004) Attending a patient's funeral. Minn Med 87(1): 32–33

Phipps S (2005) Commentary: contexts and challenges in pediatric psychosocial oncology research: chasing moving targets and embracing "good news" outcomes. J Pediatr Psychol30(1):41–45

Prchal A, Landolt MA (2009) Psychological interventions with siblings of pediatric cancer patients: a systematic review. Psychooncology18(12):1241–1251

Redinbaugh EM, Sullivan AM et al (2003) Doctors' emotional reactions to recent death of a patient: cross sectional study of hospital doctors. BMJ 327(7408):185

Reuter K, Harter M (2004) The concepts of fatigue and depression in cancer. Eur J Cancer Care (Engl) 13(2):127–134

Rini A, Loriz L (2007) Anticipatory mourning in parents with a child who dies while hospitalized. J Pediatr Nurs 22(4): 272–282

Robison LL, Mertens AC et al (2002) Study design and cohort characteristics of the Childhood Cancer Survivor Study: a multi-institutional collaborative project. Med Pediatr Oncol 38(4):229–239

Sahler OJ, Fairclough DL et al (2005) Using problem-solving skills training to reduce negative affectivity in mothers of children with newly diagnosed cancer: report of a multisite randomized trial. J Consult Clin Psychol 73(2):272–283

Schultz KA, Ness KK et al (2007) Behavioral and social outcomes in adolescent survivors of childhood cancer: a report from the childhood cancer survivor study. J Clin Oncol 25(24):3649–3656

Shemesh E, Bartell A et al (2002) Assessment and treatment of depression in medically ill children. Curr Psychiatry Rep 4(2):88–92

Slavin LA, O'Malley JE et al (1982) Communication of the cancer diagnosis to pediatric patients: impact on long-term adjustment. Am J Psychiatry 139(2):179–183

Sloper P (2000a) Experiences and support needs of siblings of children with cancer. Health Soc Care Commun 8(5): 298–306

Sloper P (2000b) Predictors of distress in parents of children with cancer: a prospective study. J Pediatr Psychol 25:91

Speechley KN, Noh S (1992) Surviving childhood cancer, social support, and parents' psychological adjustment. J Pediatr Psychol17(1):15–3 1
Spinetta JJ (1978) Communication patterns in families dealing with life-threatening illness. In: Sahler OJZ (ed) The child and death. Mosby, St. Louis, xviii, 300 p
Spinetta J, Maloney J (1975) Death anxiety in the outpatient leukemic child. Pediatrics 56(6):1035–1037
Spinetta JJ, Deasy-Spinetta P et al (1981) Talking with children who have a life-threatening illness. In: Spinetta JJ, Deasy-Spinetta P (eds) Living with childhood cancer. Mosby, St. Louis, xvii, 279 p
Spinetta JJ, Masera G et al (2002) Refusal, non-compliance, and abandonment of treatment in children and adolescents with cancer: a report of the SIOP Working Committee on phychosocial issues in pediatric oncology. Med Pediatr Oncol 38(2):114–117
Spinetta JJ, Masera G et al (2003) Valid informed consent and participative decision-making in children with cancer and their parents: a report of the SIOP Working Committee on psychosocial issues in pediatric oncology. Med Pediatr Oncol40(4):244–246
Spinetta JJ, Masera G et al (2006) A prospective and retrospective view of pediatric hematology/oncology. In: Brown RT (ed) Comprehensive handbook of childhood cancer and sickle cell disease. Oxford University Press, Oxford/New York
Spinetta JJ, Jankovic M et al (2009) Optimal care for the child with cancer: a summary statement from the SIOP Working Committee on psychosocial issues in pediatric oncology. Pediatr Blood Cancer 52(7):904–907
Steele RG, Dreyer ML et al (2004) Patterns of maternal distress among children with cancer and their association with child emotional and somatic distress. J Pediatr Psychol 29(7): 507–517
Stuber ML, Christakis D et al (1996) Post trauma symptoms in childhood leukemia survivors and their parents. Psychosomatics37: 254–261
Syse A (2000) Norway: valid (as opposed to informed) consent. Lancet356(9238):1 347–1348
Tattersall MH, Butow PN et al (1994) The take-home message: patients prefer consultation audiotapes to summary letters. J Clin Oncol 12(6):1305–1311
Thornton KE, Carmody DP (2005) Electroencephalogram biofeedback for reading disability and traumatic brain injury. Child Adolesc Psychiatr Clin N Am 14(1):137–162, vii
Turner EH, Matthews AM et al (2008) Selective publication of antidepressant trials and its influence on apparent efficacy. N Engl J Med 358(3):252–260
Walkup JT, Albano AM et al (2008) Cognitive behavioral therapy, sertraline, or a combination in childhood anxiety. N Engl J Med 359(26):2753–2766
Weiner L, Noll RB et al (2010) Personal communication
Werba BE, Kazak AE (2009) Commentary: life threat, risk, and resilience in pediatric medical traumatic stress. J Pediatr Psychol34(1):27–29
Wiener LS, Steffen-Smith E et al (2008) Sibling stem cell donor experiences at a single institution. Psychooncology 17(3): 304–307
Wiener LS, Pao M, Kazak AE, Kupst MJ, Patenaude AF, Holland JC (eds) (2009) Quick reference for pediatric oncology clinicians: the psychiatric and psychological dimensions of pediatric cancer symptom management. American Psychosocial Oncology Society, Charlottsville, VA
Zebrack BJ, Zeltzer LK et al (2002) Psychological outcomes in long-term survivors of childhood leukemia, Hodgkin's disease, and non-Hodgkin's lymphoma: a report from the Childhood Cancer Survivor Study. Pediatrics 110(1 Pt 1): 42–52
Zeltzer LK, Dolgin MJ et al (1996) Sibling adaptation to childhood cancer collaborative study: health outcomes of siblings of children with cancer. Med Pediatr Oncol 27(2):98–107
Zeltzer LK, Lu Q et al (2008) Psychosocial outcomes and health-related quality of life in adult childhood cancer survivors: a report from the childhood cancer survivor study. Cancer Epidemiol Biomarkers Prev 17(2):435–446
Zwaanswijk M, Tates K et al (2007) Young patients', parents', and survivors' communication preferences in paediatric oncology: results of online focus groups. BMC Pediatr 7:35

Part VIII

Global Strategies to Improve Leukemia Care and Outcome for Children

Improved Outcome for Children with Acute Leukemia: How to Address GlobalDi sparities

12

Yaddanapudi Ravindranath, Hans Peter Wagner, Giuseppe Masera, Fulgencio Baez, Anjo.J.P. Veerman, Jacqueline Cloos, Raul Ribeiro, and Gregory H. Reaman

Contents

Y.R avindranath (✉)
Georgie Ginopolis Chair for Pediatric Cancer and Hematology, Wayne State University School of Medicine, Children's Hospital of Michigan, 3901 Beaubien Boulevard, Detroit,M ichigan4 8201, USA
e-mail:ra vi@med.wayne.edu

H.P.W agner
Schneiderstrasse45, CH3084W abern/Bern, Switzerland
e-mail:hpw agner@bluewin.ch

G.M asera
Department of Pediatrics, University of Milano-Bicocca, SanG erardoH ospital, Monza, Italy
g.masera@hsgerardo.org

F.B aez
PediatricH emato-OncologyD ivision, La Mascota Children's Hospital, Managua, Nicaragua

A.J.P. Veerman and J. Cloos
Department of Pediatric Oncology, Room 9D18, VU University Medical Center, PB7057, 1007MBA msterdam, TheN etherlands
e-mail:a jp.veerman@vumc.nl

R.R ibeiro
St. Jude Children's Research Hospital
Department of Oncology, 262 Danny Thomas Place MS 721, Memphis,TN 38105-3678 , USA
e-mail:ra ul.ribeiro@stjude.org

G.H.R eaman
George Washington University School of Medicine & Health Sciences, The Children's National Medical Center, IIIM ichiganA ve.,D .C.2 0010N W, Washington

G.H. Reaman and F.O. Smith (eds.), *Childhood Leukemia*,
DOI: 10.1007/978-3-642-13781-5_12, © Springer-Verlag Berlin Heidelberg 2011

12.1 Introduction

Modern treatment of childhood acute leukemias started with the use of methotrexate (MTX) by Farber and colleagues in 1948 (reviewed in Dawn of Chemotherapy of Childhood Cancer) (Wolff 1999). The first observations of risk categorizations came in 1949 when Wolf Zuelzer noted that in patients treated with supportive care alone, those with initial white blood cell (WBC) counts of less than 10,000/μL survived longer than those with higher WBC counts (Zuelzer 1949). Subsequently, Dr. Roger Hardisty called attention to a lymphosarcoma variant that is detectable on chest X-ray by the presence of mediastinal enlargement. In 1975, two groups of investigators (from St. Jude Children's Hospital, Memphis and Children's Hospital of Michigan, Detroit) simultaneously showed that the so-called lymphosarcoma variant is of T-cell lineage (Ravindranath et al. 1975; Sen and Borella 1975), and in 1978 Secker-Walker, Lawler, and Hardisty (Secker-Walker et al. 1978) showed the critical importance of cytogenetics in childhood common acute lymphoblastic leukemia (ALL). Shortly thereafter, immunophenotyping and cytogenetic evaluation of childhood ALL became a standard practice.

The pivotal breakthrough for recognizing that cure is achievable in children with ALL came with the introduction of the concept of preemptive central nervous system (CNS) prophylaxis in the early 1970s by Pinkel and colleagues from St. Jude (Simone et al. 1972). Subsequently, stepwise augmentation and intensification of therapy tailored to risk for relapse led to the present cure rates approaching 80% in children with ALL and in several other cancers as well. A dramatic illustration of the success can be seen in the nearly universal curability of mature B-cell ALL, a once universally fatal disease. Remarkably, in ALL, these high cure rates have been achieved with drugs discovered prior to 1980. While there have been huge successes in the treatment of childhood ALL, success with the therapy of acute myeloid leukemia (AML) has been slow; nevertheless, it has improved so that nearly 50–60% of children with AML can also achieve cure with proper treatment.

As dramatic as these achievements have been in the West, the results of therapy in both ALL and AML lag behind considerably in a vast part of the world, notably the low- to mid-income countries (LMIC) of parts of Asia (South Asia, China, Southeast Asia – excluding Thailand, Malaysia, and Singapore), Africa (excluding Republic of South Africa and Egypt) and Central America. The goal is to cure childhood cancer worldwide, but 80% of children with cancer live in parts of the world where, for a variety of reasons, they do not have access to care that is available in the economically developed countries (EDC) of Western Europe and North America.

Limitation of access to care of children with leukemia and other cancers in LMIC is due to lack of resources at multiple levels: low family income, limited governmental resources, lack of trained physicians, lack of focused centers of care for children with cancer, lack of clinical trials organizations, and insufficient advocacy on behalf of children with leukemia by physicians and the community. A common denominator is the cost of diagnostic studies and therapy, which neither the private citizen nor the budget-strapped public institutions are able to sustain. Adding to the problem is the physical separation in many "developing countries" of facilities for care of the affluent and poor. With few exceptions, the indigent and poor thus receive little benefit from the technologies in place for the evaluation and treatment of children of affluent families. In addition to disparities in cure rates, this dichotomy of care has led to lacunae in defining the epidemiology and biology of childhood cancer in large parts of the world. Nowhere is this more evident than in the reported frequencies of various risk categories of childhood ALL from large parts of Asia, Africa, and Central America. Consequently, risk-based treatment strategies are not often in place and many "low-risk" ALL children may be exposed to intensified treatments along with the consequent therapy-related morbidity. It is also likely that many low-risk children, as defined by age, low initial WBC, or ab-sence of mediastinal mass on chest X-ray (a surrogate for T-cell phenotype), receive inappropriate therapy designed for high-risk patients or do not actually receive any therapy. For example, with one of the first generation CNS-prophylaxis-based regimens, 90% 5-year survival was obtained in a group defined as low-risk using modified Children's Cancer Study Group (CCSG) defined low-risk criteria (age between 3 and 7 years, WBC <10,000/μL and absence of mediastinal mass on chest X-ray); the systemic chemotherapy was based on vincristine, prednisone, oral methotrexate, and oral 6-mercaptopurine (Zeulzer, Ravindranath et al. 1976). Treatment for low-risk ALL is inexpensive, and since about one-third to one-half the children with ALL fall into the low-risk category, cure rates of children with ALL could be improved severalfold if all such children receive therapy.

In this chapter, various attempts at improving results of therapy of childhood cancers in "low-middle income countries" will be described. Attempts have been made by individual investigators, individual institutions (e.g., St. Jude Children's Research Hospital from USA, Vrije Universteit from Amsterdam), national and international childhood cancer organizations/clinical trials groups (e.g., International Society of Pediatric Oncology (SIOP), Children's Oncology Group (COG), Berlin-Frankfurt-Münster (BFM) group, Dutch Childhood Oncology Group, Italian Association of Pediatric Hematology/Oncology (AIEOP), French African Pediatric Oncology Group), the World Health Organization and related institutions, international cancer societies (e.g., International Union Against Cancer [UICC]), governmental and semi-governmental agencies such as the US National Institutes of Health and the International Network for Cancer Treatment and Research (INCTR); all of these work with institutions in various parts of the world to increase knowledge and resources for improving the care of children with leukemia worldwide. A diversified approach is necessary because issues and needs are vastly different in various parts of the world, with some countries having an almost total lack of resources at all levels (governmental, institutional, family), others having a lack of commitment, and others having no countrywide organized delivery of care for children with cancer.

Dr. Hans Peter Wagner will describe the lead taken by the International Society of Pediatric Oncology (SIOP), Dr. Guiseppe Masera will describe his twinning experiments in Central America, Dr. Anjo Veerman will describe the Dutch–Indonesia collaborations, Dr. Raul Ribiero will describe the approach taken by St. Jude's Research Center, and Dr. Yaddanapudi Ravindranath will give an overview of the recent efforts of the Children's Oncology Group and its collaborative efforts in South America and in the Middle East with the MECCA (Middle East Children's Cancer Alliance) group.

12.2 Globalizationo ft hel nternational Society of Pediatric Oncology (SIOP)

Hans Peter Wagner, MD
Chairman, "Committee on Pediatric Oncology in Developing Countries," SIOP

The SIOP was founded in 1968 to promote pediatric oncology in Europe by establishing clinical trials and by creating an international platform for pediatric oncology. During the first 20 years, SIOP remained predominantly a European-North American Society. In 1987, the Board decided to set up Continental branches, but in 1990 only 10% of SIOP members were from resource-poor countries. Since the start of globalization in 1990, the number of SIOP members has increased from 355 to 1,470 (in 2008), and the percentage of members from emergent countries has risen from 10% to 40%.

At the 15th International Cancer Congress in Hamburg in 1990, a symposium on pediatric oncology in developing countries (PODC) was organized by N. Gad-el Mawla and G. Prindull. After this symposium, an International Working Group (IWG) for PODC was established with representatives from the European Society of Pediatric Hematology and Immunology (ESPHI), the American Society of Hematology (ASH), the US National Cancer Institute (NCI) and SIOP. The first goal of the IWG was to collect information on existing twinning projects between hospitals in resource-poor countries and centers in resource-rich countries in order to promote twinning while avoiding pitfalls.

In 1992 H. J. Riehm invited over 180 doctors from emergent countries to the 24th Annual SIOP Congress in Hannover. At this meeting, the Board of SIOP agreed to establish a SIOP scholarship program, enabling young doctors and nurses caring for children with cancer in emergent countries to participate at SIOP Congresses and Continental Meetings. Two years later, P. Hesseling organized the first SIOP Africa meeting in Stellenbosch, South Africa. A review of pediatric oncology in Africa showed that only the North and the South had some structure for pediatric oncology; in many sub-Saharan countries, pediatric oncology was practically nonexistent. Doctors from Malawi and other countries reported on the dismal outlook for African children with Burkitt's lymphoma (BL).

In 1996 S. Lie, president of SIOP, organized a strategic meeting in London to better define the role of SIOP in emergent countries. At this meeting it was decided to invest SIOP's limited resources into three new projects: the Malawi Burkitt's Lymphoma Project, the Indian National Educational Project, and the White Book project. The first two projects were successful, while the White Book project failed (Wagner 2001).

The BL project was started in Malawi with the idea that if it functioned there, it could function anywhere in sub-Saharan countries. The challenge was to develop guidelines for an affordable, short treatment with limited toxicity, yielding a survival rate of approximately 50%. In Blantyre, Malawi, a pediatric cancer unit (PCU) with doctors and nurses, diagnostic tools, drugs, supportive care, accommodation for accompanying persons, and transportation for follow-up was organized and financed at the Queen Elizabeth II Hospital.

Since 1997, seven therapeutic studies with over 500 patient enrollments and only very few patients excluded or lost to follow-up, have been designed and monitored by P. Hesseling in Malawi (Hesseling 2000; Kazembe et al. 2003; Hesseling et al. 2008). During these studies, it became evident that treatment with modified, very mild LMB-like B-lymphoma regimens developed by the Société Française d'Oncologie Pédiatrique was poorly tolerated and associated with a high (37%) initial death rate. It was therefore decided to return to monotherapy with cyclophosphamide (CP). The Malawi studies proved that oral doses of 40 or 60 mg CP/kg were as effective as intravenous (IV) doses. They also showed that three doses of 40 mg CP/kg could be given weekly and three doses of 60 mg CP/kg could be given biweekly, even if combined with intrathecal MTX and hydrocortisone. The early studies with a modified LMB protocol demonstrated that 1 g of MTX/m^2 given IV over 3 h, followed 24 h later by one 15 mg leukovorin tablet every 6 h × 7, could be safely administered without determining MTX levels. In addition, about one-third of nonresponding or relapsed patients could be rescued with three doses of 60 mg CP/kg IV or orally plus vincristine 1.5 mg/m^2 IV at 2-week intervals. Follow-up ultrasound exams demonstrated that a residual intra-abdominal mass with a volume of >30 mL after Intensification was a poor prognostic sign. The low-cost Malawi guidelines for the treatment of BL were proven to be effective in three newly established PCUs in Western Cameroon, and in the French African Pediatric Oncology Group (GFAOP) setting, with similar survival rates of around 50% and 60–65% with rescue treatment for nonresponders and relapsed patients, respectively. The newest BL Cameroon 2008 treatment guidelines (Table 12.1) are based on the aforementioned experiences. With the correct use of these treatment guidelines, up to two-thirds of all children with endemic BL in sub-Saharan countries can be cured, a significant accomplishment if one considers that BL is the most frequent childhood cancer (up to 50% or more) in sub-Saharan countries.

The GFAPO, alluded to above, was founded in 2000 by J. Lemerle in Paris. The group was established to develop cooperation between France and Africa for the study and treatment of childhood cancers. So far, this group has established 12 PCUs in nine African countries. Since 2000, four protocols have been adapted to the resource-poor environment: one for nephroblastoma, one for BL, one for Hodgkin lymphoma and one for leukemia; each of these has been tested and used, and two more are in preparation (Harif et al. 2008). Among the over 1,500 patients treated in African GFAOP centers, 68% are survivors.

SIOP's Indian project, officially designated as Indian National Training Program in Practical Pediatric Oncology (INTP-PPO), was conceived entirely by Indian investigators, but was initially financed by and through SIOP (Agarwal et al. 2001). The goal of the project is to train pediatricians, practitioners, and surgeons to avoid late referrals and to be actively involved in the diagnosis and treatment of children with cancer, underscoring the fact that childhood cancer is curable. In 1997 the first national trainer's workshop was organized under the auspices of SIOP and the Pediatric Hematology Oncology Chapter of the Indian Academy of Pediatrics (IAP) in Mumbai. A 2-day standard training module was adopted by 44 pediatric oncologists from all over India with input from a foreign faculty, and a reference manual and slide sets were approved as information for teaching and practical demonstrations (skill stations). Between 1998 and 2001, 19 INTP-PPO courses (workshops) were held throughout the country. In 2002, a second national teacher's review meeting took place in Mumbai and a consensus was reached to modify the training module and to revise the reference manual and the slide sets. Beginning in 2003,

Table 12.1 Burkitt's lymphoma Cameroon 2008 treatment guidelines

Phase	Patients	Drugs	To be given on days
Induction	All	CP 40 mg/kg IV or oral	1,8,15
		MTX 12.5 mg intrathecal	1,8,15
		Hydrocortisone 12.5 mg intrathecal	1,8,15
Intensification	Stages I and II in CCR	CP 60 mg/kg IV or oral	29
Risk Group 1			
Intensification	Stage III	CP 60 mg/kg IV or oral	29,43
Risk Group 2	Or exact stage unknown in CCR with good ultrasound response (remaining tumor volume <30 mL)		
Intensification	All stage IV	CP 60 mg/kg IV or oral	29,43,57
Risk Group 3	Stages I, II, III and exact stage unknown who have a poor ultrasound response (>30 mL remaining tumor volume)	Vincristine 1.5 mg/m^2 IV	29,43,57
		MTX 1.0 g/m^2 IV[a]	29
		Leukovorin 15 mg tablets: one tablet every 6 h for seven doses starting exactly 24 h after the onset of the MTX infusion	30–31

CCR complete clinical remission, *CP* cyclophosphamide, *MTX* methotrexate

[a]Instructions for methotrexate administration for Cameroon 2008 BL protocol:

WBC > 1.0 × 10^9/L before starting treatment; normal kidney and liver function; commence treatment on a week day, early in the morning. The patient must be well-hydrated before starting the MTX infusion by giving intravenous fluid (Dextrose and Darrows or 5% Dextrose in water) for 4 h at a rate of 3 L/m^2/24 h (= 125 mL/m^2/h)

Sodium bicarbonate (4% $NaHCO_3$) 30 mL is added to each liter of IV fluid to keep the urine alkaline. This infusion must be continued for 48 h after the onset of the MTX infusion. Urine output must be recorded 6 hourly and should be not less than 3 mL/kg/h (18 mL/kg every 6 h)

MTX is reconstituted with sterile water (if in powder form) and added to 5% Dextrose in water or 0, 9% NaCl to a total volume of 200 mL. This is then given as a constant intravenous infusion over 3 h

ten additional teaching courses in the revised format were held in India, as well as three additional courses in Nepal, Bangladesh, and Oman. In addition, a short half-day module was tested and became popular among busy pediatricians and practitioners. Starting in 2009, 25 half-day courses with 75 participants each were planned for the next 5 years. An important aspect of INTP-PPO was the bringing together of a large body of pediatric cancer specialists from all parts of India and the establishment of an Indian National Pediatric Oncology Group (INPOG).

SIOP has also been active in defining standards; they have published "Requirements for the Training of a Pediatric Hematologist/Oncologist" and "Recommendations for the Organisation of Paediatric Cancer Unit (PCU)." The venues of the last ten SIOP Congresses (Amsterdam, Brisbane, Porto, Cairo, Oslo, Vancouver, Geneva, Mumbai, Berlin, and Sao Paulo) demonstrate that SIOP has evolved over the last two decades into a truly global medical society.

12.3 The "La Mascota" Twinning Program Between Monza (Italy) and Managua (Nicaragua): A 23-year Experience

Giuseppe Masera
Department of Pediatrics, University of Milano-Bicocca, San Gerardo Hospital, Monza, Italy
Fulgencio Baez
Pediatric Hemato-Oncology Division, La Mascota Children's Hospital, Managua, Nicaragua

The great progress in pediatric oncology over the last 30 years has led to an increasing gap in survival between children with cancer living in low-middle income countries (LMIC) and those in economically developed countries (EDC). Moreover, it has to be remembered that 85% of childhood cancer cases diagnosed every year are in LMIC. Since the early 1990s, SIOP has acknowledged the increasing importance of cancer as a cause of childhood mortality in LMIC and has promoted a series of initiatives through the Pediatric Oncology in Developing Countries Committee (Wagner and Antic 1997; Masera et al. 2004).

There has been much debate regarding the most appropriate strategy for promoting the progress of pediatric oncology in LMIC. How can national and international institutions be involved? How can SIOP contribute, and which contributions could come from pediatric oncologists, oncology centers, and non-profit institutions (parents' associations, foundations) (Wagner 2001). In 1997, SIOP approved the document "Montevideo Statement" that proposes "systematic implementation of center-to-center cooperation as a concrete contribution to the respect of the neglected rights of children" (The Montevideo Document1997).

In 1986, pediatric oncologists in Monza (Italy) and their colleagues in Managua (Nicaragua) had the opportunity to activate a long-term twinning program. Nicaragua, Central American Republic, has 5.5 million people and is one of the poorest countries in Latin America; at the time the twinning program was established, it did not have the resources to give adequate treatment to children with cancer.

This twinning program, known as "La Mascota Program" (LMP), has evolved quite well and now, after 23 years, the lessons learned from a global, long-term twinning program can be summarized. Details of the project have been previously published (Masera eta l. 1998;D 'Angio 2009;M asera 2009).

A. A twinning program between Pediatric Cancer Units (PCUs) of EDC and LMIC should be based on the clearly defined intention to "cooperate for change," with the main aim of contributing to bridging the mortality gap by offering the best feasible treatment to all children with cancer regardless of the ability to afford treatment .

La Mascota Program: In 1986, a call for help came to Monza from Dr. Fernando Silva, poet and Director of "La Mascota" Hospital in Managua, the only pediatric institution in Nicaragua. Without waiting for improbable funding from governmental institutions, Monza responded with the support from the Parents' Association "Comitato M.L. Verga" and the Foundation for Research "Tettamanti," expressing a profound sensitivity and spirit of solidarity with the families and children of a little country, far away.

B. A long-term program should be based on a bilateral agreement, with periodic reassessments and adjustments of strategies and needs. Management responsibilities should be given to local professionals, in particular to the Director of the PCU. The reciprocal respect of autonomy, culture, and local traditionsa ree ssentialtos uccess.

LMP: After more than 20 years, the cooperation between the two PCUs is excellent, with reciprocal esteem, respect, and even friendship. The management responsibilities have been with the Director of "La Mascota" PCU from the beginning. An active, noninvasive, supervisory, and scientific advice relationship has been assured with annual site visits and frequent contacts by email for particular problems.

C. A program for childhood cancer may become a trigger for the development of similar programs in other medical specialties, and may also help to promote a closer relationship between specialized centersa ndpe ripheralhos pitals.

*LMP: Important improvements have been achieved in the following services in La Mascota in particular: laboratory of hematology, pathology, and infectious diseases. After a few years, Franco Cavalli (Bellinzona, Switzerland) and the Ayuda Medica a Centro America (AMCA, a Swiss association of medical help to Central America) joined the program, as well as Franca Fossati of the National Cancer Institute of Milan. In 2004, a program for Neonatology was started at the "Hospital de la Mujer Bertha Calderon." Since 1997, a twinning program for Nephro-Urology has been established between La Mascota and the Pediatric Clinic "De Marchi" of the University of Milan, with excellent results (*Edefonti et al. 2010*). More recently, a network involving La Mascota (Oncology, Nephro-Urology) and five peripheral hospitals has been activated.*

D. A "therapeutic alliance" should be established among health professionals, parents, and volunteers in order to sensitize institutions and health authorities, mobilize resources, and effectively identify needsa ndprioritie s.

LMP: In Italy, the Parents' Association "Comitato Verga," the Research Foundation "Tettamanti," and the Zegna Foundation gave their support to the program; the AMCA from Switzerland, the Liga Nacional Contra la Leucemia y Cancer en el Niño from Nicaragua, the Comision Nicaraguense de Ayuda al Niño con Cancer (CONANCA), and the Asociacion de Padres (MAPANICA) contributed to the program as well.

E. The program should start with the training of physiciansa ndhe althprofe ssionals.

LMP: The staff now working in the PCU includes 8 Pediatric Hemato-Oncologists, 1 Pediatric-Oncology Surgeon, 1 Anesthetist, 17 Nurses, 2 Laboratory Scientists, 1 Psychologist, 1 Social Worker, and 1 "Clown-Psychologist." Some of them have been trained in Monza; in particular, the eight Pediatric Hemato-Oncologists each spent 1 year in Monza (and, in part, at the National Cancer Institute of Milan). All eight continue to work at La Mascota.

F. Structuralf acilitiess houldbe c reatedorimpro ved.

LMP: Structural facilities have been established through the program: 1991: ten bed ward for Hematology (financed by Tettamanti Foundation. and Liga Contra Leucemia y Cancer); 1992: ten bed ward for Oncology (financed by AMCA-Bellinzona, F.Cavalli); 1993: Playroom (financed by the President of the Republic of Nicaragua); 1995: Residence for families (with the support of Alessandria Town Council, Italy); 1999: 12 bed ward for Oncology (provided by Dukedom of Luxembourg); 2005: Day Surgery (financed by CONANCA); 2007: New outpatient clinic (provided by a company from Costa Rica).

G. Protocols for diagnosis and therapy should be tailored to the local situation, starting with ALL, the most frequent type of childhood cancer and the one with more favorable results. Later, protocols for the other common pediatric tumors should be developed, with the supervision of experts.

LMP: The program started with ALL, with annual monitoring at La Mascota. Afterwards, other protocols were activated, in collaboration with the Asociacion de Hemato-Oncologia Pediatrica de Centro America (AHOPCA); these included protocols for AML, APL, HL, NHL, Wilms tumor, retinoblastoma, osteosarcoma, and rhabdomyosarcoma.

During this collaboration, it has become evident that a protocol has to be tailored to the experience of the health-care providers and to the local organizational possibilities in order to avoid excessive toxicity and severe, fatal, complications in Induction and Maintenance. The application of the treatment protocol must also be tailored to the clinical condition of the child.

H. Financial support is best assured through a consistent pool of donors. A number of diverse sources favors the independence, long-term security, and flexibility of the project. A policy of absolute transparency on all project activities, with periodic reporting to supporting groups, guarantees trust and promotesmore a ctivepa rticipation.

LMP: The funding was (a) international, from 14 sources in Italy, Switzerland, Luxembourg, USA, Canada, and Austria;(b) national, from the CONANCA, the Liga Nacional Contra la Leucemia y Cancer en el Niño, MAPANICA (Parents' Association), the Asociacion Hogar de Esperanza, and the Ministerio de Salud.

I. A holistic approach should be taken with psychosocials upport.

LMP: From the program's inception, great attention has been paid to the psychological and social aspects of the child and the family. A multidisciplinary team has been created, including two psychologists, one social worker, and one clown-psychologist. Specifi c initiatives that have been activated are: (a) adoption of adapted SIOP psychosocial recommendations; (b) "Enseñando a pescar" ("Teaching to fish") program for long-term survivors supported by MAPANICA; (c) Program Payaso (clown Dr. Kelocura);(d) an educational program for parents to improve compliance with treatment; (e) a laboratory of poetry (coordinated by Ernesto Cardenal, poet- writer); (f) a laboratory of painting;(g) a program for reading.

J. Refusal or early abandonment of treatment should be controlled, in order to avoid it as a relevant cause off ailure.

LMP: Psychological and economic support was provided to the families through the "Support-a-child" program from Italy and Switzerland. Since its beginning in 1994, about 1,400 children have entered the program. Patient dropout rate has dramatically improved from 35% 20 years ago, to about 8–10% most recently.

K. Formal research projects aimed at broadening and strengthening the cultural interest and the original initiatives of the collaborating teams should be promoted. Priority should clearly be given to topics of interest for LMIC centers, and the visibility of their contribution (e.g., in publications) must be assured.

LMP: From 1990 to 2008, 2,667 patients have been treated at La Mascota Hospital. The experience and the progress made with limited resources has been documented and published in international journals such as: The Lancet, Annals of Oncology, Medical& Pediatric Oncology, Pediatric Blood & Cancer, and International Journal of Pediatric Hematology-Oncology.

12.3.1 Long-Term Impact of La Mascota Program

The positive results of the LMP developed in the early 1990s as a new idea by the Director of Pediatric Oncology in Managua (Fulgencio Baez) and by Giuseppe Masera, have been extended to other Latin America countries with the collaboration and activation of other twinning programs. Thus, Monza's International School for Pediatric Hematology/Oncology (MISPHO) was created, and since 1996, meetings for discussion and training have been organized, lasting about 1 week each, in Milan or Monza; these meetings took place yearly from 1996 to 2003, and were then begun in Latin America (Bogota, Tegucigalpa, San José). The training was financed by grants from the CARIPLO Foundation (Milan) in the first 8 years, and, afterwards, from the Zegna Foundation (Biella, Italy). About 40 pediatric oncologists from 15 countries (Bolivia, Colombia, Costa Rica, Cuba, Ecuador, El Salvador, Guatemala, Honduras, Nicaragua, Panama, Paraguay, Peru, Dominican Republic, Uruguay, and Venezuela) attended the meetings, with experts in different fields coming from Italy, USA (St. Jude Childrens' Research Hospital of Memphis), and Canada.

Some other twinning programs were activated in the countries belonging to MISPHO: Honduras, El Salvador, and Guatemala with St. Jude; Paraguay with Modena and Madrid; Colombia with Boston; and Dominican Republic with the University of Colorado College of Medicine. In 1998, pediatric oncologists from Central America created the "Asociacion de Hemato-Oncologia Pediatrica de Centro America" (AHOPCA), with the participation of all the Central American countries and of the Dominican Republic, and the collaboration of the International Outreach Program of St. Jude, the Pediatric Oncology Group of Ontario (POGO), and MISPHO. In November 2009, the Pan American Health Organization (PAHO) activated a working group PAHO-AHOPCA to promote a Pediatric Oncology program for 2010–2011.

Data on patients are collected in an online pediatric oncology networked database (POND) developed by St. Jude Children's Research Hospital, and are analyzed in Monza by the Statistical Office for Pediatric Hemato-Oncology in Low-Middle Income Countries (SOPHOLIC).

12.3.2 Conclusions

The La Mascota Program exemplifies that a global, long-term twinning program is feasible, rewarding, and encourages the creation of new opportunities and new collaborations. Now, the PCU of Managua is a concrete reality, included in the regional pediatric oncology network and in tight connection with the Pediatric Hemato-Oncology center of Monza-Milan and with St. Jude Children's Research Hospital. Figure 12.1 shows the great progress that has been achieved.

The concept can be underscored that "an attempt to reduce the gap in mortality from childhood cancer, and particularly acute leukemia, between developed and less developed countries should become an integral part of the care and research activity of a hemato-oncological department of a developed country and not simply an exercise in solidarity" (Masera et al. 1998; Rohatiner 2005). It is essential to define a mutually shared strategy that has as its main focus access to adequate therapies for all children with cancer, regardless of the country in which they reside.

An old Chinese saying provides conclusion: "Go in search of your people: love them, learn from them, plan with them, serve them; begin with what they have, build on what they know. But of the best teachers when their task is accomplished, their work is done, the people all remark: 'We have done it ourselves'" (Werner andB ower 1982).

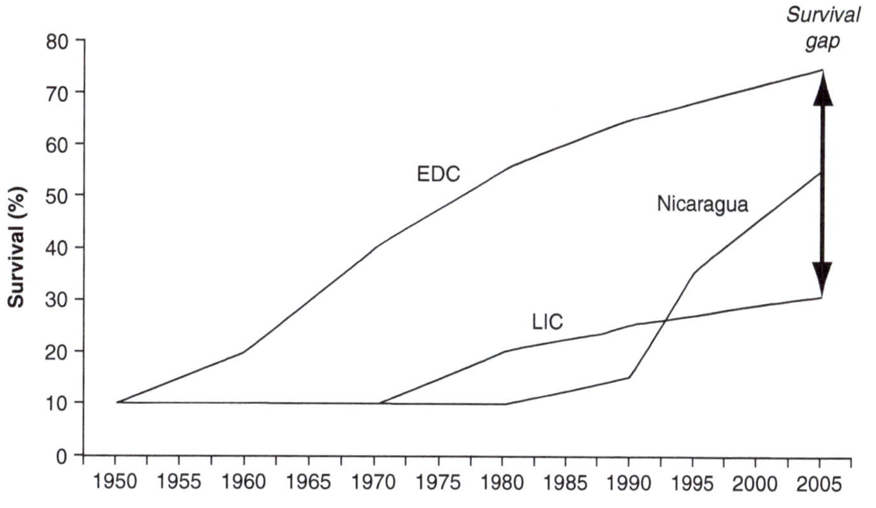

Fig. 12.1 Survival of children with cancer in economically developed countries (EDC), in low-income countries (LIC), and in Nicaragua

12.4 Twinning:T heV U-Netherlands-UGM-Indonesia Experience – Staff Education, Protocol Development, and Research

A. J. P. Veerman
VU University Medical Center, Amsterdam, The Netherlands and
Visiting Professor, Universitas Gadjah Mada, Yogyakarta, Indonesia
J.C loos
VU University Medical Center, Amsterdam, The Netherlands

From the many examples of successful twinning, the one between the Netherlands and Indonesia seems to have several specific characteristics. First of all, as a background, these two counties have a long common history; they fought, separated, and came to good understanding again. Indonesia is an island state (consisting of about 20,000 islands); it is the fourth most populated country in the world with 220 million inhabitants, 40% of whom are children. It also has the largest Muslim population of any country, about 200 million. One of the characteristics of the twinning between VU University Medical Center in Amsterdam and Gadjah Mada University in Yogyakarta was human resource development; staff and students were exchanged, and worked together on research projects (Veerman et al. 2005). Most of this took place in Indonesia, so that the whole local team would benefit. Seminars and workshops were therefore organized locally, rather than having the Indonesians taught in the Netherlands.

Protocols were developed in the twinning program, as were associated research questions to be answered in randomized clinical trials. One of the primary achievements of the twinning program was the design of a national Indonesian protocol for ALL, the Wijaya Kusuma ALL-2000 (WK-ALL) protocol, introduced in all academic hospitals treating children with cancer. The results of ALL treatment in Indonesia, although improving, are seemingly still lower than in low-income countries in Central and South America. Basic protocols can cure more than 50% of children and more than 80% in low-risk ALL (Hunger et al. 2005).

In a randomized study on the use of simple medication diaries, the very basic WK-ALL protocol was shown to produce 3-year event-free survival (EFS) in 62% of children of well-educated mothers, while only 22% of children of less educated mothers had 3-year EFS on the same protocol (Sitaresmi et al. 2009). The more highly educated mothers benefitted from having a diary, with 62% 3-year EFS (as previously stated), while the control group, more educated mothers without a diary, had a 3-year EFS of 29%, barely higher than the less educated group, in whom the diary made no difference. Literacy levels and socioeconomic status are linked. Children with ALL from households with a monthly income of less than the equivalent of US$80 fared worse (EFS actuarial 11%) than the so-called prosperous group (EFS actuarial 45%; $p < 0.001$) (Mostert et al. 2006). This analysis counted deaths from all causes as failure, including resistant disease, relapse, noncompliance, not starting therapy, as well as abscondence (dropout) later in the course of therapy. Reasons for failure differed between socioeconomic groups; in the poorest group, dropouts amounted to 45% but in the prosperous group to only 2%. Toxicity related deaths in Induction and after complete remission were less different, with 25% in the poor and 18% in the prosperous group. Thus, the main reasons for failure of treatment were not resistant disease or relapse, but noncompliance and (toxic) death.

Studies of ALL in the Netherlands during the same time span identified treatment-related death as a significant problem, more so with a dexamethasone-based protocol than with a prednisone-based protocol (Slats et al. 2005; Te Poele et al. 2007). In resource-rich Western countries, however, the gain in relapse-free survival greatly exceeds the (nonstatistically higher) toxic mortality of 3–4% (Mitchell et al. 2005; Veerman et al. 2009). In low-income countries, where the toxic death rate is already high, a doubling in toxic deaths may mean an increase from 15% to 30% mortality. Therefore, protocols have to be adapted to local situations (Hunger et al. 2009). The local factors that influence prognosis include not only supportive care facilities, but also malnutrition, poverty, and distance (travel time) to the hospital. In the Yogyakarta region, which is a rather densely populated area on the island Java, the median travel time was found to be more than 3 h (Sitaresmi et al. 2009, psycho-oncology in press) and was far longer for patients traveling from outer islands. Cultural issues play a role as well.

Several leukemia biology studies were conducted with the WK-ALL protocol in Yogyakarta. These studies proved that it is possible to introduce randomized questions in Indonesia. One laboratory study focused on differences in genotype between Western and Asian populations that might influence drug metabolism (Giovannetti et al. 2008). For instance, the thymidilate synthase enhancer region occurs as a 2-repeat or 3-repeat, the latter associated with higher enzyme activity. Asians have a higher frequency of 3-repeat promoter, show faster methotrexate metabolism, and worse prognosis. Another Indonesian study tried to find apoptotic cells in the circulation during the first few days of steroid treatment, but was not successful, probably because apoptotic cells are marginalized and thus not present in the circulation (Widjajanto and Sutaryo 2006). Immunophenotyping has now been introduced in Indonesia, and facilitates the confirmation of a diagnosis of ALL versus AML (Supriyadi, to be published).

Ciprofloxacin prophylaxis and dosage of L-Asparaginase were both tested in clinical studies within the WK-ALL protocol. The first study involved a blinded randomized trial of ciprofloxacin prophylaxis in Induction. Unexpectedly, more patients died in the ciprofloxacin group than in the placebo group, and this was correlated with a lower nadir of WBC in the ciprofloxacin group (Widjajanto, manuscript in preparation). Another study was an open, randomized trial of three extra doses of L-Asparaginase during the 6 weeks of Consolidation following complete remission after Induction; the study showed no difference between the treatment arms, while the toxicity was quite significant in the arm with three additional doses of L-Asparaginase. The cost of L-Asparaginase, the most expensive drug in the armamentarium, was also a serious drawback.

The WK-ALL study also evaluated whether the dexamethasone-based protocol, although superior in high-income countries (Veerman et al 2009, Mitchell et al 2005), would indeed be too toxic in the low-income situation in Indonesia. In the Indonesia ALL-2006 protocol, patients were randomized to receive dexamethasone or prednisone. Preliminary evidence, presented at the St. Jude-VIVA Forum in Singapore in March 2009, indicated that indeed, the toxic mortality rate with prednisone in Induction phase was lower than that in the dexamethasone group. Although the size effect was considerable, statistical significance was not reached, so the randomization was continued. Finally, the previously mentioned randomized trial in which some patients were provided with a medication diary gave a surprising result. Even while some parents in the control group copied the diary from the intervention group, the outcome was superior in the diary group, although only among the better-educated parents. In the less educated group, some diaries were not used, or were used as a sketchbook for the patient. These clinical studies emphasize that in low-income situations there is a need for local randomized studies.

The situation there demonstrates that results of Western trials are not, or at least not always, applicable in low-income countries. Protocols in low-income countries need to be tailored to the local situation (Hunger et al. 2009).

The research program in Yogyakarta, and now also in other cities in Indonesia, is also important because it demonstrates the necessity of good data management to monitor the results of treatment. Currently, data management in Yogyakarta is excellent, because there is a very dedicated and compulsive data manager, who also monitors adherence to protocol-based therapy. He sees to it that for every patient a shadow file (research file) is created. The clinical files are often lost, but because of this shadow file, all essential data regarding diagnosis, protocol, and follow-up are available in hard copies. Data are extracted from the shadow files and managed in simple excel files. A statistical packet (SPSS) can be used to analyze these data. This database has become invaluable after more than 10 years of data sampling. Feedback to patient care is therefore an important spin-off from the research program.

Many questions remain to be answered in Indonesia. For instance, why are the reported results of treatment of ALL in Central and South America better than those in Indonesia? Do genetic factors such as polymorphisms in drug metabolizing enzymes play a part? Some evidence points in this direction. Do different degrees of poverty or malnutrition, which is rampant, impact prognosis? Other potential factors include lack of insurance, lack of drug availability (sometimes essential medication is just not available in Indonesia), lack of support from health-care officials for this rare and expensive disease, lack of belief in the possibility to achieve cure (Mostert et al. 2008; Sitaresmi et al. 2009), selection bias due to the fact that the more affluent patients tend to come for care, and bias in reporting abscondence.

Although much still remains to be done, the progress in the last 10 years, including the development of local protocols and the increased expertise of doctors, nurses, and technicians are great achievements. The increased self-supporting nature of research and development is very important as well. A new generation of pediatric oncologists has been trained, and they can act on their own with only limited support from external advisors. Cooperation now is more on a bidirectional level, as opposed to unilateral help. There is hope for a better future for new children with leukemia in low-incomec ountries.

12.5 Strategiest ol mprovePedi atric Cancer Care in Low- and Mid-Income Countries: The Experience of the St. Jude International Outreach Program

Raul C. Ribeiro, MD
Department of Oncology and International Outreach Program, St. Jude Children's Research Hospital, Memphis, TN, USA and the Department of Pediatrics, University of Tennessee Health Science Center, Memphis, TN, USA

This work was supported in part by a Cancer Center Support Grant (CA21765) from the National Institutes of Health and by the American Lebanese Syrian Associated Charities (ALSAC).

12.5.1 The Status of Pediatric Oncology Worldwide

Survival of children with cancer has increased dramatically in high-income nations, from essentially zero in the early 1950s to rates approaching 80% today (Jemal et al. 2007). This success is due in part to disease-adapted multimodality treatment, including surgery, chemotherapy, and radiation, that has been refined through a series of multi-institutional clinical trials. Parallel gains in supportive care, particularly in the management of infectious complications, have made it possible to escalate the intensity and thus the efficacy of these therapies. However, an estimated 80% of the 160,000 children diagnosed with cancer each year lack access to modern treatment and thus have dismal outcomes (Barr et al. 2006). In a recent survey of ten low- and mid-income countries (LMIC) that participated in the "My Child Matters" program, postulated survival rates varied from less than 10% to 60%, depending on the country. In four of the ten countries, only about 15–37% of cases would have even been seen by health-carepro viders(R ibeiroe ta l. 2008).

12.5.2 Implementing Pediatric Cancer Care in Low- and Mid-Income Countries

In 1994, the St. Jude International Outreach Program (IOP) was created with the mission of improving the survival of children with cancer in LMIC by sharing knowledge and organizational skills and supporting the implementation of pediatric oncology units in public pediatric hospitals in selected countries. These "twinning" initiatives were envisioned as culturally sensitive demonstration projects that would be integrated with and adapted to the local health-care systems.

The St. Jude twinning programs are defined as long-term, close relationships with centers in LMIC. These programs have eight essential components called "the critical Cs" (Table 12.2). Strong leadership at different program components is essential. Leadership creates a sense of purpose by encouraging team building and sharing the ownership of the process among participants. This consistent mutual recognition of the efforts made by different team members and their inclusion in the decision-making process enables commitment, active participation, and mission-oriented pursuits. Strong leaders are necessary among health-care providers (physicians, nurses, psychologists, nutritionists, social workers) and nongovernmental foundation members. These individuals must understand the needs of children with cancer, including physical, social, and spiritual, as integral components of the chain of care. Moreover, the twinning activities have to take into

Table 12.2 The St. Jude twinning program's "critical Cs" for childhood cancer care in low- and mid-income countries

Critical" C"	Components	Content	Constraints
Commitment by EDC partner	1. Leader in EDC (willing to devote time and effort to the program) 2. Institutional commitment	A committed leader is necessary to define, develop, initiate, implement, and maintain the program. The leader facilitates intra- and interinstitutional communication and engages the hospital to mobilize resources (human, technical, and financial).	Lack of leadership in EDC makes a twinning program unlikely to succeed.
Commitmentby LMIC partner	1. Leader in LMIC (willing to devote time and effort to the program) 2.I nstitutional commitment	A committed leader is necessary to define, develop, initiate, and implement the program. The leader facilitates intra- and interinstitutional communication and must engage the hospital and community to mobilize resources (human, technical, and financial).	Lack of leadership in LMIC makes a twinning program unlikely to succeed.
Communitya dvocacy and fundraising in LMIC	1.N onprofit, nongovernmental foundation to solely support childhood cancer care 2. One cancer foundation per geographic area	Members of the supporting foundation should include influential members of society, professionals, and parents/relatives of patients. The foundation works with both government and the medical team to effect change. Credibility of foundations established yearly by independent auditing agencies.	If multiple foundations develop in a single region, their message is diluted and their ability to raise money and advocate are diminished.

Table 12.2 (continued)

Critical" C"	Components	Content	Constraints
Collaborative spirit	1. Respect 2.T rust 3.H umility 4.C ollegiality	Twinning must be a culturally sensitive relationship of equals who are willing to learn from one another. In the best programs, the association is beneficial and enjoyable on both sides.	A focus on individual accomplishments is less helpful than a focus on the shared mission to cure patients with cancer.
Communication	1. Effective	1. Rapid, honest, in the same language	Absent or dishonest communication makes a twinning program impossible.
	2. Comprehensive	2. Addresses programmatic aspects (contracts, financial matters, documentation of activities), patient care (individual cases, supportive care, protocols), continuing education, and hospital infrastructure	
	3. Multimodal	3. E-mail, online meetings, phone conversations, exchange visits of key personnel	

EDC economically developed countries, *LMIC* low- to mid-income countries

account social and cultural values and available resources and needs. Treatment plans must be based on medical evidence and integrated with other programs already existent in the health-care system. The vision is that implementing a pediatric cancer unit within a hospital not only benefits children with cancer but also other sick children and the hospital itself. Specific goals include improving cure rates and access to care for children with cancer, producing generalizable knowledge that has global benefits, and demonstrating to the local community that progress in pediatric cancer care is both necessary and feasible. Although the benefits of twinning are almost always bidirectional, twinning programs must be distinguished from contractual or commercial partnerships for mutual gain and from research collaborations that focus on a specific project. Therefore, the St. Jude twinning model emphasizes a horizontal distribution of resources, rather than restricting the activities to single diseases such as those of the Global Fund for HIV/AIDS, tuberculosis, and malaria (http://www.theglobalfund.org/en/about/).

St. Jude twinning programs have been established in Amman, Beijing, Shanghai, Beirut, Casablanca, Rabat, Caracas, Maracaibo, Culiacán, Guadalajara, Tijuana, Davao, Guatemala City, Quito, Recife, San Jose, San Salvador, Santiago, and Tegucigalpa. The St. Jude IOP also enters into agreements with institutions in developed countries that have specific training needs or that wish to actively participate in the development of twinning sites. These include Our Lady's Hospital for Sick Children in Crumlin, Ireland; Russian Children's Clinical Hospital in Moscow; the National University Hospital in Singapore; Ospedale S. Gerardo and Universita` di Milano-Bicocca in Monza, Italy; and Rady Children's Hospital in San Diego, USA. The St. Jude IOP has also facilitated the formation of twinning programs by other medical organizations. These include the Keira Grace Foundation with the Hospital Infantil Dr. Robert Reid Cabral (Santo Domingo, Dominican Republic); the American Society of Hematology International Consortium on Acute Promyelocytic Leukemia (Ribeiro and Rego 2006) with institutions in Brazil, Mexico, Uruguay, and Chile; and the Dana Farber Cancer Institute with the National Cancer Institute in Bogotá, Colombia. The latter project is supported by a 5-year grant from the World Child Cancer Foundation (http://www.worldchildcancer.org/). Finally, the St. Jude IOP has worked in collaboration with global health agencies, such the International Agency for Atomic Energy (http://cancer.iaea.org/index.asp), to develop specific pediatric cancer control and nutrition projects in member states and has collaborated with the International Union Against Cancer (UICC) http://www.uicc.org/) and the Humanitarian Department of Sanofi-Aventis (http://en.sanofi-aventis.com/sustainability/people/sponsorship/situation-policy.asp) to develop the "My Child Matters" program, which funds specific pediatric cancer programs in LMIC.

12.5.3 Components of Pediatric Cancer Care in Low- and Mid-Income Countries

Optimally, patients are cared for in a dedicated pediatric cancer unit that combines the necessary professionals, expertise, and infrastructure. Expertise is the most crucial programmatic component. Therefore, the pediatric cancer units become the focus of intense education for direct caregivers, including pediatric hematologists/oncologists, nurses, surgeons, pathologists, radiotherapists, infectious disease specialists, and acute care physicians. Further, continuing education, including subspecialty nursing education (Day eta l. 2008),is ne eded.

In many LMIC, the pediatric cancer units must also be the focus of intense educational efforts to reduce death from infection and abandonment of therapy (defined as missing 6 or more consecutive weeks of treatment). Death from infection is a greater risk in LMIC, partly because of a delay in starting antibiotics and other supportive measures.

The St. Jude IOP has adopted a stepwise approach to implement interventions. This takes into consideration local resources and needs. At most of the partner sites, ALL is the initial disease to be addressed, as it is a common childhood malignancy and is highly curable with relatively accessible and inexpensive drugs and evidence-based guidelines. However, successful management of ALL requires the integration of several components of care, including diagnostics, supportive care, delivery of multiagent chemotherapy, adherence to treatment, and long-term follow-up. Treatment protocols should be based on published evidence and developed with specific local conditions in mind, including the availability and affordability of the chemotherapy agents, the expected requirements for supportive care, and the availability of support services needed to deliver the therapy. The goal is to quickly achieve a 60% event-free survival rate and then to target the most common causes of failure for improvement. For example, if abandonment of therapy and toxic death are the most common causes of failure, improved hospital supportive care and social/economic help for the families are the logical priorities.

The above points are elegantly demonstrated by the experience in Recife, Brazil, in which the rate of abandonment was reduced to less than 1% and the rate of toxic death to less than 10% (Howard et al. 2004;Ribeiro and Pui 2005). Toxic death was reduced through a combination of improved supportive care and individualization of the treatment protocol according to each patient's clinical condition. For example, patients with a large tumor burden and associated morbidity, such as infection and malnutrition, received gentle tumor reduction, treatment for infection, and nutritional support for several days before the intensity of anti-cancer therapy was escalated. Individualized protocol adaptation is facilitated by weekly case discussions among the local and St. Jude physicians via the www.cure4kids.orgw eb-conferencetool.

The infrastructure created to treat ALL can support the successful management of lymphomas, promyelocytic leukemia, and other cancers that can be cured with chemotherapy alone. With the availability of trained pediatric surgeons and radiotherapists, Wilms tumor, favorable-prognosis rhabdomyosarcoma, neuroblastoma, Ewing sarcoma, osteosarcoma, and retinoblastoma can also be adequately treated. In some countries, chemotherapy-only protocols have been developed for childhood Wilms tumor and Hodgkin lymphoma because of the unavailability of radiation therapy (Baez et al. 1997). Management of AML and brain tumors remains challenging at many partner sites.

12.5.4 Outcome Measures

To measure the progress of partner sites' cancer units, several quantitative variables were established and individualized for each program. An increase in the survival rate is the absolute indicator of success. Other outcome indicators are the number of children treated, the number of children who finish treatment, the number of children who remain in follow-up, the number of disease protocols (evidence-based guidelines) activated, and the number of health-care providers dedicated to pediatric oncology. Finally, an important consideration is to determine whether a partner achieves self-sustainability. The amount of the St. Jude direct financial contribution relative to the entire pediatric cancer unit is one of these indicators. For example, in many partner sites, the St. Jude contribution represented the largest portion of the pediatric cancer unit budget at the start of the program. However, as the programs developed and financial support from nongovernmental and governmental sources became available, the relative St. Jude contribution to the entire cancer unit budget decreased to about 3–4% of the total expenses.

Careful documentation of the outcome of children managed uniformly on protocols is crucial to detect areas that need improvement (Ribeiro and Pui 2005; Mostert et al. 2006; Howard et al. 2007). Weekly data manager training sessions are held via www.Cure4kids.org in both English and Spanish. A database specifically designed for pediatric oncology (Pediatric Oncology Networked Database [POND], www.Pond4kids.org) is available at no cost in English, Spanish, Portuguese, French, and Chinese. It can easily be customized to accommodate tumor registry and cancer-specific nutritional, psychosocial, and socioeconomic information. The data are stored on a dedicated server, encrypted, password-protected, and backed up every 10 min. Treatment protocols can be shared via a global library so that other sites can use them. POND is currently used at 44 sites in 30 countries, and more than 20,000 patients have been registered. POND is also used as the database for the American Society of Hematology's international acute promyelocytic leukemia protocol and could potentially serve the needs of other international study groups.

12.5.5 Program Sustainability

The sustainability of the pediatric oncology units has been an important consideration since the inception of the twinning concept. The public sector is an unlikely funding source for these initiatives. In most countries in which St. Jude IOP establishes partnerships, government health budgets are barely adequate to fund the management of common communicable pediatric diseases. In addition, government officials in these countries often lack the experience needed to implement a national pediatric cancer program; hence, pediatric cancer care emerges as an individual or private-sector initiative.

Fortunately, individuals whose child has been treated elsewhere for cancer can often be persuaded, after they return to their countries, to establish nongovernmental organizations (NGOs) to support the local pediatric cancer units. A local NGO has been developed at almost all St. Jude IOP partner sites where pediatric cancer treatment is not government-funded, to provide the support needed for the diagnosis and treatment of childhood cancer. The NGOs are also an important vehicle for community education and fundraising for additional services, such as bone marrow transplantation, clinical investigation, and continuing education of clinicians. The key leaders of the local NGOs are trained by American Lebanese Syrian Associated Charities (ALSAC), the St. Jude fundraising organization. Importantly, all funds raised in partner countries are used within that country.

Some key members of the partner-site multidisciplinary teams receive salary supplementation from the St. Jude IOP to allow them to work full-time in the pediatric oncology unit. Although the amount varies among the different partner sites, annual salary supplementation is commensurate to the salaries of the physicians working in pediatric hematology and combining academic and private activities. This strategy aims to retain these individuals in the public hospitals, which serve large patient populations and have insufficient personnel, medications, and infrastructure.

12.5.6 Conclusions

The St. Jude IOP twinning programs have demonstrated that it is feasible and relatively inexpensive to rapidly improve the cure rates of children with leukemia in LMI countries and to improve their access to care in public hospitals. To expand the St. Jude experience, academic cancer centers in economically developed countries must work collaboratively with global health and development agencies and local governments to establish broad-based cancer control projects inLM IC.

12.6 InternationalC linicalT rials for Children with Cancer – Hurdles and Solutions: The Children's Oncology Group (COG) Approach

Yaddanapudi Ravindranath, Gregory H. Reaman

International collaborative clinical trials in childhood cancer have become increasingly necessary due to the great success achieved in North America and Western Europe. These trials are needed (1) to export technology and to offer geographically and culturally appropriate curative options to children with cancer in low- to mid-income countries and (2) to develop new curative strategies for certain rare childhood cancers, which requires international trials for sample size and disease incidence considerations. International clinical trials pose many challenges due to the varied regulatory requirements and linguistic/cultural barriers in various countries. The following is a brief description of the hurdles faced and solutions adopted by clinical trial groups in the USA and Europe in developing transcontinental clinical trials in children with cancer.

The Children's Oncology Group (COG) and its predecessor groups in the USA (Children's Cancer Group, Pediatric Oncology Group, International Rhabdomyosarcoma Study Group) are clinical trials organizations primarily funded by the US National Cancer Institute (NCI). As a federally funded entity, COG must comply with certain rules and regulations regarding the use of federal funds in its collaborations with institutions in foreign countries. All institutions of COG, including participating full-member foreign institutions, must comply with the regulatory requirements for human subjects participating in any clinical trials as governed by the Office of Human Research Protection (OHRP) of the department of Health and Human Services (HHS) and must submit to on-site audits as required by the US NCI's Clinical Trials Monitoring Branch. The participating institutions must obtain Federal Wide Assurance (FWA) numbers certifying compliance with guidelines regarding human subject research governed by the US Code of Federal Regulation. The current membership of COG includes institutions from Canada, Mexico, Switzerland, The Netherlands, Australia, and New Zealand.

The limitations in extending this approach to institutions from other countries are the availability of federal funds for total support of COG efforts and compliance with the auditing and regulatory requirements at international sites. Recently, COG has expanded international collaborations utilizing guidelines for international collaborations from the Cancer Therapy Evaluation Program (CTEP) of NCI. Establishing formal agreements for international collaborations between clinical trial groups across countries and continents provides an opportunity for shared responsibility for compliance with all of the regulatory requirements and the conduct of audits. Briefly, in this model, the coordinating center of the collaborating clinical trial group must have an FWA number and is responsible for assuring compliance with their national regulatory requirements as well as those of the USA and for conducting the necessary audits; there is no exchange of US federal funds for patient care or diagnostic services between COG and the participating foreign institutions. The clinical trial of interest is conducted by each of the groups; all clinical, outcome, and toxicity data are shared between COG and the international clinical trials group(s) following formally executed agreements detailing data submission, management, and analysis. Currently, several trials in metastatic osteosarcoma and Ewing's tumor are underway utilizing this mechanism between COG and various European clinical trials organizations.

This model also helps to address the language barrier, which is another important hurdle in conducting international clinical trials; many Latin American countries require that not only the consent form but the entire protocol as well all contractual documents be submitted in the language of the country. Large-scale translations become the responsibility of the collaborating group. With this in mind, COG is exploring disease-specific collaborations; examples are international clinical trials in rare cancers such as retinoblastoma and adrenocortical carcinoma. To facilitate this model, COG has focused outreach efforts to assist and promote the development and support of regional clinical trials by local organizations. Examples include (1) the development of GALOP (Groupo America Latina de Oncologia Pediatrea) in Latin America – investigators from GALOP and COG attend meetings of each other's groups and provide scientific support for the development of regional and international clinical trials – and (2) the Scientific Advisory Board of the Middle East Childhood Cancer Alliance (MECCA). In addition, COG provides opportunities for representative, established investigators from foreign institutions to be associate members of COG at no cost, with privilege to access COG protocols and attend COG meetings.

12.7 SummaryandC onclusions

The educational efforts, the twinning programs, and collaborative international clinical trials described above demonstrate that it is feasible and relatively inexpensive to rapidly improve the cure rates of children with cancer, particularly ALL, in LMIC and to improve their access to care in public hospitals through locally developed protocol-based clinical trials. It is possible to envision the clinical and research benefits of a formal international oncology training program at academic cancer centers in the economically developed countries, the availability of competitive funding for specific twinning projects from several countries and international cancer organizations, and academic career opportunities in international pediatric and medical oncology. Hopefully, international oncology will become an academic discipline within pediatric and medical oncology, with the goal of exchanging knowledge with colleagues in LMIC and preventing unnecessary death and suffering caused by cancer.

References

Agarwal BMR, Kurkure P, Choudhry V, Dalvi R, Johnsolomon P et al (2001) Indian National Training Project in Practical Pediatric Oncology (INTPPPO): evaluation of progress and lessons for the future. Med Pediatr Oncol 37(3):163

Baez F, Ocampo E et al (1997) Treatment of childhood Hodgkin's disease with COPP or COPP-ABV (hybrid) without radiotherapy in Nicaragua. Ann Oncol 8(3):247–250

Barr RD, Ribeiro RC, Agarwal BR et al (2006) Pediatric oncology in countries with limited resources. Lippincott Williams and Wilkins, Philadelphia

D'Angio GJ (2009) The La Mascota project. J Pediatr Hematol Oncol31(10):709

Day SW, Dycus PM et al (2008) Quality assessment of pediatric oncology nursing care in a Central American country: findings, recommendations, and preliminary outcomes. Pediatr Nurs34(5):367–37 3

Edefonti A, Montini G, Castellon M (for the Nicaraguan Network of Pediatric Nephrology – NINEPEN) (2010) comprehensive cooperative project for children with renal disease in Nicaragua. Clin Nephrol (in press)

GiovannettiE,UgrasenaDGetal(2008)Methylenetetrahydrofolate reductase (MTHFR) C677T and thymidylate synthase promoter (TSER) polymorphisms in Indonesian children with and without leukemia. Leuk Res 32(1):19–24

Harif M, Barsaoui S et al (2008) Treatment of B-cell lymphoma with LMB modified protocols in Africa–report of the French-African Pediatric Oncology Group (GFAOP). Pediatr Blood Cancer50(6):1138–1142

Hesseling PB (2000) The SIOP burkitt lymphoma pilot study in Malawi, Africa. Med Pediatr Oncol 34(2):142

Hesseling PB, Molyneux E et al (2008) Treating Burkitt's lymphoma in Malawi, Cameroon, and Ghana. Lancet Oncol 9(6):512–513

Howard SC, Pedrosa M et al (2004) Establishment of a pediatric oncology program and outcomes of childhood acute lymphoblastic leukemia in a resource-poor area. JAMA 291(20): 2471–2475

Howard SC, Ortiz R et al (2007) Protocol-based treatment for children with cancer in low income countries in Latin America: a report on the recent meetings of the Monza International School of Pediatric Hematology/Onco logy (MISPHO) – part I. Pediatr Blood Cancer 48(4): 486–490

Hunger SP, Winick NJ et al (2005) Therapy of low-risk subsets of childhood acute lymphoblastic leukemia: when do we say enough? Pediatr Blood Cancer 45(7):876–880

Hunger SP, Sung L et al (2009) Treatment strategies and regimens of graduated intensity for childhood acute lymphoblastic leukemia in low-income countries: a proposal. Pediatr Blood Cancer 52(5):559–565

Jemal A, Siegel R et al (2007) Cancer statistics, 2007. CA Cancer J Clin 57(1):43–66

Kazembe P, Hesseling PB et al (2003) Long term survival of children with Burkitt lymphoma in Malawi after cyclophosphamide monotherapy. Med Pediatr Oncol 40(1): 23–25

Masera G (2009) Bridging the childhood cancer mortality gap between economically developed and low-income countries. J Pediatr Hematol Oncol 31(10):710–712

Masera G, Baez F et al (1998) North-South twinning in paediatric haemato-oncology: the La Mascota programme, Nicaragua. Lancet 352(9144):1923–1926

Masera G, Baez F, Biondi A et al (2004) Bridging the childhood cancer mortality gap between economically developed and low income countries: lessons from the MISPHO experience. In: Tannenberg S, Cavalli F, Pannuti F (eds) Cancer in developing countries. The great challenge for oncology in the 21st century. Verlag, Muenchen-Bern-Wien-New York, Zuckschwerdt, pp 42–60

Mitchell CD, Richards SM et al (2005) Benefit of dexamethasone compared with prednisolone for childhood acute lymphoblastic leukaemia: results of the UK Medical Research Council ALL97 randomized trial. Br J Haematol 129(6): 734–745

Mostert S, Sitaresmi MN et al (2006) Influence of socioeconomic status on childhood acute lymphoblastic leukemia treatment in Indonesia. Pediatrics 118(6):e1600–1606

Mostert S, Sitaresmi MN et al (2008) Parental experiences of childhood leukemia treatment in indonesia. J Pediatr HematolO ncol30(10):738–743

Ravindranath Y, Kaplan J et al (1975) Significance of mediastinal mass in acute lymphoblastic leukemia. Pediatrics 55(6): 889–893

Ribeiro RC, Pui CH (2005) Saving the children – improving childhood cancer treatment in developing countries. N Engl J Med 352(21):2158–2160

Ribeiro RC, Rego E (2006) Management of APL in developing countries: epidemiology, challenges and opportunities for international collaboration. Hematol Am Soc Hematol Educ Program1:162–168

Ribeiro RC, Steliarova-Foucher E et al (2008) Baseline status of paediatric oncology care in ten low-income or mid-income countries receiving My Child Matters support: a descriptive study. Lancet Oncol 9(8):721–729

Rohatiner A (2005) Keynote comment: not just an exercise in solidarity. Lancet Oncol 6(11):818–819

Secker-Walker LM, Lawler SD et al (1978) Prognostic implications of chromosomal findings in acute lymphoblastic leukaemia at diagnosis. Br Med J 2(6151):1529–1530

Sen L, Borella L (1975) Clinical importance of lymphoblasts with T markers in childhood acute leukemia. N Engl J Med 292(16):828–832

Simone J, Aur RJ et al (1972) "Total therapy" studies of acute lymphocytic leukemia in children. Current results and prospects for cure. Cancer 30(6):1488–1494

Sitaresmi MN, Mostert S et al (2009) Chemotherapy-related side effects in childhood acute lymphoblastic leukemia in Indonesia: parental perceptions. J Pediatr Oncol Nurs 26(4): 198–207

Slats AM, Egeler RM et al (2005) Causes of death – other than progressive leukemia – in childhood acute lymphoblastic (ALL) and myeloid leukemia (AML): the Dutch Childhood Oncology Group experience. Leukemia 19(4):537–544

Te Poele EM, de Bont ES et al (2007) Dexamethasone in the maintenance phase of acute lymphoblastic leukaemia treatment: is the risk of lethal infections too high? Eur J Cancer 43(17):2532–2536

The Montevideo Document (1997) SIOP News 17:32

Veerman AJ, Sutaryo S et al (2005) Twinning: a rewarding scenario for development of oncology services in transitional countries. Pediatr Blood Cancer 45(2):103–106

Veerman AJ, Kamps WA et al (2009) Dexamethasone-based therapy for childhood acute lymphoblastic leukaemia: results of the prospective Dutch Childhood Oncology Group (DCOG) protocol ALL-9 (1997-2004). Lancet Oncol 10(10): 957–966

Wagner H (2001) Alliances in pediatric oncology: where do we go from here? Med Pediatr Oncol 36(2):310–311

Wagner HP, Antic V (1997) The problem of pediatric malignancies in the developing world. Ann N Y Acad Sci 824: 193–204

Werner D, Bower B (1982) Helping health workers learn. Hesperian Foundation, Palo alto, CA

Widjajanto PH, Veerman AJP, Sutaryo (2006) apoptotic cell identification: An *in vivo* study during induction treatment of childhood acute lymphoblastic leukemia. Paediatrica Indonesiana46: 195–198

Wolff JA (1999) Chronicle: first light on the horizon: the dawn of chemotherapy. Med Pediatr Oncol 33(4):405–407

Zeulzer WW, Ravindranath Y et al (1976) IMFRA (intermittent intrathecal methotrexate and fractional radiation) plus chemotherapy in childhood leukemia. Am J Hematol 1(2): 191–199

Zuelzer WW (1949) Current trends in hematology. Pediatrics 4(3):269–276

Part IX

Perspectives and Future Direction

Future Challenges and Opportunities to Improve Outcomes for Children withL eukemia

13

Gregory H. Reaman and Franklin O. Smith

The past 50 years have seen remarkable progress in improving the survival of children with cancer (Smith et al. 2010). Among the greatest of these successes are the outcomes for children with acute leukemia. To better understand the incidence and survival for children with all cancers, including leukemia, a comprehensive analysis was recently performed in the United States using the Surveillance, Epidemiology, and End Results 9 (SEER 9) Registry (Smith et al. 2010). This data showed an increased incidence rate for all cancers in children less than 20 years of age during the years 1975 through 2006 (Fig. 13.1). The incidence rates for lymphoid leukemia increased significantly during this time period, with an annual percentage change of 0.8%. Mortality rates for all childhood cancers combined declined by more than 50%, with an estimated 38,032 childhood cancer deaths averted in the United States during this 31-year time period (Fig. 13.2). Remarkably, there was a 64% reduction in mortality rates attributable to leukemia. However, despite these significant reductions in leukemia-specific mortality rates, death due to leukemia remained the leading cause of cancer death in children in both 1975 and in 2006.

G.H.R eaman (✉)
George Washington University School of Medicine & Health Sciences,
The Children's National Medical Center, III Michigan Ave. D.C. 20010, NW, Washington
e-mail: greaman@childrensoncologygroup.org

F.O. Smith
Cincinnati Children's Hospital Medical Center (CCHMC), Burnett Avenue, 3333 University of Cincinnati College Medicine, Cincinnati, OH, USA
e-mail: frank.smith@cchmc.org

Five-year survival rates for children with acute lymphoblastic leukemia (ALL) less than 15 years of age improved from 61.0% in 1975–1978 to 88.5% in 1999–2002 (Fig. 13.3). Improvements in survival were also seen in adolescents 15–19 years of age, although survival rates were less good overall, with only 50.1% surviving at 5 years. Similarly, infants with ALL had a significant improvement in survival at 5-years, improving from 22% in 1975–1978 to 62% in 1999–2002, although as with adolescents with ALL, these results remain suboptimal. These improvements in the survival of children and adolescents with ALL reflect numerous refinements in therapy and importantly, the transition to the use of risk-adjusted therapy within the context of refined risk classification as described in thiste xt.

Significant improvements have also been seen for children less than 15 years of age with acute myeloid leukemia (AML), with 5-year survival rates improving from <20% in 1975–1978 to 58% in 1999–2002 (Fig. 13.4). For adolescents 15–19 years of age, improvements were also seen, with 5-year survivals increasing from <20% to 40%. This progress can be attributed to a number of therapeutic advances, including intensified approaches to the treatment of AML, the selective use of allogeneic hematopoietic stem cell transplant (HSCT), improved supportive care, and in a manner similar to ALL, the increased use of disease-and risk-directed therapy, best exemplified by alternative treatment approaches for children with acute promyelocytic leukemia and children with Down syndrome and AML.

These dramatic improvements in survival for children and adolescents with cancer in general, and leukemia in particular, are attributable to a number of important factors. First, due to the infrequent nature of childhood cancer, it was recognized in the 1950s that no single institution would have a sufficient number of

G.H. Reaman and F.O. Smith (eds.), *Childhood Leukemia*,
DOI: 10.1007/978-3-642-13781-5_13, © Springer-Verlag Berlin Heidelberg 2011

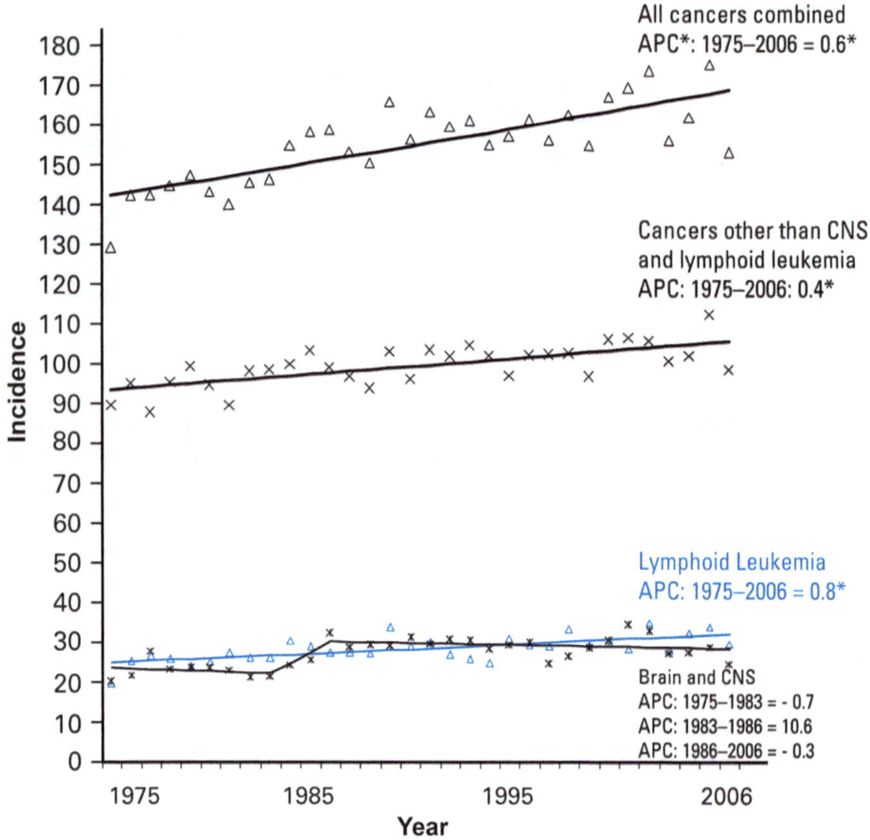

Fig. 13.1 Incidencera tesf or all cancers combined, cancers other than CNS and lymphoid leukemia, and brain and CNS cancers among children younger than 20 years of age, according to data from Surveillance,Epide miology, and End Results 9 (SEER 9) Registries,1975 through 2006. (*) The slope of the join point regression trend line is significantly different from zero ($p \leq 0.5$) . (Reprinted from Smith et al. 2010w ithpe rmission)

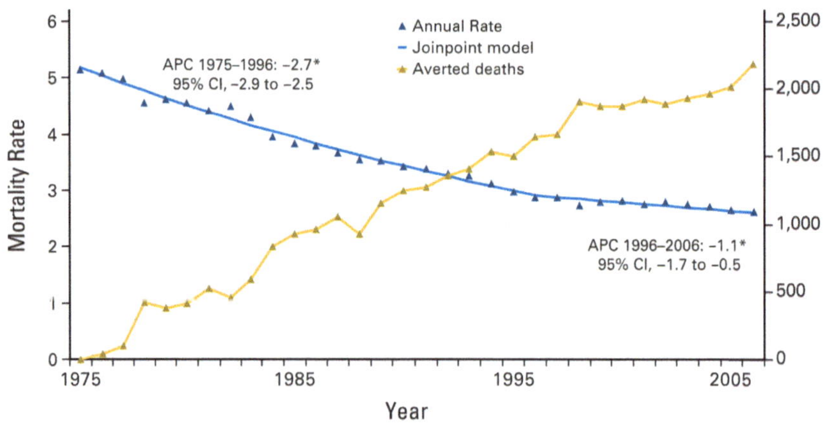

Fig. 13.2 Age-specific mortality trends for all malignant cancers combined among children younger than 20 years of age in the United States from 1975 to 2006. An estimated 38,032 childhood malignant cancer deaths were averted from 1975 through 2006, assuming that the 1975 baseline rate persisted through 2006. (*) The slope of the join point segment is statistically different from zero ($p < 0.5$). APC, annual percentage change. (Reprinted from Smith et al. 2010 with permission)

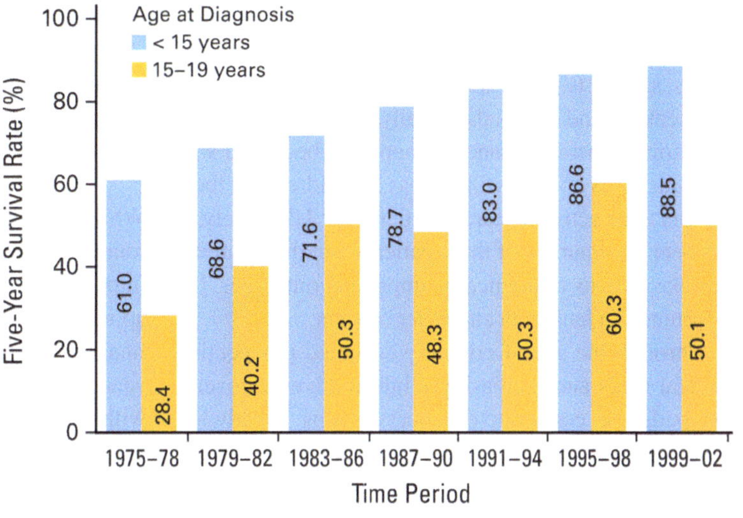

Fig. 13.3 Five-year survival rates for acute lymphoblastic leukemia. (Reprinted fromSmithe ta l. 2010 withpe rmission)

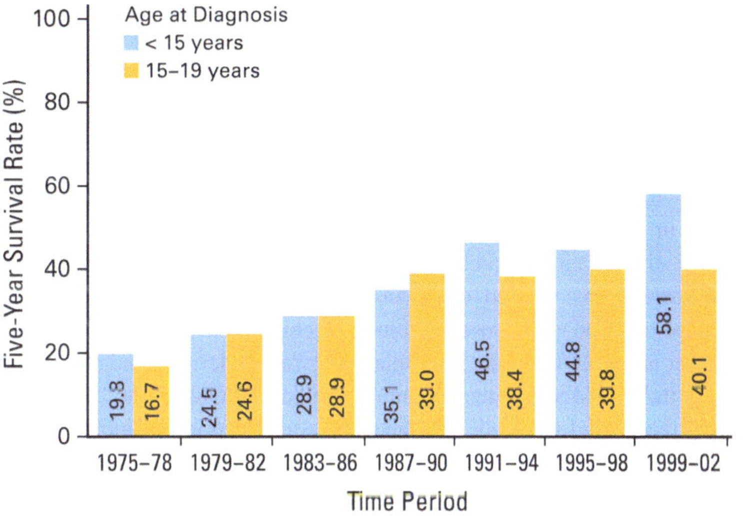

Fig. 13.4 Five-year survival rates for acute myeloid leukemia. (Reprinted from Smith eta l. 2010w lthpe rmlsslon)

patients to allow for meaningful clinical trials. Therefore, cooperative cancer groups arose in the United States and throughout the world with a goal to enroll children on multicenter, prospective clinical trials. In the United States, this led to four federally funded pediatric cooperative cancer groups that merged into a single group, the Children's Oncology Group (COG) in 2000. The COG now includes over 200 member institutions in North America, Australia, New Zealand, and Western Europe. The COG is dedicated to clinical, translational, and epidemiology research in childhood cancer.

The COG and other pediatric cooperative groups and clinical trial networks have achieved success in understanding leukemia biology and improving treatment approaches largely due to highly collaborative and multidisciplinary research supported by consolidated infrastructures that are efficient and cost-effective, lack of duplicative research efforts, a focus on the most compelling and clinically important research questions, and increasingly, prospective clinical trials that are informed by biological understandings of the disease and the host. The success of these groups has resulted in a culture that values collaborative research. This culture includes pediatric cancer health care providers, scientists, governments, payers, academic medical centers, and hospitals. Finally, the success of the pediatric cooperative cancer groups has been and will continue to rely on the willingness of children and their parents to be active research participants. Ultimately, it has been the courage of these patients and their parents that has led to dramatically improved outcomes for children with leukemia and other cancers.

Through the use of critically designed prospective clinical trials and increasingly informative discovery, the pediatric cooperative cancer groups worldwide have continually refined the use of standard, conventional chemotherapy, HSCT, surgery and radiation as the major approaches to the treatment of cancer. However, while further small and incremental improvements may still exist using these therapeutic modalities, it is more likely that there will be few significant improvements in outcome using these traditional approaches to therapy. This conjecture is exemplified and supported by recent data from the SEER Registry (Smith et al. 2010). For example, in this analysis, children with sarcomas appear to have had little improvement in survival over the past 15–20 years, despite the same significant research efforts. Therefore, it is increasingly recognized that transformative changes will be required to improve outcomes for children with cancer and even for acute leukemia going forward.

In the United States, the Institute of Medicine (IOM) recently studied the National Cancer Institute's cooperative cancer group program (adult and pediatric cooperative cancer groups) and issued four broad recommendations to improve the cooperative cancer group clinical trials process (Institute of Medicine 2010):

- Improve the efficiency and reduce average time for the design and launch of innovative clinical trials by consolidating functions, committees, and cooperative groups; streamlining oversight processes; facilitating collaboration; and streamlining and standardizing data collection and analysis.
- Adequately support those clinical trials that have the greatest possibility of improving survival and the quality of life for cancer patients, and increase the rate of clinical trial completion and publication.
- Incentivize the participations of patients and physicians in clinical trials by providing adequate funds to cover the costs of research by reimbursing the costs of standard patient care during the trial.
- Incorporate innovation in science and trial design, for example, in studies identifying biomarkers that canpre dictthe rapeuticre sponse.

While the effective implementation of each of these four broad recommendations is likely to be critically important if the collaborative, multicenter research approach is to remain effective going forward, it is the final recommendation that will be of the greatest relevance to improvements in the outcomes for children with leukemia. Specifically, leukemia biologists and clinical researchers will increasingly need to focus on developing innovative therapies that are directed toward cellular pathways that promote tumor growth and survival, inhibit cell death, and block differentiation. These novel agents will, for the foreseeable future, likely be additive to current conventional therapies. However, as targets that are critical to the development and survival of leukemia cells are increasingly identified and effective drugs are developed to target these pathways, it is possible that the use of multiple new targeted agents, alone and in combination, will begin to replace toxic conventional therapies.

A rapidly expanding array of technologies are being developed that will allow scientists to better define the cellular, molecular, and genetic signatures of leukemia and the host. These platforms include sequencing of the whole genome, exome, transcriptome, tyrosine kinome, and microRNAs, expression arrays, proteomics, methylation, phosphorylation, copy number, gene polymorphisms, and leukemia cell growth in xenograft models, to name but a few. While the ability to effectively analyze enormous amounts of high throughput data from each of these platforms will challenge current biomedical informatics systems and infrastructures, future success will require novel models of disease that will integrate data from multiple platforms in meaningful ways. As these new informatics methods are developed, the resulting models of leukemia will undoubtedly identify new and critically important pathways that can be targeted.

A recent example of the power of this approach is the addition of imatinib mesylate to intensive chemotherapy in children with t(9;22)/Philadelphia chromosome positive (Ph+) ALL (Schultz et al. 2009). Ph+ ALL accounts for only 3–5% of pediatric ALL, but unlike most ALL in children, children with Ph+

ALL have a very poor outcome, with only 40% of children surviving despite aggressive therapy, including allogeneic HSCT (Arico et al. 2000; Gaynon et al. 2000; Maloney et al. 2000). Leukemia biologists have demonstrated that the BCR-ABL oncoprotein that results from the t(9;22) translocation has tyrosine kinase activity and that imatinib mesylate has selective tyrosine kinase inhibition (Druker et al. 2001; Mauro et al. 2002; Savage and Antman 2002). Based on these results, the COG conducted a prospective clinical trial with escalating doses of imatinib added to intensive ALL chemotherapy and allogeneic HSCT. Patients receiving the highest doses of imatinib (cohort 5) had a 3-year event-free survival (EFS) of 80% ± 11% (95% CI, 64–90%), more than twice the 3-year EFS for a historical control group (35 ± 4%; $p = 0.0001$) (Fig. 13.5). Importantly, no significant toxicities were seen with the addition of imatinib to ALL chemotherapy.

With this experience in Ph+ ALL as "proof of principle," significant efforts are now underway to identify cellular, molecular, and genetic targets that are critical for the survival of leukemia cells that could potentially be targeted by new drugs. For ALL, several new targets have recently been identified, with efforts now underway to develop and test drugs directed to these targets. Specifically, it has been shown that B-cell-progenitor ALL cells characterized by deletions in the

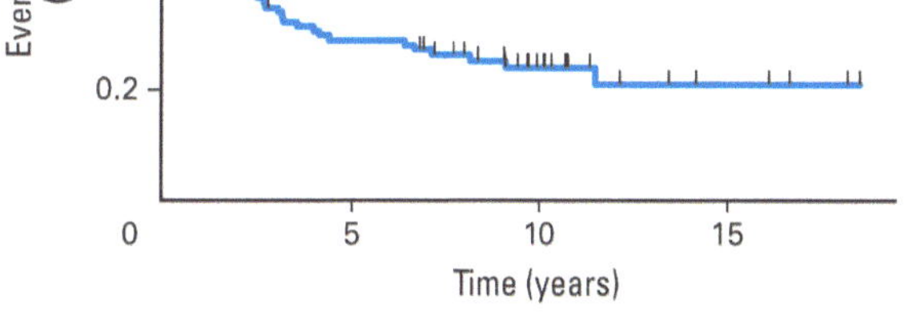

Fig. 13.5 Early event-free survival (EFS) in Philadelphia chromosome-positive acute lymphoblastic leukemia patients treated with imatinib. Treated patients in cohort 5 ($n = 44$) were compared with patients previously treated on Pediatric Oncology Group (POG) protocols ALinC 14, 15, and 16 from January 1986 through November 1999 ($n = 120$). (Reprinted from Schultze ta l. 2009w ithpe rmission)

lymphoid transcription factor IKAROS (*IKZF1*) have BCR-ABL1-like activated kinase signaling and these children have a poor prognosis (Mullighan et al. 2008, 2009b). Similar exciting results have also been recently reported for children with ALL with mutations in the Janus kinases (*JAK*) 1, 2, and 3 genes (Mullighan et al. 2009) and cytokine receptor-like factor 2 (*CRLF2*) gene (Mullighan et al. 2009a, c; Harvey et al. 2010). Early investigations of a small molecule JAK inhibitor are underway in ALL.

Future opportunities will require similar translation of important biologic findings to clinical trials. In the United States, the National Cancer Institute has created a pathway that supports new target identification, *in vitro* and xenograft testing of drugs, pediatric Phase I drug testing, and subsequent Phase II and III clinical trials. Specifically, using the biology platforms described above to define cancer signatures, the Childhood Cancer Therapeutically Applicable Research to Generate Effective Treatments (TARGET) initiative (http://target.cancer.gov/) seeks to catalog genetic abnormalities in childhood leukemia and other cancers. The Pediatric Preclinical Testing Program (PPTP) (http://ctep.cancer.gov/MajorInitiatives/Pediatric_Preclinical_Testing_Program.htm) is evaluating new agents against pediatric leukemias and other cancers. The National Cancer Institute supports the conduct of Phase I studies of new drugs and Phase II and III clinical trials by the COG. These key resources and infrastructure are proving to be highly effective.

However, one of the many consequences of increasingly defining subgroups of leukemia patients on the basis of demographic, clinical, cellular, molecular, and genetic factors is the increasingly small number of patients with identifiable abnormalities, alone and taken together. This is particularly true in AML, which is defined by its genomic complexity. These increasingly small groups of patients with increasingly "personalized" therapies will create challenges and opportunities to create new and innovative models for clinical trials and biostatistical analytic plans.

At the present time and for the foreseeable future, progress in improving the outcomes for children with leukemia will require: transformative changes in how leukemia biologists perform discovery research; greatly improved abilities by biomedical informatics specialists to analyze and integrate vast amounts of data; more rapid development of new drugs directed to newly identified targets; novel and innovative clinical trial designs; reassessment of the increasingly complex regulatory environment, and finally, new economic and policy models that will more effectively support these efforts. These are significant challenges. However, scientists and clinicians who care for children with leukemia and other cancers are passionately optimistic about improving the outcomes for these children. The culture of highly collaborative research and clinical care that has been created in pediatric oncology over the past 50 years will surely find solutions to these challenges so that in the near future, all children with leukemia will bec uredofthe irdis ease.

References

Arico M, Valsecchi MG et al (2000) Outcome of treatment in children with Philadelphia chromosome-positive acute lymphoblastic leukemia. N Engl J Med 342(14): 998–1006

Druker BJ, Sawyers CL et al (2001) Activity of a specific inhibitor of the BCR-ABL tyrosine kinase in the blast crisis of chronic myeloid leukemia and acute lymphoblastic leukemia with the Philadelphia chromosome. N Engl J Med 344(14):1038–1042

Gaynon PS, Trigg ME et al (2000) Children's Cancer Group trials in childhood acute lymphoblastic leukemia: 1983–1995. Leukemia14(12):2223–2233

Harvey RC, Mullighan CG et al (2010) Rearrangement of CRLF2 is associated with mutation of JAK kinases, alteration of IKZF1, Hispanic/Latino ethnicity, and a poor outcome in pediatric B-progenitor acute lymphoblastic leukemia. Blood 115(26): 5312–5321

Insitute of Medicine (2010) A national cancer clinical trials system for the 21st century: reinvigorating the NCI cooperative grouppr ogram

Maloney KW, Shuster JJ et al (2000) Long-term results of treatment studies for childhood acute lymphoblastic leukemia: Pediatric Oncology Group studies from 1986–1994. Leukemia 14(12):2276–2285

Mauro MJ, O'Dwyer M et al (2002) STI571: a paradigm of new agents for cancer therapeutics. J Clin Oncol 20(1): 325–334

Mullighan CG, Miller CB et al (2008) BCR-ABL1 lymphoblastic leukaemia is characterized by the deletion of Ikaros. Nature453(7191):110–114

Mullighan CG, Collins-Underwood JR et al (2009a) Rearrangement of CRLF2 in B-progenitor- and Down syndrome-associated acute lymphoblastic leukemia. Nat Genet 41(11):1243–1246

Mullighan CG, Su X et al (2009b) Deletion of IKZF1 and prognosis in acute lymphoblastic leukemia. N Engl J Med 360(5): 470–480

Mullighan CG, Zhang J et al (2009c) JAK mutations in high-risk childhood acute lymphoblastic leukemia. Proc Natl Acad Sci USA 106(23):9414–9418

Savage DG, Antman KH (2002) Imatinib mesylate – a new oral targeted therapy. N Engl J Med 346(9):683–693

Schultz KR, Bowman WP et al (2009) Improved early event-free survival with imatinib in Philadelphia chromosome-positive acute lymphoblastic leukemia: a children's oncology group study. J Clin Oncol 27(31): 5175–5181

Smith MA, Seibel NL et al (2010) Outcomes for children and adolescents with cancer: challenges for the twenty-first century. J Clin Oncol 28(15):2625–2634

Index

B

C

MIX
Papier aus verantwortungsvollen Quellen
Paper from responsible sources
FSC® C105338

If you have any concerns about our products,
you can contact us on
ProductSafety@springernature.com

In case Publisher is established outside the EU,
the EU authorized representative is:
Springer Nature Customer Service Center GmbH
Europaplatz 3, 69115 Heidelberg, Germany

Printed by Libri Plureos GmbH
in Hamburg, Germany